THE
PRACTICE OF
OCCUPATIONAL
THERAPY

THE PRACTICE OF OCCUPATIONAL THERAPY

AN INTRODUCTION
TO THE TREATMENT OF
PHYSICAL DYSFUNCTION

EDITED BY

ANN TURNER DipCOT TDipCOT SROT

Senior Tutor, St Loye's School of Occupational Therapy, Exeter

Foreword by Katherine Ingamells DipCOT TDipCOT SROT

Principal, St Loye's School of Occupational Therapy, Exeter

CHURCHILL LIVINGSTONE
EDINBURGH LONDON MELBOURNE AND NEW YORK 1981

CHURCHILL LIVINGSTONE
Medical Division of Longman Group Limited

Distributed in the United States of America by Churchill
Livingstone Inc., 1560 Broadway, New York, N.Y. 10036,
and by associated companies, branches and representatives
throughout the world.

First published 1981
  Reprinted 1984

ISBN 0 443 01878 2

British Library Cataloguing in Publication Data
Turner, Ann
  The practice of occupational therapy.
  1. Occupational therapy
  I. Title
  615'.8515   RM735   80-40814

Printed in Hong Kong by Sheck Wah Tong Printing Press Ltd.

Foreword

Occupational therapy is the treatment of the whole person by his active participation in purposeful living. As an increasingly recognised member of the treatment team the occupational therapist is the one therapist who uses solely purposeful activity and the activity chosen by the therapist is with the aim of regaining maximal independence. These activities are, therefore, closely related to the person being treated, to his particular needs and the life to which he wishes to return. Activities can range from icing a cake to scrubbing the floor; from laying cement to mowing the lawn; from carpentry to cards.

Occupational therapy, however, is the youngest and smallest of the rehabilitation professions. Although the Egyptian priests were using the principles of occupational therapy in 2000 BC, the first Association of Occupational Therapy was not founded until 1917 and the first courses of training until 1927. State registration occurred in 1961. There are now 16 schools of occupational therapy in Great Britain with approximately 500 students qualifying each year, and a total professional membership of 6215 (April 1978). Despite all this growth and increasing respectability little is known about the practice of occupational therapy, little research is done and few texts are written.

This book is the work of occupational therapists who have had the enthusiasm to start and, even more creditable, the perseverance to continue and complete a detailed text on the physical side of our work. It aims to cover the general practice of occupational therapy within the experience of the authors and attempts to give enough medical background to remind the therapist of the conditions being treated. It is no 'bible', more a document for discussion. It increases the number of our specific texts by 25 per cent.

I hope this book contributes to the teaching of students, to the practice of occupational therapy and to the enthusiasm of others to write its psychiatric sister.

Exeter, 1981   Katherine Ingamells

Preface

It is, I suppose, rather strange to say that a book has grown up as a result of lack of time but this is certainly so in this case. Having taught occupational therapy for medical and surgical conditions (commonly abbreviated to 'Applied Physical') for two years at St Loye's it became obvious that lack of time prevented the students from receiving both a theoretical background and practical experience in the basic skills required by an occupational therapist. Equally, in cases of sickness or other absence, or where practical experience in a particular field had been lacking during hospital practice, students found there was little information available to serve as reference for these skills.

In addition, several qualified therapists had commented that if they had been unable to attend refresher courses or visit departments in order to discuss ideas and techniques, or if they were referred a patient who had a condition which they had not treated since college days, an outline of principles from which to work was not always available.

It is with these two groups in mind that this book has been written. It does not attempt to be a medical textbook but gives an outline of conditions to 'set the scene' for treatment. Clearly, in these days of ever widening knowledge and expertise, no one person can have experience or confidence in all aspects of a subject as diverse as occupational therapy. For this reason I am especially indebted to those who have contributed expert knowledge by writing chapters on their speciality; a special mention must go to Mrs Anne Capon for her section on the Rehabilitation Lathe; Miss Dorothy Conder for her section on Upper Limb Amputees and Dr Claire Whitehead for her introduction to the chapter on Hemiplegia.

My special thanks also go to Miss Lynn Cheshire, Miss Jill Freston, Miss Ruth Green, Dr C.E. Halliday, Mr D.L. Harris, Mrs Vivien Hollis, Mr C. Jefferiss, Miss M. Keily, Dr J.K. Lloyd, Miss G. Lubbock, Miss Alicia Mendez, the staff of the occupational therapy departments at Ashford Hospital, Middlesex; Mount Vernon Hospital, London; The National Hospital, London; and the Robert Jones and Agnes Hunt Orthopaedic Hospital, Oswestry, Salop. I also extend my thanks to Mrs Rosemary West, Dr W. Wright and Miss Tricia Yetton for their time spent in checking and correcting many of the chapters. I am indebted to Mr Sidney J. Lock for the use of extracts from his *Larvic Rehabilitation Lathe Manual*.

Lastly, but by no means least, I must thank Mrs Rosemary Dent for her excellent typing of the script; Mrs Ruth Morgan for her secretarial work; Mrs Avril l'Anson for the tremendous effort put into the numerous and most effective illustrations; Miss Lynn Eveleigh for hours spent holding awkward poses; the staff of Exeter ALAC, Nomeq, Akron and Carters for their kind assistance with providing photographs; and Mrs Vivien Hollis for helping me get the idea off the ground in the first place. The staff and students at St Loye's deserve special mention for their support and encouragement, in

particular Katherine Ingamells and Sybil Hopson
who have borne the brunt of my temper, exaspera-
tion, gloom and obsession!

And at the end of all, I must give my love and
thanks to my husband for all the effort he has put
into producing photographs and for the support
and encouragement he has given me during the
preparation of this book.

Exeter, 1981   A.T.

List of Contributors

Gill Arnott DipCOT SROT
Senior Occupational Therapist, Spinal Injuries Unit, Robert Jones and Agnes Hunt Orthopaedic Hospital, Oswestry, Salop

Anne Capon DipCOT SROT
Head Occupational Therapist, Ashford Hospital, Middlesex

Dorothy Conder DipCOT SROT
Senior Occupational Therapist, Princess Elizabeth Orthopaedic Hospital, Exeter, Devon

Margaret Foster DipCOT SROT
Tutor Derby School of Occupational Therapy. Formerly Head Occupational Therapist at Derbyshire Royal Infirmary

Hilary Grime DipCOT SROT
Tutor at Dorset House School of Occupational Therapy, Oxford. Formerly Community Occupational Therapist, Oxford

Sybil Hopson DipCOT TDipCOT SROT
Dual posts of Assistant County Occupational Therapist, Devon County Council and tutor at St Loye's School of Occupational Therapy, Exeter

Katherine Ingamells DipCOT TDipCOT SROT
Principal, St Loye's School of Occupational Therapy, Exeter

Janet Jones DipCOT SROT
Designated District Occupational Therapist, Battle Hospital, Reading, Berkshire

Susan M.L. Pearce DipCOT SROT MRSH
District Occupational Therapist, Robert Jones and Agnes Hunt Orthopaedic Hospital, Oswestry, Salop

Ella Webber DipCOT SROT
Occupational Therapist, St Rose's Special School, Stroud, Gloucestershire

Claire Whitehead MA MB BChir(Cantab) MRCP(UK)
Consultant Physician in Rehabilitation, West Berkshire District

Susan Whiting DipCOT SROT
Sector Head Occupational Therapist, Rivermead Rehabilitation Centre, Abingdon Road, Oxford

Contents

Appendices

Index

Techniques and treatment media in occupational therapy

First, do no harm

HIPPOCRATES 460 – 365 BC

1

The principles of assessment

Record keeping is often seen as an encroachment on the time spent with patients, for therapists are essentially practical people and therefore often consider writing reports as unnecessary, especially when the patient's treatment programme and progress are well known to them.

The aspiring therapist may well ask why assessment is necessary when the patient's problem can be seen and his* diagnosis is known. Also, what difference does record keeping make to treatment and why is it necessary to write facts down in such detail?

The aim of this chapter is to show the basic principles of referral of patients for treatment, interviewing, assessing, recording and reporting, and why these are so important to a comprehensive treatment programme.

REFERRAL

When working in a hospital or for the social services department the therapist may first hear about the person to be treated from one of the following sources:

1. *Clinics.* In hospital the first information about a patient may often come from an outpatient clinic. The therapist may attend such a clinic in order to receive information about new patients and also to report on the progress of those already being treated in the department. In many hospitals occupational therapists regularly visit

---

*Throughout 'she' has been used to refer to the therapist and 'he' to the patient/client

clinics such as those run by orthopaedic surgeons, rheumatologists and physical medicine consultants not only for this reason but also to update and extend their knowledge in a particular field.

2. *Ward rounds.* Where the therapist has responsibility for the occupational therapy given to patients on a particular ward, it is usual for her to attend the ward round. This is most frequently conducted by the consultant, his team of doctors, the ward sister/charge nurse and other paramedical personnel concerned with the ward. During such a round it is not only possible to find out relevant information about new patients but also to ask questions and give reports on those already being treated.

3. *Case conferences.* Many hospitals are now using this form of meeting for the exchange of information instead of the traditional ward round. In this case only the consultant, his team of doctors and the senior nurse will visit each patient for examination and discussion of their medical treatment. Later a conference is held which can involve not only all medical and paramedical staff who have contact with the patients, but also others such as the community nurse or the patient's relatives, who may be asked to attend all or part of the discussion. In this way there is no need for a huge 'army' of white-coated personnel to descend at the patient's bedside, and it is easier to discuss progress reports and queries freely in private.

4. *Patient's notes.* Each patient's medical history is recorded in a personal folder which, while the patient is in hospital, is kept on the ward and, on discharge, is filed in the hospital's records department. If the therapist is not present at the time of referral for occupational therapy, a request may be written in the patient's notes.

5. *Referral forms.* Most occupational therapy departments design their own referral forms and these are kept on the wards, in departments or in clinics, so that they can be used when it is considered necessary to refer a patient for treatment. In the community the patient's general practitioner may contact the therapist directly.

6. *Other medical personnel.* In some cases other personnel may refer the patient to the occupational therapist prior to his next appointment with the doctor. This may happen where the patient is seen by a physiotherapist, nurse or social worker who feels that he would now benefit from occupational therapy. However, it should be emphasised that in such cases it is essential to obtain the doctor's consent before treatment is commenced, for it is the doctor who is responsible for the patient's overall treatment. In some areas, especially on wards where the majority of patients receive treatment from the occupational therapist, it is not uncommon to find that a 'blanket' referral is given. In this case the occupational therapist has permission to begin treatment with any of the patients when she feels it is necessary without having to notify the doctor in each individual case.

7. *The general public.* In the community especially, the therapist may frequently receive requests to see clients from members of the public. Such a request may come from the client himself or from others such as a neighbour, relative, priest or friend.

THE INITIAL INTERVIEW

Having received a referral for the treatment of a patient the therapist should obtain as much basic information about him as possible around which to conduct the initial interview. This may well have been supplied at the time of referral, otherwise it may need to be obtained from the patient's notes. At the minimum, it should consist of:

1. *the patient's name.* Both the surname and forenames are necessary, and the marital status.

2. *address/ward* and any other identification such as the record number. This is essential if the therapist is to make contact with the patient and will also enable her to obtain any additional information that may be necessary.

3. *date of birth.* Not only will this help to identify the patient but, combined with the diagnosis, may give some indication of the likely history and prognosis of the condition.

4. *diagnosis.* Both the primary and any secondary diagnoses or precautions should be known. For example, is a stroke patient incontinent or an amputee also diabetic?

5. *patient's doctor.* In the hospital the consultant in charge of the patient's treatment should be known, whilst in the community the general practitioner's name and address are essential.

6. *date*. All referrals should be dated so that an accurate record of progress can be kept.

7. *signature*. This is important as the referee may not be the patient's doctor.

Other useful, although not essential, information to obtain at this stage includes:

(a) *the patient's occupation*. This will give a guide to the general level of function required in order for the patient to return to work. It may give a guide to the patient's level of intelligence, although this is not always so; it will, however, give no indication as to his motivation to get better!

(b) *treatment required*. Some therapists will be asked to treat a particular area, joint or problem of the patient. This, may, however not be so in all cases and the therapist is therefore expected to plan the patient's treatment from her own assessment.

The initial interview usually takes place in the occupational therapy department, on the ward or in the client's home. The therapist must remember that especially the elderly, the young or the very disabled, will feel more relaxed and secure if they are approached on their 'own ground', that is by the bedside, in the day room or in other familiar surroundings, rather than in a strange department. With such patients it is often advisable to see them only briefly prior to the first interview just to introduce oneself and arrange the next meeting. In this way the patient is not taken unawares by a complete stranger bombarding him with a barrage of rather personal questions and it is also possible to arrange a time when both the therapist and the patient are free.

The initial interview should be conducted in as private a place as possible so that both the patient and the therapist feel free to ask and answer questions. The therapist must remember that this first contact with the patient is important, for first impressions last and too formal or casual an approach can hinder the relationship being formed. The therapist should be neat, tidy, well prepared and unhurried. She should be able to address the patient by name, have any information about him to hand, any necessary equipment for assessment ready and be aware of the appointment time. This first interview may be an emotional experience for the patient, especially if he has

been seriously ill, as this may be the first occasion on which he has been asked to face the facts about the results of his illness. The therapist must be prepared to cope with emotional outbursts such as crying or aggression, which may result from the frustration of having to accept, and beginning to overcome, any residual disability.

The purpose of the initial interview is threefold. Both the therapist and the patient will be required to:
1. give information
2. receive information
3. establish rapport

Giving information

It is always wise for the therapist to introduce herself at the beginning of an interview in case the patient has forgotten or misheard her name. This is especially important when visiting the client's home for the first time, as he may be expecting several 'new' visitors because of his illness. It is also advisable to explain why she is there, and how she hopes to help the patient, especially as occupational therapy is a long, and frequently misunderstood, label! The therapist may also find it appropriate to explain to the patient how he was referred, as he may wonder from where the therapist's information was obtained.

The therapist's introduction may, therefore, be along the following lines: 'Hello, Mr Jones, my name is Miss Thompson and I'm the occupational therapist. Dr Johnson has asked me to see you, as I hear you fell and hurt your leg last week. I hope that now you're getting about a bit we can make things a little easier for you to manage.'

In this way the therapist not only introduces herself and briefly explains her role, but also informs the patient of how his problem was made known to her.

During the first interview, the therapist should also confirm or arrange times for treatment sessions and their frequency and duration. She should remember that these have to be fitted not only in to her own routine, but also round the ward routine, other treatment schedules, the patient's work or school hours (if applicable) and available transport. An appointment card should be completed for him and any necessary transport arrangements made or confirmed. If the patient is still in hospital the ward staff should be informed of the times he is required for treatment.

Receiving information

The therapist will need details from the patient in addition to a confirmation of his name, date of birth and address. It is necessary to discover during this initial interview how much the patient understands about his condition and what his attitude to it is. The therapist should never assume that the patient is aware of his diagnosis — especially as the doctor may not yet have revealed it to him — so that shocked statements such as 'Well, the doctor didn't tell me I had multiple sclerosis.' or 'Do you mean that Billy is a spastic?' don't occur.

The therapist should offer the patient the opportunity to reveal his knowledge and attitude towards his condition by asking, for example 'How long have you had difficulty with walking?' This may disclose an open 'Well, the doctor told me last month that I had multiple sclerosis but I'd had my suspicions for a year or so,' or a wary 'Oh, it's been awkward for a month or two but it's getting better.'

The therapist should also enquire about the patient's home and work circumstances, where these are relevant to treatment, and should assess the extent of the injury or condition. Where the problem is limited to one particular area, as in a crush injury to the hand or a fracture at the ankle, a full physical assessment can be carried out at this stage, but if the patient has more extensive problems (as in the case of someone suffering from rheumatoid arthritis or a stroke) only a general assessment will be made initially and a more detailed one should follow. It is necessary to check what other treatments the patient is receiving so that sessions do not clash, or the patient does not arrive too tired to benefit from treatment. The date of the next clinic appointment should be noted so that reports can be prepared in time.

Establishing rapport

This is a vital, though often forgotten aspect of the initial interview, as it is during this first meeting that an understanding is built up between the therapist and the patient. A good relationship will lead to mutual trust and respect so that both parties can feel at ease and secure during treatment sessions. (These may seem ideal sentiments but they form the basis of a successful partnership.)

Whether the interview is conducted in a department or on the patient's own 'territory', it is the therapist who arranges and directs the proceedings and it is therefore her responsibility to ensure that the interview is as successful as possible.

Positioning is important. The patient should feel comfortable and secure without feeling hemmed in. The therapist and patient should sit at the same level so that either can take the initiative to make or break eye contact. The patient should not feel dominated by a therapist who stands over him or lurks behind a large, untidy desk with books and telephones creating a barrier to the free exchange of information (Fig. 1.1). The therapist should not sit so close to the patient that he feels uncomfortable and any direct contact which is needed during lifting or measuring should be made confidently and positively. Again, it is important for the therapist to explain her role and how she hopes to help the patient. She should show empathy, that is understanding without over-involvement. This can be shown by the non-verbal techniques mentioned above and also, for example, by the early suggestion of one minor treatment technique, such as how to tie a shoelace with one hand. The explanation of a relevant remedial activity will demonstrate to the patient an understanding of the condition and reassure him as to the techniques to be used during treatment sessions.

Empathy comes through observation, knowledge, experience and a desire to help, and any good therapist will find more understanding through time and, where possible, through the personal experience (perhaps best gained early on during training) of 'becoming handicapped' for a while and having to cope herself with the problems encountered. The therapist should use language and terminology which the patient understands, although this does not mean treating the patient like a child. Her voice should be clear and natural, never patronising or demanding. Gesture, either conscious or unconscious, can assist or detract from the establishment of a relationship. Obviously the therapist should display the normal

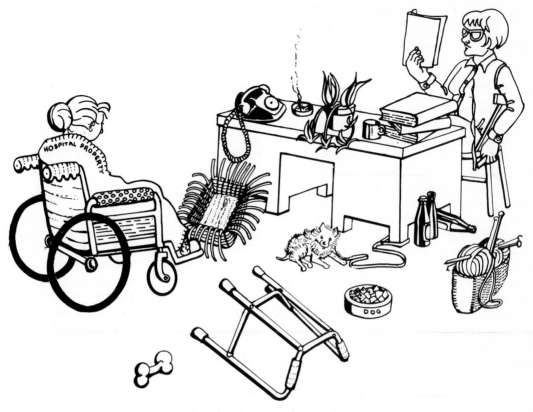

Fig. 1.1   '. . . lurks behind a large, untidy desk . . .'

social graces and not blow cigarette smoke over her patient or scratch her feet! Unconscious gestures such as constantly checking the time, avoiding eye contact or stifling a yawn can indicate to the patient that his problem is a bore and his presence undesirable. Conversation should be based on topics relevant to the situation. Although some informal exchange about the weather, pets or the ability of the local rugby team may help to relax the atmosphere, an interview which rambles off the point for too long can be both tiring and puzzling to the patient.

ASSESSMENT

Taking and recording information in a way that is clear, relevant and unobtrusive is an art gained through experience, observation and practice. To be too consciencious and write down every word that is spoken will make the patient feel uncomfortable and less likely to give information, while being too casual may make him wonder why all his personal information is so important in any case.

The reasons for assessing and recording can be summarised as:
1. forming a basis on which to plan treatment
2. showing progress, or lack of progress, to the therapist, the patient and the doctor
3. showing the exact extent and effect of the injury and/or disability
4. showing the expected level of recovery in a unilateral condition by using the unaffected side as a guideline.

Whatever is being assessed it is important for the therapist to bear the following in mind:

What is she assessing?

Will the activity being used tell her what she wants to know? For instance, does a week spent working in the heavy workshop really assess the capability of a milkman to return to work; or does a session in a strange remedial kitchen making a Swiss roll form a fair basis for deciding whether a housewife is ready to cope at home?

What is she assessing for?

For whom is the assessment meant and for what purpose? Again, is a full work assessment really necessary if the Disablement Resettlement Officer is sending the patient on to an Employment Rehabilitation Centre (ERC) where another assessment will be carried out; or would it be more relevant to simply establish whether the patient can cope with the demands of the ERC and not fail miserably because his stamina, concentration or motivation had not been checked?

The types of assessment undertaken by a therapist working with physical disabilities fall, in the opinion of the author, into four types:

Physical assessment: to show the strength and range of movement within a limb.

Work assessment: to show the patient's physical (and to a lesser extent psychological) capabilities in relation to his work or his potential for retraining.

Personal assessment: to show the level of independence reached by the patient in the activities of daily living/home management. Home visits can be included here.

Specific others: these include level of function in a particular field such as prosthetic training, hand assessment or wheelchair assessment.

Assessment forms will vary according to the case load, functioning of the department and the preference of the therapist. However, whatever the layout of the assessment form certain basic information should be included:

1. *Unit or department:* for the information of other departments.

2. *Patient's name, ward/address, date of birth and record number:* for easy reference.

3. *Diagnosis and referee:* this should also include the name of the patient's consultant or general practitioner if he is not the referee.

4. *Date of first and any subsequent assessments:* for ease and speed of noting progress.

5. *A list of items being assessed:* to assist in remembering all relevant items to be recorded. A space for comment may be appropriate.

6. *Space for general comment:* for recording any additional information not catered for on the form.

7. *Therapist's signature:* If you lack the courage to sign it, don't write it!

Each type of assessment form is discussed below and an example shown. (The reader will note that some forms allow space for the assessment to be recorded only a few times. If more space is required a continuation sheet will be necessary.)

Physical assessment

Forms for these assessments (Fig. 1.2) are usually used within the department and the results are then summarised for inclusion in a report. Assessments of joint range, muscle strength and related information such as the degree of swelling and skin condition must be made and recorded regularly if they are to be of use. In some cases, for example when treating one particular joint within a limb or hand, it may be relevant to assess the range of movement at the beginning and end of each treatment session. It is especially important that such assessments are clearly written and laid out and also that each set of figures is initialled by the therapist who performed the assessment, as individuals may well vary in their recording of a joint's movement. For further details see Chapter 2.

Work assessment

The information required for a work assessment will vary enormously according to the type of disability and occupation of the patient. However, in broad terms a work assessment aims at estimating both general and specific skills necessary for a return to previous employment or, where this is not possible, the potential skills for training or retraining (Fig. 1.3). Work assessment is often not repeated as regularly as other types of assessment as significant change is less likely over short periods. For further details see Chapter 12.

Personal assessment

These assessments (often referred to as 'Activities of Daily Living' — ADL — assessments) are

| | REHABILITATION UNIT
GENERAL HOSPITAL, SOMETOWN | | Upper
limb
assessment | | |

Name .... Diagnosis .... Doctor ....

Date of birth .... Address/ward ....

Record No. ....

Unaffected limb		Date	Date	Date
	Shoulder Elevation through Abduction			
	Elevation through Flexion			
	Extension			
	Adduction			
	Medial Rotation			
	Lateral Rotation			
	Elbow and Forearm Flexion/Extension			
	Pronation			
	Supination			
	Wrist Flexion			
	Extension			
	Radial Deviation			
	Ulnar Deviation			
	Hand Span			
	Grip strength			
	INITIALS OF THERAPIST			

Comments

Note: This form would be one of a series used for a full physical assessment. A detailed hand assessment – if required – would be carried out on a separate form.

Fig. 1.2 Physical assessment form

REHABILITATION UNIT
GENERAL HOSPITAL, SOMETOWN

Work
Potential

General
Ability

Name ....   Diagnosis ....   Doctor ....

Date of birth ....   Address/ward ....

Record No. ....

Previous occupation ....   Employer ....

	Date			Date			Date		
	Good	Average	Poor	Good	Average	Poor	Good	Average	Poor
Punctuality									
Personal appearance									
Work standard									
Ability to work with others									
Ability to work alone									
Ability to drive									
Ability to work at heights									
Ability to work outdoors									
Ability to work with dust & fumes									
INITIALS									

Comments

Note: This form would not be used in isolation to assess the patient's work potential. Some assessment of physical and intellectual function would also be necessary.

Fig. 1.3 Work assessment form

**REHABILITATION UNIT
GENERAL HOSPITAL, SOMETOWN**

**Personal
Dressing – men**

Name .... Diagnosis .... Doctor ....

Date of birth .... Address/ward ....

Record No. ....

Rating Guide

0:Impossible
1:Accomplished with difficulty
2:Accomplished with minor difficulty
3:Independent with use of aid
4:Independent

Activity	Date	Comment	Date	Comment
Put garment over head				
Take off garment over head				
Put on garment round shoulders				
Take off garment round shoulders				
Put garment over feet				
Take off garment over feet				
Fasten belt				
Manage buttons				
Manage fly fastening				
Put on shoes – tie laces				
Take off shoes – untie laces				
Put on socks				
Take off socks				
Fasten tie				
Secure braces				
INITIALS				

Comments

Note: This form would be one of a series available for dressing assessment.

Fig. 1.4 Personal assessment form

REHABILITATION UNIT
GENERAL HOSPITAL, SOMETOWN
ARM TRAINING REPORT

V. Good	3
Average	2
Poor	1

Dr. ....

Name .... No. ....

Age .... Site of amputation R ....

Address .... L ....

Cause of amputation and date ....

Pre-amputation occupation ....

Relevant hobbies ....

Dominant hand .... Commencement of arm training ....

	Tolerance to prosthesis
	Putting on prosthesis
	Dressing
	Toilet
	Feeding

	Use of kitchen utensils
	Peeling vegetables
	Washing-up
	Control of cooker
	Baking

	Writing
	Technical drawing
	Typing
	Use of telephone

	Laundering
	Housework

	Metalwork
	Woodwork
	Assembling electric fitments
	Gardening, digging
	Gardening, long-handled tools
	Gardening shears

	Sewing
	Knitting

	Ability to manipulate controls of a car

Appliances ordered

Resettlement

Special comments

Completion of arm training

Date .... Signed ....

Fig. 1.5 Assessment form for arm training following upper limb amputation

perhaps the most extensively used by the occupational therapist working in general medicine (Fig. 1.4). They cover all those activities which the patient needs to complete in order to become personally independent. For this reason a wide variety of forms (both in content and in layout) will be found, as each will be drawn up to cover the particular needs of the group of patients with whom the therapist is working. The amount of information required may vary from the specific and detailed as, for example, in the dressing assessment of a spinal injury patient, to the general, for instance a simple recording of the few difficulties encountered by a patient who has suffered a Colles fracture.

As with the forms for physical assessment, most are for departmental use only, a summary being taken for inclusion in a report. Following the initial personal assessment the therapist may find that she is treating the patient daily because of the difficulties encountered. She should ensure that progress is recorded regularly, even though familiarity with the patient's progress may make this seem unnecessary. For further details see Chapter 3.

Specific others

In some centres occupational therapists will find that the forms mentioned above do not cover the type of assessment which needs to be carried out. In this case individual forms must be drawn up to act as a guide and record of these specific assessments. Some of the more common types of assessments which require specific forms have been mentioned and an example of an upper limb training form is given (Fig. 1.5). The sheet illustrated was drawn up for use in the occupational therapy department of an orthopaedic hospital, which has an Artificial Limb and Appliance Centre.

Assessment technique

An assessment may be completed in a few minutes or over a period of several days or weeks and the therapist must remember several points which are common to all, whether formal or informal.

1. It is important to tell the patient what is being assessed and why. Not only is this courteous, it will also take away part of the mystery surrounding some of the rather strange or seemingly pointless activities he is asked to perform.

2. The therapist should always encourage the patient to perform activities to the best of his ability, especially when measuring joint movement, as this will help to ensure that all attempts are the result of equal effort.

3. The assessment session should be as relaxed and short as possible. Many patients become embarrassed or reluctant to focus for too long on their specific disability. They are also likely to tire easily from great effort or if pain results from performing the assessment tasks. However, the session should not be hurried to the point where normal conversation is neglected.

4. When recording the result of activities it is often appropriate to comment on them, for points written down in front of the patient accompanied only by a mumbled 'Hmm' (or worse still a surprised 'Well! Well!' or a low whistle) will do little to put the patient at his ease. A short remark such as 'Now, that's better than last time.' or 'That's not too bad; let me write it down.' will help to reassure him.

5. For all assessment the activities required should be well organised and any necessary equipment available and in full working order. A goniometer that loses a screw when moved or a dynamometer whose bulb pops off when pressed will do nothing for the confidence of the patient or the therapist. The assessment should be done in a private area as a patient who is required to divulge rather personal information will do so more readily if he is both out of the sight and hearing of others. Naturally, the therapist should ensure that the patient is as comfortable as possible, that the room is well lit, heated and ventilated.

RECORDING AND REPORTING

Knowing what to write down in order to record the result of a performance or how to summarise a series of remarks into a clear and succinct report is an art which requires much practice. However, some pointers can be given.

For both recording (notes made from day to day to chart a patient's performance) and reporting (the

	REHABILITATION	
NAME Mrs M T		**No.**

DATE	THERAPISTS INITIALS	TREATMENT AND PROGRESS
3 July Thurs	Sue	Mrs T worked on the wire twister for 10 mins today. She seemed happier. Wire twister 10 mins. Putty.
8th July	S A C	Started making a stool – putting on the top. Green and yellow cord.
22/6		Nearly finished stool. Saw Dr N in clinic on ~~Hosp~~ Friday. Putty 5 mins and printing – notepaper (for Sister S – Willard Ward)
23 July	Anne	Physio says she is progressing well. They've measurements shows an increase of 15° at the elbow. Mrs T wants to make a tray next.
Monday	Pat	Elbow sore and looks a bit red. Mrs T only stayed for 20 mins and made a cup of tea.
29th July	S A C	Sister says Mrs T was discharged from OPD today. She will call in next week to collect her tray.

A

Fig. 1.6   Examples of recording. (A) Incomplete, untidy recording (B) Clear, relevant recording

REHABILITATION

NAME Mrs D   B

No. 361/9774

DATE	THERAPISTS INITIALS	*Continued* TREATMENT AND PROGRESS
9/4/	S. Williams	Perceptual testing shows loss of ability in Figure background discrimination. Body image. Visual apraxia. (see attached form.) Treatment activities to now include:— Body puzzles and outline (body image) Mosaic and picture description (figure background) Object recognition (apraxia.) Dressing— Mrs B now manages to sit on the side of the bed unsupported but topples when clothes are put on or taken off over her head. She is beginning to remember dressing sequence but still has difficulty finding the appropriate garment.
11/4/	S.C.W	Perceptual activities commenced. Mrs B was very labile during the 10 minute session but managed to complete the facial puzzle with a little verbal prompting.
12th April	T. Smith (student)	Dressing— Mrs B's balance continues to improve. She can transfer unaided from bed to chair. Her daughter has now brought in her shoes although the left is a little tight owing to some swelling in her foot and ankle. Suggested that a Tubigrip is applied to left lower limb before getting up in the morning.
13/4/	C. Boyce (aide)	Group activity — Mrs B participated well in group cookery session. She coped well with weighing ingredients using a spoon and initiated conversation with other patients. She says her niece from Woking will visit this weekend and she was pleased to be able to explain this to me.
	S. Williams	Perceptual activities continued. Mrs B still very upset by her lack of ability at figure background. Mosaic session not successful — Mrs B could not distinguish shapes on the plan related to the tiles. To try simple objects on plain background and relate to picture of object.

B

OCCUPATIONAL THERAPY

Type of Assessment/Report.................................Date *Wednesday 27th*

Name *Mr S.B.* D.O.B Hospital No

Address Ward/Unit

Diagnosis *Trauma to knee* Consultant *Dr C*

In the O.T.D. we have been trying to assist Mr Brown to recover after injury to his lower limb.

Mr Brown has been attending the HWS for some time and has completed several articles of woodwork including a stool and letter rack, which were both of a high standard.

His legs seem to be moving much more freely and he can stand for much longer than originally. I can still feel swelling around his knee after certain activities.

He gets on fairly well with the other patients and talks about his wife. He seems to be missing his home and work, and wants to get back to them as soon as possible, though I don't think that he should be discharged for a while.

We have assessed Mr Brown and found that he has 25° of flexion in the mid-range. He is almost fully independent in ADL.

May L. MacDonald.

A

Fig. 1.7 Examples of reporting. (A) Untidy report, lacking important information (B) Clear, concise report

OCCUPATIONAL THERAPY

Type of Assessment/Report. Clinic................................Date. 12:3:...........

Name. Mrs Mary S .... D.O.B. 24:1:44......Hospital No. 369/A....

Address. 39, Smith Street, Sometown ....Ward/Unit. O.P.U.......

Diagnosis. Right Colles Fracture ....Consultant. C..........

This lady has been attending this department 3 times a week for 6 weeks.

Wrist (Right)

R.O.M. (active) – Extension – full
                 Flexion   – limited in last few degrees

Fingers and thumb (Right)

R.O.M. – full

Grip (Right hand)

On initial assessment the grip was weak, but this has improved and the patient appears to have more confidence in using the wrist and hand. However, she still complains of pain over the dorsum of the wrist on activities requiring a strong grip.

DATE	RIGHT	– GRIP –	LEFT
15th Jan	$\frac{1}{2}$ lb		7 lb
27th Feb	$5\frac{1}{2}$ lb		7 lb

Conclusion:

She now has functional use of wrist and hand and we feel that she should discontinue treatment.

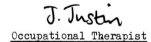

Occupational Therapist

B

Table 1.1 Recording and reporting techniques

	Recording	Reporting
When	After each treatment session or when a significant change is noted.	As required for clinics, ward rounds, case conferences, etc.
What	Changes or upgrading in activity. Specific details related to the patient's condition and/or performance, e.g. pain, swelling, progress, regression, attitude and difficulties encountered.	A relevant summary of progress/regression since the last report. An opinion, conclusion or request where relevant.
Who	The therapist in charge of the treatment programme. Other staff, e.g. an aide, student or technician who has conducted the major part of the treatment session.	The occupational therapist in charge of the treatment programme.
Why	As a memory aid. For information to others if the therapist is absent. As an exact record of progress/regression.	To enable the doctor to form an accurate overall picture of the patient from this and other reports. As a permanent record of the patient's state. As a written statement/conclusion/opinion/request if the therapist is absent.
How	Short, relevant, legible information.	Clear, concise and correct information.

Note: *All* reports and records should be signed and dated.

summary made of daily records) certain rules apply and the following chart may help to form a basis from which to begin.

Recording

Although it is tempting to scribble a hurried record which is legible only to the writer, it is important that all records can be easily read by others and are laid out in a clear and quickly summarised manner. Standard abbreviations are acceptable, such as POP for plaster of Paris, but the therapist should ensure that any abbreviations used are universally understood.

Some examples of good and bad recording are shown in Figure 1.6. Figure 1.6A shows untidy recording, not signed or dated in places, with some irrelevant information while at the same time leaving out necessary information such as noting what happened during the clinic appointment. Figure 1.6B, on the other hand, shows a clear layout, dated and signed. The information is relevant and will be easy to scan for report writing.

Reporting

Where possible reports should be typewritten for legibility. They should, as already stated, be clear, concise and correct. A long, complex and muddled report will more than likely remain unread in a busy clinic.

A good report should state clearly where it comes from. It should give the patient's name and a brief summary of his progress to date. It should not include information on, for example, any items made during treatment or of specific activities used.

Examples of good and bad reporting are given in Figure 1.7. Figure 1.7A shows a report that is not clear or concise and contains irrelevant information regarding articles made during treatment and the patient's wish to return home. It also uses specific and unnecessary abbreviations and is non-informative about the patient's progress. Finally, the basic information is incomplete and the signature is illegible. Figure 1.7B, however, shows a short, well composed and conclusive report.

It can be seen that, with practice, the therapist can become proficient at assessing, recording and reporting her patient's progress. If done regularly and with care, these tasks will soon become a matter of routine requiring less effort and being more accurate than those 'written up' in haste at the end of the week.

2

Measurement techniques

Measurement is an essential part of the overall assessment of most disabilities and when regularly repeated and recorded gives an accurate picture of the effectiveness of a treatment programme. However, the therapist has to remember that in addition to the purely physical factors related to her patient's condition she must also record other aspects of his recovery, such as his functional ability to use the affected limb and his willingness to do so. In addition to this she must be aware of the level of function required by the patient in order to resume his normal lifestyle as soon as possible and of any factors which may, either physically or psychologically, prevent him from using his limb to its full potential.

PRINCIPLES OF MEASUREMENT

Whenever any form of measurement is to be undertaken the therapist should bear certain principles in mind which will make the process as efficient and comfortable for the patient as possible.

1. All necessary equipment should be to hand and in working order. The therapist should be familiar with the equipment so that she can use it confidently. Any other accessories which may be needed, such as record cards or a firm chair or stool (on which the patient can sit while his measurements are being taken) should also be available.

2. The place in which the measurement is to be carried out should be well lit, warm and spacious

enough to allow the patient and therapist to move freely. The area should also offer sufficient privacy to allow the procedure to be carried out without the patient becoming embarrassed by the presence of others. This is especially important during the first measurement session when the required movements are being explained and the patient may be apprehensive about moving the affected area.

3. The therapist should tell the patient what she is going to do and why. Often a simple and short explanation of the method and importance of the measurements to be taken will put the patient at his ease and make the procedure quicker and easier.

4. As well as knowing how to use the equipment correctly the therapist must know exactly which measurements she is going to take and the methods required to take them. She should handle and move the patient's limbs with confidence, thus causing him minimal discomfort, and she should be able to explain clearly any movements she wishes the patient to perform. It is usually helpful to demonstrate the movements.

5. Any tight clothing which may restrict the movements to be measured should be removed or loosened.

6. Whenever possible, measurements of any one patient should be carried out by the same therapist, as people vary in their handling of equipment and therefore no single measurement taken by two different people will be exactly the same.

7. Where possible, measurements should be taken at the same time of day, and at the same time relative to treatment. For example, the movement and dexterity of the hand of a patient suffering from rheumatoid arthritis will vary considerably from early morning (when he is at his stiffest) to mid-day (when his drugs are beginning to take effect and he has 'loosened up'). Similarly, the movement of a joint will vary from the beginning to the end of a treatment session and any measurement, therefore, should be taken either consistently before treatment or afterwards, but not at random.

8. With each measurement the therapist must not only record the result of that measurement but should also note the following:

(a). The skin colour of the limb or area being measured: Is there any bruising? Reddening may indicate the presence of infection, pallor may point to poor circulation in the affected area. Navy or blackened skin may indicate the onset of gangrene.

(b). The skin temperature: Skin which feels hot may point to the presence of infection, whereas skin which feels cold to the touch may indicate poor circulation or the fact that the patient has been reluctant to move the part.

(c). The condition of any wounds: This should be checked to see if they are healing well and that there is no sign of pus, dirt, foreign bodies or tissue breakdown. Although invariably tender to the touch a wound should not be excessively painful when the limb is at rest. Any scarring should be noted as its presence around a joint may inhibit movement.

(d). Pain: This is invariably present following injury, but the therapist should note if the pain becomes excessive during movement or if the patient complains of a throbbing or stabbing pain when the limb is at rest.

(e). Swelling: This may inhibit joint movement or cause pressure on surrounding tissue or structures.

(f). Sensation: Any loss or abnormality in the level of sensation can lead to further injury — especially in the lower limb — or it may inhibit the use of the part, especially in the upper limb.

9. All measurements must be taken regularly and recorded accurately and clearly.

10. The therapist must remember that the measured range of movement, power or muscle bulk of a limb does not indicate its functional ability. It is important, therefore, that as well as measuring the limb the therapist also considers factors such as gait, balance, coordination and dexterity.

METHODS OF MEASUREMENT

In order to measure a limb or joint following injury or disease, the therapist can carry out an investigation of the power, range of movement, swelling and muscle bulk of the affected part.

Measuring muscle power

Control of a particular joint. During the early stages of treatment muscular control around a joint may be weak owing to:

(i) Muscle wasting during a period of inactivity.

(ii) The loss or lowering of innervation following a disturbance to the nerve supply.

(iii) Other mechanical disturbances such as damage to a tendon or tendon sheath.

Due to this weakness it is often not possible to move the joint in the normal manner, i.e. against gravity, in order to measure its range of movement. During the later stages of treatment the therapist will not only want to know whether the joint can be moved against gravity but also whether the muscles which control it are strong enough to move the joint against resistance. Ultimately, she will want to know whether the power on the affected side has reached that of the unaffected side.

For this reason a standard method of manually estimating the muscle power around a joint has been developed. This method is known as the 'Oxford five point scale'. The patient is asked to move the affected joint as far as possible and in a particular plane, so that the muscular power around the joint can be assessed. The power is graded on a scale from 0 to 5 in the following way (an example using the wrist joint is given in brackets):

0 (Zero): No muscular contraction or joint movement is evident. (With the elbow flexed and the forearm supported in mid-position to isolate the movement, no muscular contraction or joint movement is evident.)

1 (Trace): A flicker of muscular contraction is seen or felt but no joint movement is evident. (With the forearm supported as above a flicker of muscular contraction — in the flexors or extensors — is seen or felt but no joint movement is evident.)

2 (Poor): A full range of movement is possible when gravity is eliminated. (With the forearm supported as above, i.e. with gravity eliminated from wrist movement, a full range of movement is possible.)

3 (Fair): A full range of movement is possible against gravity. (With the forearm supported in pronation — for wrist extension — and in supina-

tion — for wrist flexion — a full range of movement is possible.)

4 (Good): A full range of movement is possible against gravity and some manual resistance. (With the forearm supported as in 3 above a full range of movement is possible against some manual resistance, for example with two fingers of the tester's hand pushing across the patient's metacarpals.)

5 (Normal): A full range of movement is possible against gravity and the maximum amount of resistance which allows the unaffected side — or a comparable joint if both sides are affected — to perform fully. (With the forearm supported as in 3 a full range of movement is possible against maximum resistance, for example with four fingers of the tester's hand pushing across the patient's metacarpals.)

Grip strength. A variety of equipment is available for assessing grip strength of the hand (Fig. 2.1):

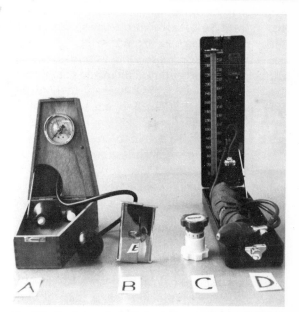

Fig. 2.1   Equipment for assessing grip strength. (A) Bulb-type vigorometer (B) Spring-type vigorometer (C) Torquometer for measuring twist grip (D) Sphygmomanometer adapted to assess grip

(i) The vigorometer (or dynamometer). The bulb type vigorometer (Fig. 2.1A) consists of a pressure gauge to which one of three different sizes of bulbs can be attached. With both needles of the gauge set at zero the patient is asked to grip the bulb securely and squeeze it as hard as he can using his whole hand (where possible) and then to relax. A reading is then taken from the red needle (which will remain static at the furthest point reached) and this needle is then reset to zero. This process is repeated three times in all and the average of the three readings is taken and recorded. The therapist should note that a) each vigorometer will have its own variation in reading making it difficult to give an 'average' normal grip strength, and b) the smaller bulbs can be used to measure pinch or tripod grip if required.

(ii) The spring-type vigorometer (Fig. 2.1B) consists of a metal rectangle, approximately ½" thick, inside which springs are attached to a numbered scale. With the scale set to zero the patient holds the instrument in his hand and squeezes as hard as possible and then relaxes. A reading is taken from the metal pointer, the scale reset to zero and the action repeated twice. An average of the three readings is recorded. The therapist should note that a) this type of vigorometer offers more resistance than the bulb type and is therefore most commonly used on those with a normally strong grip and b) that it requires little participation from the thumb. Should it be necessary to note the effect of the thumb during grip, e.g. when treating patients with a fracture of the first metacarpal or phalanx, or a median nerve injury, the bulb type vigorometer is preferable for assessment.

(iii) The torquometer (Fig. 2.1C). This consists of two short cylinders with a grooved hand grip at each end and a numbered scale, formed and marked by a pointer, in the centre. The white (static) end of the instrument is held by the therapist and the coloured (mobile) end is held by the patient. With the pointer set to zero the patient grips and twists the coloured end as far as possible and then relaxes. As before the average of three readings is taken and recorded.

This instrument is designed to test both twist and grip of patients who experience particular difficulties with this movement, such as those suffering from a forearm or elbow injury, or from rheumatoid arthritis.

(iv) The sphygmomanometer (Fig. 2.1D). Although not designed to test grip strength the sphygmomanometer can be adapted to test the power of those whose grip is especially weak, for example following severe hand injuries. The sphygmomanometer is designed to measure small changes in pressure and can, therefore, more easily detect any minor change in grip strength. This is especially useful in patients who would be unable to make any impression on the other types of vigorometer, as it allows small improvements in the weak grip to be recorded.

The sphygmomanometer is adapted by rolling up and taping the cloth cuff which will act as a hand grip for the patient. The cuff is inflated (using the attached rubber bulb) up to a standard pressure (for example 20 mmHg) which acts as a base line for the readings. The assessment of grip strength is then taken from the average of three readings, as before. The therapist should note that the pressure should be released from the cuff when the instrument is not in use.

Measuring range of movement

The range of joint movement may be assessed in a variety of ways. For each measurement the therapist should check both the active and the passive range within the joint. This will not only allow her to demonstrate to the patient the movements he will have to perform himself, it can also point to the cause of any limitation of movement. For example, a joint which moves freely through a passive range of movement but is limited when moved actively, will indicate that muscle weakness is inhibiting joint movement although the joint itself is free to move. On the other hand, a joint which is limited in both its active and passive range may indicate that other factors, such as contractures, swelling, soft tissue damage or scar formation near or around the joint, may be responsible for the limitation in movement. The therapist must be aware, however, that a discrepancy in the expected active movement of a joint, based on the observation of its passive range and muscle strength, may be due to other factors such as a misunderstanding by the patient of the action required; pain or the fear of producing pain through movement. It may also be due to inhibition, conscious or unconscious, of the joint's movement by the patient (often referred to as compensationitis). This latter phenomenon may occur when a patient is awaiting an assessment of the level of his acquired disability pending an insurance claim or when, for some other reason, he does not wish to use the limb. When moving a joint through a passive range the therapist must always support the limb both above and below the joint. The joint should never be forced to move beyond the range which can be easily achieved.

The active range of movement can be measured using the various pieces of equipment described below.

Principles of measuring joint range of movement

(a). *Starting position.* The most widely used method of recording joint movement today is one in which all joints are measured from a specifically defined starting position which is taken as zero (0°). In the majority of joints this zero starting position is the anatomical position of the joint. For example, at the elbow the starting position is in extension (Fig. 2.2).

(b). *Measuring joint movement.* The joint's movement is measured in degrees from the starting position (0°) to the furthest point of travel. For example, at the elbow joint the measurement is taken from 0° to the point of greatest flexion (Fig. 2.3).

(c). *Measuring a limited range of movement.* If the joint cannot be placed in the starting position (0°), measurement should be taken from the nearest angle to this that can be reached. For example, in Figure 2.4 the measurement of movement at the elbow joint would be taken from (a) to (b).

(d). *Measuring a joint which hyperextends.* Should the joint fall into hyperextension then this extra movement can be recorded as a 'minus' reading. In Figure 2.5, for example, at the elbow joint the measurement would be taken from the furthest point of hyperextension (a) through to the furthest point of flexion (b).

(e). *Measuring a unilateral disorder.* When measuring a patient with a unilateral disorder

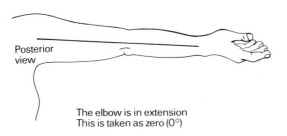

Fig. 2.2 Starting position for elbow measurement

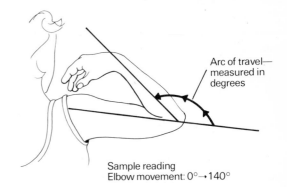

Fig. 2.3 Measuring joint movement at the elbow

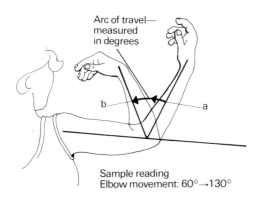

Fig. 2.4 Measuring a joint which is unable to reach the normal starting position

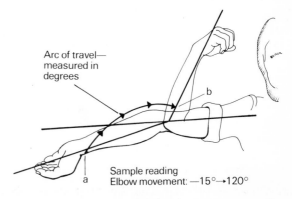

Fig. 2.5 Measuring hyperextension

Table 2.1 Points of reference for joint measurement

Joint	Starting position	Fixed line	Axis	Mobile line	Average range of movement
Shoulder	Anatomical position	Line parallel to the spine	Acromium process	Shaft of the humerus	Elevation through flexion 0°–158°. Elevation through abduction 0°–170°. Extension 0°–53°
Elbow	Anatomical position (with the shoulder flexed for ease of measurement)	Shaft of the humerus	Lateral (or medial) epicondyle of humerus	Shaft of radius (or ulna)	0°–146°
Wrist	Anatomical position (with elbow flexed) for flexion. Forearm in pronation (and elbow flexed) for extension	Shaft of ulna	Ulnar styloid	Shaft of fifth metacarpal	Extension 0°–71° Flexion 0°–73°
Metacarpal phalangeal joints of fingers	Anatomical position	Shaft of metacarpal	Over dorsum of MCP joint	Shaft of proximal phalanx	0°–90°
Proximal inter-phalangeal joints of fingers	Anatomical position	Shaft of proximal phalanx	Over dorsum of PIP joint	Shaft of middle phalanx	0°–100°
Distal inter-phalangeal joints of fingers	Anatomical position	Shaft of middle phalanx	Over dorsum of DIP joint	Shaft of distal phalanx	0°–80°
Carpo-metacarpal joint of thumb	Anatomical position	Parallel to metacarpal of middle (3rd) phalanx	Base of 'Anatomical snuffbox', that is over base of 1st MCP	Shaft of 1st metacarpal	Extension 15°–45° Abduction 0°–58°
Metacarpal phalangeal joint of thumb	CMC joint of thumb in abduction	Shaft of 1st metacarpal	Over dorsum of joint	Shaft of 1st proximal phalanx	0°–53°
Inter-phalangeal joint of thumb	CMC and MCP joints of thumb in extension	Shaft of 1st proximal phalanx	Over dorsum of joint	Shaft of 1st distal phalanx	0°–81°
Knee	Anatomical position, that is extension (patient seated on plinth with knee at the edge of the plinth)	Shaft of femur (or in line with the greater trochanter)	Lateral condyle of femur	Shaft of fibula (or in line with the lateral malleolus)	0°–134°
Ankle	Anatomical position (patient seated on table with knee bent over edge)	Shaft of fibula (or in line with head of fibula)	Lateral malleolus (or the indentation just below it)	Shaft of the fifth metacarpal	Dorsiflexion 0°–18° Plantarflexion 0°–48°

Note: The reader will notice that several joints/movements are not mentioned in the above table. This is because, in the experience of the author, they are not usually measured with a goniometer by the occupational therapist. The measurement of these joints/movements is discussed later. Those which do not appear at all, for example the movement of the toes, are rarely measured by the occupational therapist.

measurements of the unaffected side should always be taken as a guide to the expected level of recovery. Where both sides are affected the average range of movement of the joint should be used as a guide (see Table 2.1). The therapist should remember, however, that these can only give a rough guide to the expected level of recovery as they depend on age, build, race and occupation of the patient.

(f). *Handling the patient.* Moving an affected joint is often painful for the patient and, therefore, all measurements should be made as quickly as possible.

(g). *Compensatory movements.* It is important

to remember that the patient may be making compensatory movements when asked to perform a certain joint motion. This may be conscious or unconscious and usually takes the form of an apparent exaggeration in the movement performed which is the result of a sympathetic movement of a joint close to the one being examined. For example, when the patient is asked to abduct the arm he does this in conjunction with side flexion of the spine, thus exaggerating the shoulder movement (Fig. 2.6).

This compensatory movement can be overcome by:

(i) telling the patient he is doing it (frequently he will be quite unaware of this) and correcting the movements he is making.

(ii) asking the patient to perform shoulder movements bilaterally, so that the spine remains static.

(iii) supporting the part which is not required to move if possible, either manually or by resting it on a firm surface so that it remains still.

(iv) asking the patient to perform the action in front of a mirror so that he can check his own compensatory movements.

If these methods are not successful the therapist should make allowances for the additional movement when she is measuring the joint.

Joint measurement using the goniometer

The goniometer is the most commonly used instrument for measuring the exact range of movement

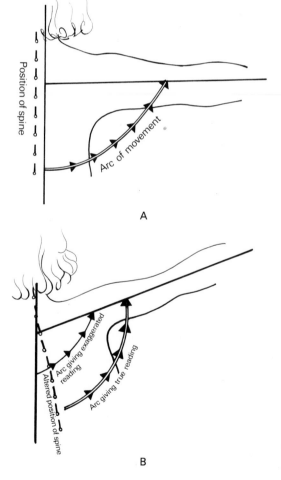

Fig. 2.6 Allowing for compensatory movement around a joint. (A) Correct movement (B) Compensatory movement of the spine exaggerating shoulder movement. (Note: the fixed arm of the goniometer must remain parallel to the spine to give a true reading)

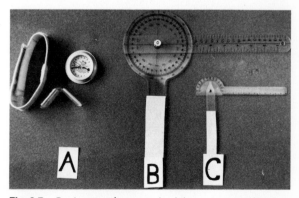

Fig. 2.7 Goniometers for measuring joint movement. (A) Swedish OB goniometer 'Myrin' (B) Standard-size goniometer for measuring large joints (C) Small goniometer for measuring joints in the hand

at a joint. Several different designs are available and the standard goniometer consists of
1. a central protractor marked in degrees
2. a fixed arm
3. a mobile arm

Figure 2.7 shows a standard large goniometer for general use (B), a standard smaller instrument specifically designed for measuring the joints of the hand (C) and a newer model capable of measuring most joint movements (A).

To use the standard goniometer the therapist must first find three points related to the joint to be measured:

(i) *The axis (or fulcrum).* This is the point on the body surface which most closely responds to that around which the joint movement occurs.

(ii) *A fixed line.* This is a line close to the joint which acts as a reference point from which the movement occurs.

(iii) *A mobile line.* This is a line close to the joint which acts as a reference point to show the arc of movement of the joint.

For example, at the wrist joint the axis can be

the ulnar styloid, the fixed line can be the shaft of the ulna and the mobile line can be the shaft of the fifth metacarpal. With the joint held in the starting position (see Table 2.1) the goniometer is lined up with the relevant reference points (Fig. 2.8A). The patient is then asked to perform the required movement while the therapist, ensuring that the fixed arm of the goniometer remains parallel to the fixed line on the body surface, moves the mobile arm to lie along (or level with) the mobile line (Fig. 2.8B). The central screw (if there is one) is then tightened to secure the reading and the patient is allowed to relax while the therapist reads and records the movement obtained.

Table 2.1 shows the starting position, fixed line, axis, mobile line and average range of movement of those joints most commonly measured with a goniometer by the occupational therapist.

Joint measurement using a joint outline

The range of movement at a joint is measured either by drawing around the outline of the joint or by tracing the joint outline with a soft, thin wire

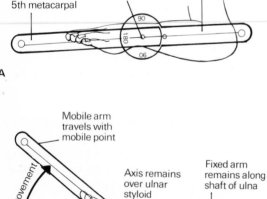

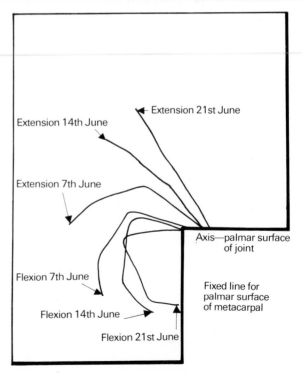

Fig. 2.8 Using the goniometer at the wrist. (A) Starting position (B) Position to read movement

Fig. 2.9 Measuring joint movement with an outline chart

(this latter method appears to be less frequently used).

For the former method, the therapist must locate the fixed point, axis and mobile point near the joint which is to be measured. The fixed point and axis are then placed over the area marked on a prepared piece of card and the patient is asked to move the joint through its maximum range of movement while the therapist marks the furthest point reached (Fig. 2.9).

This method is usually used for measuring the joints of the fingers where a composite reading is required.

Joint measurement using a tape measure/ruler

In cases where it is difficult or inappropriate to measure the range of movement of a joint or series of joints in degrees, a tape measure or ruler can be used. For example, in the hand the span, that is the combination of abduction of the fingers and extension of the thumb, is frequently measured as the maximum distance between the tips of the little finger and the thumb (Fig. 2.10).

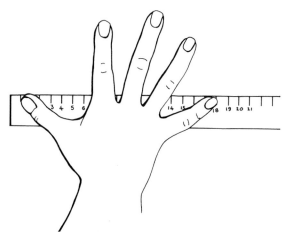

Fig. 2.10 Measuring span of the hand with a ruler

Other joints which can be measured in this way include:

1. Joints in the hand. Composite movement of finger flexion can be measured as the distance between palm and finger tip (Fig. 2.11).

2. Joints in the spine. Composite movement of the joints involved in forward flexion can be measured by recording the distance between the

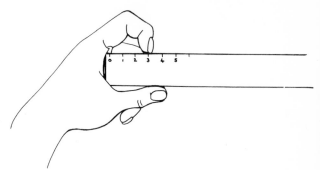

Fig. 2.11 Measuring composite movement of a finger with a ruler

spinous processes of C7 and S1 first with the patient standing erect and then when he is bending forward in flexion.

Visual assessment of joint movement

The patient is asked to perform a specific movement whilst the therapist makes a visual assessment of the range of movement at the joint. Under these circumstances, the movement cannot be recorded in specific units of measurement such as degrees or centimetres; it is therefore often expressed as a percentage or fraction of the patient's normal range of movement (for example that achieved on the unaffected side). The recording may, for instance, show that a joint can move through 50 per cent (or a half) of the expected range.

Visual assessment is often used to estimate movement in:

(a). *the spine.* Cervical flexion, extension and rotation; spinal side flexion, extension and rotation (see Ch. 16).

(b). *the thumb.* Opposition is frequently measured in this way. When full opposition is possible most people can manage to place the thumb pulp on the base of the fifth finger. The degree of opposition can, therefore, be measured by asking the patient to touch the tip of each finger in turn and lastly the base of the fifth finger. The result is then recorded. The therapist must ensure that the thumb has been turned round into opposition and not slid across the hand by a combination of flexion and adduction.

(c). *the shoulder.* Medial and lateral rotation at the shoulder can be assessed by noting the limit in

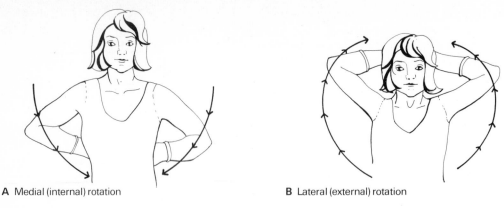

A Medial (internal) rotation   **B** Lateral (external) rotation

Fig. 2.12   Estimating movement at the shoulder. Method 1

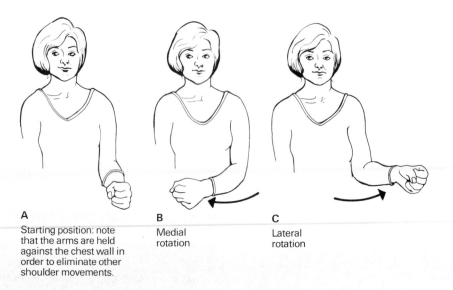

A
Starting position: note
that the arms are held
against the chest wall in
order to eliminate other
shoulder movements.

B
Medial
rotation

C
Lateral
rotation

Fig. 2.13   Estimating movement at the shoulder. Method 2

the range of movement when the patient is asked to touch the small of his back (medial rotation) and then the back of his neck (lateral rotation) — see Figure 2.12. Alternatively the method shown in Figure 2.13 may be employed.

Adduction can be estimated by assessing the amount of pressure which can be exerted on the therapist's hand when placed between the patient's arm and chest wall or by noting the distance travelled by the upper limb across the front of the body.

(d). *the forearm.* Pronation and supination can be estimated by assessing the amount of movement obtained when the patient is asked to tuck his arms into his side and, with his elbow flexed to

90°, rotate his forearm to bring his palms to face upwards (supination) and then downwards (pronation) — see Figure 2.14.

(e). *the wrist.* The amount of radial or ulnar deviation can be estimated by asking the patient to perform those movements.

(f). *the thumb.* Adduction can be assessed by estimating the amount of resistance offered when the therapist pulls on a piece of card placed between the thumb and the lateral surface of the second metacarpal (Fig. 2.15).

(g). *in the hip.* The movements at the hip can be assessed as described in Chapter 16. Note: a full description of visual assessment of movement in all joints is given in that chapter.

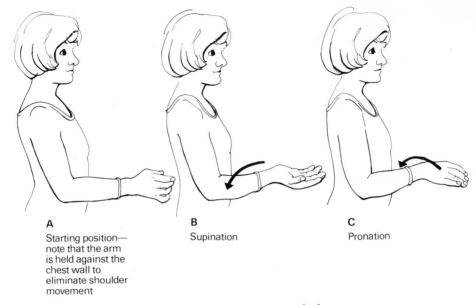

A
Starting position—
note that the arm
is held against the
chest wall to
eliminate shoulder
movement

B
Supination

C
Pronation

Fig. 2.14   Estimating movement in the forearm

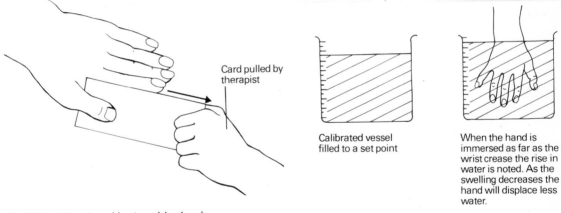

Card pulled by
therapist

Fig. 2.15   Estimating adduction of the thumb

Calibrated vessel
filled to a set point

When the hand is
immersed as far as the
wrist crease the rise in
water is noted. As the
swelling decreases the
hand will displace less
water.

Fig. 2.16   Measuring swelling in the hand by immersion in water

Measuring swelling

It is often necessary to measure swelling around a joint, as this can hinder movement. The therapist should note whether the swelling is reducing as a result of treatment and the healing process or whether it has failed to disperse and thus continues to hinder movement.

Measuring swelling with a tape measure

The simplest method of assessing swelling is by measuring the circumference of the swollen joint with a tape measure. The tape must always be placed around the same point of the limb for accuracy. If swelling is present in the hand this is measured by placing the tape around the palm just proximal to the metacarpophalangeal joints.

Measuring swelling by immersion in water

It is possible, though less common, to estimate the amount of swelling in the whole hand (rather than around the level of the palm) by measuring the amount of water displaced by the hand when it is immersed up to the wrist crease (Fig. 2.16).

Measuring muscle bulk

The muscle most commonly measured in this way is the quadriceps group. These muscles waste very quickly during a period of inactivity and their rate of recovery can be checked by measuring the muscle bulk. The measurement is usually made with a tape measure and the circumference around the thigh is taken at a set point each time (for example 6 inches above the proximal border of the patella). Other muscle groups may also be measured in this way.

Recording measurement

It is important to record all measurements neatly, accurately and in a manner which is easily read. Many therapists prefer to design their own record cards and an example of such a card can be used for recording the measurements of the range of movement of the joints in the upper limb is shown in Chapter 1.

Clearly, the occupational therapist who is working with patients suffering from physical dysfunction will be required, at some point, to measure the extent of that dysfunction. However familiar she may be with the various instruments and methods available to do this, she must always remember that there is no substitute for practical experience in their use.

REFERENCES AND FURTHER READING

American Academy of Orthopedic Surgeons 1976 Joint motion, method of measuring and recording. Churchill Livingstone, Edinburgh

Trombly C, Scott A 1977. Occupational therapy for physical dysfunction, Williams & Wilkins, Baltimore.

Zimmer Orthopaedic Ltd SFTR measuring and recording method, Zimmer Orthopaedic Ltd, Bridgend, Glamorgan (N.B. This is a chart of illustrations)

3

The principles of activities of daily living

The purpose of this chapter is to give the student or newly qualified therapist an understanding of the principles involved in the treatment of patients in 'Activities of Daily Living' (ADL). Since it is not possible, within this chapter, to discuss each illness or condition and offer solutions to problems, only the principles of treatment and such points as mobility, dressing and toilet management are dealt with.

Activities of daily living consist of those tasks which all of us undertake every day of our lives in order to maintain our personal levels of care. To the disabled person the ability to perform these tasks may mean the difference between being independent or dependent. One disabled person has been recorded as saying that ADL are 'all those little things' which, frustratingly, he cannot manage.

ADL comprise an important area of habilation or rehabilitation (see Ch. 8), particularly for those who are suffering from the more disabling conditions as for example multiple sclerosis. A normal life of work, recreation and family activity may be impossible for these patients and they therefore need, both physically and psychologically, to be able to achieve and maintain their optimum potential in mobility and personal care. The therapist's work will also involve the treatment of patients with short-term conditions, such as fractures or peripheral nerve lesions, and the patient may require advice regarding his temporary inability to manage certain aspects of daily living.

Skill in personal care is acquired gradually throughout childhood; it improves with practice and is finally taken for granted. Consider yourself and the process of getting up each morning and preparing to go to work. On waking you automatically stretch, get out of bed, put on a dressing gown, walk to the bathroom and toilet. You wash, dress and prepare breakfast, all without as much as a second thought. But, imagine the thinking ahead and preparation required if you relied on a wheelchair or calipers for mobility. It is then that the simple tasks which are taken for granted by the able-bodied take on vastly different proportions for the disabled.

Some patients re-learn skills through practice, in spite of their disability, and others learn new ways in which to perform skills. The therapist who guides this learning must rely on her ability to break down and analyse complex sequences of movement and adapt them to meet the individual's needs.

When considering the individual, his condition and his abilities and inabilities in ADL, therapists must remember that the ultimate success of a programme of treatment often lies in long, strenuous practice and exercise to strengthen weak muscles and improve coordination and agility, which may cause frustration, anxiety, depression and lack of motivation. The number and nature of self-care activities which a person can manage will depend very much on his own standards and those of his family or community group.

Impairment of any part of the body may hinder self-care. Spinal immobility, for example, may make it impossible for the patient to reach his feet, leading to difficulty in washing and drying them and putting on shoes and socks. However, self-care activities are carried out principally by the upper limbs and involvement of one or both contributes considerably to any difficulties experienced.

Activities of daily living rehabilitation involves the patient and his family, doctors and therapists, and this team work cannot be over-emphasised. In addition to personnel, ADL will revolve round the patient's natural environment, his personality, mental state, hobbies, work, outdoor pursuits and interests.

Maximum independence in ADL is important because most people do not want to be dependent upon others for personal care, and their inability to perform a task may make the difference between constantly needing help and managing alone. If the patient is independent in the self-care activities which are important to him, he may be encouraged to greater efforts, for example purposeful work or a particular leisure pursuit.

ADL are also important for the following reasons:

1. Knowledge of a person's level of performance can act as a baseline from which future progress or deterioration may be measured.

2. They are a guide to any changes which need to be made in a person's routine and functional techniques.

3. They may add to both diagnostic and/or prognostic data, in addition to providing information regarding the patient's level of physical impairment.

4. They enable therapists to plan treatment, habilitation or rehabilitation programmes.

5. Competence in ADL is affected by self-confidence, intellectual capacity and motivation, in which physical and psychological factors are very closely linked.

6. They enable therapists to distinguish between the patient's optimum, that point at which any condition is most favourable, and his maximum potential, that point at which he reaches his highest possible level.

7. Independence contributes to the quality of a person's life.

8. By planned 'salvage operation' the therapist can help the patient to adjust to his new role brought about by disability.

ASSESSMENT

The basis of all modern occupational therapy is functional assessment. Physiotherapists are concerned with range and strength of movement, whereas occupational therapists use that range and strength for the performance of essential activities. Functional capabilities have to be expressed in a practical way, that is, in terms of normal activities, and assessment will include social, clinical, educational and domestic aspects, either over a period of a few days or as the start of a comprehensive, progressive treatment programme.

Points which should be considered include:

(a) Patient's age, diagnosis, social circumstances, reactions, dependence, cooperation and adaptability, particularly to his disability.

(b) Motivation, attitudes and emotions.

(c) Experience of doing ordinary everyday tasks.

(d) Residual physical abilities and their exploitation.

(e) The physical and psychological factors arising from his condition and/or disability.

(f) The patient's actual and potential function with or without aids, appliances or equipment.

(g) General condition of the patient:

(i) acute or chronic stage

(ii) local joint condition

(iii) degree of deformity and consequent functional disability

(iv) extra-articular features and complications

(v) concurrent illness, physical and/or psychological.

(vi) muscle weakness, wasting, spasm

(vii) sensory and/or proprioceptive loss.

(h) The patient may only need an opportunity to try activities in a suitable environment and it will become obvious to him, his family and the therapist that he has retained former skills.

(i) Check lists for ADL (Fig. 3.1) usually specify activities which are used to assess the patient's ability in various tasks. However, in practice these activities cannot be isolated. Mobility is essential for them all, as is skilful use of the upper limbs.

To summarise, assessment takes place in three stages:

1. To ascertain which self-care activities the patient can perform and which not.

2. To evaluate the extent to which self-care ability can be improved, that is, which additional activity the patient may be able to perform alone as a result of treatment.

3. To decide which methods the patient may be able to use to achieve his potential, and how to manage his self-care.

Prior to considering aims and treatment of the patient, the 'how, when and where' aspect of ADL assessment should be noted.

How?

1. By being realistic, taking the patient's overall condition, home circumstances and prognosis into consideration.

2. Knowing the patient as a person, especially if his condition is going to involve long-term planning and treatment, and how his condition affects him and his family.

3. Assessing relevant activities at the 'normal' time of day, for example eating and drinking at meal times, dressing in the morning and undressing later in the day.

4. Adjusting assessment to the patient and his condition, that is, considering whether it is short-term or long-term.

5. Ensuring that the patient has privacy, whether he is being assessed on the ward, in the department or at home.

6. By not taking a patient too literally in his own assessment of his independence. It is a good idea to let him perform certain activities in the normal course of events, for example having a cup of coffee and then going to the toilet. The therapist can then observe for herself whether or not he can manage.

When?

1. On the first day the patient attends for treatment.

2. Patients with short-term disabilities should undergo a brief ADL assessment during their initial treatment session, so that the therapist can isolate any difficulties and advise, teach a temporary alternative method or provide a temporary aid. In this way the patient can be made independent and can assist in his own recovery.

3. Patients with long-term problems may fall into one of two categories, (i) those with a static condition, for example paraplegia caused by an accident, or (ii) with a progressive illness which deteriorates with time, as multiple sclerosis.

In the first group the patient will be assessed at the post-traumatic stage and assisted towards independence. Thereafter reassessment may be irregular. For example, as the patient grows older he may develop secondary problems and seek advice on how to avoid undue stress and strain on, for example, osteoarthritic shoulders secondary to his paraplegia.

In the second group of patients assessment will

BLANKSHIRE SOCIAL SERVICES
OCCUPATIONAL THERAPISTS ASSESSMENT RECORD FORM

Name ....

Age .... Occupation ....

Is able to contact help/community services

Marital Status

	M	S	W	D
*Housing	H	F	B

| H | F | B | W | C | R | O |

Other interested in this case:

DHSS	CN	HV	HH	SW	Warden	Vol. bodies	Minister	Meals on Wheels	Armed Forces	

Attends:

Hospital	Clinic	Club	Centre	Place of Worship

Support given by family/community:

Details of disability:

Treatment programme:

Structural alterations:

Aids required:

Therapeutic activities/occupation:

Comments/recommendations:

Signature of Therapist .... Date ....

*H = House   W = Warden dwelling   If other type of housing (e.g. caravan) occupied, please state.
F = Flat   C = Council house or flat
B = Bungalow   R = Rented accommodation   O = Owner occupied

Fig. 3.1 Activities of daily living (ADL) assessment form

1 manages alone; 2 manages with assistance from another; 3 manages with aids; 4 cannot manage

Bedroom

☐ Turns over

☐ Can raise up

☐ Get onto bed

☐ Get off bed

☐ Manages bedclothes

Mobility

☐ Can stand

☐ Walk indoors

☐ Manages steps

☐ Manages stairs

☐ Can sit down

☐ Can get up from chair

Wheelchair
Able to:

☐ transfer

☐ manoeuvre indoors

☐ manoeuvre outdoors

☐ Type of chair

Personal
Can wash:

☐ face

☐ body

☐ feet

☐ Can brush teeth

☐ Can brush hair

☐ Bath

☐ Dry self

☐ Trim nails

☐ Dress hair

☐ Use make up/shave

☐ Can dress fully

☐ Manages: underwear

☐ top clothes

☐ outdoor wear

☐ shoes

☐ stockings

☐ socks

☐ manages toilet

☐ Manages elastic stockings

☐ Manages appliance

☐ Maintains neat appearance

General
Can manage:

☐ shelves

☐ cupboards

☐ drawers

☐ doors

☐ locks

☐ windows

☐ curtains

☐ taps

☐ switches

☐ meters

Kitchen

☐ Caters for self/family

☐ Prepares food

☐ Serves food

☐ Can feed self

☐ Can drink

☐ Manages kettle/saucepan

☐ Handles equipment

☐ Washes/dries dishes

☐ Can dispose of refuse

☐ Deals with dustbin

☐ Can fill hot water bottle

Laundry

☐ Can use equipment

☐ Hand washing

☐ Can wring

☐ Can hang out clothes

☐ Can iron

☐ Can mend

Housework

☐ Can use equipment

☐ Clean windows

☐ Clean shoes

☐ Can keep house tidy/clean

Communication
Able to:

☐ talk

☐ write

☐ read

☐ use typewriter

☐ use telephone

Outdoors

☐ Garden available

☐ Can care for garden

☐ Can use equipment

☐ Can get into car

☐ Can drive

☐ Type of car

☐ Can use public transport

Handicapped Mother

☐ Can care for children

Pets

☐ Can care for pets

Social/leisure activities

☐ Participates physically

☐ Participates mentally

☐ Can fill leisure time

Help re work/office

be continuous. After the initial assessment and treatment the patient will require reappraisal as deterioration occurs.

4. The time of day at which an assessment and subsequent practice take place has already been mentioned, but since it is so important it is reiterated. A patient will be far more cooperative and better motivated if he sees a reason for undertaking an activity, for example undressing prior to hydrotherapy. To perform any task at an inappropriate time of day is extremely frustrating for the patient and often a waste of time, and unreasonable requests like this do nothing for the therapist's credibility.

Where?

ADL assessment may take place wherever it is appropriate, for example:

1. In the patient's own home: in *his* bathroom and toilet, bedroom, kitchen, at his front door, in his garden.

2. In the ADL unit of the hospital's occupational therapy department which has all the necessary facilities.

3. On the ward. ADL assessment is often carried out on the ward and generally includes mobility, toilet use, feeding, and dressing.

4. In rehabilitation centres to which patients are referred for very specific concentrated treatment.

5. In special units, for example the Disabled Living Unit at Mary Malborough Lodge, Oxford.

When considering the 'where' of an assessment, the therapist must decide whether it is best for the patient to be seen in familiar surroundings, such as the ward or his home or in strange surroundings, such as the occupational therapy department or a special unit.

Recording assessment results is vital. The therapist should note her findings both during and after assessment in a way that is meaningful to all concerned, including the patient. In the treatment of severely handicapped patients a clearly set out assessment of functional ability is far more informative as a record of achievement than the form which illustrates a patient's range of movement and muscle strength.

Aims in ADL

The therapist concerned with ADL should always remember the general aims of treatment:

(a). Establishing and/or maintaining the independence of each patient in all basic relevant activities of daily living and developing his potential abilities.

(b). Training the patient according to his ability, disability, level of motivation and home situation. If success is not forthcoming, assisting the patient by using an easier or alternative method, or supplying an aid or piece of equipment.

(c). Assessing the degree of independence — which will vary for each patient — and deciding what kind of help might be needed by a patient who does not reach full independence and when and where it will be necessary.

(d). Conditioning the patient physically and psychologically in order to improve his mobility, dexterity and coordination, and encouraging positive attitudes towards his own independence.

(e). Finding solutions to practical problems. This may mean:

(i) avoiding the cause of the problem if possible, i.e. not to wear a particular garment if it is difficult to put on and/or take off

(ii) trying alternative methods

(iii) using an aid, a piece of equipment or an appliance

(iv) making a specific aid for a patient if no other solution is available.

(f) Educating the patient's family:

(i) to be realistic about the patient's level of independence

(ii) to help him only when necessary and not because it is quicker or the patient is demanding, as some children or elderly people can be.

Finally, therapists must remember that patients often find their own solutions to difficulties and these should be noted for future reference.

Planning a treatment programme

The therapist will plan a treatment programme whether she has made a complete or partial assessment. She will take into consideration the patient's diagnosis, his immediate needs, his future needs, his home environment, his family and his physical and psychological condition. She must determine the priorities and decide whether he needs to become fully independent in ADL (if the patient lives alone) or whether he should concentrate on specific activities such as toilet use and mobility, as his spouse will assist him to dress, leaving him with sufficient energy to cope with a day at work.

Treatment programmes usually follow a similar pattern:

Mobility and transfers: walking, toilet management, in/out of bed, up/down from a chair.

Personal ADL: toilet management, eating and drinking, dressing, washing.

Household/domestic: preparing a meal, shopping, housework.

Other: handling money, keys, communications, use of telephone, recreation, work.

Treatment

Following her assessment and organisation of a programme aimed at meeting the patient's needs, the therapist will consider whether or not it is worthwhile to attempt to make a patient independent in a specific activity. For example, a patient with a progressive illness may have the neuromuscular potential to feed himself, but incoordination and weakness in his upper limbs may make meal times frustrating. So he gains no pleasure at all from eating and just struggles to get his food into his mouth. In these circumstances training is not rehabilitative but torturous. Self-care is valuable only if it gives the patient pleasure, dignity and the feeling of achievement. A severely disabled person who has had an adequate assessment and has full understanding of his problems should always be given the choice of being assisted.

As performance and attitude vary so much from one person to another, it is impossible to generalise in ADL treatment. A therapist cannot say that 'this is the way in which an arthritic man should put his socks on' any more than she can say 'the hemiplegic should fasten his buttons this way'. It is natural that the therapist will think along similar lines for patients with similar diagnoses until she knows each patient individually. She must remember that a patient's difficulties are individual to him, yet they may resemble those of others and be alleviated in similar ways. With experience, therapists also find that patients with dissimilar conditions present with identical or similar difficulties to which similar solutions may be applied.

When carrying out a programme it is useful to remember the points below:

Give the right help at the right time.

Utilise the overlap between occupational and physiotherapy to the patient's advantage.

Give advice on how to avoid pain and fatigue, on general health and fitness, on how to maintain ideal body weight and on activities using minimal effort.

Teach the patient measures or methods which will prevent deformity or additional deformity. Figure 3.2 shows alternative ways of holding a plate, opening a jar and squeezing a dish cloth for

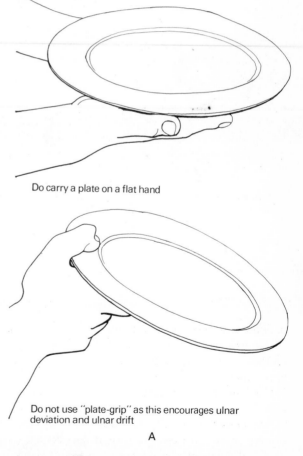

Do carry a plate on a flat hand

Do not use "plate-grip" as this encourages ulnar deviation and ulnar drift

A

Fig. 3.2 The prevention of hand deformity in rheumatoid arthritis. (A) Carrying a plate (B) Opening a jar (C) Squeezing a dish cloth

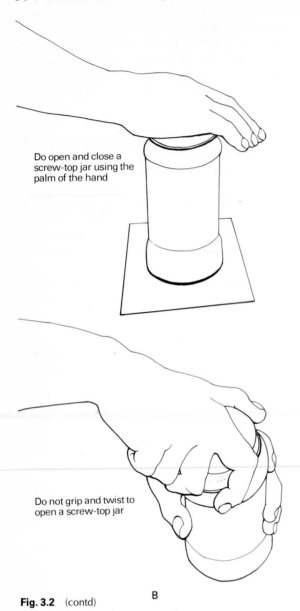

Do open and close a screw-top jar using the palm of the hand

Do not grip and twist to open a screw-top jar

Fig. 3.2 (contd)

B

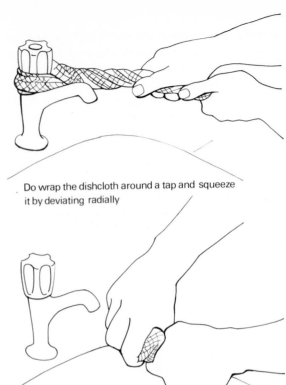

Do wrap the dishcloth around a tap and squeeze it by deviating radially

Do not grip and twist a dishcloth in both hands

C

patients with rheumatoid arthritis.

Use exercise and specific remedial treatment to increase strength, mobility, coordination, when appropriate.

Use alternative methods before considering aids.

Any activity can be broken down into its component parts and exercises should be selected to enable the patient to perform specific movements. Therefore, it is necessary to analyse the movements of a given activity, for example getting up from a chair, and practise each movement as a separate exercise until the entire action is possible.

Practise in a real life setting.

Do not encourage exhausting effort from a patient when the assistance of a helper or an aid would preserve energy for something more important, such as playing with the children. However, remember that there are exceptions: patients with arthritis, for example, need the effort in order to maintain function.

Many patients' conditions vary from day to day, therefore their programme must be flexible. The therapist should be adaptable and able to identify the cause of a poor performance and to initiate treatment which will improve the patient's chance of success.

She must be able to clarify points with the patient's doctor and her other colleagues, and use the appropriate team members for assessment and treatment. Thus a patient with communication difficulties may be helped further by speech therapy, or another whose balance is too poor for the occupational therapist to commence full dressing practice by physiotherapy.

Where applicable, a home visit should be undertaken early in the treatment programme and contact made with the appropriate community services.

Involve the family as much as possible, for example by teaching them how to feed the child with cerebral palsy.

Know what to expect from the patient in the early stages of treatment. For those who lack motivation it is important to achieve something during the first session, however small or unimportant it may seem, for example combing his hair, turning the pages of a book or communicating by gestures.

Consider the patient's pre-morbid personality, i.e. his personality prior to his illness or accident. If the patient has always been dependent upon his spouse, he will not be enthusiastic about independence following his illness.

The outlook of the patient and decisions made by him and his family must be respected by therapists.

The content of a treatment programme must be appropriate for the physical environment and home circumstances. For example, prior to admission to hospital the elderly arthritic widow may have had a home help, the community nursing service and meals on wheels; therefore it is likely that she will need these same services following discharge, so that the inclusion of certain domestic activities, bathing or cutting toe nails, may not be necessary.

The therapist must be inventive and able to compromise. The more ways she knows of completing an activity the better. She should try methods for herself and be ready to learn from patients. She should also be able to demonstrate, slowly and efficiently, any technique which the patient has to learn with her right- or left-hand. The ease with which she does this may influence the patient's attitude towards his difficulties.

Methods as such are not important, but each method chosen must be effective and safe for the patient who uses it.

Specific activities

The general principles of specific activities of daily living are considered below.

Mobility

Mobility in some form or another is essential to us all. To achieve mobility is of considerable importance to the small child, the elderly person or the disabled person, for much of their total independence relies on it. Broadly speaking, mobility serves three purposes. Firstly, it serves a physical purpose by preventing disuse atrophy, contractures, infection and pressure areas. Secondly it is psychologically important as it stimulates and motivates the patient. Thirdly, it is rehabilitative, enabling the patient to carry out all essential activities.

In the context of activities of daily living, mobility is concerned with moving in bed, all transfers, standing, sitting and walking safely. In a treatment programme mobility progresses through three stages: first, the ability to move in bed and on and off the bed; second, the ability to move about a room and/or the home; third, the ability to be mobile within the environment.

General principles of moving in, and on and off, the bed. Patients who have difficulty in moving in bed tend to assume their most comfortable position, but they must be encouraged and taught to change position in order to avoid general stiffness, flexion contractures and pressure sores. Patients who are immobile because of their condition, for example quadriplegia or severe rheumatoid arthri-

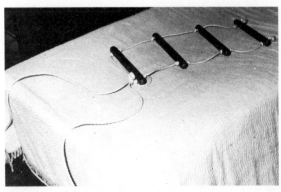

Fig. 3.3 A rope ladder

tis, often need positioning by a helper; a hemiplegic who has the potential to be mobile may need special instruction. To encourage mobility, the patient will be taught exercises by the physiotherapist which will enable him to perform specific manoeuvres, such as turning from prone to supine lying. For those who are unable to move themselves or for whom help is not readily available, there are various aids, for example an overhead lifter, a hoist, a rope ladder (Fig. 3.3), a grab rail or an electrically or manually operated bed, such as the Egerton.

When assessing and teaching the patient it is important to consider the following factors. The bed should be of a suitable height, neither too low nor too high, and have a firm mattress or fracture boards underneath the mattress. This will support the patient while moving about the bed, or on and off it. The use of smooth sheets, such as nylon, will

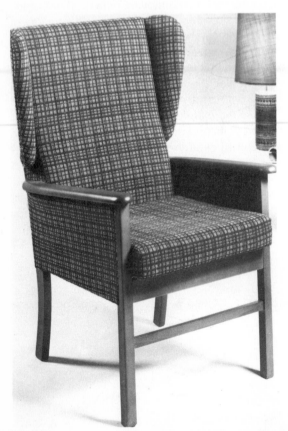

Fig. 3.4 A high seat chair (photograph reproduced by kind permission of J S Smith)

facilitate movement, but some people find them uncomfortable and hot to lie on. Bed cradles which support the weight of the bedclothes so that the patient's lower limbs are unrestricted, may be useful in aiding mobility.

Transfers. These are dealt with specifically in Chapter 4, but it is essential to note certain points within the context of ADL. Transfers are only possible for many severely disabled people if, for example, chairs, toilets, bath rims and car seats are of a suitable height for them. Chairs must be carefully chosen and selection will depend upon how often the patient uses the chair and what he uses it for, apart from resting. Generally, a chair should give support to the thighs so that the patient's feet are flat on the floor, provide good lumbar support, offer support for the head and neck and a comfortable functional position for the upper limbs (Fig. 3.4). As therapists, we find that it is the seat height which often causes difficulties for our patients. The patient with weak quadriceps muscles or stiff hips will be unable to rise from a chair if his hips, knees and ankles are at right angles. He needs a chair whose seat is level with his buttock crease when he is standing, or which will lift him to an upright position mechanically, as does the 'Powell' range of chairs and seats.

Walking. Patients with limited walking ability should be given the opportunity to walk, even if it is only for a few moments each day. Walking has practical advantages compared with wheelchair mobility, in that the ambulant patient has access to areas which are too small or narrow for a wheelchair and he can negotiate slopes, steps or stairs. However, even if the patient is able to walk, it may not be advisable for him to use this method to the exclusion of all others. Factors which should be considered when advising the individual whether to walk or not, and to what extent, include:

1. Safety. The patient must be sufficiently adept in order to avoid falling.

2. The effort required to walk. This may be too much for some patients, a few steps making them breathless and exhausted.

3. The possibility of further damage to joints and the surrounding tissues.

4. The efficiency of walking compared with wheelchair mobility in relation to the patient's daily living tasks. It is often advisable for the

they may be descended backwards or with hand rails on both sides.

Some patients, for example wheelchair users, find it impossible to negotiate steps and stairs and in such circumstances ramping may be the only means of allowing access to the house. The patient's safety is the most important consideration, and the assessor must estimate the available space and recommend the required incline, the maximum gradient being 1 : 12. When ramping is impractical within the home a lift between floors or a stair lift may provide alternative access.

For additional information regarding mobility refer to Chapters 4, 5 and 6 and those dealing with specific conditions.

Dressing, undressing, clothing, footwear and grooming

Anyone may draw attention to himself because of his appearance and the disabled person is no exception. Deformity, paralysis or unnatural movement may all attract attention, particularly if they are exaggerated by clothes. Disguising and/or compensating for any difficulties may be of considerable importance to the individual and by careful selection and adaptation of clothing, or method of dressing the situation can be eased.

The ability to undress, dress and generally make our appearance presentable and pleasing to ourselves and others requires certain skills and these include balance and coordination, the ability to reach, that is joint mobility, strength, dexterity, insight into the task to be undertaken, sensation and a degree of spatial awareness.

General principles. All patients should be encouraged to change into day clothes rather than to spend every day in their nightclothes and slippers, even if the reason for this is primarily a psychological one. Boosting the patient's morale and enabling him to look 'normal' is important.

Assessment of undressing and dressing ability should be made as soon as possible and remain realistic regarding the patient's likely level of independence. It will establish areas in which he is independent and those in which he needs practice and/or teaching. His ability and speed should increase gradually and many patients will achieve independence given time and correct teaching.

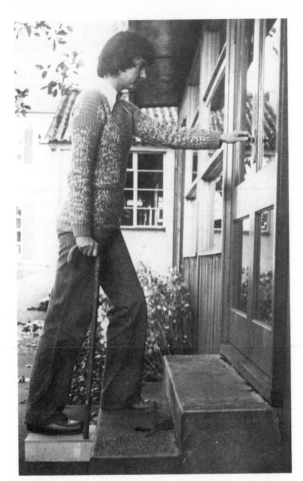

Fig. 3.5　A half step and stick

patient to use his wheelchair for certain activities, for example preparing meals, and walk at other times, for example in the bathroom and toilet where space may be limited.

Steps and stairs cause many difficulties for the disabled and each situation needs careful assessment. A single step may be ascended or descended sideways if the normal forward method is impossible. Grab rails, strategically placed, will assist those who are unable to negotiate steps or stairs safely. Half-steps sometimes help the patient with stiff lower limb joints, or the half-step incorporating a walking stick (Fig. 3.5) may help where the installation of a handrail is impossible. Flights of stairs, such as those to the upper storey of a house, may be ascended and descended one stair at a time with the patient seated on his bottom;

Undressing is easier than dressing. It is less tiring and should be tackled first. It is usually done at a time which is less taken up by routine, either in hospital or at home. There is no need to rush and this will contribute to success. Advise or teach a patient to start by taking off his upper garments, then his lower ones and finally his shoes. Footwear is left until last in case the patient has to stand for any reason, as he is safer in shoes than in socks or stockings.

The patient must be encouraged to think ahead whilst undressing and try to remember that undressing is more than just removing clothes. It is preparation for dressing and the clothes to be worn again should be left right side out and in the order for putting them on.

Ideally, he should undress and dress in the same part of the same room each day, so that clothing is close at hand. The room should be warm, comfortable and afford him adequate privacy. This applies to the hospital ward, his bedroom at home or the occupational therapy department. Privacy is something which we all expect and patients are no exception.

When planning a patient's treatment for undressing and dressing, make every effort to use suitable techniques for him, rather than special garments, adapted clothing or aids.

The dressing sequence needs careful consideration; for example, calipers and shoes must be put on before the patient can stand, or pants and trousers before he can transfer into a wheelchair.

Time a patient's routine to fit in with the rest of the family's routine, especially if he requires help.

Allow ample time for dressing and attempt a little at a time during treatment.

Timing is also important when considering the patient's early morning routine. The therapist should note the time at which the patient has breakfast and goes to the toilet, for this is all part of 'getting up'.

A patient should practise dressing first his upper half and then lower half with the therapist observing, advising and assisting when necessary. She must decide at what stage he should accept help, considering his pain, stiffness, slowness and weakness. He may only require help temporarily, particularly if suitable clothing and the most efficient way of organising and putting it on can be devised.

Patients should be encouraged to persevere in trying to attain standards which are acceptable to them and to achieve these unaided.

Patients with different conditions or difficulties will often find positions which are particularly helpful when undressing or dressing and the therapist should help the individual in finding this optimum position for each stage. A patient may need a well-balanced starting position, for example sitting on a firm chair — with arms and a seat of ample width — with his feet flat on the floor. He must be well balanced to cope with the strain of twisting, reaching up and leaning forward. Another patient may find that lying on the bed is best to dress his lower half, whilst he can sit on a chair to dress his upper half. Once the optimum position has been ascertained the patient should use it for practice.

Particular methods of putting on or taking off clothes must be suited to the individual's needs and those which have been worked out by the patient himself are usually the best ones for him, so encourage and learn from him.

A final point concerning dressing: the level of independence aimed for should take into account the individual's circumstances and needs. Maximum or total independence may be possible but unrealistic. Remember that it is sometimes more important to save a patient's energies and time for more interesting, stimulating and rewarding activities.

Clothes. Generally speaking, it is best to select clothes from those currently available in the shops. It is almost always possible to choose garments which are suitable for the patient's age, taste and capabilities and which will conceal wasted muscles, deformities and/or appliances. Clothes can be specially made, but if they are they should be skilfully designed to disguise infirmity or deformity and produced in contemporary materials and colours.

Shopping for clothes is often difficult, tiring and frustrating and patients may find that the larger stores are more accessible, have larger fitting rooms and a wide range of all types of clothing and footwear. If shopping locally is impractical, reputable mail order firms may provide a solution, as clothes can be tried at home and returned if unsuitable.

Evaluation of each patient's needs, circumstances and disability is essential when choosing suitable garments. Particular attention should be paid to comfort as some patients have to spend many hours in the same position.

There are several points to remember when choosing a garment: Ideally it should be simple and loose fitting with a minimum of fastenings and/or ample openings and/or gussets. Loose, simple styles are also more comfortable and smarter than clothes which are tight. Elasticated waists, cuffs and shoulder straps are often easier to manage. Many patients need warmer clothing than most of us because they are inactive physically and they should be advised to choose warm fabrics rather than wearing many layers of clothing. This last point is very important, for more items mean more effort in undressing and dressing, and patients usually wish to avoid this.

Particular garments need careful selection bearing in mind the patient's abilities.

1. All *underwear* should be easy to take off and put on, give the required support and facilitate toilet use. Bra's and corsets present some patients with great difficulty, therefore the therapist must be able to advise them about suitable alternatives, for example front fastening bra's, or adaptions to garments so that the patient or helper can manage easily. All-in-one garments, such as the Liberty bodice, may still be worn by older patients and these give adequate support and warmth. Pants can be altered to suit individual needs.

2. *Socks, stockings and tights* also cause considerable frustration to patients and the therapist can give advice as to suitable types of hose and methods of coping with them. If a patient wears a corset she must wear stockings to keep it in position and this means she has to be able to fasten and unfasten suspenders. If she does not need to wear a corset she may wish to try tights or stockings with grip tops. For those who have difficulty with socks natural fibre ones (made from wool or cotton) may be easier to put on, as they have more 'give'.

3. *Skirts* should be 'A' line or flared, as straight ones restrict movement and tend to slide up.

4. *Garment sleeves* should permit freedom of movement, particularly around the shoulders. Wheelchair users find raglan rather than inset sleeves best. Their sleeves often need to be short or three-quarter length to prevent over-soiling on the wheel rims. If, however, the patient has to wear long sleeved garments, some form of protection can be worn over the cuffs to prevent excessive soiling and wear. On the other hand, patients walking with axilla crutches find that inset sleeves are less likely to ride up than raglan ones.

5. A *size* larger in an outer garment may be suggested if it helps the patient's function. This applies particularly to trousers for wheelchair users, because they need additional room in the seat and crutch for comfort.

6. *Braces* for ambulant men are better than belts, as they keep the trousers well positioned, will expand at the shoulders with movement and will assist some patients in clothing management when using the toilet.

7. *Two-piece outfits* for women prevent the problems which dresses sometimes cause, for example riding up whilst sitting and moving in a wheelchair. They may also be easier to put on and take off and are more adaptable.

8. *Pockets* are very useful additions to clothing, but they must be suitably positioned. They are most useful on the front of the garment rather than the side and they enable the patient to carry small items about with him, so leaving both hands free for walking aids, handrails or wheelchair propulsion.

9. Finally, remember that garments will require extra *laundering* if a patient is incontinent, so the fabric must be washable, and quickly and easily dried.

Fastenings. Following assessment the therapist has to decide whether the patient is going to dress himself completely, whether he will receive help with certain items, or whether he will be dressed, for this will influence both the choice of fastening and its position on a garment.

For the patient who dresses himself fastenings — if any are required — should be kept to a minimum. They should be on the front of the garment and near the mid-line or middle of the trunk, because the less able patient will have difficulty with fastenings below hip level and at shoulder level.

Where fastenings are a necessity they must be of a type which the patient opens and closes easily.

Examples include Velcro and 'D' rings rather than hooks and eyes on underwear and waistbands; zips rather than buttons on trousers and jackets; large buttons instead of small ones, Velcro dabs on shirts and blouses to eliminate buttoning and unbuttoning.

If the patient needs help to dress or has to be dressed, it is sometimes more convenient for the helper if fastenings are sited on the back of garments.

Adaptations to clothing. These have to be considered when difficulties are experienced with ordinary clothes and nothing suitable can be made. The most common alterations are:

Enlarging an opening, for example a neck line, to ease putting on and taking off over the head.

Additional openings, for example a zip inserted into an inside trouser leg seam to facilitate access to a urinary appliance for emptying, or to assist the patient to get his trousers on and off if he wears a caliper or prosthesis.

Moving fastenings so that the patient or helper can reach them, for example back or side fastenings on bra's or corsets can be brought to the front.

Changing to a more suitable fastening, for example using Velcro instead of a hook and eye or button on a waistband; buttons instead of a zip for the patient who is only able to use one hand, or a zip for those with reach and coordination difficulties.

Elastic will aid dressing and keep a garment in position, for example shirr elastic in cuffs, elastic in the shoulder straps of a bra'.

Reinforcing some garments against excessive wear by a caliper or prosthesis, for example inside knee patches.

The comprehensive series of booklets published by the Disabled Living Foundation illustrates these fastenings and alterations in more detail.

Fabrics. A therapist should not add to a patient's difficulties by using or recommending clothing which restricts movement and is uncomfortable. The choice of fabric will therefore be as important as the style of the garment.

Generally, lightweight warm fabrics are best, so that only a few garments will be needed, which makes undressing and dressing simpler and quicker. For example, a lined skirt dispenses with the need for a petticoat, a quilted anorak is easier to put on, more comfortable and warmer than a tweed jacket.

Stretch fabrics are useful for loose-fitting over garments as no fastenings are needed.

Slippery materials or linings to garments facilitate dressing, but they do increase the tendency to slip forward in a chair. However, as a general rule, they are of great value to patients for whom lack of movement and weakness present problems.

Underclothes should be well fitting and made of absorbent fabrics, especially if the patient is prone to develop pressure sores or is incontinent. They should be made of natural rather than man-made fibres, for example cotton pants rather than nylon ones.

Easy care fabrics which are washable and dry quickly are invaluable and some of the more popular ones in use today are mentioned below:

(i) Cotton — easy to wash, soak or boil, particularly if the garment is likely to become stained or soiled.

(ii) Crimplene — crease resistant, washes well, dries quickly and needs little or no ironing. It is a stretchy fabric, lightweight, warm, keeps its shape and is available in a very wide range of weaves of varying weights, warmth and texture.

(iii) Terylene — garments comprising terylene and another fabric, for example cotton, are also crease resistant, lightweight, warm and usually washable.

(iv) Wool or wool jersey — warm and lightweight, but needs care if it has to be washed regularly.

Note: Man-made fibres tend to build up static electricity which is especially noticeable when wheelchair users wear too many nylon garments. In addition, some patients are unable to wear man-made fibres for other reasons. In these cases, natural fibres should be recommended.

Footwear. Appropriate footwear is imperative. Patients should be persuaded to wear 'sensible' supportive shoes rather than slippers, as these are much safer, particularly for those with impaired mobility. Patients may argue that their slippers are much more comfortable, and so they may be, but they are more likely to trip or slip in well worn slippers than in supportive shoes. If the patient cannot wear the standard types of shoe available, he may need special footwear. If the therapist is

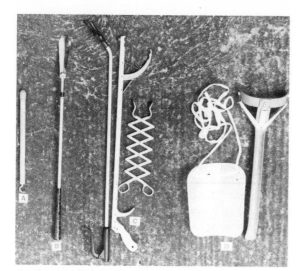

Fig. 3.6 A selection of dressing aids including A) A dressing stick B) A long handled shoehorn C) Long handled reachers D) A stocking/sock aid

unable to assist, for example with plastazote boots/shoes or 'DRU' shoes (orthopaedic bootees which provide correction, comfort and support), then the patient should be referred to his consultant who will ensure that he is assessed and fitted by the Appliance Officer and his team.

Simple dressing aids. Simple dressing aids should be considered if alternative methods and/or alterations to clothing and footwear are insufficient to make the patient independent. One or more dressing aids may be necessary. They should be lightweight, portable, easily cleaned, durable, have no rough edges and be cheap to make or readily available. Figure 3.6 shows some of the examples given below:

(a). A dressing stick for pulling on or pushing off clothing, as used by patients with severe shoulder joint limitations. ·

(b). Long-handled shoehorns for those who cannot reach their feet to pull the backs of their shoes over their heels.

(c). Button hooks are often helpful to the one-handed who find it easier to use the hook than to do up a button with their fingers, or to the bilateral upper limb amputee who cannot manipulate buttons with his split hooks, but can hold a button hook.

(d). Long-handled pick-up sticks are usually used to pick up items beyond a patient's reach, but can be equally useful in pulling pants and/or trousers over his feet.

(e). Stocking, sock or tights aids, of which there are a variety available, can assist those who find it impossible to use an alternative method.

(f). Elastic shoe-laces for the one-handed who cannot master one-handed shoe-lace tying or for those who cannot reach their feet. Shoes fastened with elastic laces are usually put on with a long-handled shoehorn.

Appliances. Appliances should be mentioned here, for they too have to be put on and taken off. Some patients will have to wear calipers, prostheses, surgical corsets or splints, and the fastenings should be positioned bearing the individual's capabilities in mind. If possible, a therapist should be present at the initial assessment by an Appliance Officer, so that consideration may be given to the following: the direction of 'pull' to do up and undo the fastening, whether the patient is right- or left-handed, the optimum position of a fastening with regard to particular problems, for instance the grip and dexterity of the individual.

Grooming. Grooming is a necessary part of anyone's daily routine. It is important to encourage the patient to take pride in his/her appearance, for first impressions are often lasting.

Hair should preferably be kept in a manageable style, that is short and simple, unless the patient has a helper who does not mind coping with a more complicated style every day. Hair washing, setting and drying is often difficult and for those who cannot manage at home or visit a local hairdresser, a mobile service can usually be contacted.

Proper care of finger and toe nails is essential for reasons of hygiene and appearance, and the care of the latter is closely linked with mobility. Nail files and clippers can be attached to small boards to assist stability when caring for finger nails. Toe nails often present insurmountable problems and it is advisable to obtain help from the family, the community nursing service or a chiropodist, particularly if the feet and toe nails need professional attention, for example those with diabetes.

Make-up application may need to be taught to female patients. A woman may have had previous experience of skin care and the use of cosmetics, but due to her present condition may be physically unable to follow her former regime. She may require assistance with the repositioning of a mirror, provision of adequate lighting or change of containers for her beauty preparations. The younger patient may find that sessions in skin care and the use of cosmetics given by a beauty consultant or therapist are invaluable, for she may have missed opportunities to learn earlier on.

If impaired vision is partly responsible for inadequate grooming magnifying mirrors may help the patient.

Techniques. Techniques of undressing and dressing are set out briefly below. For difficulties arising from a patient's specific condition consult the appropriate chapter.

Continuous practice will gradually reduce the time taken to undress and dress and safety is an important consideration in positioning the patient.

1. *The one-handed.* Having chosen the most suitable clothing the patient should be taught one process at a time.

(i) Ensure that fastenings are accessible.

(ii) Place everything required, in order, on the affected or unaffected side or in front of the patient and ensure that it is right side out — exact positioning depends on the treatment regime used.

(iii) Ensure that the patient is in the optimum position, i.e. on the bed or in a chair.

(iv) Use a long mirror if this helps.

(v) Dress one half of the body at a time, for example the upper half first and then the lower half, for this saves effort and the patient is less likely to become cold.

(vi) When undressing remove the unaffected limb from a garment first.

(vii) When dressing place the affected limb into a garment first. These methods ensure that the patient's most mobile limb is free from clothing when manoeuvring a garment around or up and down his body, thereby making the procedure easier.

2. *The two-handed.* The patient has to learn to manage the lower half of his body, for the upper half should pose no problems and may be dressed and undressed first.

(i) Decide on the optimum position for undressing and dressing, i.e. on the bed or in a chair.

On the bed: sit/lie on the bed to put on socks, pants and trousers and pull them up as far as possible. The patient lies on his side and pulls the free sides of his pants and trousers over his iliac crest to waist level. He rolls over and repeats the procedure. He lies supine to fasten the garment at the waist and then puts on his shoes.

In a chair: the patient places his feet flat on the floor to assist his balance. He places the openings of garments which go over his feet at his feet and pulls them up over each foot. Trouser legs will then be 'gathered' between his shoe and knee, and holding himself off the seat with one hand he will pull up his pants and trousers on one side with his free hand and repeat this for the other side.

(ii) Women wearing button-through skirts or dresses will probably find it simpler to move onto the garment when it is laid out on a chair seat or they may roll onto the garment whilst on the bed.

The methods described above serve as a guide only in undressing and dressing techniques. Each can be adapted or used in similar ways for patients with similar difficulties. For example, the hemiplegic, the unilateral upper limb amputee or the patient with severe osteoarthrosis of one shoulder joint will use techniques for the one-handed, whereas the multiple sclerosis sufferer, double lower limb amputee or paraplegic may employ any of the methods described for the two-handed person.

Toilet management

It is more difficult to feel confident in the toilet than anywhere else, yet it is often the one place where the patient really wants to be independent. For the severely disabled patient using the toilet is the most difficult aspect of self-care, and often the most crucial for attaining personal independence and resettlement at home.

The therapist who is treating a patient with toileting problems must heed the following:

Generally, the more disabled the patient the more space he will require in which to manoeuvre. The toilet is usually the smallest and most inaccessible room in the home and even a toilet combined with the bathroom does not always provide adequate space. The majority of problems are architectural and prior to treatment in hospital it is necessary to either make a home visit or obtain details of the patient's own toilet from the family and/or community therapist. Access is hindered by narrow corridors, awkward corners, narrow doorways and steps and stairs; outside toilets pose additional problems. Non-slip flooring, gentle ramps or shallow steps with handrails and good lighting are essential. Access can often be improved by rearranging furniture and fittings, for example reversing the hang of a door or fitting a sliding one. Ideally there should be a wash-hand-basin in the toilet, if this is separate from the bathroom, to save additional mobility and exertion, particularly where perineal and anal cleansing may be difficult due to lack of adequate facilities in the right place. For details of design and dimensions refer to '*Designing for the Disabled*' by Selwyn Goldsmith.

To improve access to both the toilet and bathroom, reconstruction to integrate the two is often necessary. The removal of a dividing wall for better manoeuvrability may solve the major difficulty.

The position of the toilet pedestal is crucial and if rails are needed, they should be installed to suit the patient.

Wheelchair users find that a sideways transfer is often facilitated by setting the pedestal further out from the wall than is usual.

The majority of less able patients prefer a pedestal seat which is higher than usual. Ideally this preferred height is 21 inches (53 cm). The type of seat may make a considerable difference to the comfort and ability of the patient, for example the

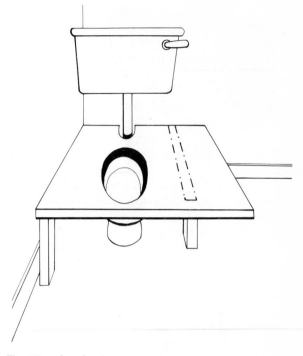

Fig. 3.8 A bench toilet seat

horse-shoe shape (Fig. 3.7) which is open at the front makes perineal cleansing easier for some, but may be unstable for others. The old fashioned wooden bench type seat (Fig. 3.8) is very stable and also acts as a sliding or transfer board. Inclined seats (Fig. 3.9) can be used by patients with stiff joints in their lower limbs, particularly their hips. For increasing the height of the seat various raised toilet seats are available, with or without

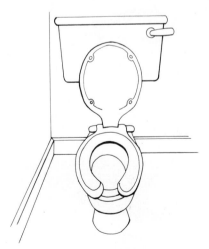

Fig. 3.7 A horse-shoe shaped toilet seat

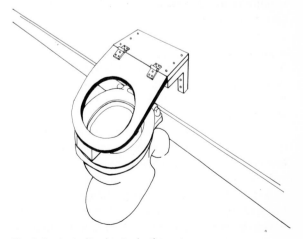

Fig. 3.9 An inclined, raised toilet seat

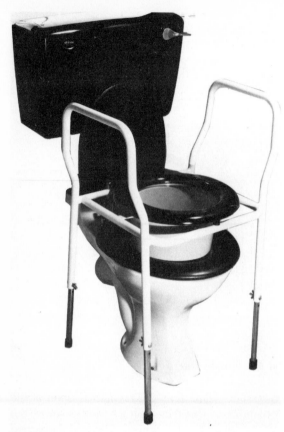

Fig. 3.10 A combined raised toilet seat and rails (photograph reproduced by kind permission of Llewellyn & Co. Ltd.)

handrails incorporated into the design (Fig. 3.10).

The size and positioning of grab rails is extremely important and is a matter of individual preference and need. Horizontal and vertical rails are usually more stable than inclined ones, although some patients find inclined rails of great assistance when rising from the toilet, for this latter type will support their forearm as well as provide a firm grip for their hand. A matt finish is easier to grip than chromium plate and a rail of 1½ to 2 inches (3.75 to 5.00 cm) in diameter is more serviceable than a slimmer one.

Specific techniques are dealt with in Chapter 4, but it is important to mention certain aspects of transfers related to toileting here.

1. A patient who uses a wheelchair for some activities, but not all, can often be taught to stand up, take one or two steps and turn round and sit down. If he can do this, many problems may be solved and if at all possible this is worth aiming

for, because it enables the patient to care for his own toileting needs in many situations, that is, at home, when visiting friends or in the day hospital.

2. Permanent wheelchair users need techniques adapted to suit them and the toilet/s to be used. Sliding boards and bench type seats are common solutions to transfer difficulties, but some patients will be able to transfer sideways directly from their wheelchair on to the toilet seat by using the mobility and strength in their upper limbs, shoulder girdle and trunk. Other patients will have to transfer backwards. The wheelchair back canvas should have a zip fastening, but this may cause difficulties as zips are not designed to take the stresses and strains imposed on a wheelchair back and may break. In addition, many patients with upper limb dysfunction will find it difficult or impossible to unfasten and fasten the zip. However, for some paraplegics the zip-back canvas is an ideal solution.

3. Certain patients will make forward transfers onto the toilet and function sitting back to front. Double lower limb amputees, who rely on wheelchair mobility, frequently use this method.

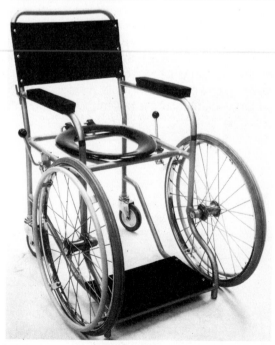

Fig. 3.11 A self-propelling Sanichair (photograph reproduced by kind permission of Surgical, Medical Laboratory Manufacturing Ltd)

4. For those who cannot transfer from their wheelchair to the toilet, sanichairs are available (Fig. 3.11) and these can either be propelled by the patient or wheeled by a helper and positioned over the toilet pedestal.

Undressing, cleansing, washing and dressing must all be assessed in conjunction with actual use of the toilet. The therapist must remember that these activities are usually undertaken within a confined space, thereby adding to some patients' difficulties. Alterations to clothing, especially underwear, and instruction in alternative methods can make a patient independent. If a patient is no longer able to stand or balance, he may be taught to slide forward on the toilet seat and wipe himself from the back, or to slide back on the seat and clean himself with his legs apart. For other patients a simple aid will help (Fig. 3.12). For the severely disabled the use of a bidet or electrically-operated toilet such as the 'Clos-o-mat' or 'Medic-loo', which dispense warm water followed by warm air, may solve cleansing difficulties.

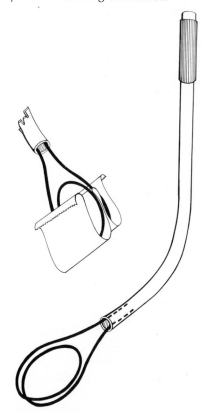

Fig. 3.12 A cleaning aid

The assessment should also include a patient's night-time management. Frequently a completely different arrangement has to be made, taking into account relatives' or helpers' needs. This is imperative, for they require an uninterrupted night's rest if they are heavily committed to a caring role during the day. Alternatives to the toilet include urinals, commodes or non-mains toilets such as the Perdisan range. These are often easier and safer to use at night and save the individual much exertion.

Menstruation causes much discomfort, embarrassment and depression to disabled women. Periods are often painful with a heavy loss of blood and the patient may need medical advice and treatment to suppress or regulate menstruation. Therapists should assist patients to manage as easily as possible and may be able to offer advice, particularly to younger patients, about the most suitable and easily managed forms of protection, for example sanipants with tuck-in pads. They should also emphasise the need for perineal hygiene to prevent odour.

Two final points must be mentioned and should be borne in mind by the therapist at all times, both when assessing and treating the patient. She must ascertain *why* he has to use the toilet, for he may not use it in the conventional manner, he may just wish to empty a urine bag. She must also ensure that methods she advises and teaches are, above all else, safe for that patient.

Incontinence. This is a symptom of several conditions and is occasionally the sole cause of admission to hospital. Therapists treating elderly people, or those with multiple sclerosis, paraplegia, diabetes or emotional disturbances will have to consider incontinence management within their treatment programmes. The therapist must be understanding, for incontinence of urine and/or faeces causes patients acute embarrassment, misery and discomfort. They lose their self-respect and may be a burden on caring relatives and staff. Therapists can contribute to management in very practical ways, initially by adhering to the regime introduced by nursing staff and additionally by advising patients, relatives and colleagues.

The *environment* is often the primary cause of incontinence, particularly for the immobile patient. The toilet should be within easy walking or wheelchair propelling distance; it should be easily accessible, warm and afford privacy. A commode may be the solution to night-time toilet use.

Training in a particular regime is important, whether the patient is wearing an appliance which needs emptying at regular intervals or if frequency of micturition is the problem. Worrying only makes the situation worse, so patients need help in timing their visits to the toilet. This is very individual; some patients may need to express their bladder every hour, while others may have to go to the toilet after meals and mid-morning and afternoon drinks. Some patients are advised to curtail their intake of fluids in the latter part of the day, but medical advice must be sought in this instance, as some patients must maintain a regular fluid intake throughout the day. Any regime should become an integral part of a patient's treatment programme. With increasing mobility the patient's incontinence may decrease or he may become continent again.

A variety of *appliances* are available for dealing with urinary incontinence. Men are able to manage incontinence more readily, for their anatomy makes the wearing of appliances or the use of a catheter easier. Most women prefer to wear some form of absorbent pad inside protective pants and several types are available. Some pants are the simple pull-on variety, while others have drop-front panels or open out flat.

Clothing need not be a problem. It may be advisable for patients to wear separate upper and lower garments. Upper garments need to be short to avoid the possibility of soiling and lower garments should be kept to a minimum and be made of easy-care fabrics.

Skin care and odour control are essential for the comfort and self-respect of the patient and therapists will work with nursing staff so that the patient's regime is continued when he is not in the ward.

Therapists are often able to advise colleagues about the range of suitable commodes, urinals and bedpans available. Their recommendations take into account safety, the mobility of the patient and his degree of independence in personal hygiene.

For more detailed information refer to *Incontinence* by Dorothy Mandelstam and *Management for Continence* by Bob Browne.

Personal hygiene

Washing and bathing is another area of self-care in which the majority of patients have a great desire to be independent and the following points should be considered:

1. Safety, above all else, for bathrooms are potentially dangerous places.

2. Most patients can manage to wash their own hands and face, provided they have access to hot water, soap, flannel and towel. They do not necessarily have to go to the wash-basin which may be inaccessible, of an unsuitable height or inconvenient to their early morning routine. It is often easier to take a bowl of warm water to the patient whilst he is still in bed. The bowl should be made of good quality firm polythene and placed at a suitable height in a convenient position, for example on a stable overbed table.

3. It is unrealistic to expect a patient with upper limb dysfunction to be able to wash himself all over without help and even if he can do so, the effort will be exhausting and he may become cold. To assist both the patient and his family help may be obtained from the community nursing service. If this is not possible the patient must be helped to work out a routine of washing different parts of his body on certain days, that is, working in rotation. Items which may assist those with impaired function of their upper limbs include long-handled sponges and brushes, hand held shower sprays, flannel mittens to enclose a bar of soap and loofahs. 'Trick' methods are often a great help, for example using one foot to soap the other; using a forearm instead of a hand to soap the other arm, or thigh.

4. Bathing is difficult and strenuous for elderly and slightly disabled patients; for the more severely disabled it is often extremely dangerous as well. Bathrooms are often small, with awkward access and potentially slippery surfaces and the hot and steamy atmosphere may precipitate faints and fits. Considerable agility and strength, including the ability to stand on one leg, is needed to get in and out of the standard bath safely, and assessment and practice should be made realistically, that is, with the patient taking a bath.

Lack of space is a tremendous problem and it is often difficult or impossible to alter a patient's bathroom at home. However, prior to making any recommendations the therapist must ensure that the patient is capable of using the facilities safely.

Bathrooms designed or altered for use by an elderly and/or disabled person should include certain features in addition to standard fittings. Floors should be non-slip when wet. Grab rails must be well placed and are best sited horizontally and/or vertically about three or four inches (7.5 to 10 cm) above the bath rim and two to three feet (60 to 100 cm) long. A combination of horizontal and vertical rails enables most patients to pull up and forward, to push up or to hold onto and to steady themselves when getting in and out of the bath. Some patients will manage well with the small grab handles incorporated in the rims of modern baths, or with one appropriately positioned grab rail with which to steady themselves. Although older baths with high sides present access difficulties for the ambulant, they do facilitate the use of mobile hoists, for they usually have more space underneath than their modern counterparts.

In teaching a patient to bath himself the therapist must consider the height, size, type and depth of the bath he uses at home, and its accessible side. It is of no use whatsoever for a patient to be able to manage to bath alone in the department or ward, if he cannot do so at home.

The height of the bath is critical for the wheelchair user and the rim, ideally, should be the same height as the wheelchair seat, or slightly lower, if the patient is to be independent with or without aids.

If a helper is needed, his needs must also be considered. The bath rim may need to be higher than usual to facilitate lifting and to prevent backache and strain. If a hoist is to be used, access to the side or end of the bath is vital and side panels may need to be removed and/or the bath raised if no other solution is available.

Non-slip mats or surfaces to baths and showers are essential.

Transfer in and out of a bath may be straightforward over the side, sideways, over the end or with the use of a chair, or board and/or seat. In all cases, a bath which is shorter than usual is safest, because the patient is less likely to slip under the water.

Teaching a patient to get in and out of the bath unaided may be possible, but accurate assessment is absolutely essential, for he must be safe and physically and mentally capable of coping when both he and the bath are wet.

Taps and other fittings should be of a design and in a position which facilitates their use. Patients should be discouraged from using taps, inset soap dishes and the wash-basin as additional grab rails, for the stability of these fittings may be suspect. If a patient cannot operate conventional taps, lever taps or a tap turner may assist him. Soap, flannel, sponge, nail-brush and other accoutrements should be within easy reach and suitably positioned bath bars, trays or shelving will assist.

5. For many patients a well designed and positioned shower provides a safer and more suitable method of washing than a bath. It is also easier to manage and more economical. However, bathing is warming, whilst showering can be a cold task if the room is unheated and for certain patients, for example arthritics, a soak in a warm bath will ease their stiff, aching joints. When recommending shower installation consider a patient's capabilities. He may manage quite safely with a shower spray attached to the taps, but generally speaking thermostatically controlled showers are safer for the elderly and/or disabled. A compromise is often the only solution and a suitable shower installed over the bath is helpful for the patient who can step over the bath rim. He can then sit on a board or seat with his feet in warm water and use the shower to wash himself. This method requires less effort than straightforward bathing and it is easier to clean the bath afterwards. The position of the shower rose is important and those fixed overhead are generally unsuitable for the disabled person who is likely to be sitting on a seat. The rose needs to be at chest height and movable to allow all-over washing from a seated position, as many patients do not like showers of water directed at their head or face. Where separate shower units are installed, the tray will have to be negotiated and, again, handrails will assist the ambulant. The non-ambulant, for whom showering is essential, will need to be lifted into the shower. However, it is sometimes feasible to have a shower tray flush with floor level and sloping away to a drainage point. This type facilitates the use of wheeled

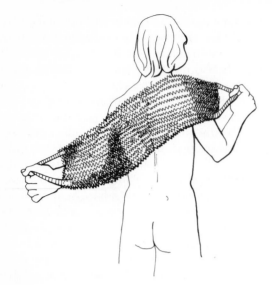

Fig. 3.13   A towel with tape loops

shower chairs on which the patient can be moved into the cubicle. If shower chairs or plastic garden chairs are used only by the patient, these should have rubber ferrules, such as those used on walking aids, attached to the legs to prevent them slipping. If built-in shower seats are used, these should be positioned to suit the individual's needs. They may have to be hinged so that they can be hooked up against the wall so as not to hinder able-bodied family members.

6. Drying the body requires grip and coordination, that is, the ability to control the towel and to reach the extremities, and the ability to apply sufficient pressure to dry that area. A warm room and facilities on which to warm a towel or bath robe are most useful. The patient who is wrapped or wraps himself in a warm robe or bath towel will dry effectively with a minimum of effort. Roller towels with tape loops at each end (Fig. 3.13) facilitate drying of the back and legs, and thick soft towelling mittens can be used by patients with severely impaired grip.

7. To clean his teeth efficiently the patient must be able to do it himself, particularly if the teeth are natural as opposed to dentures. Tooth-brush handles can be enlarged to assist patients with weak grip, or lengthened and/or angled to assist those with impaired upper limb mobility. Electrically operated tooth-brushes may be essential for the more severely disabled patient who wishes to retain his independence in oral hygiene.

8. Most men like to shave themselves, for no-one else can shave them satisfactorily, unless he is a trained barber. If the patient has always 'wet shaved' and is now unable to do so, he may be advised to use an electric or battery operated razor, if only for reasons of safety rather than any other. The razor should be positioned at a convenient height if the patient is unable to hold it and it may be held by a suitable bracket at the required angle; it can also be fitted into a leather socket with firm elastic handloops. Patients with severe upper limb impairment can often use this latter method in conjunction with mobile arm supports.

Many of the more disabled patients treated by occupational therapists have difficulties with personal hygiene and it is imperative to help them to attain a level of independence which is acceptable to them, to those in a caring role and to their friends and workmates.

Eating and Drinking

It is generally accepted that meals are eaten with a knife, fork and spoon, and drinks taken from a cup or glass. Most patients are able to do so, but for a few specially designed or adapted cutlery and crockery may be necessary.

When assessing feeding difficulties the therapist must consider whether the patient has any muscle weakness, tremor, spasm or incoordination and whether he has chewing and swallowing difficulties. She must consider the positioning of the patient's head, arm and hand in relation to his food and drink, the choice of tableware and furniture, accessibility to the dining area used by the family and also suitable protective garments, such as a towelling apron, if this should be necessary.

When considering *the dining area* and furniture the therapist needs to ascertain whether the patient will sit at the table on an ordinary chair, whether he will sit in his wheelchair at the table, whether he will use a tray on his wheelchair or whether he will be having his meals in bed, in which case he must have a stable overbed table of the correct height.

If he is to sit at the table in the normal way, does he need a slightly higher table and chair to accommodate his stiff lower limbs? Does he need a heavy table placed in a corner of the room or against a wall if he is incoordinated or suffers from spasticity? Is the existing furniture potentially suitable for his use?

The wheelchair user requires clearance under the table apron and the table must be very stable in case he inadvertently knocks against it with his wheelchair. Domestic armrests will facilitate his use of the table, but if he cannot use the dining table, he may have to use a cantilever table or a detachable tray, so that his meal can be positioned appropriately for him.

In normal use *cutlery* is held like a small tool with the handle pressed into the palm and stabilised by thumb pressure against the middle finger. It is stabilised and guided from above by the index finger and additional downward pressure is exerted by flexion of the wrist joint. If any of these abilities is absent, as in a median nerve lesion, in quadriplegia or in rheumatoid arthritis, efficiency is reduced considerably. The therapist must identify the deficit and suggest an alternative method of holding the cutlery or provide or recommend a substitute, for example padding for the handle of the knife, using a splint to place the thumb in opposition to the fingers, so that normal grip and action may be achieved.

If cutlery handles are thin and slippery and the patient's grip and/or control is poor, if he is in pain, or when heavy cutlery is not suitable, he should use lightweight enlarged grips such as those provided by Rubazote, the Melaware manoy range, or handles specially designed in perspex to meet his specific needs. For one-handed patients there are several alternatives to having their food cut up for them and eating it with a fork or spoon. The Nelson knife, Dinafork, 'spork' or 'splayd', or a sharp cheese knife can be used, and illustrations of the more readily available ones will be found in Chapter 19. Cutlery such as this has a sharp cutting edge with a fork incorporated into the design and therapists must ensure that the patient and his family are aware of the potential risk of cutting the side of the mouth. For those with a severely restricted range of movement in their upper limbs, angled and lengthened cutlery may be the solution and this must be tailor-made for them. Swivel cutlery is also available and compensates for lack of elbow and wrist movement.

Suitable crockery may help a patient to become independent. Deep-rimmed plates, which are usually quite heavy, are currently available, but their weight may make them unsuitable for those living alone and/or having to do their own washing up. The Manoy range of tableware includes dishes which are useful for the severely disabled person, as the shape of the dish assists in the pushing of food onto a fork or spoon. Plateguards may be used in the same way and fit any average-sized dinner or breakfast plate.

Stabilising crockery is relatively simple and can be achieved by using a cork table mat or the oil skin cloth so popular many years ago. These are easy to clean, pleasant to look at and do not attract attention to the patient. Other types of stabilising materials include dycem netting and mats and pimple rubber. Even a damp cloth will serve to steady a plate. For severely incoordinated patients a rimmed table or tray with a non-slip surface may be necessary.

A winged headrest to his chair may assist a patient with a mild head and neck tremor to control his head whilst eating, but if his tremor is very severe independent eating may be an unrealistic goal for him and he will need to be fed.

Where *weakness of the hand and forearm* is the primary cause of difficulty, it may be helpful to stabilise the wrist with a splint and provide adapted cutlery.

Drinking difficulties may be alleviated by only part-filling a cup, mug or glass, by using lightweight beakers, flexistraws or plastic tubing clipped to the cup or glass. For severely disabled patients beakers on a stand which can be angled ease drinking problems. Bottle carriers used by cyclists can be adapted for the wheelchair user, the carrier and bottle being attached to the side of the chair and fitted with a long piece of plastic tube. Children's non-spill training beakers can be used in some cases, for example the very severely disabled patient who cannot control the amount of liquid taken and who tends to spill the contents of a cup or glass. Insulated beakers prevent cooling of hot drinks when patients are very slow.

Preparation and presentation of the patient's diet may obviate some of the difficulties occurring at meal times. For example, the rheumatoid arthritic with severe limitation of his tempero-mandibular joint may find it difficult and painful to open his mouth, or the patient with upper limb ataxia or incoordination may have difficulty with solid foods such as slices of meat, which should therefore be served in minced or very tender form rather than in slices which require cutting, biting and chewing. Well shredded salads can be eaten with a fork or spoon and certain foods can be liquidised to provide nutritious soups which can be served in a cup or beaker rather than in a bowl. Ensure that a patient's diet is nutritious and includes adequate fibre and vitamins, protein and carbohydrate, but if in doubt consult the hospital dietician.

Simple snacks will be easier and quicker to prepare for the patient spending most of his day at home alone and he will be able to eat his main meal of the day with the family. For those who live alone and have considerable difficulty in meal preparation, therapists may need to consider services such as meals on wheels or home help for weekday provision.

Communication

Our ability and skill in communicating with others is acquired throughout infancy and childhood, and as we mature we become more adept at expressing our opinions or needs by various means. It is a skill which is taken for granted until it is lost. A proportion of the patients treated by occupational therapists have communication difficulties of one sort or another. The elderly patient may suffer from impaired hearing, the hemiplegic may be dysphasic, the partially sighted person will be unable to read as he once did, the rheumatoid arthritic may be unable to use his telephone and the patient with motor neurone disease will be unable to turn the pages of his book or to write. In conjunction with the speech therapist there is a great deal that the occupational therapist can offer to her patients in the way of aids to communication.

The solutions to particular difficulties are not discussed in depth in this chapter, but some examples are given below. For additional information refer to *Equipment for the Disabled — Communication* and Dr Philip Nichols' books *Living with a Handicap* and *Rehabilitation of the Severely Disabled*.

Speech. Liaise with the speech therapist and emphasise her treatment methods whilst the patient is in your department. This may involve the use of the written word, pictures and signs and the 'Lightwriter'.

Hearing. Liaise with the speech therapist, the social worker for the hearing-impaired, the Post Office regarding telephone apparatus and the Royal National Institute for the Deaf. If the patient wears a hearing aid make sure that he knows how it operates, where he should obtain new batteries, how to look after it and, above all, that he wears it! Flashing light alarm bells or door bells are available for the patient's use at home.

Reading. For patients with impaired vision advice may be sought from the Royal National Institute for the Blind. Aids available include large-print books, magnifiers, talking books and tapes, and Braille and Moon publications. For patients with motor impairment which hampers their ability to handle newspapers or books such items as newspaper or book stands, rubber thimbles and electric page turners will be of use.

Writing. Everyone needs to be able to write, even if only to sign their name. Once again the speech therapist's advice may be sought, depending on the patient's problems, but the occupational therapist can assess for and provide penholders, a tilting table, a magnetic board or splints. If writing is impossible, a patient may need to use a typewriter and the electric variety can be part of an environmental control system such as Possum, for use by very severely disabled people.

Domestic tasks

Assessment of a patient's domestic abilities — where applicable — is an integral part of a full ADL assessment and will include such tasks as house cleaning, shopping, meal preparation, cooking and serving meals, sewing and mending, laundry, budgeting and planning meals and other essential requirements for running a home. Assessment and retraining of the disabled homemaker is an area in which the occupational therapist can make a considerable contribution and the major aspects of that contribution are set out below. Further details will be found in such publications as *Kitchen Sense for Disabled or Elderly People*.

Training must be realistic and undertaken with full knowledge of the patient's home situation, that is, the type of home, its design and organisation, how many there are in the family, what help is available from the family and/or outside agencies and whether appropriate reorganisation of any of these will make the patient more independent.

The therapist can assist the patient to re-establish a routine and regain confidence if he/she has been in hospital for some time.

She can help the patient to build up physical stamina, improve his/her physical skills and recommend appropriate safe and labour-saving techniques.

Training in specific areas may be necessary, such as balancing on a kitchen stool, safe mobility in the kitchen, optimum working positions or lifting techniques.

Where the patient is unable to continue using his previous methods, new ones need to be tried and the most appropriate ones adopted. He/she will need practice in these new techniques, for example using different utensils, holding a kettle in a different way, storing food at an accessible height, compensating for slowness and/or lack of agility and mobility by reorganising the kitchen, coping with shopping from a wheelchair.

It is important to plan the day so that necessary tasks may be completed comfortably, allowing for rest periods and time spent with the family.

The therapist may help the patient to organise the family so that each of its members has his/her own duties, for example bed making, cleaning their own bedroom, preparing vegetables for the evening meal, doing the shopping, or taking the dog out.

The therapist who is also a housewife may have more empathy towards the disabled homemaker and should use her own experience in the treatment of her patients. If she puts her own treatment principles into practice at home, she will know from first-hand experience which labour-saving methods may be most suited to the individual patient and which kitchen or household 'gadgets' are most reliable and easiest to use.

Work and recreation

An overall ADL assessment will include evaluation of a patient's capabilities and interests in both work and leisure pursuits. Work is dealt with in detail in Chapter 12, therefore this section will concentrate on recreation.

Leisure time pursuits are an important part of any person's daily life and frequently even more important in the life of disabled people who may be unable to work. Leisure activities and involvement in local organisations are a substitute for work and provide opportunities to participate in creative activities, increase social contacts, introduce broader areas of interest and compensate for the lack of status which unemployment may give.

Initially, leisure activities may help the more severely disabled or elderly person to adjust to a new lifestyle, but later on these activities may become more than a time filler. They may encourage the individual to strive for more knowledge and skills than he had time for previously. Individual needs differ considerably and, yet again, the therapist advising a patient must 'know' him before she can guide him towards fulfilling his needs. She needs to take into account his previous hobbies and interests, for these may still be pursued quite easily. Some patients may be able to seek alternative employment if they undertake further study first, for example correspondence or Open University courses. However, not all patients want or need intellectual fulfillment and they may need guidance from the therapist, their family, friends and local groups on how to express their particular talents in other ways. Once the therapist is aware of the patient's interests and capabilities she can help him to explore the very wide range of sports, social activities and practical pastimes.

Comprehensive information is available from the Disabled Living Foundation, *Equipment for the Disabled — Leisure and Gardening* and the many guides for the handicapped regarding facilities in a specific town.

1. Practical pastimes: sewing, model making, gardening, photography.

2. Intellectual pursuits: further education courses, study and appreciation of music or art, reading.

3. Active participation in sport or games: table tennis, chess, cards, darts, archery, swimming, riding.

4. Making collections can be an absorbing interest: stamps, coins, particular types of records or books.

5. Activities requiring little or no active participation: the theatre, radio, television, music, following a particular sport through the media.

6. Social outlets are very important and should be encouraged: local clubs/organisations catering for particular interests, entertaining at home, visiting friends, art galleries or museums and special clubs such as PHAB (Physically Handicapped and Able Bodied), riding groups for the disabled.

Personal relationships and marriage

Personal relationships are imperative if man is to survive and function at all in today's world. Without contact with other human beings life can become meaningless. Some people do not wish to participate in the 'social whirl', but even so they should be discouraged from becoming complete recluses and encouraged to participate actively in family life and to maintain contact with their friends.

For those who become disabled in their later years, relationships with others are more straightforward. They have built up a circle of friends over a period of time and have usually married and had families prior to the start of their disabling condition. The younger person who was born with a limb deficiency or has suffered illness or trauma since birth which resulted in disability, has entirely different circumstances to contend with. He may never have had an opportunity to mix at school or socially with his able-bodied peers and he may need careful guidance from those who care for him, teach him or employ him.

Modern society still tends to look upon serious personal relationships, love or marriage between a disabled and an able-bodied person, or two disabled people, with some concern, as if it were unnatural for two people of opposite sexes to want to spend time together. Like the able-bodied, the less able do have feelings and a need to be liked, loved and cared for, and it is often left to the professionals involved to help and guide them in this situation, for their families will not, or feel they cannot do so, as they see deep personal relationships between disabled people as 'wrong'.

Occupational therapists working with the more disabled people, particularly young men and women, will realise that they need opportunities which will add to the quality of their lives. They need private and intimate companionship; if they live in an 'institution' their privacy should be respected. They need sex education and may need genetic counselling. They want to know about contraceptives or whether sterilisation should be considered. They want to know whether they are physically able to bear children. But even a marriage without children will bring companionship, a sharing of interests and building a home together. Prior to marriage they may wish to live together to find out whether or not they are compatible and they should be given this opportunity.

Facilities for disabled couples are still very limited and some couples continue to need a great deal of assistance and support. Practical trials are often necessary to establish the degree of help required for independent living, be it within a unit or in a flat.

The person who married prior to the onset of his/her disabling condition is generally accepted by society, but young disabled people often have to live with and suffer indignities. The disabled couple usually understand one another's feelings and needs far more than anyone else.

Understanding the stresses and strains of married life and caring for one another often makes each individual strive for greater independence. Why? Because they have an aim in life, the happiness of their partner.

Special equipment

When assessing and treating the severely disabled patient the need for special equipment is likely to arise, but aids, appliances or equipment should only be recommended after comprehensive assessment and trials of other methods. The therapist must ensure that recommendations are appropriate to individual needs, for disuse or misuse is usually a result of inadequate assessment and/or misunderstanding.

Throughout the text references have been made to 'aids', 'appliances' and 'equipment' and the meaning of each term is enlarged upon below.

1. An *aid* is 'any small easily handled item prescribed to assist functional ability', for example adapted cutlery or clothing, a dressing stick, typing stick.

2. An *appliance* is 'any device made to fit an individual patient in order to correct or prevent deformity and/or increase function', for example hand splints, mobile arm supports, calipers, urinary appliances, prostheses.

3. *Equipment* is 'any standard article, not usually portable by the patient, prescribed to assist functional ability; any standard item adapted to fit the needs of the individual patient', for example a wheelchair, special bed, hoist, electric typewriter, telephone equipment, Possum.
(British Medical Association Planning Unit Report No. 3.1968)

Provision of any item in these three categories is complex and must be preceded by a detailed assessment of a patient's needs and his environment. Many of them are expensive and require expertise to make, fit and/or install.

Other points of note are:

(a). The therapist must know the names of suppliers of aids, appliances and equipment.

(b). She must know where specialist help is available for patients who may benefit from such items as Possum, mobile arm supports or a particular make and model of wheelchair.

(c). She should maintain contact with organisations such as the Disabled Living Foundation, her professional association, the Royal Association for Disability and Rehabilitation and others.

(d). She should have sufficient understanding of the design of commonly used 'equipment' to be able to assess immediately whether it will be suitable for a particular patient and his environment.

(e). Finally, each department should have its own supply of small aids and relevant appliances. These are used both for assessment of patients and for loan or purchase. Such items might include dressing sticks, stocking/sock/tights aids, raised toilet seats or bath seats.

Therapists must realise that many of the daily problems faced by the disabled are associated not with their condition but with the design and construction of the environment in which we all live. Their own homes may not be suitable architecturally and public buildings, the homes of friends, roads and pavements may hinder access and proper function.

Although this chapter has dealt primarily with assessment and treatment of the patient, it is apparent that it is often necessary to assess and treat the environment too. There are circumstances, as you will find, in which treatment of environmental factors would obviate the need to treat a patient. Many medical conditions are incurable and therapists may not be able to alter a patient's situation or solve all his difficulties. However, a 'cure' is potentially possible for the environment. All therapists, as practical, down-to-earth people, have a responsibility to the less able, to assist them in campaigning for availability of information, signposting of facilities and the education of those who plan, design and build our environment.

Acknowledgements

Mrs Hazel Burrows, Senior Occupational Therapist, St Martin's Hospital, Bath, for reading and commenting on the manuscript.

REFERENCES AND FURTHER READING

Buchland Lawton E 1963 Activities of daily living for physical rehabilitation. McGraw-Hill, New York
Goble REA, Nichols P J R 1971 Rehabilitation of the severely disabled — evaluation of a disabled living unit. Butterworths, London
Gull J G, Hardy R E 1974 Rehabilitation techniques in severe disability (Case studies). Thomas, Illinois
Macdonald E M 1976 Occupational therapy in rehabilitation, 4th edn. Balliere, Tindall & Cassell, London
Nichols P J R 1971 Rehabilitation of the severely disabled — management. Butterworths, London
Nichols P J R 1976 Rehabilitation medicine — the management of physical disabilities. Butterworths, London
Wilshere E R Clothing and dressing, 4th edn. Communication, 4th edn. Disabled child, 3rd edn. Disabled mother, 4th edn. Hoists & walking aids, 3rd edn. Home management, 4th edn. Housing & furniture, 3rd edn. Leisure & gardening, 4th edn. Outdoor transport, 4th edn. Personal care, 3rd edn. Wheelchairs, 4th edn. All from a series: Equipment for the disabled, Oxfordshire Area Health Authority, Oxford

4

Transfer techniques

Our body weight is 'transferred' a thousand and more times a day, as we move from foot to foot, chair to feet or sitting to lying. The unthinking ease with which we do this is halted by even a minor injury, but with a major injury or disability independent transfers become difficult if not impossible. In order to lead even a reasonably independent life, however, a person needs to be able to transfer himself from bed to chair and to the toilet or commode. The therapist, therefore, needs to try and enable the patient to achieve independence in transfer. Where this is not possible an assisted transfer, which should be taught to the patient and his assistants is the next most satisfactory method. Where neither independent nor assisted transfer is possible or in conditions where they prove inappropriate, methods of lifting the person, either manually or with the help of a hoist, must be taught.

In the following pages various ways of moving a patient from one place to another and of teaching him to move himself, are described. There is no 'correct' way for any particular person or condition, nor are all ways suitable for every lifter or patient and the choice of method should come from the therapist who has a detailed knowledge of the patient's disability and the type of assistance available.

During the teaching of transfers, methods should be selected with an eye to progression from assisted to independent manoeuvres. It is also worth considering that, as ours is an ageing population, many disabled people fall into the category of those with a short memory and poor retention of new knowledge. It follows, therefore, that once a suitable method has been found, this should be used consistently and the teaching accompanied by simple commands given one at a time. Similarly, where assisted or lifting techniques are necessary it is important to explain to the patient how best he can help (by positioning his body or maintaining his posture, for example) and also what is unhelpful. Where more than one assistant is necessary one of them should be 'in charge' in order to give the instruction of when to lift, where to turn and so on.

The four sections are discussed separately:

1. Independent transfers
2. Assisted transfers
3. Lifting
4. The use of hoists.

INDEPENDENT TRANSFERS

Principles

1. The surfaces for transfer should be stable and, for horizontal transfers, of the same height. Where a wheelchair is used the brakes must be applied before the transfer is attempted. It may also be necessary to remove one or both arms from the chair and to lift, retract or remove the footrests.

2. The surfaces should be as close together as possible. Where a gap exists this may be bridged with a transfer board.

3. Although there is no 'correct' method of transfer for any one person, that which is easiest and safest for the individual should be employed.

4. When teaching transfers the therapist must be sure that her instructions are clear and satisfy herself that she has been understood.

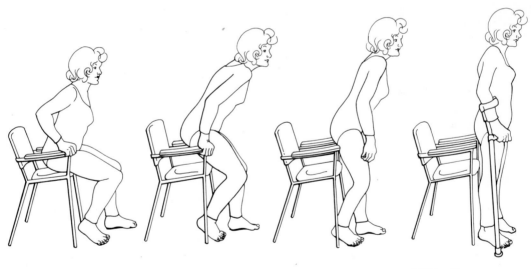

Sit well forward on the chair with both feet on the floor and the weight taken through the stronger (rear) foot—if this is applicable. Hold the arms of the chair firmly. Keep the head up.

Push up with the hands and feet, with the head well forward.

Transfer weight evenly onto both feet, and adjust balance.

Collect aids

Fig. 4.1   Transfer from sitting to standing

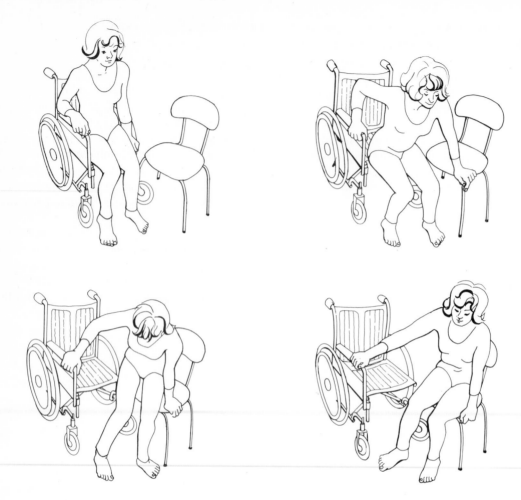

Fig. 4.2 Corner transfer

5. Balance must be retained throughout the transfer.

6. Independence in transfer should be taught at the most appropriate time related to the patient's condition. It is important not to attempt it too soon, so that the patient develops a fear of failure or falling, nor to continue helping too long so that he loses the desire to move himself.

7. It is important to show the patient how to use his body weight to advantage.

Transfers to and from a chair

Standing from sitting (Fig. 4.1)

Ensure any aids needed for walking are to hand. Move to the front edge of the chair.

Lean forward, hold onto the arms or seat of the chair. The feet should be well back, apart and with the whole foot on the floor. It may be helpful to place one foot in front of the other and this should be the weaker one, where applicable.

Push up with the arms and feet. *Never* encourage a patient to pull up onto a walking aid or grab at a nearby surface as it may be unstable.

Collect aids and establish balance.

Sitting from standing

Back up to the chair until it can be felt with the back of the legs.

Put aids aside, hold onto the arms or seat of the chair.

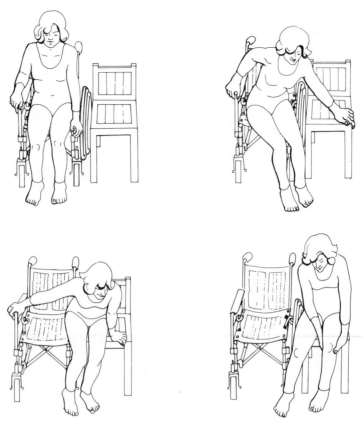

Fig. 4.3 Side transfer

Lower *slowly* into the seat.

Note: For those with difficulty rising from or sitting down on a chair the following points may help:

A high seated chair is easier to transfer to and from than a low seated one.

The chair seat needs to be firm. This can be done by putting a wooden board under the cushion.

Any loose or additional cushions should be removed from the chair.

A chair with arms is easier to push out of when rising and also to hold for support when sitting.

An ejector seat or chair can give the extra impetus needed to help the person rise independently. Many designs are available.

Chair to chair

Note: The chair on which the person is sitting is referred to as the first chair; that onto which he will transfer is referred to as the second chair.

Method 1: Corner transfer (Fig. 4.2). The chairs should be angled to each other as shown. Where a wheelchair is used the arm between the two chairs can be removed.

The patient moves to the front of the chair and places his feet well back. The hand nearest the second chair grasps the furthest arm or side of that chair while the other hand grasps the arm of the first chair. For the patient who cannot use his legs it is helpful if he lifts them over towards the second chair before transferring.

The patient pushes up with his arms (and feet where possible). He swings his hips round until he is over the second chair.

Both hands now grasp the arms of the second chair and the feet are adjusted to retain the balance.

The patient lowers himself slowly onto the second chair.

Method 2: Side transfer (Fig. 4.3). The chairs are

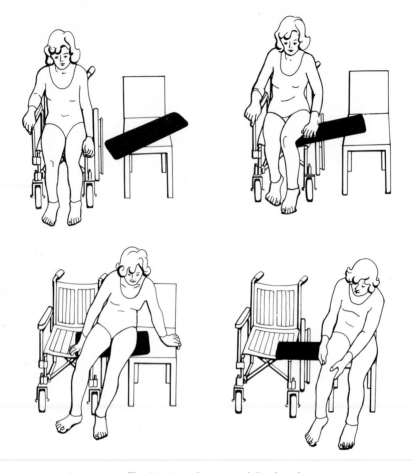

Fig. 4.4   Transfer using a sliding board

placed side by side as shown. If a wheelchair is used the arm rest between the two chairs should be removed.

The patient leans over towards the second chair and grasps the furthest arm or the far edge of the seat. The other hand holds the arm of the first chair.

The patient moves his hips across from the first to the second seat and then adjusts the position of his feet.

Method 3: Sliding board transfer (Fig. 4.4). Note: This method is useful where the heights of the surfaces vary or where there is a gap.

The chairs are placed side by side. If a wheelchair is used the arm between the two chairs is removed.

The sliding board is placed across the two chairs and the patient sits on one end of it as shown.

The patient slides across the board by holding onto the board and the chairs.

He then adjusts his legs and the sliding board is removed.

Method 4: Front transfer (Fig. 4.5). Note: This method is useful for transfer in confined spaces.

The chairs face each other with the first chair slightly to the right (or left) of the second. If a wheelchair is used the leg rests should be swung aside or removed. The chair arms need not be removed.

The patient swings his legs to the right (or left) of his chair and the chairs are moved as close together as possible.

The patient slides to the front of the chair. He places his left (or right) hand on the arm of the first chair and his right (or left) hand on the back of the seat of the second chair.

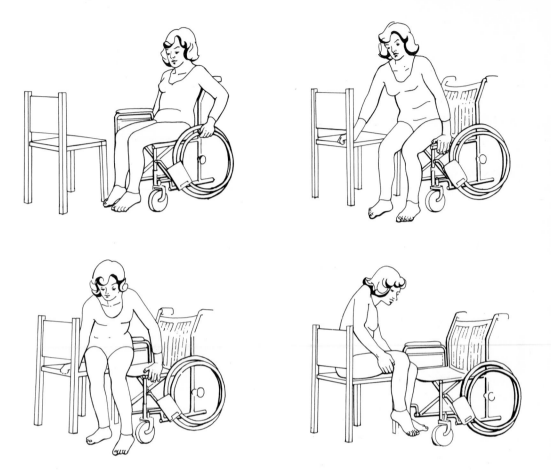

Fig. 4.5   Front transfer

He lifts his hips by pushing down on both hands and then swings round to sit on the second chair.

The first chair is pushed away from the second chair (if a wheelchair is used, this is moved away). The patient adjusts his legs and hips to a comfortable position.

Note: If the patient is fairly agile he can move onto a chair with fixed arms.

Transfers to and from a bed

When transferring onto or off a bed several points should be noted that will help make the transfer easier.

The bed frame. For many disabled people a standard divan bed is too low to allow easy transfer. Where possible the height of the bed, i.e. from floor to mattress *when compressed*, should be as near as possible to the height of the chair seat onto which the patient will move. For standing up from the bed the mattress should be at the optimum height to allow easy transfer. The height of the bed can be altered by lengthening or shortening the bed legs or by the use of *secure* bed blocks. In some cases it may be advantageous to remove the castors from the bed legs, as these may cause the bed to move during transfer.

The mattress. This should be as wide as the bed frame. A firm edged mattress is easier to rise from. If the mattress edge is soft, boards can be placed between the mattress and the bed frame to provide a firm base for transfers. Ideally the boards should cover the whole width of a single bed and at least half the width of a double bed so that the patient does not have the problem of rolling on and off the board.

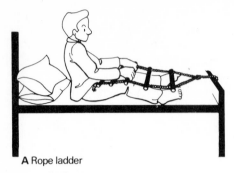

A Rope ladder

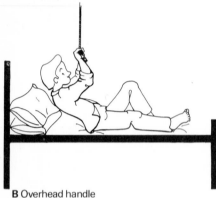

B Overhead handle

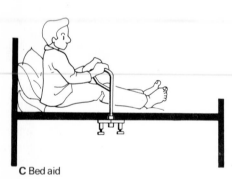

C Bed aid

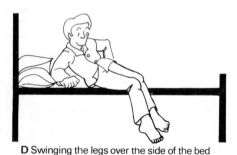

D Swinging the legs over the side of the bed and pushing up with the arms

Fig. 4.6 Sitting up in bed (A) using a rope ladder (B) using an overhead handle (C) using a bed aid (D) swinging the legs over the side of the bed and pushing up with the arms

Positioning. Where the person needs to transfer to a chair or walking aid there must be sufficient space at the side of the bed for these manoeuvres.

Sitting up in bed (Fig. 4.6)

The following methods can be adopted:
(a). Use of a rope ladder attached to the base of the bed.
(b). Use of a lifting pole.
(c). Use of a bed aid.
(d). The patient moves to the side of the bed, swings his legs over the edge of the mattress and pushes himself up into a sitting position on the edge of the bed. Note: Always advise the person to push up from lying rather than pull on the bedclothes.

Sitting over the edge of the bed (Fig. 4.7)

The following methods can be adopted:
(i) Hooking one leg over the other (the weak over the strong if this is applicable) and swinging them over the side of the bed. The patient then sits up by pushing on his elbow and hand.
(ii) Patients with a stiff and/or weak leg can hook a walking stick or crutch handle round the foot and then lift the leg over the edge of the bed.
(iii) A bed aid, lifting pole or rope ladder can give support while legs are swung over the edge of the bed.

Getting up from a bed

The same principles apply here as for getting up from a chair. If additional support or help is needed the use of a bed aid, head or foot board or *stable* piece of furniture, such as a chest of drawers placed permanently by the bed, can be used for the patient to push up on.

Sitting down on a bed

The same principles apply here as for sitting down on a chair.

Bed to chair/chair to bed

The following methods can be employed:

1. Corner transfer (Fig. 4.1)
2. Side transfer (Fig. 4.2)
3. Sliding board transfer (Fig. 4.3)
4. *Forward transfer (Fig. 4.8)*

The chair is brought up to face the side of the bed as shown. The footrests should be swung sideways and/or removed.

When a little away from the bed the patient lifts his legs onto the mattress. The chair is then brought up to the bed and the brakes locked on.

The patient slides forwards onto the mattress pushing first on the arms of the chair and then on the bed.

The patient then turns round to sit lengthways in the bed.

The process is reversed for getting off the bed.

Note: a sliding board placed between the bed and the chair seat may help.

5. *Backward transfer (Fig. 4.9)*

Note: a chair with a zipped back opening is required. If a chair with rear-wheel drive is used a sliding board may be needed to bridge the gap.

The chair is brought up backwards to the side of the bed as shown.

The back of the chair is unzipped and the patient slides or hitches backwards onto the bed.

The patient lifts or swings his legs clear of the chair and sits lengthways on the bed. The sliding board is removed.

Transfers to and from a toilet

When transferring to and from a toilet several points should be borne in mind:

Many toilets, especially modern ones, are quite low and the seat may, therefore, need raising in order to allow easy transfers. Various designs of seat raises are available, and the therapist must ensure that these fit *securely* before issuing them. Ejector and sloping seats are also available.

Grab rails fixed to the wall near the toilet, or toilet frames fixed round the toilet, will provide a firm grip for transfer. Again many designs are available, including those which combine toilet frame and raised seat. A lifting handle attached to the ceiling above the toilet may be helpful.

The patient must be able to cope with clothing, toilet paper and flushing the toilet as well as the transfer.

Where toilet transfer presents great problems because of disability, lack of space, distance to the toilet or other difficulties, alternatives such as commodes, urinals, sanichairs or sanitary facilities in wheelchairs must be considered.

If a wheelchair is used the type selected should allow easy and close access to the toilet.

Standing up from and sitting down on the toilet

The same principles are applied as for 'Standing from sitting' and 'Sitting from standing'.

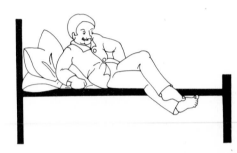

Hooking the weak leg over the strong leg

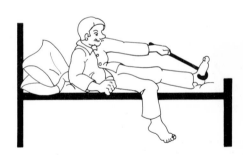

Lifting the weak leg with the aid of a stick handle

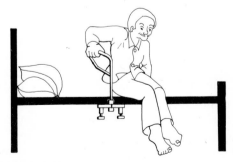

Using a bed aid

Fig. 4.7 Sitting over the edge of the bed

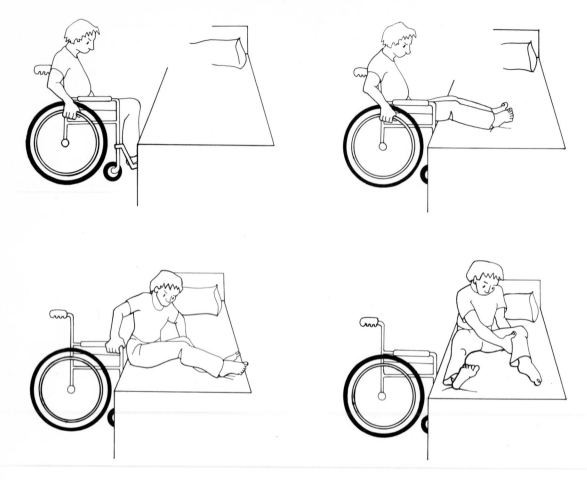

Fig. 4.8 Forward transfer onto a bed

Chair to toilet

The following methods may be employed:

(a). Corner transfer (Fig. 4.2)

(b). Side transfer (Fig. 4.3)

(c). Front transfer (Fig. 4.5)

(d). Forward transfer (Fig. 4.8). Note that for this transfer (for example for double lower limb amputees) the patient uses the toilet facing the cistern with his feet on either side of the pan. Toilet rails are essential to assist transfer.

(e). Backwards transfer (Figure 4.9). Note that for this transfer the sliding board is not used. A chair with front-wheel drive is best, as this can be wheeled right up to the pan. For both forward and backward transfers chairs with a single cross-brace frame can be pushed nearer to the toilet.

Transfers into and out of a bath

Independent transfers into and out of the bath will require much practice and frequently considerable upper limb strength of the disabled person. Whenever bath transfers are being attempted it is advisable that the person is supervised so that assistance can be given should a problem arise, for in a hot and steamy bathroom a wet and slippery patient may get into difficulties, especially when getting out of the bath after washing. Where bath transfers create a great problem the therapist and patient must decide whether an alternative method, such as a shower, all-over wash or bed bath, is preferable for the sake of ease and safety.

Where aids such as bath boards, bath seats or grab rails are needed these should always be

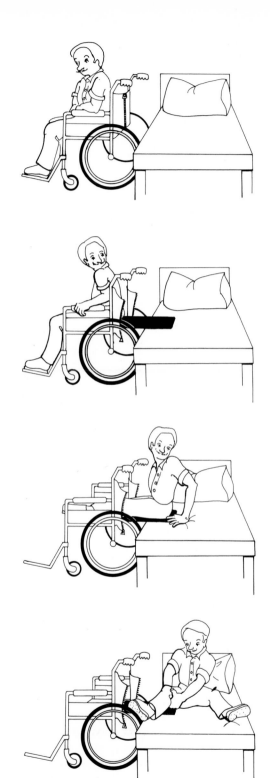

Fig. 4.9 Backward transfer onto a bed

checked for security and safety and should have a non-slip surface. It is also advisable that a non-slip bath mat be placed in the bottom of the bath. The therapist must, in addition to showing the patient how to transfer into and out of the bath, check that he can also cope with undressing, washing, drying and dressing.

Getting in and out of the bath from standing

1. *Use of grab rail or pole (Fig. 4.10).* Many types of grab rails and poles are available to help those who require a little support when getting in and out of the bath. Some of these aids are illustrated in Figure 4.10.

2. *Method for those with one-sided weakness (Fig. 4.11).* Note: the patient must be able to rise from the floor through sitting.

The patient stands with the strong side next to the bath. He holds the side of the bath with his strong hand and steps into the bath first with his strong and then his weak leg.

He leans forward and holds onto the sides of the bath with both hands if possible and then sits down.

After bathing the water should be drained. The patient holds onto the side of the bath behind him with his strong arm.

He swings round towards the sound side, ending in a kneeling position.

The patient pushes up into a standing position using the strong leg and holding onto the side of the bath.

Holding the side of the bath he steps out with the strong and then the weak leg.

Getting in and out of the bath from a sitting position

Transfers from a chair, stool, wheelchair, extended bath board, side of bath or other seated position are described.

1. *Side transfer with standard bath board or extended bath board (Fig. 4.12).*

The patient sits on the wheelchair or stool which is placed next to the bath as shown. Note: for those with unilateral weakness it is advisable to have the stronger side nearest the bath.

By holding the side of the bath, a wall mounted

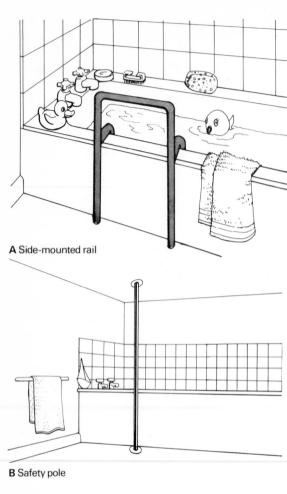

A Side-mounted rail

B Safety pole

C Tap-mounted rail

Fig. 4.10 Grab rails for the bath. (A) Side-mounted rail (B) safety pole (C) Tap-mounted rail

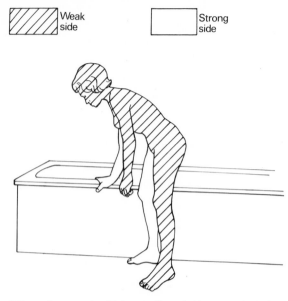

A The patient stands with her unaffected side next to the bath Holding on to the side of the bath with the strong hand she steps in first with her strong leg then with her weak one

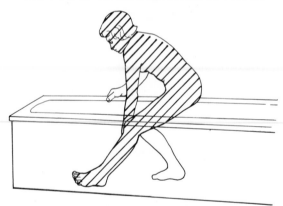

B Holding on to the far side of the bath with the strong hand and taking weight through the strong leg, the patient sits down in the bath

Fig. 4.11 Independent bath transfer for those with one-sided weakness

grab rail or the bath board he transfers to the edge of the bath board and slides across to sit over the centre of the bath.

His legs are brought over the side of the bath. (An all-over wash or shower may be taken from this position.)

The patient lowers himself into the bath *or* first onto a bath seat and then into the bath if this is more appropriate.

Note: for the more agile patient the provision of

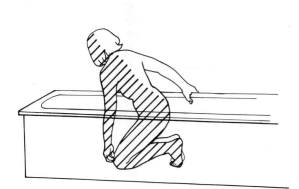

C After bathing, the water should be drained. The patient holds the side of the bath behind her with her strong arm

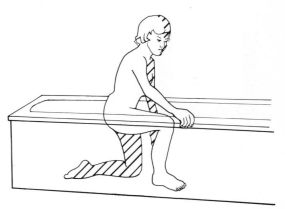

E The patient pushes up into a standing position using the strong leg and holding on to the side of the bath

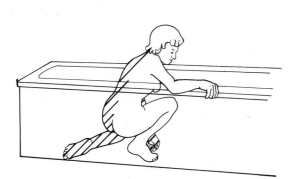

D The patient swings round towards the sound side ending in a kneeling position

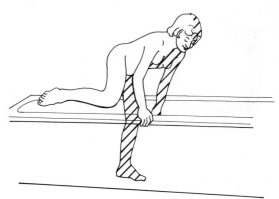

F Holding the side of the bath with the strong hand she then steps out

a seat by the side of the bath plus an inside bath seat may suffice. In this instance the patient slides to sit on the edge of the bath before bringing his feet over the side. If getting up from the bottom of the bath poses a problem the therapist may advise that the patient baths from a bath seat (as described), from a kneeling position or that he uses a bath aid such as the Sunflow Sitinbath which fits over the top of the bath and reduces its depth.

2. *Side transfer without aids (Fig. 4.13).* Note: a grab rail fixed to the wall is advisable.

The patient sits to the side of the bath as shown. If a wheelchair is used the arm nearest the bath must be removed.

His legs are lifted over the side of the bath.

He holds onto the grab rail or far side of the bath and moves to sit on the edge of the bath.

Holding the grab rail and edge of the bath or

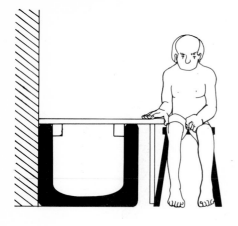

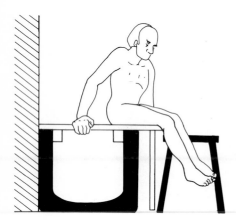

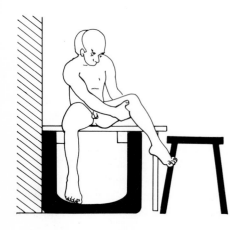

Fig. 4.12 Side transfer using a board

chair he lowers himself slowly into the bath. Getting out is the reverse action.

3. *Forward transfer without aids (Fig. 4.14).*

The chair is wheeled to face the side of the bath as shown.

The patient swings his legs over the edge of the bath and then moves the chair right up to the bath and locks the brakes.

He pushes forwards to sit on the edge of the bath.

By holding the far edge of the bath (or grab rail) and the near edge of the bath (or chair arm) he swings his hips forwards and lowers himself slowly into the bath.

ASSISTED TRANSFERS

For those whose disability does not allow them to move independently, assistance with transfer is often necessary. The therapist must be aware that these patients will rely implicitly on her help and, therefore, she must be sure of the basic principles involved in assisted transfer as well as the exact method she is going to employ before giving assistance. The principles listed below apply to any type of assistance which may be given.

1. Before giving assistance the therapist must be aware of the amount of help the patient himself is able to give and the type of assistance she is going to give.

2. In some cases the handicapped person will be able to tell the therapist how he is usually moved. She should listen to him and take heed.

3. The handicapped person should help the therapist as much as possible, when and where he is able.

4. Giving assistance during transfer often demands considerable physical effort. Therefore, the therapist should learn, practise and cultivate skill and technique rather than strength.

5. The 'force' for assistance comes from the leg muscles. The therapist must ensure that before and during the movement her hips and knees are bent, her spine is straight and her head erect, her feet are spaced to give a firm base and that her balance is maintained throughout.

6. Prepare the way. Ensure that any aids necessary for mobility are to hand, that the patient

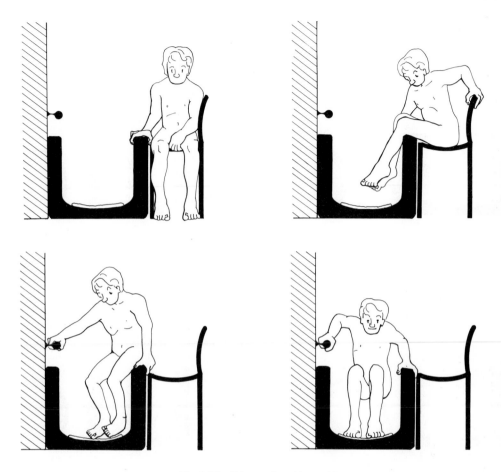

Fig. 4.13 Side transfer without aids

knows where he is moving to and that this place is prepared. There should be an obstacle-free passage through which he can walk.

7. Prepare yourself. The therapist should know exactly what help she is going to give and stand in the appropriate place to give it. She should ensure that she is suitably dressed, for example, that her shoes give firm support, that her clothing allows adequate movement and that her hair or jewellery do not dangle across the patient. It should be unnecessary to mention that her personal hygiene will not cause offence!

8. Prepare the patient. The therapist should tell the patient what she is going to do and how he can help. She should ask him to move into the position required to start the transfer or move him into that position if he cannot manage alone.

9. To initiate movement the therapist may rock the patient backwards and forwards in the chair to help him gain enough impetus to stand.

Assisted standing from sitting

As with independent transfers there is no 'correct' way of giving assistance. Some basic holds are described below.

1. The pelvic hold (Fig. 4.15)

(a). The patient prepares for transfer by sitting to the front of the chair, leaning slightly forward and placing one foot (the stronger where this is applicable) slightly behind the other. His feet should be apart.

(b). The therapist faces the patient and places one foot and knee against the patient's forward leg

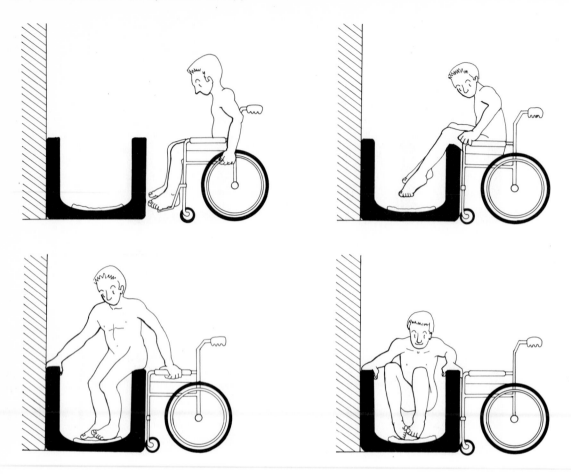

Fig. 4.14 Forward transfer without aids

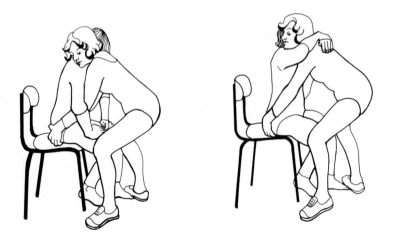

Fig. 4.15 Pelvic hold

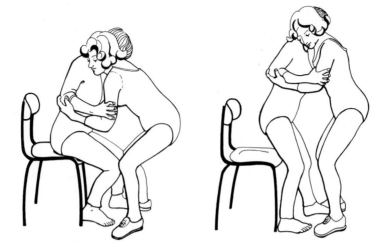

Fig. 4.16 Forearm hold

and knee in order to 'block' it and prevent it from slipping. Her other foot is placed so that her feet are well apart to give a firm base.

(c). With her knees bent and back straight, she passes her arms under the patient's arms and places her hands under his hips as shown. If she cannot reach them, she may place one hand only under the hips with the other grasping firmly onto the patient's clothing at waist level. For the patient's comfort the lift should never be attempted by holding the clothing only!

(d). To execute the lift the therapist and patient stand together on command from the therapist. Where transfer to another seat is required the therapist helps the patient to swing his hips towards the second seat before he sits down.

There are several variations to the basic hold.

(i) The therapist places one hand on the patient's hips and the other over his scapula.

(ii) The therapist places both her hands round the patient's ribcage or locks them together behind his waist.

(iii) The patient holds round the back of the therapist's neck with both hands during the lift.

2. The forearm hold (Fig. 4.16)

(a). The patient prepares for standing as before.

(b). The therapist faces the patient and blocks one leg as before. With her knees bent and back straight she asks the patient to hold both her arms just above the elbow while she in turn holds the patient's arms underneath his elbows and presses his arms into his side.

(c). The patient is asked to keep his elbows bent and on command from the therapist they stand together, the therapist lifting the patient from under his elbows. Again, if transferring from one seat to another the therapist helps the patient to swing his hips towards the second seat before he sits down.

3. The arm-link hold (Fig. 4.17)

(a). The patient prepares for standing as before.

(b). The therapist stands to the side of the

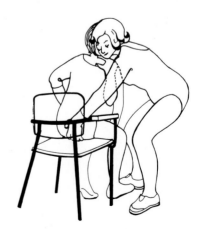

Fig. 4.17 Arm-link hold

patient (the weak side where this is applicable) and blocks his knee and foot as before. She asks the patient to place his hands on the arms of the chair (where this is possible) before pushing up with them to stand; she then links her arm which is nearest to him through his arm and places her hand over his scapula as shown. The therapist's other arm (i) stabilises the patient's elbow, (ii) pushes on the back or arm of the chair or (iii) helps to lift the patient from under his hips.

(c). Both stand on command from the therapist.

Note: upward pressure should not be exerted on the axilla because of the danger of possible damage.

4. Supporting behind the scapula (Fig. 4.18)

This method is particularly useful where the 'bilateral approach' to treatment is being used.

(a). The patient sits to the front of the chair with his feet placed as before. With elbows extended he clasps his hands together between his knees, ensuring that the affected thumb is uppermost.

(b). The therapist faces the patient and blocks his forward leg as before. She reaches behind his shoulders and places the palms of her hands over each scapula.

(c). On command from the therapist both stand together. Using this method the therapist is able to protract the patient's affected scapula thus reducing the onset of spasm on effort.

LIFTING THE HANDICAPPED PERSON

Where the person's disability does not allow him to support his own weight during transfers, the therapist must take the whole weight of the patient and lift him from one place to another.

The same principles apply when lifting the patient as when giving assistance. However, the therapist must ensure that when two or more helpers are involved in the lifting, one must take overall charge and give the command to the group. Good timing is essential during lifting so tthat effort is synchronised.

Before executing a lift the patient should be asked to
● relax, have confidence in the lifters, and not 'fight' against them on the lift
● look ahead, not at the floor or the lifters
● endeavour, if possible, to maintain his body in the position in which it has been lifted, i.e. a sitting, lying, or recumbent posture.

1. The standard or chair lift (Fig. 4.19)

Note: For this lift the patient requires some trunk balance and control.

(a). The patient prepares himself for being lifted as before where this is possible.

(b). The two helpers stand one either side of the patient, facing each other and with their feet apart, knees bent, backs straight and heads erect. They

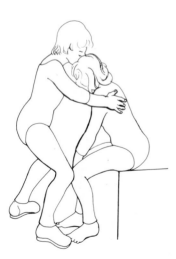

Fig. 4.18 Scapular hold

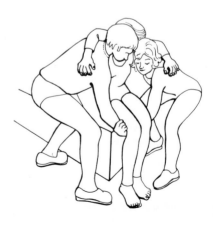

Fig. 4.19 The 'chair' lift

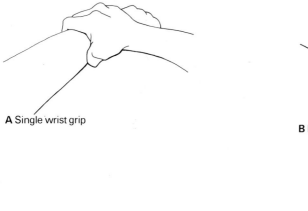

A Single wrist grip

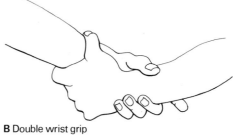

B Double wrist grip

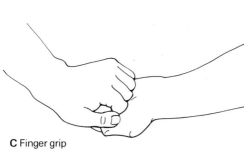

C Finger grip

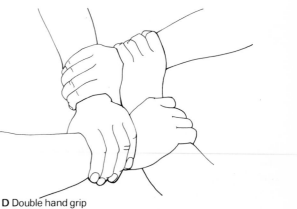

D Double hand grip

Fig. 4.20 Grips for the chair lift. (A) Single wrist grip (B) Double wrist grip (C) Finger grip (D) Double hand grip

each place one hand under the patient's thighs as near to his hips as possible and grasp each other's hands by one of the methods shown (Fig. 4.20 A, B, C, D). Their other hand, if free, supports the patient's back or shoulders. For this lift the patient's arms may be placed round the lifters' shoulders if preferred.

(c). On command from the lifter in charge the lifters raise the patient up by straightening their knees and hips, i.e. the effort comes from the leg muscles and not from the back. Once the lifters have gained an upright stance they can transfer the patient to the required position.

2. The through-arm lift (Fig. 4.21)

(a). The patient prepares himself for being lifted by sitting as upright as possible, crossing his arms in front of him and grasping his own forearms if possible.

(b). One lifter stands behind the chair (or kneels behind the patient on the bed), links her arms through under the patient's axillae and then grips his forearms. The second lifter places her hands under the patient's legs, one under his thighs and one under his calves, in order to support them during the lift.

(c). On command from the lifter in charge (preferably the one holding the patient's arms) the patient is lifted and moved to the required position.

Note: The arm lift alone is especially useful for lifting a patient back into a more upright position if he has slumped down on the bed or chair.

3. The shoulder or Australian lift (Fig. 4.22)

(a). The patient prepares himself by sitting as upright as possible and holding his arms out to the side as shown.

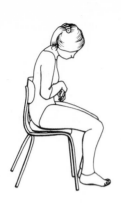
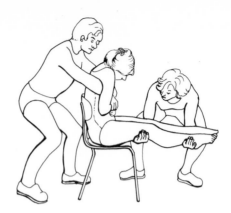

The patient crosses her arms in preparation for lifting

The helpers lift as shown

Fig. 4.21 The 'through-arm' lift

(b). The lifters stand to either side of the patient, facing towards his back, with their knees bent, feet apart, backs straight and heads erect. They press the shoulder nearest to the patient against his chest wall under his axilla so that his arms rest across their backs. This same arm is then placed under the patient's thigh and they grasp hands using one of the grips illustrated in Figure 4.20.

(c). The lifters' free hands can be used to support the patient's back, to push up on the chair/bed during the lifting process or to open doors if the patient is being moved over a long distance.

(d). Both rise on command from the lifter in charge. Once upright this lift can be used to transport patients over a considerable distance.

Many other methods of lifting and assisting patients exist and, as already mentioned, there is no 'correct' way to lift any one person. However, the therapist should be aware of some of the basic methods used so that she can try several different ways until one is found which suits both her and the patient.

Whenever lifting or assisting a patient to move

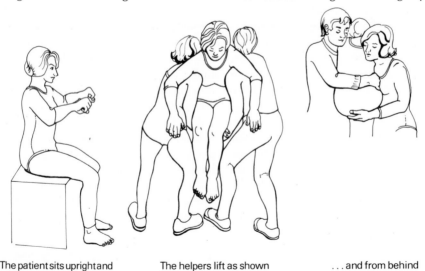

The patient sits upright and raises her arms in preparation for lifting

The helpers lift as shown from the front

. . . and from behind

Fig. 4.22 The 'Australian' lift

the therapist must obey the basic rules of using skill rather than strength, leg rather than back muscles and maintaining balance throughout the movement.

HOISTS

A hoist is a mechanical lifting aid designed to transport and/or lift an individual by means of suitable slings or a static seat from one place to another, for example from bed to commode or into the bath.

A hoist may be used by severely disabled patients who have difficulties with transfers.

As there is often only one helper available in the patient's home, lifting the disabled person can be difficult and dangerous for both helper and patient. In this situation hoists can be used to great advantage, provided that those who use it are taught to use it correctly. With proper techniques all manoeuvres should be easy and comfortable for the patient, whereas unsuitable slings and inexperienced handling may hurt him and make him apprehensive about future use.

Assessment

A comprehensive assessment of the user, his family and environment should be made by someone who has medical knowledge and an understanding of the problems of disability. The following information should be included in the assessment:

1. The user's clinical condition and prognosis, so that the most suitable hoist may be recommended. His physical and mental capabilities to assess whether he can operate the hoist himself, or whether he could tell a helper how it should be operated. His height and weight must also be recorded, so that the correct size slings may be ordered for the hoist.

2. Can the user be taught to transfer safely and independently and can this be achieved with minimal help or simple alterations in the home? Re-arranging the furniture or providing a more suitable wheelchair (for example one with detachable armrests to facilitate the use of a sliding board) may often solve his problem.

3. How capable is the helper? Does he find it difficult, dangerous or impossible to lift the patient or help him transfer, and has he been taught how to do so?

If independent transfer is not safe, or is becoming difficult, the assessor should recommend mechanical assistance, i.e. a suitable hoist. It is often better to advocate the use of a hoist before the family crisis point is reached and the helper can no longer manage without the risk of injury to herself.

4. The choice of hoist will also be affected by the space and storage area available. Hoists are most commonly used in the bedroom, bathroom and toilet, for it is here that most lifting and transferring takes place. Therefore, the width of doorways, available turning space and the size and the layout of appropriate rooms must be recorded.

If a fixed-track hoist is to be recommended, the structure of the home should be checked to see whether suitable tracks could be installed. Someone with technical or building knowledge should advise the assessor on this point.

5. Once it has been decided that a hoist is necessary is there a competent helper to operate the hoist or can the user operate it safely himself?

6. Practical trials are essential if the most suitable techniques and hoist are to be chosen.

7. Once the selection has been made the assessor must ensure that both the user and helper are trained in the use of the equipment and that they are capable and confident in the chosen techniques. They should also be taught how to care for hoist and slings and should be given a contact in the event of difficulties or breakdowns.

Finally, the assessor must remember that if any piece of equipment, and this applies in particular to hoists, is to be accepted by the user and his family, it must prove itself in the overall management of daily living.

Types of hoist

Once the assessor has established that a hoist is required, she must decide which of the basic types is most appropriate, bearing in mind that a compromise may have to be made, depending on the need for stability and/or manoeuvrability.

There are three basic types:

1. Mobile hoists

These are constructed in round or rectangular steel tube and the user is lifted either by slings or a static seat. They are:

(a). guaranteed by the manufacturers to lift up to 20 stone (127 kg) in weight for the smallest models and up to 35 stone (220 kg) for the largest models.

(b). helper-operated; the operator needs to be reasonably fit in order to manoeuvre the hoist from room to room, especially if carpets, corridors and so on have to be negotiated.

(c). available with two types of control: (i) an hydraulic system (Fig. 4.23A) in which the boom is raised by operating the pump handle and lowered by slowly opening the release valve, allowing the helper to place the user in the required position (ii) a hand-wound screw mechanism (Fig. 4.23B) in which the single handle is turned to raise and lower the boom.

(d). equipped with castors attached to the chassis of the hoist. A range of sizes is available; large castors, for example, facilitate moving the hoist over carpets or small thresholds. The larger the castors the greater the clearance required for the hoist chassis. Basic chassis heights vary, so the space available under the bed, bath or car must be known. Chassis widths also vary and certain makes, operated by a ratchet or winding system, can be narrowed and widened. Hoists which have fixed chassis widths can be ordered with a base of the required width to facilitate use around chairs and so on.

(e). easily transportable, for they can be dismantled. However, some models are lighter and easier to handle than others.

In addition it should be mentioned that some mobile hoists may not be suitable for the severely disabled person as they tend to be of the completely rigid type.

2. Hoists fixed to the floor (Fig. 4.24)

These hoists may either be permanently fixed to the floor or may be a mobile type whose upright can be detached from the chassis and inserted into a floor socket.

The floor socket must be sited so that — when

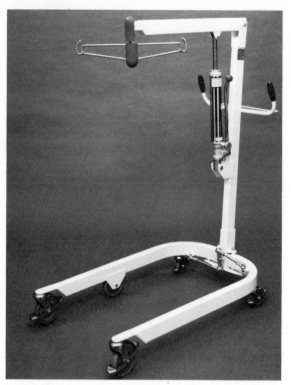

A

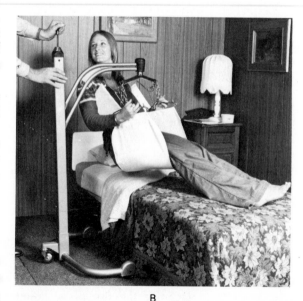

B

Fig. 4.23 Mobile hoists. (A) Hydraulic hoist (B) Hand-wound screw mechanism

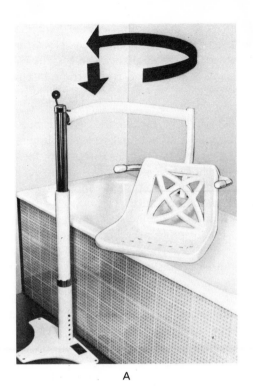

A

fitted — the hoist with the user can be lifted over the bath rim, rotated and lowered into the bath or pool. (Fig. 4.24A, B)

They are useful where space is limited or the bath unsuitable for use with a mobile hoist.

Different models can be operated either by the user or the helper, for example the Autolift, whereas others, for example the floor-mounted Oxford hoist, can only be operated by a helper.

3. Fixed overhead hoists

These hoists are either fixed in a permanent position or attached to straight or curved overhead tracks of varying lengths (Fig. 4.25).

They are operated either manually or electrically.

They can be operated either by the user or by his helper, usually by means of nylon cords. The simpler controls have two cords, one which raises and another which lowers the user. A more com-

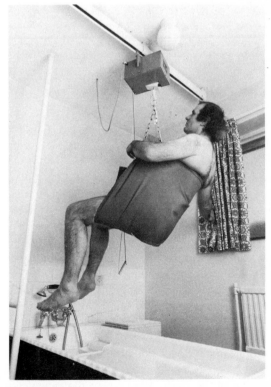

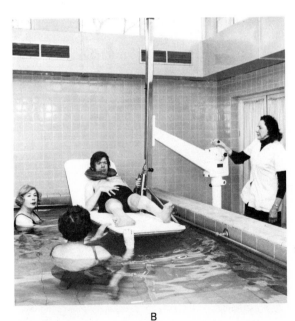

B

Fig. 4.24 Hoists fixed to the floor (A) Autolift (B) Pool hoist fixed to the floor (photograph reproduced by kind permission of Mecanaids Ltd)

Fig. 4.25 Hoist attached to straight overhead track (photograph reproduced by kind permission of Wessex Medical Equipment Co. Ltd)

plicated system, which involves an electrical traversing unit, enables the user to move himself sideways as well. This movement is controlled by two additional cords, one to move left and the other to move right. However, when assessing the potential user and/or helper, one must remember that it can be difficult to learn how to operate this system, so assistance may be required. Cords must be within reach, especially as this system is used by those with severely limited upper limb function, therefore 'parrot perches' or knobs need to be attached to the cords (Fig. 4.26). In addition to the cord systems, hand-wound screw mechanisms are used on certain hoists, for example the Hewatson.

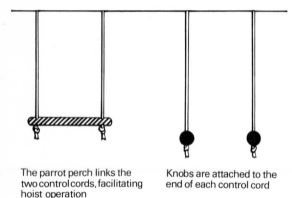

The parrot perch links the two control cords, facilitating hoist operation

Knobs are attached to the end of each control cord

Fig. 4.26 Cord control systems with electrically operated hoists

Installation of fixed overhead hoists should be carried out either by the manufacturer or by a person experienced in this type of work.

(i) The permanently fixed type must be secured to weight-bearing beams or joists; if this is not possible, it must be attached to bearers inserted between the beams.

(ii) For some of the overhead hoists ceiling tracks must be installed. A short track will usually be contained within one room and more than one may be installed. The longer, continuous tracks can connect several rooms and would be used in circumstances where a mobile hoist is unsuitable and/or impractical. However, tracking from room to room involves considerable architectural alterations, such as leaving gaps above doors to allow passage of the track. Because of the many difficulties with this type of installation, few people recommend room to room tracking.

It is worth mentioning at this point that the structure of the user's home needs careful assessment prior to installation of tracking. Ceilings often need to be strengthened and in some instances a rolled steel joist can be fitted into weight-bearing wall brackets if the ceiling cannot be used.

When ordering tracking the assessor must provide the following information to the supplier: the purpose for which the hoist is required; the maximum weight to be carried; a plan of the track with dimensions, including the distance between floor and the proposed track.

(iii) If an overhead hoist is only required in one room, for example a bedroom, a gantry can be used (Fig. 4.27). These are portable frames which in certain circumstances, for example in short-term use for terminal care or for baby care, will solve installation difficulties as they obviate structural alterations. However, they occupy considerable floor space.

(iv) If the hoist is a 240 volt electrically-operated model and is to be used in a bathroom and toilet, an isolating transformer is necessary. This ensures that the hoist can be used safely in a potentially dangerous, i.e. damp or wet, area. The Electricity Board must be consulted in such situations. Some electric hoists now run on 24 volts and therefore always need a transformer.

It is worth mentioning car-top hoists at this point. These are fixed to a car roof by steel clamps

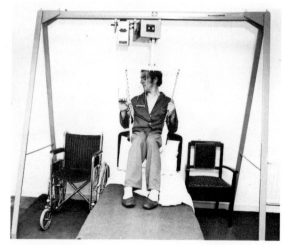

Fig. 4.27 Hoist attached to a free-standing gantry (photograph reproduced by kind permission of Wessex Medical Equipment Co Ltd)

and are attendant-operated by hydraulics. When considering the use of a hoist for getting in and out of a car, the assessor must check that the car door is wide enough and high enough to allow easy access. As the use of these hoists is very limited, their advantages and disadvantages should be weighed up carefully and compared to those of a mobile hoist.

Slings

It is important that the assessor has a comprehensive knowledge of the types of slings available so that she can select the most suitable type for the user, taking into consideration his height, weight, diagnosis and physical and mental capabilities.

Slings are available in a variety of materials, sizes and designs. Materials include PVC, canvas, nylon weave, polyester and terylene. Sheepskin linings are now also available. The British Standards Institution advises that all slings must be made of rot-proof material, as must the thread used for stitching. All slings are washable.

A great number of slings are available, and for convenience only the three basic designs are described here:
1. Two-piece slings
2. All-in-one slings
3. Three-piece slings.

All these are available in three sizes, i.e., small, medium and large.

Two-piece slings

These are either of the strap type (Fig. 4.28A) or consist of wider bands (Fig. 4.28B). The straps, although simple to use, have limited application and are poorly tolerated by users in pain or with sensitive skin. Band slings are used in the same manner as straps, but, being wider, they spread the user's weight more evenly. However, for the more severely disabled person with widespread weakness or paralysis these slings are not suitable, as he may 'jack-knife' between the two slings.

All-in-one slings

These are also known as 'hammock' slings and are used to lift the more severely disabled, as they

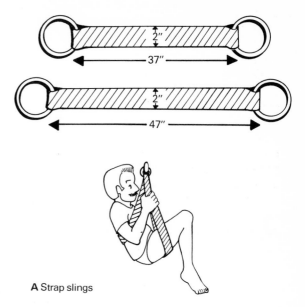

A Strap slings

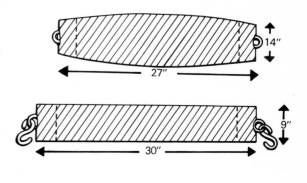

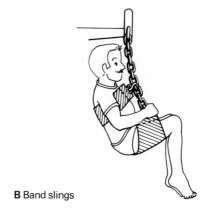

B Band slings

Fig. 4.28   Two-piece slings. (A) Strap slings (B) Band slings

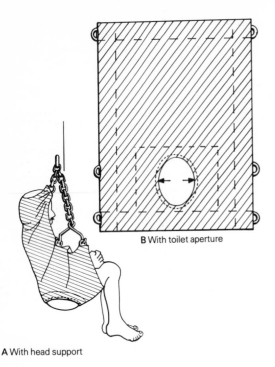

A With head support

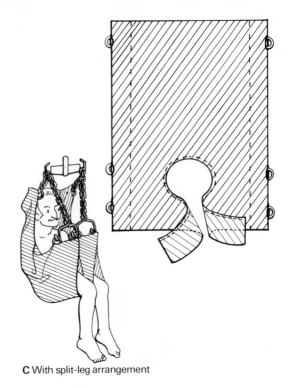

B With toilet aperture

C With split-leg arrangement

support the trunk, pelvis and thighs. Various designs are available including those with a head support (Fig. 4.29A), a commode or toilet aperture (Fig. 4.29B), a split-leg arrangement (Fig. 4.29C) or a full hammock. A complete hammock sling is safe and comfortable once the positioning of attachments has been adapted to the user's needs. The one-piece sling with split or divided leg pieces is easier to use than a hammock sling. Methods of use include:

(a). holding each leg separately

(b). holding both legs together with a strap under both thighs

(c). holding each thigh separately, with the sling fastened to the opposite side, in a criss-cross fashion (Fig. 4.29D).

Methods (a) and (c) facilitate hip abduction for toilet use and cleansing purposes. All types are easily removable so that the user does not have to sit in them all day.

Hammock slings for children are of a very simple design, easy to use and support the child completely. With training, a child may be able to roll himself onto the sling which can be placed either on the bed or the floor. When considering the special needs of the child, the assessor must

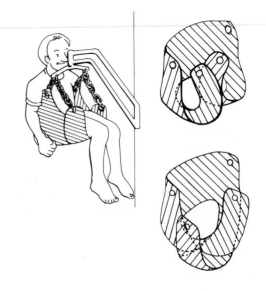

D Used in criss-cross arrangement to support lower limbs

Fig. 4.29 All-in-one sling adapted for different uses

liaise with the parents, the school and health departments, and plan for the future.

One other all-in-one sling worth mentioning is a harness consisting of narrow straps of terylene webbing with a quick-release buckle, similar to a car safety harness (Fig. 4.30). This can be left in position with little or no discomfort to the user. It is of particular value for those who because of their disability have to remain in the sling all day. They do not cover such a large body area and therefore are generally more comfortable. Some harnesses are used because they are easily removed and re-inserted.

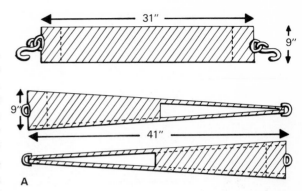

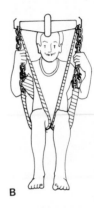

Fig. 4.31 Three-piece sling. (A) Parts of the sling (B) Sling in position

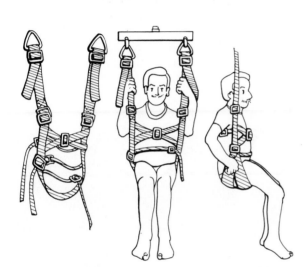

Fig. 4.30 Harness sling

Three-piece slings

These have a back band and two leg slings (Fig. 4.31). They are easy to use and, again, facilitate toileting, cleansing and clothing management.

General points regarding slings:

(a). Alterations to slings should only be undertaken by the manufacturers. They should *never* be made on a domestic sewing machine or without the manufacturer's knowledge.

(b). The user's position during hoisting should be the most comfortable for him and should induce a feeling of security.

(c). Correct positioning of slings will prevent the user from swinging about. For additional infor-

mation the reader should refer to Bell: *Patient Hoist Biomechanics.*

(d). Always choose the most appropriate and easiest method of inserting and removing slings, so that the user feels safe (Fig. 4.32A–L).

(e). Each user should ideally have a minimum of three slings/sets of slings, one in use, one 'in the wash' and a third set ready for use, i.e. in case of soiling, broken stitching and so on.

(f). As already mentioned, all slings should be washable not only to keep them looking fresh, but also for hygienic reasons. Most metal attachments are removable to facilitate laundering, but if there is any difficulty in removing sling bars the whole sling can be placed in a pillowcase for washing.

(g). The assessor should remember that a user may need a different arrangement of slings for different activities.

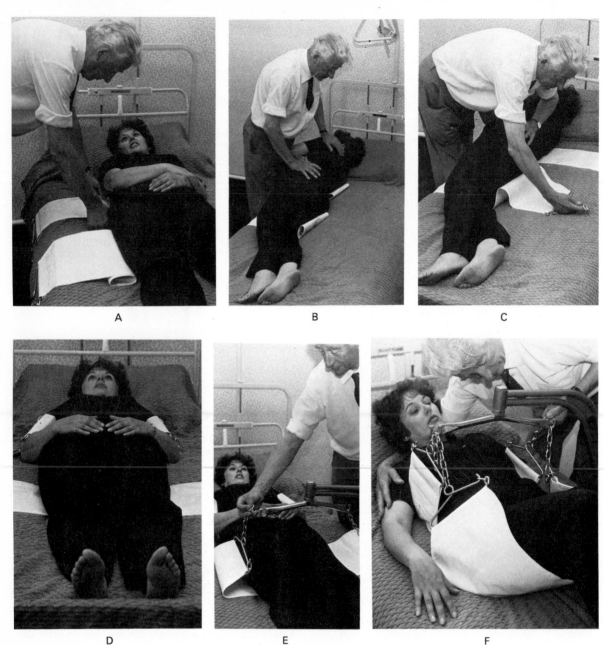

Fig. 4.32 Using a Mecalift

Fig. 4.32A The patient lies supine on the bed, slings rolled with hardware inside and positioned as required. The rolled ends of the slings are pushed under the patient's body as shown.

Fig. 4.32B The patient is turned towards the assistant so that the rolled ends of the slings are free and ready to unroll

Fig. 4.32C The assistant supports the patient with one hand and forearm, whilst her free hand unrolls the slings

Fig. 4.32D The patient is returned to the supine position on top of the unrolled slings

Fig. 4.32E The hoist is moved to the bedside and the seat band sling is attached to the spreader bar

Fig. 4.32F The assistant supports the patient whilst attaching the back sling to the spreader bar

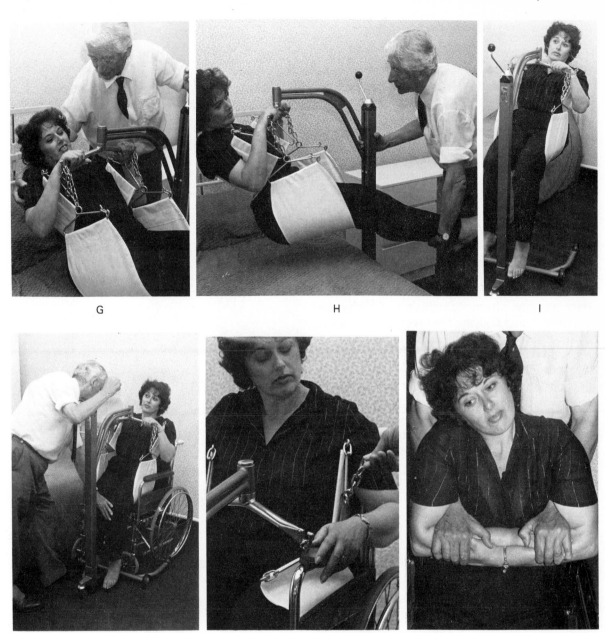

G

H

I

J

K

L

Fig. 4.32G The patient is raised slowly whilst the assistant ensures that the slings are supporting the patient adequately

Fig. 4.32H When the patient's bottom is clear of the bed, her legs are lifted over the edge of the bed, as shown

Fig. 4.32I To aid comfort and balance, the patient's legs are placed one on either side of the mast

Fig. 4.32J The hoist is manoeuvred to the wheelchair, as shown. The assistant presses back on the patient's knees, whilst lowering the boom, to effect a good sitting position

Fig. 4.32K The assistant removes the sling chains from the spreader bar once the patient is seated in the chair

Fig. 4.32L If the patient is not sitting well back in the chair, the assistant uses the through-arm grip to move the patient back into the chair

Metalwork attached to slings

All slings have some form of metalwork for attachment either to chains or directly to the spreader bar of the hoist. Here are some examples:

(a). Sling bars are inserted into the end of band slings or the sides of hammock slings (Fig. 4.33A).

(b). Side suspenders as for sling bars above (Fig. 4.33B).

(c). S-hooks are inserted into some band slings and attached to the chains (Fig. 4.33C).

(d). D-rings attached to strap slings (Fig. 4.33D).

(e). Chains are attached directly to sling bars, side suspenders or to a sling and hooked over the ends of the spreader bar (Fig. 4.33E).

The spreader bar is the 'coat hanger' — like metal bar attached to the hoist's boom (Fig. 4.34). It separates the chains to which the slings are attached, thereby giving the user optimum lifting position. They are available in several sizes and it is important to use the correct size. The width of the spreader bar determines whether the slings grip or chafe the body during lifting. Generally, the bar should be the smallest one which can be used without chafing, as this will ensure that the slings grip the body well, with little possibility of any slipping. However, some independent electric hoist users dispense with a spreader bar, preferring to attach narrow band straps with large D-rings at the end which loop directly over a hook at the base of the lifting tape.

Attachment of slings to the spreader bar

As spreader bars on the various models of hoists differ, the attachment of slings varies also. Attachments include:

(a). dog clips (Fig. 4.35A). These must be of manageable size. If they are too small they are difficult to open.

(b). S-hooks and suspender just hook over the spreader bar (Fig. 4.35B).

(c). D-rings on webbing straps hook onto the spreader bar.

(d). chains attach slings to the spreader bar and trial will show the assessor which link in the chain should be attached to the bar for a particular sling. The carrying angle can easily be adjusted by

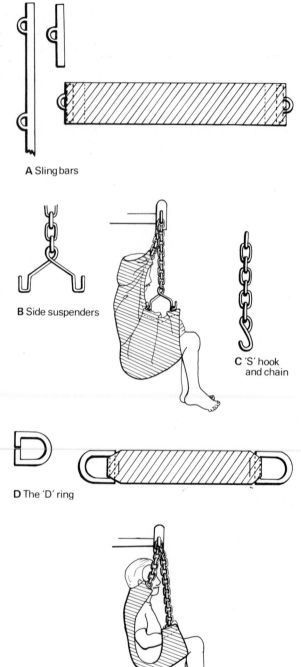

A Sling bars

B Side suspenders

C 'S' hook and chain

D The 'D' ring

E Chains attached to sling bars

Fig. 4.33 Metalwork attached to various types of slings

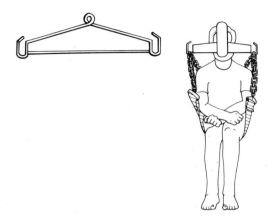

Fig. 4.34 The spreader bar

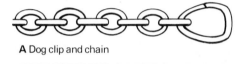

A Dog clip and chain

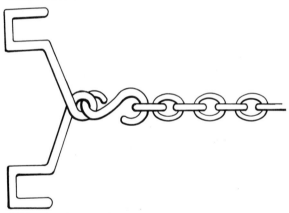

B 'S' hook and suspender

Fig. 4.35 Attachment of slings to spreader bar

selecting the appropriate chain link. Once the most comfortable position for an individual has been found, the appropriate link may be marked, for example with coloured thread or tape.

Provision of hoists

Hoists for use in a disabled person's home may be supplied by Local Authority Social Services Departments, Health Authorities or by voluntary organisations.

Insurance

In the opinion of the author all hoists should be insured by the issuing authority and only in certain circumstances, for example travel abroad, by the user himself. However, few authorities insure their hoists, the person/s using it or the assessor. Those who do, ask that once the user and his family or helper have been taught how to use and care for the equipment, they sign an indemnity. This usually provides them with insurance cover within their home county or borough. Staff who use hoists in the course of their duty should also be included in insurance arrangements. Occupational therapists who are members of the British Association of Occupational Therapists have insurance cover for all aspects of their work and certain employing authorities will ensure that staff involved in this type of work are insured against any accidents.

Maintenance

It is essential that hoists be checked and maintained at regular intervals, starting on the day of delivery to the user's home. The frequency of inspection should be related to the type of hoist and the amount of use it gets. For example, a hoist which is used in a unit caring for 20 chronically sick young people will require far more regular checking and maintenance than one being used by someone in his own home. The assessor and technician of the issuing authority should undertake regular checks and maintenance; in some instances local contractors or the manufacturer's representative will do this. The insurance company will also carry out 'spot checks' on hoists covered by the issuing authority's policy.

To check whether a hoist is in good working order and safe, the following should be noted:

(a). the condition of harnesses/slings: the state of the material, stitching and fastenings, as well as their general appearance.

(b). the seals in the hydraulic system.

(c). the condition of chains, wires and/or cords.

(d). the tightness of all nuts and bolts.

(e). the wear and distortion of suspension members.

Issuing authorities should make arrangements for a 24 hour emergency service so that, in the event of a breakdown or accident, the user and his family or helper receive immediate assistance.

The issue of a hoist can relieve much of the stress and strain on a family caring for a severely disabled person, but for maximum benefit its limitations and use must be fully understood.

Acknowledgements
Miss C Tarling, M.B.A.O.T., Newcastle Aids Centre, for her invaluable advice, for permitting reference to her text 'Hoists and their use', and for reading the manuscript. Surgical Medical Laboratory Manufacturing Ltd, for the use of their comprehensive illustrations of slings.
The following for the loan of photographs:
  Mecanaids Ltd.
  F J Payne & Son Ltd.
  Wessex Medical Equipment Co. Ltd.
  Hewitt Watson Equipment.

REFERENCES AND FURTHER READING

Bell F 1979 Patient hoist biomechanics. British Journal of Occupational Therapy 42 (1) January: 10–16

British Standards Institute 1978 British standard specification for manually operated mobile patient lifting devices (mechanical safety). British Standards Institute, London

Buchwald E 1952 Physical rehabilitation for daily living. McGraw-Hill, New York

The Chartered Society of Physiotherapy 1975 Handling the handicapped. Woodhead Faulkner, Cambridge

Foott S 1977 Handicapped at home. The Design Council, London

Goldsmith S 1976 Designing for the disabled, 3rd edn. RIBA, London

Jay P 1974 Coping with disablement. Consumer's Association, London

Johnstone M 1976 The stroke patient – principles of rehabilitation. Churchill Livingstone, Edinburgh

Kamenetz H L 1969 The wheelchair book. Thomas, Illinois

Macdonald E M 1976 Occupational therapy in rehabilitation, 4th edn. Balliere, Tindall & Cassell, London

Mattingly S 1977 Rehabilitation today. Update Publications, London

Nichols P J R 1971 Rehabilitation of the severely disabled – management. Butterworths, London

Nichols P J R 1973 Living with handicap. Priory Press, London

Rudinger E 1974 Coping with disablement. Consumer's Association, London

Trombly C, Scott A 1977 Occupational therapy for physical dysfunction. Williams & Wilkins, Baltimore

Wilshere E R 1974 Hoists & walking aids, 3rd edn. From a series: Equipment for the Disabled. Oxfordshire Area Health Authority, Oxford

5

Walking aids and their use

Where the mechanism of walking is impaired due to disease or injury a variety of mechanical aids is available, ranging from large stable aids such as gutter frames to less stable ones such as walking sticks.

This chapter aims to describe the walking aids in common use, how to measure and check them, and the walking patterns which can be used with them. In Great Britain most people who need walking aids obtain them either through the National Health Service or their local social services department. They may, of course, be bought privately.

The occupational therapist will notice that in most hospitals walking aids are supplied from the physiotherapy or out-patient departments. However, it is essential that she knows how each aid should be used in order that good walking patterns can be encouraged and how to check its suitability for use in the patient's home. Occupational therapists working in the community are frequently required to assess for, issue, and then teach the client to use, a walking aid.

THE ISSUE AND CARE OF AIDS

The main parts of a walking aid are illustrated in Figure 5.1. All aids should be checked before issue and at regular intervals thereafter and the therapist should take particular notice of the following points:

(a). Is the ferrule complete? If the tread is badly worn or the ferrule perished or split it should be

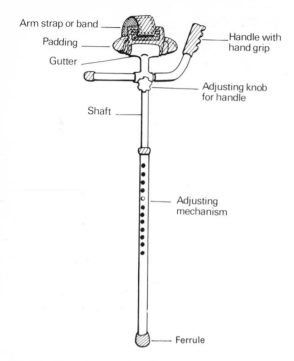

Fig. 5.1 The main parts of a walking aid

replaced immediately as the aid is unsafe to use in this state.

(b). Does the ferrule fit properly? Many different sizes of ferrule are needed to fit the wide variety of aids available and a ferrule should be of the correct size. A ferrule that is too large and has been 'padded' with elastoplast wound round the stick, or one that is too small and has been split to fit the stick, is not safe for permanent use.

(c). Does the adjusting mechanism work easily? With a sprung-knob type of mechanism it is important that both knobs should spring out easily and that the outer shaft moves freely over the inner one.

(d). Is the padding complete? Padding which is split, perished or missing should be replaced in order to avoid discomfort or damage to the patient.

(e). Does the aid stand square and upright if free-standing?

(f) Are all the wooden parts of the aid free from splinters?

(g). Are all the joints secure?

(h). Where there are handgrips are they complete and not too loose? Handgrips which swivel round the handle can be difficult to hold securely.

(i). Is the aid suitable for the environment in which it is to be used? If it is to be used at home it is important to check that there is sufficient space for it to be used with ease. It should pass easily through all doors and passageways and the patient should be able to manoeuvre it over all types of surfaces. The therapist should make sure that if there are steps and stairs in the house the aid(s) can be easily carried up and down, or that a second one be supplied for use upstairs. The patient should also be taught to use the aid outside on rough ground where appropriate. If it needs to be transported in a car the aid should be small enough to fit inside easily.

(j). Has the patient been taught to use the aid correctly and can he, or his relatives, check it for safety?

The walking aids in common use are listed below and their measurement and uses discussed.

WALKING STICKS

There are several types (Fig. 5.2) of walking stick available and these include:
(a). a crook handle wooden walking stick
(b). an adjustable metal walking stick
(c). a 'Bennett' type walking stick
(d). a 'Fischer' type walking stick
(e). those of individual design.

To measure the aid

Walking sticks can be measured either:
1. By asking the patient to stand erect with his weight evenly distributed on both feet, looking forward and with shoulders and arms relaxed. The therapist should ensure that the patient is not leaning forward or to one side and that he is wearing shoes of similar height to those he normally wears. If he requires support to stand the therapist must check that he is standing symmetrically. With the wooden or Fischer type walking stick the ferrule is removed, the stick turned upside down and the handle placed on the floor. Holding the stick vertical the shaft is marked at the point level with the ulnar styloid (Fig. 5.3). The shaft is then sawn off at this point and the ferrule replaced. For the adjustable walking stick the measurement

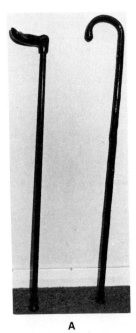

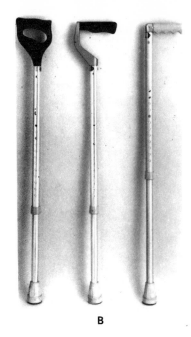

Fig. 5.2 Walking sticks (A) (left) Fischer walking stick (right) Standard wooden stick (B) Adjustable metal sticks (left) Bennett (centre) Swan neck (right) Standard

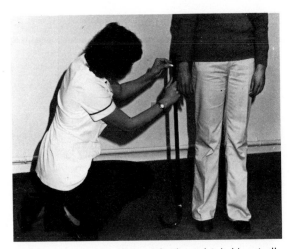

Fig. 5.3 Measuring a walking stick. The stick is held vertically and a mark is made on the shaft at the level of the ulnar styloid

measurement obtained will give the overall height of the stick.

With the stick measured correctly the user should be able to maintain an upright posture with the elbow slightly flexed. In this way he is able to lift his weight by fully extending his elbow as he pushes down on the stick when walking (Fig. 5.4).

Points of use

The user's wrist and grip must be strong enough to allow him to bear weight through this area when using the stick. If this is not possible an alternative aid, such as gutter crutches, should be chosen. When using the stick the person should be taught to look where he is going rather than at the ground and an even heel-toe gait should be encouraged.

Occasions when walking sticks may be used

Walking sticks are used for a variety of reasons and may be required:

(a). to supplement power where there is muscular weakness, for example in cases of poliomyelitis or nerve injury to the lower limb

(b). to relieve pain as in osteoarthrosis or following a fracture within the lower limb.

is taken as above, but there is no need to turn the stick upside down as the adjustable shaft allows alterations to be carried out *in situ*.

2. By asking the patient to lie straight with his hands at his side and measuring the distance between the ulnar styloid and the bottom of the heel. An inch is then added to this measurement in order to allow for the height of the shoe. The

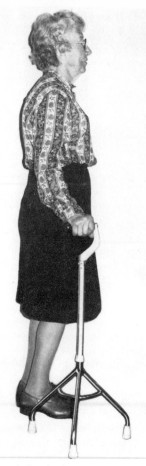

Fig. 5.4 A correctly fitted aid

(c). to widen the walking base in conditions of impaired balance, for example following a head injury or in those with multiple sclerosis

(d). to protect weak bones or damaged joints, for example in cases of osteoporosis or following a meniscectomy

(e). to compensate for deformity, for example where there is scoliosis or limb shortening

(f). as a feeler, for example for the blind or some patients with hemianopia

(g). for social reasons, for example to warn others of the user's slowness or lack of confidence in walking or — occasionally — as a 'fashion aid'.

THE QUADRUPED (Fig. 5.5)

This is a more stable version of the walking stick

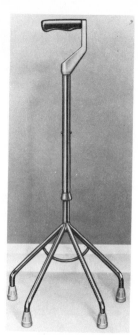

Fig. 5.5 A quadruped

having a four-footed base. Tripods with a three footed base are also available but are considered by some to be rather unstable.

To measure the aid

These aids are measured in the same way as an adjustable walking stick. The therapist should ensure that, when the aid is in use, the open end of the handle is facing backwards and the flat side of the rectangle made by the feet is nearest the user as shown in Figure 5.4.

Points of use

These are as for the walking stick, but it is particularly important to ensure that the aid is neither too close to the patient so that he leans over it to balance when taking weight, nor too far away so that the aid will tip inwards when weight is taken on it.

Occasions when quadrupeds may be used

These are usually issued singly for a weakness of one lower limb or a unilateral weakness of the whoe body where more support is needed than can be obtained from the use of a walking stick, for example in some cases of hemiplegia. N.B. The therapist may note that, where the 'bilateral' approach to treatment is followed the use of such aids is not encouraged. Quadrupeds may also be issued in pairs following bilateral amputation of the lower limbs or to young sufferers of cerebral palsy or spina bifida.

CRUTCHES

Elbow Crutches (Fig. 5.6)

These aids, which are usually issued in pairs, provide an armband support which fits round the forearm thus bracing the wrist when the aid is in use.

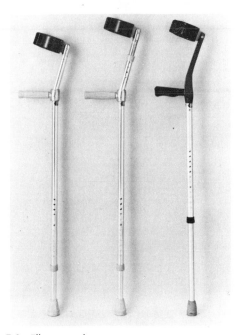

Fig. 5.6 Elbow crutches

To measure the aid

The height of the aid from the floor to the handle is measured as for the adjustable walking stick. The forearm band should be neither too tight so that the aid is difficult to remove, nor too loose so that it does not give enough support. The band should hold the forearm at a point slightly above midway

between the wrist and elbow, for if it is too low it will not give sufficient support and if too high it may block the action of the elbow and/or rub on the ulnar nerve, causing bruising and subsequent tingling or loss of sensation in the fourth and fifth digits.

Points of use

The points of use of these aids are as for those of the walking stick. However, as elbow crutches can be awkward to handle the patient may need some practice in putting on and taking off the aids as well as in walking with them. It is essential that the user has good strength throughout his upper limbs as they support much of the body weight when walking on these aids.

Occasions when elbow crutches may be used

As elbow crutches offer a great deal of support to the lower limbs they can be used when the patient's strength or balance have been severely affected. Elbow crutches may be issued in cases of:
(a). bilateral weakness and/or incoordination of the lower limbs, for example following spinal injury or in some cases of spina bifida
(b). unilateral weakness of a lower limb when the patient is not permitted to bear his full weight through the injured limb, for example in the early stages following a Potts fracture or meniscectomy
(c) bilateral severe weakness and/or incoordination affecting the whole body and/or where the upper limbs are unable to provide sufficient support using walking sticks. This may occur in some cases of a progressive paralysis such as muscular dystrophy, or following brain damage.

Forearm or gutter crutches (Fig. 5.7)

This is another variety of a single stick aid, but one in which the weight is borne along the length of the forearm rather than through the wrist and hand.

To measure the aid

The user should stand as upright as possible with

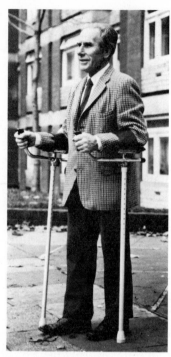

Fig. 5.7 Forearm or 'gutter' crutches

posture. It is important to ensure that the user's balance and coordination are adequate before he attempts to walk unsupervised, because the aids are strapped over the forearms and so cannot be discarded quickly in a crisis.

Occasions when forearm crutches may be used

These are usually issued in pairs and can be used for unilateral or bilateral weakness in the lower limbs in cases where the upper limbs are unable to bear weight through the wrists and hands. The most common example is the patient with rheumatoid arthritis. Other examples include persons who, because of injury to both the lower and the upper limbs, find weight bearing through the wrist and hands impossible.

Axilla crutches (Fig. 5.8)

These are aids in which weight is borne through the wrist and hand. The axilla pad, which is pressed against the chest wall, is not an area

his arms and shoulders relaxed, looking forward and with his weight evenly distributed on both feet. Measurement is taken from the floor to the olecranon process. In some cases the patient may have to be measured lying down, as he may have difficulty in standing without the use of an aid. The measurement should then be taken from the olecranon process to the bottom of the heel and an inch added to allow for the height of the shoe. In both cases the measurement obtained will give the distance required from the ferrule to the bottom of the gutter padding.

When adjusting the handle the therapist should check that there is sufficient space between the front of the gutter and the handle to leave the wrist free from pressure, especially over the ulnar styloid. Similarly, the therapist should check that the elbow is free at the back so that the gutter does not press onto the ulnar nerve which, at this point, lies just under the skin with little protection from pressure.

Points of use

The crutches should not be placed too far in front of the body as this can unbalance the upright

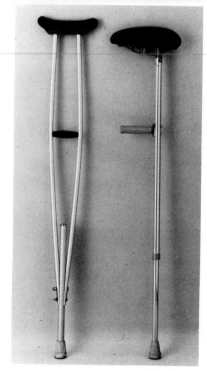

Fig. 5.8 Axilla crutches

through which weight is taken but helps to stabilise the shoulder.

To measure the aid

The height of the hand grip is measured as for the walking stick, that is, it should be level with the user's ulnar styloid. The axilla pads should be adjusted so that there is a gap of approximately two inches (or three fingers' width) between the top of the pad and the axilla. If the aids are too long there is a danger of putting pressure on the brachial plexus thus affecting the nerve supply to the upper limb. If they are too short posture will be affected during walking and the user will find difficulty in keeping the pads pressed against the chest wall for they will tend to slip out.

Points of use

It is essential that the user appreciates the importance of bearing weight through the handles of the aids and of not leaning on the axilla pads because of the danger of putting pressure on the brachial plexus. The axilla pads should be pressed against the chest wall in order to give support by bracing the shoulder and upper limb. The crutches should be used at an angle of approximately 15° to the side of the body.

Occasions when axilla crutches may be used

These aids are issued in pairs and may be used where there is unilateral weakness of the lower limb through which only partial or no weight may be taken, for example following a fracture of the tibia and fibula or after a bone graft to a previously ununited fracture. The aids may also be used where there is a bilateral dysfunction of the lower limbs when a reciprocal gait is inappropriate, for example if the hips or spine are fixed in a hip spica plaster or if other supports fixing the hip are worn.

WALKING FRAMES

The lightweight walking frame (Fig. 5.9)

This is the simplest style of walking frame and is often referred to as a 'pulpit' or 'Zimmer' frame. A

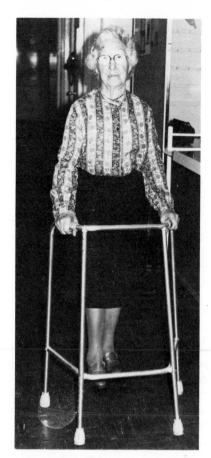

Fig. 5.9 A lightweight walking frame

hinged version, known as a reciprocal walking frame, is also available.

To measure the frame

The height is measured as for the walking stick.

Points of use

It is important to ensure that the user does not step too closely into the frame as there is a danger that he may tip backwards. Where this is a persistent problem it has been found practical to tie a piece of coloured tape or elastic across the back legs of the frame at knee level (not below, as this may trip those with poor sight or a high stepping gait) to prevent the user stepping in too closely to the frame. Similarly, the frame should not be placed too far in front of the user when walking, for this may not only upset his balance but can also cause the frame to tip if all four legs are not placed firmly on the floor when weight is taken onto it.

Occasions when a lightweight walking frame may be used

This is a very popular aid and can be used for:

(a). unilateral weakness or amputation of the lower limb where general weakness or infirmity makes the greater support offered by the frame necessary, such as in osteoarthritis or a fractured femur in the elderly.

(b). bilateral weakness and/or incoordination of the lower limbs or whole body, whenever a firm, free-standing aid is appropriate, as for example for those suffering from multiple sclerosis or Parkinsonism.

(c). general support to aid mobility and confidence, for example following a period of prolonged bedrest and sickness in the elderly.

Although not as commonly used as the standard walking frame the reciprocal frame is useful for those who require a firm, free-standing aid for use with a reciprocal gait. Where there is additional weakness in the upper limbs the use of a reciprocal frame frees the user from having to lift the whole weight of the frame at once.

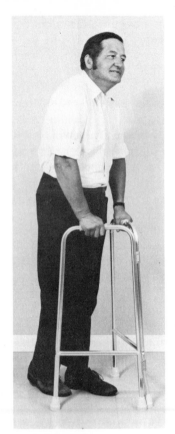

Fig. 5.10   An Alpha folding frame

Folding frames such as the three-point walking frame (Fig. 5.10)

This is a compact, folding variety of the lightweight walking frame and may be referred to as an 'Alpha' frame.

To measure the frame

The height is measured as for the walking stick.

Points of use

See lightweight walking frame.

Occasions when the three-point frame may be used

This aid is issued for the same reasons as the lightweight walking frame, but in cases where space is restricted. For example, it may be more appropriate in a small house or flat; if the standard frame will not fit into the patient's car; or for especially small patients who find the standard frame too cumbersome. Owing to its design this aid requires a little more balance by the user.

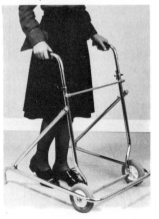 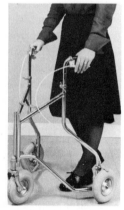

A   B

Fig. 5.11   Wheeled frames (A) Rollator (B) Delta aid with brakes

Wheeled frames

This section includes aids such as the rollator (Fig. 5.11A) which is a frame-type aid with two wheels at the front and two ferrules at the back which act as brakes. Several versions are available including those with seat or carrying baskets attached. A similar aid is the three-wheeled or 'Delta' version of the rollator which, on some models, has a brake system attached to the handgrips (Fig. 5.11B).

To measure the frame

The height is measured as for the walking stick.

Points of use

Although simple to use, most wheeled frames can be awkward to manoeuvre in confined spaces as they require a fairly large area in which to turn. This is especially true of the rollator. When issuing such an aid the therapist should ensure that the patient is able to control the braking system so that the aid presents no hazard when used on a slope or camber. Because of its design and mode of use, the rollator is not easy to use out of doors.

Occasions when the wheeled frames may be used

The rollator. Because this aid does not require the user to remember any particular walking pattern or to have sufficient strength and/or balance to lift it off the floor during use, it can be issued to those who cannot use a lightweight frame. Although useful, therefore, for the elderly infirm or for those with spina bifida, it needs a large turning area and the therapist must make sure that enough space is available for this.

The three wheeled aid. This aid, like the rollator, is used where a pick-up aid is unsuitable and also where space is restricted.

Frames with forearm rests

Of this group the forearm walker and the standing aid are the most widely used. The forearm walker is a chest high version of the walking frame which has gutter attachments fixed to the upper bars of the frame as shown (Fig. 5.12A). The frame is

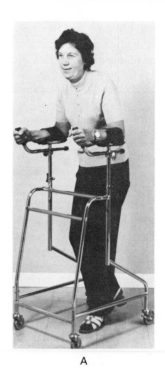

A

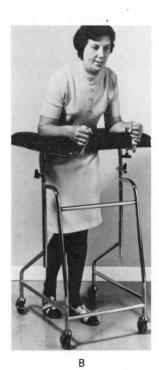

B

Fig. 5.12 Forearm resting frames (A) Stand aid with forearm gutters (B) Stand aid

usually moved on castors. The standing aid is another chest high walking frame which has a padded resting platform on which the forearms are placed when walking (Fig. 5.12B).

To measure the aids

Both aids are initially measured as for the forearm crutches. However, depending upon the severity of disability of the user, some adjustment may have to be made in order to allow the most appropriate and comfortable posture.

Points of use

As both aids are rather cumbersome they can be difficult to manoeuvre in confined spaces or out of doors. However, many patients are restricted to them as their only means of mobility and, therefore, will be obliged to adapt their activity to the limited manoeuvrability of the aid.

Occasions when forearm rest frames may be used

The forearm walker can be used in cases where a lightweight frame or gutter crutches are appropriate, but where weakness of the lower limbs, combined with weakness and/or incoordination of

the upper limbs, make them impractical. The aid is suitable, therefore, for some advanced cases of rheumatoid arthritis or where injuries to both upper and lower limbs have been sustained, making weightbearing through the wrist or hand impossible.

The standing aid may be used instead of the forearm walker, when gutter attachments are inappropriate, for example in cases of upper limb deformity.

The therapist will notice, when looking through manufacturers' catalogues, that many variations and combinations of these aids are produced.

WALKING PATTERNS

All walking aids must be used correctly in order to provide adequate support and allow the patient to maintain good posture, balance and gait. Walking aids, like all other aids, should never be issued unless full instruction for their use is provided. The walking patterns illustrated below cover the use of aids already discussed. The therapist may find that the names given to the gaits vary from place to place. The types of aid with which each gait can be used are given in brackets.

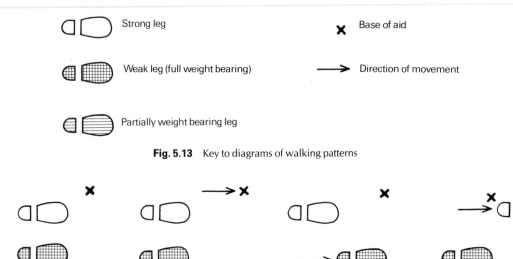

Fig. 5.13 Key to diagrams of walking patterns

Fig. 5.14 The use of one walking aid in the early stages of recovery (tripod, quadruped or walking stick)

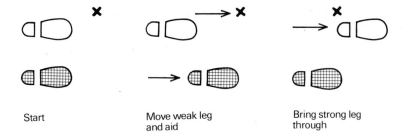

Fig. 5.15 The use of one walking aid in the later stages of recovery (tripod, quadruped or walking stick)

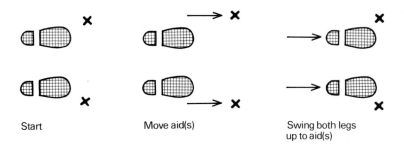

Fig. 5.16 The swing-to gait (axilla crutches or pick-up frame)

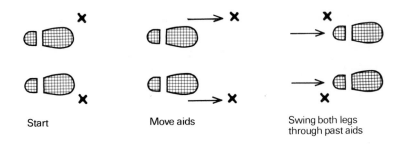

Fig. 5.17 The swing-through gait (axilla crutches)

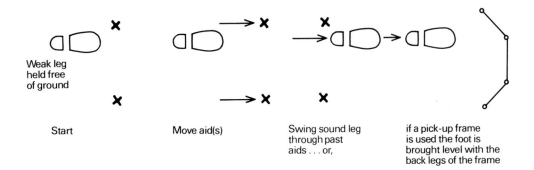

Fig. 5.18 The non weight-bearing gait (axilla crutches or pick-up frame)

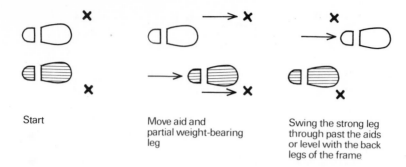

Start

Move aid and
partial weight-bearing
leg

Swing the strong leg
through past the aids
or level with the back
legs of the frame

Fig. 5.19   The partial weight-bearing gait (axilla crutches, pick-up frame or elbow crutches)

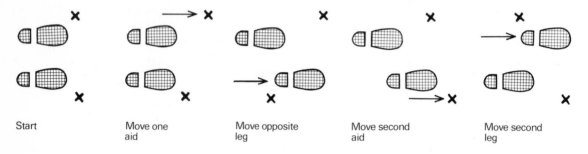

Start

Move one
aid

Move opposite
leg

Move second
aid

Move second
leg

Fig. 5.20   The four-point gait used in the early stages of recovery (gutter crutches, axilla crutches, elbow crutches,
walking sticks or reciprocal frame)

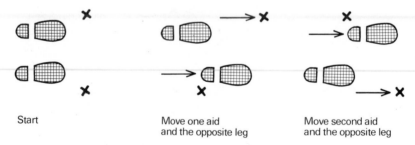

Start

Move one aid
and the opposite leg

Move second aid
and the opposite leg

Fig. 5.21   The four-point gait used in the later stages of recovery (aids as above)

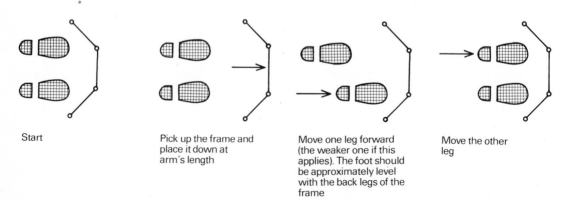

Start

Pick up the frame and
place it down at
arm's length

Move one leg forward
(the weaker one if this
applies). The foot should
be approximately level
with the back legs of the
frame

Move the other
leg

Fig. 5.22   Using the pick-up aids

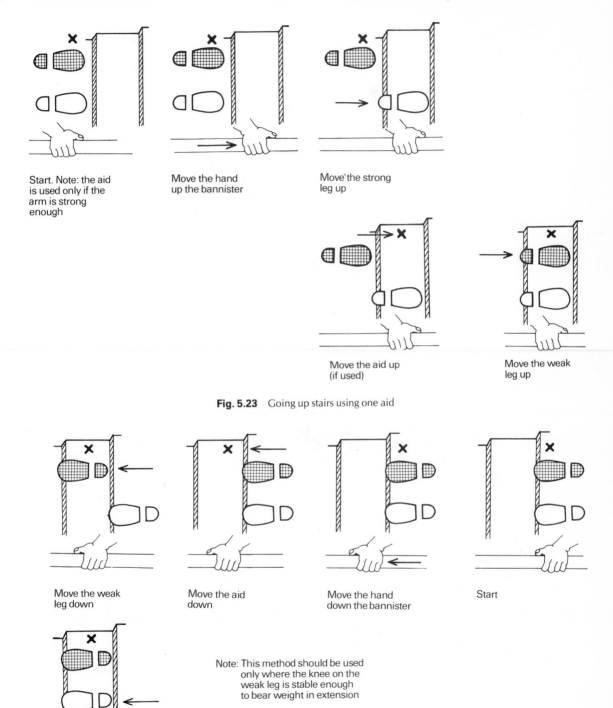

Fig. 5.23 Going up stairs using one aid

Fig. 5.24 Going down stairs using one aid

Start. Note: the aid is used only if the arm is strong enough

Move the hand up the bannister

Move the strong leg up

Move the aid up (if used)

Move the weak leg up

Move the weak leg down

Move the aid down

Move the hand down the bannister

Start

Move the strong leg down

Note: This method should be used only where the knee on the weak leg is stable enough to bear weight in extension

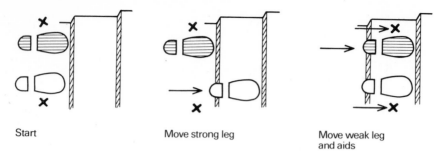

Start

Move strong leg

Move weak leg and aids

Fig. 5.25   Going up stairs using two aids (partial weight-bearing)

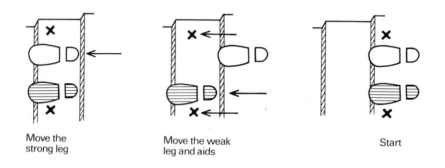

Move the strong leg

Move the weak leg and aids

Start

Fig. 5.26   Going down stairs using two aids (partial weight-bearing)

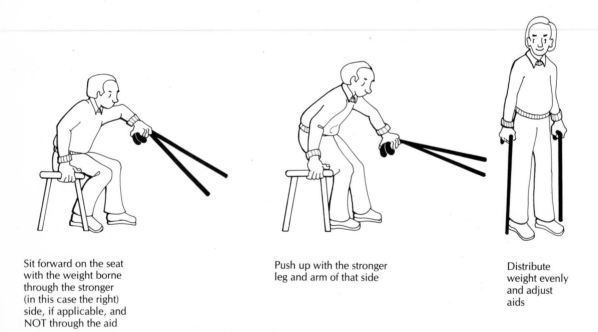

Sit forward on the seat with the weight borne through the stronger (in this case the right) side, if applicable, and NOT through the aid

Push up with the stronger leg and arm of that side

Distribute weight evenly and adjust aids

Fig. 5.27   Standing with a non-free-standing aid

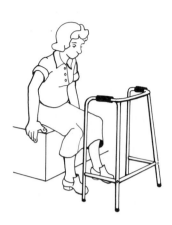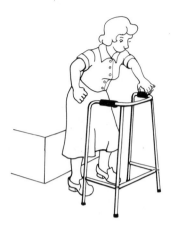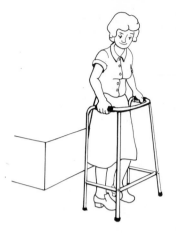

Sit forward on the seat with the weight borne through both arms and legs (or the stronger side if this is applicable)

Push up, transferring weight evenly onto both feet

Transfer hands to the frame to help support weight and assist balance

Fig. 5.28 Standing with a free-standing aid

Information regarding the range of walking aids produced may be obtained from manufacturers' catalogues. A list of a selection of firms producing walking aids in Great Britain is given below:

Carters (J & A) Ltd, Alfred Street, Westbury, Wiltshire

Cooper & Sons Ltd, Wormley, Godalming, Surrey (Manufacturers of the Cooper Fischer walking stick)

Day's Medical Aids, Llandow Industrial Estate, Cowbridge, Glamorgan

Edward Doherty & Sons Ltd, Eedee House, Carlton Road, Edmonton, London N9

Ellis Son and Paramore Ltd, Spring Street Works, Sheffield S3 8PB

Remploy Ltd Orthopaedic Division, Remploy House, 415 Edgware Road, London NW2

Seaco Products Ltd, 144 Old South Lambeth Road, London SW8

R H Stock, 71 High Street, Hardingstone, Northampton

Acknowledgements

My thanks to Carters (J & A) Ltd for supplying many of the photographs used in this chapter.

6

Wheelchairs and outdoor transport

There is more to wheelchairs than meets the eye! When first year students at St Loye's Occupational Therapy School are asked to spend a day in a wheelchair in order to gain firsthand experience of disability, their initial reaction is usually one of eager anticipation. However, the reports of their experience invariably show that the novelty soon wears off (often around lunch time, when fellow students tend to get fed up with their slowness and incompetence) and they often sheepishly confess that their 'day' finished at around 6 p.m. when they could stand the wheelchair no longer. Many have been astonished at their own, and other people's, reactions. Some have been ashamed to admit to wanting to throw the wheelchair into the River Exe; others have been asked to leave restaurants, refused entrance to pubs, been patted on the head, given sweets by elderly matrons, stared at by children and adults and, classically, been infuriated when, upon trying to buy a pair of shoes, found the shop assistant asked their partner what size feet they have!

Despite this love-hate relationship with an object that frequently provides mobility at the cost of loss of anonymity and dignity, the occupational therapist needs to be aware of the wide variety of models, their features and accessories, as well as of the types of assistance that can be given with outdoor transport.

The types of transport available for those who need help with mobility can be divided into three main areas:

1. *Hand-propelled wheelchairs:* Many models are available, including child or adult sizes, self-

or attendant-propelled, folding- or rigid-framed types. They are available in Great Britain either on prescription or they may be bought privately.

2. *Electrically-propelled wheelchairs:* Fewer models are available in this area. They range in design from a basic dining-type chair mounted on a platform and propelled by a battery operated motor to a car-type chair complete with soft-topped canopy. A few are available on prescription and many types are available for private purchase.

3. *Assistance with outdoor mobility:* This mainly includes mobility allowances and parking concessions, all of which can be obtained through various Government departments. Private cars can be adapted at the driver's own expense by a number of specialist firms.

ASSISTANCE AVAILABLE THROUGH GOVERNMENT DEPARTMENTS

Hand-propelled wheelchairs

The large selection of hand-propelled wheelchairs available on prescription can be divided into several types with certain basic features. The therapist will note that each model is a combination of some of these basic features. These must be considered before choosing the best wheelchair for the patient.

1. *Folding or rigid frame:* Folding frame chairs make transport and storage easier whereas rigid framed chairs tend to be sturdier and more comfortable for long periods of use.

2. *Self-propelled or attendant-propelled:* Self-propelled chairs have two large wheels for pushing (usually fitted with a handrim) and one or two small castor wheels. Chairs for pushing by an attendant have four smaller wheels and can generally be stored in a smaller space.

3. *Indoor or outdoor use:* Chairs for indoor use are generally fitted with solid tyres and have rigid or minimally folding frames. Those for outdoor use have pneumatic tyres, the latter being preferable if a chair is to double for indoor and outdoor use.

4. *Standard weight or lightweight:* Lightweight chairs are best for carrying in cars or Invacars for example, but tend to be slightly less stable and are not recommended for double above-knee amputees without prostheses unless specifically adapted. All lightweight chairs supplied on prescription have the letter 'L' following the model number.

5. *Size:* Not all chairs are available in all sizes (see sections 'Models' and 'Assessment')

Child size: Up to 5 stone and 4 ft tall (model C)

Junior: Up to 9 stone and 5 ft 2 in tall (model J)

Adult/Standard: Up to 14 stone and over 5 ft 2 in tall

Outsize: Over 14 stone and over 5 ft 2 in tall (model O/S)

Features and adaptations

Each basic model can be fitted with a wide variety of special features and adaptations. The therapist must remember that some of these features come as standard fittings on certain models and also that not every feature can be fitted to every model. Those features which are available and the models to which they can be fitted, are specified on the application form (AOF5G) and in the Department of Health and Social Security (DHSS) *Handbook of Wheelchairs and Self-propelled Tricycles.* These features must also be considered when ordering the wheelchair.

Frames. Folding frames can be single or double cross brace. For adults using a folding chair indoors those designed on a single cross brace make forward transfers easier as they can be pushed nearer to toilet, bed, etc., provided that the footrests can be swung free or removed. Double cross brace chairs are slightly sturdier, though heavier, for outdoor use.

Wheels. Large wheels for self-propelled adult chairs can be 18, 20, 22 or 24 inches in diameter. Although the bigger ones are easier to reach they make side transfers more difficult as they protrude higher above the seat; they also take up more space when the chair is folded.

Castors vary from 5 to 7½ inches in diameter. The smaller ones are easier to manoeuvre but more difficult to manage over ridges, bumps and kerbs. They are fitted double when at the front and single or double at the back. A single rear castor can make a chair more difficult to control yet easy to manoeuvre.

Tyres can be solid (best for indoors and easy maintenance by the elderly or very disabled) or pneumatic. The latter will absorb the jolts from uneven surfaces more easily if maintained at the right pressure.

Handrims in metal or wood are a standard feature on most self-propelled chairs. Variations include (a) capstan rims for those with a weak grip who cannot manage to grasp a standard rim or (b) one-arm drive where both handrims are fitted to the wheel on the non-affected side. With practice these can be steered in a straight line, or to the right or left, depending upon how the rims are moved.

The position of the wheels can be altered for double lower limb amputees; the large wheels can either be set back 3 inches to counterbalance the loss of weight at the front to prevent the chair from tipping backwards or they can become front propelling to throw more weight forwards and therefore act as a counterbalance.

Backrests. The rear tilt of backrests varies from 5° to 30°, the 15° tilt being the commonest. The greater angle of tilt helps patients with fixed or weak spines and hips to balance and also assists respiration of those with cardiac or chest problems. Extensions of 3, 6, 9 and 12 inches are available for those with poor head control. Horizontally folding backrests can be fitted to allow the chair to be stored in a small space such as the boot of a car. Rigid backrests can be fitted to some folding chairs in order to provide extra support. Zipped backrests may also be ordered.

Footrests. A wide range of types, adjustments and accessories is available.

(a). Types

(i) Divided: all individual footrests can be swung up for ease of transfer

(ii) Platform: a single rest to accommodate both feet

(iii) Carcason: a rigid 'hammock' type rest which reduces the overall length of the chair

(iv) Foot box: a more enclosed foot rest to give overall support.

(b). Adjustments

(i) Fixed: no adjustments are possible

(ii) Swinging (or retractable if of the platform type): for ease of transfer

(iii) Swinging and detachable

(iv) Elevating leg rests: for one or both legs to help reduce oedema or to accommodate fixed joints.

(c). Accessories

(i) Heel loops or toe loops: to prevent the foot slipping off the foot rest

(ii) Leg straps

(iii) Foot rest extension.

Armrests. All arm rests are padded and the variations available include:

1. Fixed

2. Detachable/hinged: to allow sideways transfer

3. Domestic: these are cut away at the front to enable the patient to sit closer to table, desk, etc

4. Rear cut-away to take ball-bearing arm supports

5. Provision to take a tray — the tray is also available

6. Additional padding

7. Deep arm rests: for use when a latex cushion is fitted.

Brakes. The different types available include:

(a). Push-on action

(b). Pull-on action

(c). Foot-operated by the attendant

(d). Single brake lever — left or right

(e). Lever extensions are also available.

Cushions. Cushions should be chosen with special care, as they effectively alter the height of the seat. Types available include:

(i) Foam cushions from 1–4 inches in depth

(ii) U-shaped cushion cut to accommodate a urinal

(iii) Ply-based cushion for extra support

(iv) Wedge-shaped cushions

Ripple, water, air, gel and particle filled cushions and sheepskin covers are available to help relieve pressure. An impermeable cover will help the incontinent patient but is hot and sticky for others.

Other features and accessories. The following are available only on some models:

1. Commode facilities (permanent or temporary) on models 1 and 3 only.

2. Adaptations for spastics, including footbox, ankle straps, pommel for adductor spasm, side wings to backrest and restraining harness. These are available on model 8LC, 12 and and some model 13 series chairs.

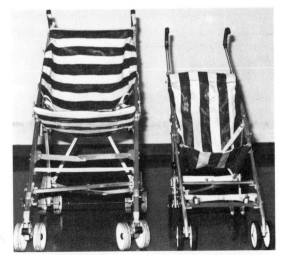

Fig. 6.7 Model 21 range: a lightweight, folding pushchair for outdoor use

propelled indoor chair which is partly folding. It can be braked only by the attendant (Fig. 6.6).

'Buggy' chairs. Various models available. These are lightweight, folding, outdoor chairs especially useful on public transport. Twin versions are available (Fig. 6.7).

Electrically-propelled chairs

Only one indoor type, the Model AC 102 battery powered 'Epic' chair (Fig. 6.8), is at present available from the Department of Health and Social Security. It is controlled by a push-bar lever and is designed for indoor use only; its very low ground clearance makes it impossible to use where there are kerbs or uneven paths. It tends to tip if used on slopes. There is only one size.

Its main advantage is the minimal physical effort needed to propel it, but this is offset by the extra attention needed to keep the battery fully charged and by the fact that its range is limited by its design and not the endurance of the pusher! As the Epic cannot be folded and is heavy to lift, an additional chair for outdoor use and for transporting in a car would be necessary. The therapist must consider, therefore, both the advantages and disadvantages of an electric chair before recommending it.

Where the Epic chair is not suitable, other electrically-propelled chairs, such as the Bec range or the 'Powerdrive' and 'Sleyride' models,

may be supplied. These models have the advantage of being compact and suitable for indoor and outdoor use. They can be adapted so that they may be propelled by even the most severely disabled, using a tiller bar, micro-switch disc or suck/blow mechanism.

Note: The therapist should be aware that these electrically propelled chairs should, not, officially, be used on the public highway. They are issued for use indoors and in the garden only.

Outdoor Transport

The various types of assistance with outdoor transport include:

The Mobility Allowance. This is a weekly, tax-free allowance aimed at assisting the disabled with the additional costs of transport. It may be used as required, for example to buy petrol, to help buy a car, pay taxi fares and so on.

Cars and Invacars. Adapted cars are available to a limited section of war pensioners. Invacars are no longer issued although there are still some in use. A mobility allowance is now issued instead.

Spinal carriage. This is a large, pram-type carriage for children or small adults who need to be in a reclining or semi-reclining position.

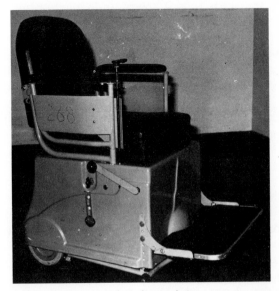

Fig. 6.8 The Epic: an indoor electric chair

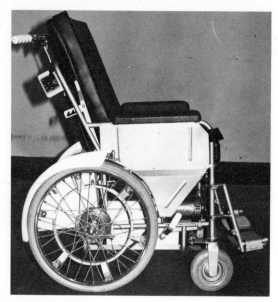

Fig. 6.9 Model 28B: an outdoor electric chair

Pedal and hand-propelled tricycles. These tricycles, although rather cumbersome and old fashioned in appearance, have a comfortable sitting position and are still popular for use in the country, at the seaside and on level ground.

Electrically-propelled wheelchair. Only one electrically-propelled chair is made by the DHSS for outdoor use. It is attendant-propelled (Fig. 6.9).

Parking discs. Orange parking discs issued by Social services departments to disabled or registered blind persons, allow the owners to park their cars in otherwise restricted areas. The scheme is operated nationwide. For example, many towns and cities with traffic-free shopping areas will allow the disabled to park in, or near, these and cars displaying the orange sticker will often get preferential treatment near cinemas, at football matches and in public car parks.

The disabled person will be provided with (Fig. 6.10):

1. a disabled person's badge to be displayed on the windscreen.

2. an orange parking disc to be displayed when parking on double yellow lines, to control the time of parking.

3. a badge for the rear of the car in order to help other motorists and officials to distinguish the car, although use of this badge is not compulsory.

The scheme *allows* the disabled person to:

(a). Park for up to two hours on yellow lines, except where there is a ban on loading or unloading at the time, in a bus lane or where the car would block traffic flow.

(b). Park without charge or time limit at parking meters.

(c). Park without time limit where limited waiting only is permitted.

However, the disabled person *may not*

(i) Park his vehicle where it will cause damage or obstruction to other road users.

(ii) Park on zig zag lines at pedestrian crossings and on or at kerbsides where there are double white lines in the centre of the road.

Motability. This is a Government-backed scheme which has been set up to help disabled people make the best use of their mobility allowance by leasing out adapted cars. For further details apply to: Motability, Boundary House, 91–93 Charterhouse St., London EC1M 6BT

Exemption from road tax. Disabled passengers who are not in receipt of a mobility allowance may be able to apply for exemption from road tax for the car in which they are carried.

Eligibility and how to apply

To sort out the mountain of information written about who is or is not eligible for help with the various types of transport is a task not to be undertaken lightly! It is made even more complex by constantly changing Government policy which affects the range of people eligible for the various types of assistance. For this reason, the information given below is a general guide only and must be checked for current alterations before an application is made.

(a). *Hand-propelled and electrically-propelled wheelchairs, tricycles and spinal carriages.* Application is made on form AOF5G which must be signed by the patient's doctor and sent to the appropriate Artificial Limb and Appliance Centre. No definite rules exist about eligibility and the decision as to who would benefit rests with the doctor.

(b). *Outdoor mobility.* Application for mobility allowance is made on form MY1 which is attached to the DHSS leaflet N1 211 *Mobility Allowance*

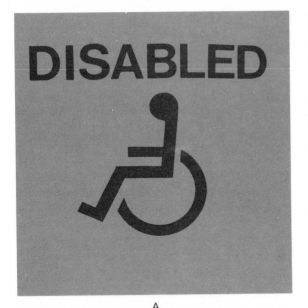

A

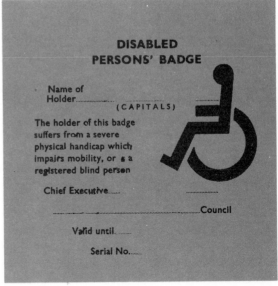

B

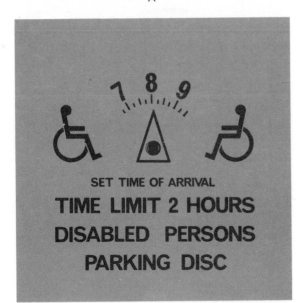

C

Fig. 6.10 The 'Orange badge' scheme A. Rear window sticker B. Front windscreen sticker C. Parking limit recorder

and is available from Post Offices. This booklet explains who is eligible to claim and how to claim. It also gives details of the allowance. The form should be completed by the patient (or his guardian if the application is made for a child) and sent to the DHSS, Mobility Allowance Unit, Norcross, Blackpool. At present (1980) the mobility allowance is payable to people between 5 and 65 years of age but proposals are being put forward to extend the upper age limit to 75 years, provided the allowance was awarded before the age of 65.

The supply of Invacars has been replaced by the mobility allowance. Patients wishing to take advantage of the Motability Scheme should apply to the address previously given.

(c). *Parking discs.* Application should be made to the local Social Services Department. The scheme is open to a person, or the driver of a person, who is suffering from a physical disability which considerably hinders mobility or who is a registered blind person. For further details refer to the booklet *Disabled Persons Badges for Motor Vehicles — Regulations 1975.*

PRIVATE PURCHASE OF WHEELCHAIRS AND ADAPTATIONS OF PRIVATE CARS

For those who prefer to provide their own aids to mobility and transport a wide range of products is available commercially, including a large selection of hand-propelled and electrically-propelled wheelchairs. There are also firms who will adapt privately owned cars to suit the disabled driver. In addition to this, many accessories for wheelchairs and cars, such as waterproof capes and car hoists, can be bought separately. The British School of Motoring make special provisions to teach disabled people to drive, either in their own adapted cars or in Invacars. Further information can be obtained from The British School of Motoring, 102 Sydney Street, London SW3. Several associations aimed at providing help and information for disabled drivers have been established and some addresses are given in Appendix I. Addresses of firms supplying wheelchairs and car adaptations are given at the end of this chapter.

When advising on the private purchase of a wheelchair, the therapist should remember that models, sizes and accessories will vary from one company to another and that servicing and maintenance costs should also be taken into consideration. The advice of the company's representative should always be sought when choosing the most suitable model to fit the patient and his needs.

ASSESSMENT FOR A SUITABLE WHEELCHAIR

In order to find the most suitable type of wheelchair for a patient, various factors must be taken into consideration. These include:

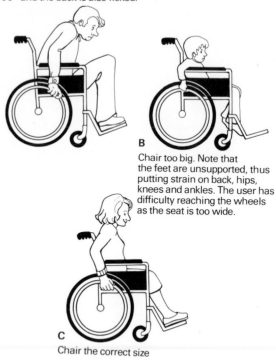

A
Chair too small. Note that the hips and knees are flexed beyond 90° and the back is also flexed.

B
Chair too big. Note that the feet are unsupported, thus putting strain on back, hips, knees and ankles. The user has difficulty reaching the wheels as the seat is too wide.

C
Chair the correct size

Fig. 6.11 Fitting a wheelchair

1. The patient himself

Age. Is he young or old and how often will he use the chair? Is he likely to use it indoors, outdoors, in the car, at work or elsewhere?

Height. When seated the patient's hip should be comfortably flexed at 90°, the back of his knees not pressed against the edge of the seat and his feet, with the ankles at 90°, resting securely on a suitable footrest. He should be able to reach the wheel rims with ease while maintaining an upright posture (Fig. 6.11).

Weight. Remember that different sizes within each range are made to take only patients up to a certain weight. If the patient is too heavy the chair will be under too much strain it will wear out more quickly, and may break down. If the chair is too heavy it will be difficult or impossible for the patient to manoeuvre it or the attendant to push.

Diagnosis. Is the condition static, progressive or likely to improve? Therefore, how long will the chair be in use? Will it serve for that period or will it have to be replaced once the patient can no longer manage it? If the chair will need to be pushed, is it suitable for the attendant? Is there incontinence, spasticity or need for help with transfer and, if so, can the model be fitted with the appropriate features to cope with this?

Physical disabilities. The patient's ability to handle the chair should be considered carefully. For example:

Can the patient, or attendant, manoeuvre the recommended model on flat and sloping ground, on rough surfaces, around corners and through doors?

Are his hands able to grip the standard rim? If not, can adaptations be fitted to that model or should an electric model be considered? How will he transfer into and out of the chair?

Can the patient manage the brakes, remove the armrests and replace them and swing the footrests without help?

Attitude and the reason for supply. Has the patient asked for the chair or has one been considered advisable?

Is the patient reluctant to accept a chair and if so, why? Will he use it if supplied?

Does he understand when to use the chair, for example that a Model 9 is supplied for outdoor use only and not to sit in all day?

Is he mentally able to understand how to use the brakes and master the one-arm drive? Will he be able to maintain the electric chair? If not, is the chair suitable for the attendant?

2. The place of use

(a). *In the home.* Consider the widths of doors, corridors and the space to manoeuvre in them.

Any steps and the possibility of ramping them should be considered.

Transfers to bed, chair and toilet, and the space and angle in which they have to be performed, must be noted. Can grab rails be fitted if necessary?

Is there room to store the chair/car when not in use? Is the store dry and the access wasy?

Are facilities available to maintain the chair/vehicle and is there someone who can carry out routine care?

Will the wheelchair fit under the sink, table or desk as required?

(b). *Outside.* Are paths, steps, gates and doors suitable for the chair or can they be made so?

Can pavements, kerbs, hills and roads be negotiated in the same chair or will another type need to be provided?

(c). *At work.* Is the chair suitable for use at work?

3. Other transport facilities

Is any other transport available or will all journeys be made in the chair?

If the chair is used in conjunction with a car, can the patient get in/out of the vehicle and can the chair be folded, lifted and stored in the vehicle?

Will a hoist be necessary for transfer?

Can the car be parked in a suitable place at home to allow easy transfer?

4. Relatives

Are relatives prepared to accept the chair or will their attitude prevent the patient from using it? If so, why?

If the patient needs help with pushing, transfer or maintenance of the chair, can and will his relatives help and are they physically/mentally able to do so?

With this information the team can now decide on the best model and size of chair, and any necessary features and accessories. Standard size chairs will be supplied much more quickly than non-standard ones.

USE, CARE AND REPAIR OF WHEELCHAIRS

As with any piece of equipment, the patient must learn how to use and maintain his wheelchair. Not only should he and his relatives be shown what and what not to do, they should also be given written instructions. The DHSS publish a small booklet on how to use and maintain chairs. The booklet varies for each model and the occupational therapist should ensure that the patient receives his copy when his chair is delivered. Another very readable booklet is published by the British Red Cross Society: *People in Wheelchairs — Hints for Helpers.* The booklet is simply written and amusingly illustrated.

Both booklets give, amongst other information, basic hints on use and these include:

Maintenance. When receiving the chair, and at regular intervals thereafter, the user should check that it is in full working order. Brakes, tyres and footrests are particularly important.

Ensure that pneumatic tyres are kept at the correct pressure (a pump is provided) and that the battery is fully charged.

Once the seat canvas sags or is split it should be replaced immediately.

Brakes. Always put the brakes on fully when the chair is stationary and before transferring. Release them fully before moving.

Footrests. Always swing and/or retract the footrests out of the way before transfer and *never* attempt to stand up on them.

Folding the chair. Remove any cushion first and

fold the chair by pulling up on the centre of the seat canvas.

Opening the chair. Push with the heel of the hands on the bars at the side of the seat, keeping the fingers towards the centre to avoid squashing them (Fig. 6.12).

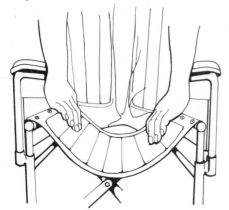

Fig. 6.12   Position of hands when unfolding a wheelchair

Self-propelled chairs. The user should sit well up and back in the chair, with his feet squarely on the footrests. He should reach back and push the wheels from 9 o'clock to 3 o'clock, thus keeping a good posture, and not push from the top of the wheel forwards (Fig. 6.13).

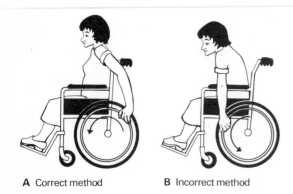

A Correct method   **B** Incorrect method

Fig. 6.13   Propelling a wheelchair

SOME DO'S AND DON'TS FOR ATTENDANTS OF WHEELCHAIRS

A comprehensive list is given in the Red Cross handbook. It includes such common sense hints as:

Helping the chair down a kerb/step. Warn the occupant what you are going to do. Hold the handgrips firmly and tip the chair back onto its rear wheels by pushing a foot on the tipping lever. Lower the chair down gently, ensuring that both rear wheels reach the road together. Lower front wheels.

Helping the chair up a kerb/step. Warn the occupant what is going to happen. Hold the chair firmly and tip it back using the tipping lever. Place the front wheels onto the pavement and push the rear wheels on behind.

Helping the chair up or down a flight of steps. This requires two helpers, one holding the chair by the handles at the back, one holding the front below the armrests (not on the footrests as these are liable to lift off). First warn the occupant what is going to happen and then tip the chair back and manoeuvre one step at a time, balancing the chair on its rear wheels. One helper should take command to ensure that the lifting is done simultaneously. Note: Whether going up or down stairs the occupant always faces towards the bottom of the stairs.

General points. Make sure that clothes, rugs and so on are tucked out of the way of the wheels. Talk with, not above, the occupant. Always warn the occupant before any move is made. Don't run when pushing the chair. Don't push the chair out into the road without looking. Beware of pushing the footplate into glass doors, walls, kerbs and shins.

THE ROLE OF THE OCCUPATIONAL THERAPIST

The role of the occupational therapist in assessment and advice regarding wheelchairs and outdoor transport will vary from area to area but she should be able to:

1. Give concise and accurate reports on the patient's physical and mental state with regard to his ability to handle the chair or vehicle.

2. Report accurately on the areas in which it will be used and arrange for any adaptations which may be necessary to aid the use of the chair or vehicle.

3. She and other members of the team should know which chairs (and other help) are available.

From her own previous information she should be able to suggest the most suitable chair for the patient. This may be done with the full support of an organised wheelchair clinic or with the responsibility resting almost entirely on the occupational therapist, for example when ordering a chair, through a general practitioner, for a patient living at home.

4. As soon as the chair is delivered, teach the user (and/or his attendant) how to use and maintain it, and how to transfer in and out of it. Ensure he is confident about its use and routine maintenance and where to get help if necessary.

5. Give advice about facilities available, both on prescription and privately, and try to find out what help/services the patient may qualify for. It is unfair to raise the patient's hopes by letting him feel he may get a mobility allowance or electric chair, for example, when this is not so.

6. Always be aware of patients who may benefit from the facilities or equipment available, especially a patient who has: (a) suddenly become disabled, for example through a stroke or spinal injury, or (b) deteriorated to a point where help with mobility will save unnecessary struggle or further advance of conditions such as multiple sclerosis, heart or chest diseases or rheumatoid arthritis.

Some suppliers of Wheelchairs in Great Britain

W & F Barrett Ltd, 22 Emery Road, Brislington Trading Estate, Bristol BS4 5PH, Avon

Biddle Engineering Co Ltd (BEC), 103 Stourbridge Road, Halesowen, West Midlands, B63 3UB

Braune Batricar Ltd, Griffin Mill, Thrupp, Stroud, Gloucestershire

Everest & Jennings Ltd, Princewood Road, Corby, Northamptonshire

Malden Care, 57a Kingston Road, Raynes Park, London SW20 8SD

Martin Creasey & Co, Bridge Works, Hasketon, Woodbridge, Suffolk IP13 6HF

Meyra Rehab (U.K.) Ltd, Unit 4, Copheap Lane, Warminster, Wiltshire BA12 0BL

Newton Aids Ltd, 2a Conway Street, London W1P 5HE

Rehab Invacare Ltd, Tondu Road, Bridgend, Mid Glamorgan, CF31 4LE

Vessa Ltd, Paper Mill Lane, Alton, Hampshire GU34 2PY

Zimmer Orthopaedic Ltd, Bridgend, Mid Glamorgan CF31 3PY

Note: Some surgical appliance shops and larger chemists shops, such as Boots Ltd, act as agents for the above companies.

Companies who will adapt cars for use by disabled people include:

Feeney & Johnson Ltd, Alperton Lane, Wembley, Middlesex, HA0 1JJ

Reselco Invalid Carriages Ltd, 262 Kings Street, Hammersmith, London W6 0SS

REFERENCES AND FURTHER READING

British Red Cross Society 1974 People in wheelchairs — hints for helpers. British Red Cross Society, London

The Chartered Society of Physiotherapy 1975 Handling the handicapped. Woodhead Faulkner, Cambridge

Department of Health and Social Security 1977 Personal handbooks for users of wheelchairs. Department of Health & Social Security, Blackpool

Department of Health and Social Security 1978 Handbook of wheelchairs and hand-propelled Tricycles. Department of Health & Social Security, Blackpool

Wilshere ER 1977 Wheelchairs, 4th edn. From a Series: Equipment for the Disabled, Oxford Area Health Authority, Oxford.

7

Home visits

When I first qualified and was working in an orthopaedic hospital I was frequently asked, or felt it was necessary, to make a home visit. Although this seemed a desirable thing to do I was always a little confused as to what exactly the aim of the visit was, beyond looking round the patient's home to 'see if he could cope'.

My main problems, as I remember, were that I was never sure exactly what I was looking for and that, if I encountered a problem which was fairly obvious, even to my inexperienced eye, I was frequently at a loss as to how to help. After all, if the patient was unable to climb upstairs to bed and if there was no room for the bed downstairs, what could be done? Having never experienced community work, I also always felt a little ill at ease in the patient's house, for suddenly the roles were reversed; this was his territory. No longer could I hide behind the security of my white uniform and expect the patient to do as I asked. Working in a country district where many families were inter-related and which was moving rather slowly into the 20th century I also discovered that my ideas, solutions, suggestions and expectations (which had, after all, taken three years of training to learn) were those of a town-bred 21-year-old and vastly different from those of a Welsh hill farmer old enough to be my grandpa!

My aim, therefore, in this chapter is to look at home visits from the hospital occupational therapist's point of view, to describe how to undertake such a visit and what to look for and to suggest some possible solutions to the more commonly encountered problems.

THE AIM OF A HOME VISIT

A home visit is usually made when the possibility of discharge is imminent or being considered. It is sometimes felt that a visit by the therapist to the patient's home will ease the transfer from hospital to community life. By visiting the patient's home the therapist will gain a much clearer picture of the circumstances in which he will have to cope after his discharge, she may also discover minor problems which could arise but would be difficult to envisage without first hand experience. The visit also gives the therapist the opportunity to see how the patient will fit into the family should he be returning home to relatives. It is easier to see exactly how a relative will cope with the weaker person when both are in their familiar surroundings. It is also possible for the therapist to see whether the methods and aids he was taught to use in the hospital can be used equally well at home — a walking frame, for instance, is relatively simple to manoeuvre around an open, flat hospital ward but not so easy to handle in a cluttered cottage with narrow stairs.

The therapist can also note the patient's emotional reaction to discharge. Hopefully, the prospect of going home will raise his morale and, surrounded once again by familiar objects and layout, the patient may well be able to cope for himself where he had to struggle in hospital because of unfamiliar surroundings and equipment. However, the therapist may find that, having finally reached home, the patient discovers that his disability is a bigger barrier than he thought and that his confident assurances of 'I'll be all right, dear, when I get home.' are suddenly dashed by the realisation that, after all, things are not as easy as he had hoped. In this case the therapist must ask the team to reconsider whether the patient is really ready for discharge.

On the other hand, an occupational therapist may plan a home visit if there is some doubt as to where the patient will be discharged. For example, for an elderly patient living alone who has suffered a stroke and regained a reasonable level of independence it may be debatable whether he is capable of functioning at home alone. Frequently the only way to try to find the answer is for the therapist to watch the patient's reaction and level of function when taken home. Similarly, if a patient has become more severely disabled and it is known that his house will need adapting and that his relatives will have to be taught how to look after him, the therapist may visit his home in order to assess the possibilities of adapting it and the willingness and/or capability of the patient's relatives to look after him. This visit may be made fairly early in the patient's treatment programme as, if there are major structural or emotional problems to be overcome, these can be worked on from an early date.

When a home visit is to be undertaken there are many points which the therapist must consider before she sets out.

Timing

Is the visit being carried out at the right time? For example, a visit carried out too early may not give a true picture of the level of independence and confidence which will eventually be reached by the patient. Alternatively, one which is carried out too late, that is, too near the discharge date, may delay discharge in order that any alterations or services can be arranged before the patient arrives home. Worse still, it may mean that the patient is discharged before such arrangements can be made. At best this may cause only a few difficulties but at worst it may mean that the patient is unable to cope at all and will have to be readmitted to hospital.

Preparation

The therapist should ensure that she has all the relevant equipment and information to hand before she carries out her visit. For example, it is essential that she should not only have the patient's correct address but also an idea as to how to get there. She must of course obtain the patient's permission to visit his house; if no-one will be at home when she calls, she must also have a key so that she can get in. Suitable transport should be arranged. The therapist may drive her own car (provided she is adequately covered with insurance for such work) or she may have to arrange a hospital car or ambulance to take her, the patient and any aids necessary. Remembering

HOME VISIT CHECK LIST

Patient's Name ....

Date of visit ....

Ward ....

Time of leaving hospital ....

Hospital Number ....

Approx. time of return ....

Address ....

Therapist ....

Items to check before leaving (tick when completed)

Patient's permission obtained
Address and directions checked
Key to house available
Transport arranged
Tape-measure, notebook and pen
Any necessary aids available

Patient's outdoor clothing
Confirmation from others who will be
at the patient's home
Tea; coffee; milk
Ward staff informed

Items to check on arrival

Comments

1. Access
Gates
Paths
Steps
Door/key
Lifts

2. Stairs
Up/down
Covering
Lighting
Height of any rails to be fixed
Existing rails/bannisters

3. Corridors and halls
Space to manoeuvre
Rugs
Floor covering
Switches
Doors
Thresholds
Telephone

4. Living room
Height of most frequently used chair
On/off chair
Floor covering
Space around, and support offered by furniture
Equipment: radio, TV, fire, etc.

5. Kitchen
Cupboards/larder
Sinks/taps
Cooker
Other appliances: kettle, fridge etc.
Work surfaces
Floor covering
Any necessary aids

6. Dining area
Ability to sit at table
Ability to bring food to table
Space to manoeuvre around table

7. Bedroom
Height of bed
On/off bed
Bedding
Heating
Lighting
Is a commode necessary/available?
Storage for clothes

8. Bathroom
In/out bath
Space for aids and appliances where applicable
Ability to reach basin

9. Toilet
On/off toilet
Any aids necessary
For outside toilet: access
                    safety
                    lighting
Commode as alternative

10. Garden/garage
Access from house
Ability to perform any gardening required
Ability to open/close garage doors
Space to manoeuvre around car
Space to use and store aids

11. Relatives/neighbours/staff of home
Help available

12. Services available
Home help
Meals on wheels
Community nurse
Others

Action to be taken

Community therapist involved:

Address

Telephone

Signed:

Occupational Therapist

Fig. 7.1   Home visit check list (Note: the patient's diagnosis does not appear on this form as it is designed for use outside the hospital)

hospital ward is warm and that the patient may still be weak, his outdoor clothes (a coat, hat and shoes) will be necessary in order to help him adapt to the change in temperature. Before the visit, the therapist must ensure that she has explained its purpose to the patient. Many people may not understand the reason for the therapist wishing to see their house and could well mistake the visit as 'poking around' or 'seeing if my house is good enough'.

During a home visit it is often relaxing for the therapist, relatives and patient to discuss any problems over a cup of tea or coffee. The therapist will have an opportunity to see how the patient copes in his kitchen (should it be relevant), if she asks him to demonstrate how well he can manage by making the drink. If the patient lives alone it will probably be wise to take the necessary supplies from the hospital in case they are not available on arrival. The therapist must check, however, whether the patient is on a special diet and provide accordingly.

Before setting out the therapist should have a clear picture of the patient's present capabilities and also an idea of the type of situation to which he is going. If the patient lives with relatives it is helpful to visit at a time when they will be at home. If any other agencies, such as the community occupational therapist, district nurse, neighbour or home help, are involved it may be necessary to arrange for them to be at the patient's house as well.

The therapist must inform the ward staff where she is going with the patient, at what time and when she hopes to return. If the visit is expected to take several hours arrangements for meals, drugs or other essentials must be made. She should also explain to the staff, the patient and his relatives the purpose of the visit in order that all can understand the reason for the questions asked and the need for the patient to demonstrate his abilities.

Finally, the author has always found that a sponge bag containing tissues and a damp flannel, plus a large towel, are very useful in case of travel sickness or other emergencies. An example of a home visit check list is shown in Figure 7.1. This ensures that no basic items have been forgotten and that all the main areas have been submitted to a check.

The patient's wishes

As already mentioned, the patient and his relatives will be in their own home and can no longer be required to act in a particular way. When discussing solutions to a problem the therapist must always remember that she can only suggest, and not dictate, a possible change in lifestyle. Her suggestions should, naturally, always be accompanied by sound reasoning and, where possible, an alternative idea, but she must remember that, ultimately, the decision to make a change lies with the patient. Ideas which are forced onto a family may be accepted at the time, possibly from politeness or because acceptance offers the line of least resistance, but will later most probably be abandoned. The therapist must avoid causing conflict in a family. It may happen, for example, that during a stay in hospital a patient has accepted the use of an aid or method which may prove unacceptable to his relatives and the therapist must be vigilant when handling such a situation.

Lastly, the therapist must be careful not to inflict her own standards or expectations onto the patient. She may be taken aback to find that the patient has coped for years with a cold tap in the garden and an earth closet in the shed, or that he allows his dog to share his plate and his cat to share his unwashed bed, but these are not her standards and she must not delay discharge by insisting that such circumstances be changed, unless they are clearly incompatible with independence or overtly dangerous to the patient's present state of health.

Services available

The therapist will be aware that many community and voluntary services are available to help the patient at home. She should know not only which services are available in her district, but also how regular they are and how to contact them. For example, to pin a patient's hopes on a discharge which relies on the services of Meals on Wheels each weekday and meals cooked by a neighbour at the weekend may be grossly unfair. The Meals on Wheels service may operate only three days a week in that patient's particular area and the therapist may well discover that the willing neighbour 'who cooks all my meals, love' may have done so in an emergency immediately before the patient's admission to hospital, but is unwilling or unable to continue to do so on a permanent basis.

Solving problems

We do not live in a perfect world and, clearly, there is no correct or ideal answer for every problem. However much both the therapist and patient may wish to overcome any arising difficulties this will not always be possible. The therapist must be aware, and must make the patient aware, that the solutions or courses open to them depend on the present circumstances and are not necessarily the most desirable. For example, a family with a severely disabled child or adult may wish to have their house extended or a stair lift installed, in order to accommodate the weak person. However, if the prognosis is poor, or the budget limited, many Social Services departments will turn down such an application as being financially unjustifiable. Similarly, if accommodating a disabled person puts a financial or social strain on the family's resources, but no other permanent solution can be found, the therapist must help the family to accept that rehousing or permanent care for the patient may not be immediately available and that adaptations or relief by holiday admissions and day centre care may be the best, if not the ideal, solution at the time.

Visiting with the patient

Depending on the timing and aim of the home visit the therapist will visit the patient's home alone, with another staff member such as the physiotherapist, social worker or the community therapist, or with the patient. Should she, for example, wish to assess the possibility of adapting the house, or to discuss with the relatives how much help they can give, it is most likely that she will go alone or with another member of staff. On the other hand, if she wishes to find out exactly how the patient can cope at home then she must take him along.

Emotional reactions

As already mentioned, the first home visit can be quite an emotional time for the patient and his relatives, especially if he has been in hospital for many months, if he is elderly, if his home circumstances have changed (for example following an accident in which a relative has been killed) or if he has become severely disabled. Under such conditions the patient may well be overwhelmed when finally brought face to face with the situation in which he has to live.

In order to help minimise these difficulties the therapist can do several things before the visit takes place. She must explain clearly to the patient and his relatives the exact purpose of the visit. If she anticipates emotional problems it may be a good idea to concentrate on only one or two points, for example the patient's ability to climb his stairs or the exact layout and space for aids in the bathroom. This gives the visit a definitive purpose and also allows plenty of time for discussion since the patient does not feel he has to rush through a great many activities. The therapist must emphasise, especially to the very young, elderly or confused, that this call will be only a visit and that both she and the patient will return to the hospital afterwards. It is not uncommon that once the patient has returned home he refuses to leave and to return to the hospital. The therapist must therefore know what procedures, both moral and legal, have to be undertaken. The therapist should give the patient plenty of opportunity to talk about his return home before the visit, for in this way most problems can be anticipated. Finally, the therapist herself should ensure that she asks the relevant questions in order to discover any likely problems. (I remember, for example, visiting the home of an elderly bilateral lower limb amputee, who was at the time just getting used to his pylons but was quite mobile in his wheelchair. On arrival I discovered that the only access to his house was along a fifty foot gravel path and up a flight of four steps. It was quite obvious that neither his elderly wife nor I were capable of manoeuvring him indoors. The visit was therefore aborted until we could return with two strong ambulance men and a supply of sturdy planking to lay over the gravel. An application for a concrete path and ramp to the door had, in the meantime, been hastily arranged! The patient, understandably, was not amused.)

COMMONLY ENCOUNTERED PROBLEMS AND POSSIBLE SOLUTIONS

The home visit assessment should start from the time the therapist and patient arrive in the vicinity of the patient's home. If he is elderly or confused the therapist should ask him to point out familiar landmarks and road names or to direct her through the last few roads up to his house in order to discover his level of orientation.

On arrival at the house the therapist should note the following items. Clearly, not all will be relevant, but a check list is useful to ensure that no item is forgotten. Some suggestions are made for possible solutions to common problems. As there are often many different ways of overcoming a problem this cannot be a definitive list. Note: The list deals only with problems caused by design and structure of the house and/or its fittings and furniture.

Access

Gate catch difficult/gate stiff or heavy: Replace with magnetic catch or bar latch. Replace gate spring with lighter model. Remove gate.

Surface of path difficult: Remove or compress gravel. Lay paving stones or other flat surface along path. Repair cracked or uneven surfaces. Supply hand rail. Lay non-slip strips on path. Replace surface with concrete.

Path too steep or steps cannot be manoeuvred: Supply half steps between existing steps. Supply grab rail. Use another entrance. Redirect path to reduce slope. Supply ramp over steps.

Door lock difficult/door difficult to open: Extend handle of key. Lower lock. Replace lock with more easily managed model. Ensure doorway is well lit. Reduce strength of door spring.

Lifts difficult to manage: Ensure user understands the use of the lift. Supply aid to help reach controls. (Apply for ground-floor flat.) Ensure controls are well lit and clearly labelled.

Stairs

Difficulty climbing/descending stairs: Fit bannisters of appropriate height and dimension. Instruct in best method to negotiate stairs and practise on a short flight of stairs initially. Supply two walking aids (one for upstairs and one for down) so that stairs can be negotiated without hindrance. Supply half step. Devise safe way of carrying any aid. Plan ahead, avoid trips where possible. Bring commonly used items downstairs. Supply commode downstairs/upstairs. Ensure lighting is good. Paint white strip on edge of each stair. Re-arrange house to avoid need to use stairs. Install stair lift. Build extension bedroom/bathroom. Apply for downstairs flat/bungalow.

Stair covering unsafe: Secure existing covering. Renew fixing stays and/or surface covering. Remove covering. Replace covering with non-slip material.

Corridors and halls

Corridor too narrow: Clear corridor/hall of all unnecessary items. Supply narrower mobility aid. Rehang doors to open into room instead of corridor.

Floor covering difficult or unsafe: Clear or secure any loose rugs. Replace or remove worn or uneven floor covering. Secure edges of any floor covering. Apply non-slip polish to lino covering.

Corridor difficult to negotiate: Ensure that lighting is good and switches accessible. Fit hand rail.

Doors difficult to open/close: Replace heavy spring on door with lighter type or remove. Replace door knob with lever type. Replace latch fastening for ball-catch fastening. Fit sliding/folding doors or swing doors. Move handle. Ensure door does not rub on frame. Remove door and replace with curtain. Remove or replace threshold. Ensure edge of carpet by door is secured. Fit automatic door.

Telephone difficult to use: Supply non-slip mat under telephone. Replace table with one of more convenient height. Supply dialling aid. Contact GPO for various aids/models to help the disabled. Move 'phone to more convenient place. Ensure 'phone is well lit.

Internal steps hard to negotiate: Supply grab rail. Supply ramp if absolutely necessary or half step.

Living room

Difficulty getting on/off favourite chair: Raise

chair height. Supply firm/additional cushioning. Supply ejector cushion/chair. Ensure access to chair is clear and that chair is secure. Remove castors. Supply hoist. Supply new chair of appropriate design.

Floor covering difficult: See under 'Corridors and Halls'. Ideal surface is uniform throughout the room, carpets should be short pile or carpet tiles.

Living area difficult to negotiate: Remove unnecessary furniture. Re-arrange furniture to give clear passage. Supply smaller mobility aid. Teach patient to manoeuvre without use of aid. Supply grab rails.

Windows/curtains inaccessible or hard to manage: Supply reaching aid to pull curtains. Fit rod/cord pulls to curtains or electro-control. Replace curtains with blind. Replace old runners/ hooks with easy-glide plastic/nylon type. Ensure clear access to window. Place stable chair/stool by window to aid balance. Enlarge handle on window catch. Lengthen stay. Ensure window frame not sticking or jamming. Fit one-handed stay mechanism. Replace opening mechanism by fan with pulley control.

Heating difficult to control: Use long-reaching aid to control appliances. Apply for controls to be moved to more convenient place. Fit automatic control switch. Install central heating. Alter/extend control handle. Replace open fires with electric-gas appliance if possible. Ensure *all* fires are well guarded. Apply to Gas/Electricity Board for details of help available.

Meters inaccessible/difficult to operate: Arrange for meter to be moved. Ask Board to fit extended handles. Remove coin operated meter and arrange for quarterly readings.

Radio/TV difficult to operate: Extend/enlarge control switches. Move appliance. Fit automatic control. If TV rented change to other model.

Dining area

Table too high/low or wheelchair will not fit under table: Lengthen/shorten legs of table. Use higher/lower chair. Supply domestic arm rests to chair. Remove arms of chair. Turn table so that apron does not impede chair. Trim section of apron. Supply appropriate table, e.g. cantilever design.

Cannot carry food to table: Move table. Supply trolley or similar aid. Build serving hatch. Create dining area in kitchen.

Kitchen

Cupboards and storage inaccessible: Keep most commonly required foods in convenient reach. Rehang high cupboards/shelves. Fit revolving cupboards. Use plastic coated wire storage racks that fit on cupboard doors, under shelves, on walls or surfaces. Make full use of hooks/magnetic strips for storing equipment. Do not encourage bulk storage.

Cannot reach sink/taps: Fit tap levers. Supply tap turners. Lower/raise sink. Raise sink with wooden stand placed on bottom. Remove doors to cupboard under sink to allow easy access. Supply tall stool.

Cannot carry equipment: Supply trolley. Use centrally placed table. Supply continuous sliding surfaces. Move appliances. Fit hose to taps to fill containers with water. Fit board across sink to hold containers being filled. Use lightweight containers. Supply tray for wheelchair users.

Plugs/switches cannot be used: Move switches. Supply long reaching aids. Supply extension lead. Change design of switch. If kettle fitting difficult either control from wall panel and fill from jug/ hose or use automatic model. Enlarge/lengthen switches on appliances.

Cooker difficult to operate: Supply sliding board to transfer food to/from oven. Enlarge cooker knobs. Raise cooker on platform. Supply table-top cooker or split level cooker. Contact Gas/Electricity Board's Home Advisory Service. Avoid use of oven. Cook by boiling, stewing, frying, grilling, pot roasting. Use automatic timer – ask helper to put food into oven.

Work surfaces wrong height: Raise/lower table legs. Move shelves/work tops. Supply tall stool. Raise surfaces by work 'platform' to fit over surface. Sit to work if surface too low.

Bedroom

Patient cannot get to upstairs bedroom: Fit stairlift or refer to other methods of negotiating stairs. Move the (matrimonial) bed downstairs. Use convertible bed/settee, Z bed or folding bed (as in caravan). Build extension to house. Apply for flat/bungalow.

Patient cannot get into/out of bed: Raise/lower height of bed. Supply firm mattress or additional mattress. Supply bed boards. Supply tilting bed. Move bed to give easy access. Supply bed aid or place grab rail/sturdy support by bed. Supply hoist. Have non-slip floor covering by bedside.

Bedding too heavy to handle: Replace heavy blankets with lightweight/cellular variety. Use 'quilt/duvet' instead of blankets. Use less bedding and electric over-blanket. Reduce bedding and wear thicker nightwear. Have bedroom well heated, reduce bedding. Use winceyette sheets, reduce bedding.

Clothes storage too heavy to handle: Ensure drawers slide well and are not overfilled. Keep clothes most frequently used in easily accessible drawers. Replace traditional storage with shelving/rails protected by curtains. Replace heavy wardrobe doors with sliding doors or curtains.

Bathroom

Patient cannot get in/out of bath: Teach different method of getting in/out of bath. Supply bath board and/or seat. Use bath mat. Fit grab rails in most convenient position. Supply hoist, bath chair. Have chair/stool by side of bath. Use shower unit fitted over bath plus bath board/seat. Fit shower. Substitute bath by wash down. Arrange for district nurse to help/give bed bath. Fit specially designed bath.

Inability to reach basin: Lower/raise basin. Extend taps. Remove any cupboard under basin. Supply stool/chair to use at basin. Replace standard basin with vanity basin. Wash from bowl or take bath/shower.

Toilet

Patient cannot get on/off toilet: Fit raised toilet seat. Fit toilet rails/grab rails. Fit ejector seat to

toilet. Use commode/commode facility to wheelchair. Supply urinal. Supply sanitary chair.

Outside toilet difficult to reach: Fit grab rails. Ensure path is flat and not slippery. Apply for toilet extension. Apply for rehousing.

Garage/garden

Garden difficult to reach/maintain: Check steps/doors/paths are negotiable. Supply long-handled, lightweight and adapted tools. Build raised gardens and flower beds. Replant flower beds/vegetable patches with plants requiring minimum care. Build patio and plant flower tubs.

Clothes line too high or difficult to use: Fit pulley unit to lower/move line along. Use 'whirligig' unit. Dry clothes on line/unit indoors. Use tumbler drier. Use laundry services. Move washing line. Build platform by washing line.

Garage too small: Extend garage to give more width/length. Clear unnecessary items from garage. If disabled person is passenger transfer when car is in drive. Obtain smaller car. Build carport.

Garage doors difficult to handle: Up-and-over doors are easiest to use. Fit counterbalance to aid closing. Have rod-extension for closing. Fit automatic closer/remote control. Build carport, remove doors.

The reader will note that the solutions vary tremendously from slight alteration and adjustments to major considerations such as building extensions, buying a different car or moving house. Obviously the patient's wishes, prognosis and financial position must be considered alongside the pure physical solutions available.

REFERENCES AND FURTHER READING

Jay P, Walker E, Ellison A 1966 Help yourselves — a handbook for hemiplegics and their families. Butterworths, London
Wilshere E R Hoists and walking aids, 3rd edn. Home management 4th edn. Housing and furniture 3rd edn. Outdoor transport 4th edn. Personal care 3rd edn. All from a series: Equipment for the disabled. Oxfordshire Area Health Authority, Oxford

8

Domiciliary occupational therapy

Bold superscript numerals ([1]) in the text refer to recent legislation, notes about which are given on page 146.

Throughout medical and social history there has been a tendency, for one reason or another, to place those who are ill, disabled or handicapped in institutions. However, in comparatively recent years there appears to have been a revolutionary change in attitudes and health and welfare services are now emphasising home or 'home-like', rather than hospital care. Occupational therapy is only one of the many services available today and it is becoming increasingly recognised as a means with which to assist the old, frail, sick and handicapped to achieve and maintain independence within their own environment.

When viewed in terms of medical history, occupational therapy as we know it today is very young and community — or domiciliary — occupational therapy is a comparatively recent innovation, most development having taken place during the last 20 or so years. The 1920s heralded the birth of domiciliary occupational therapy when voluntary organisations began to provide craft services to homebound tuberculosis sufferers. In the 1930s these services were taken over by local authority health departments. Soon other authorities who were beginning to see the value of domiciliary therapy followed suit, and gradually persons with other medical conditions were included in the service.

In 1959 the *Scheme for the Provision of Welfare Services for Handicapped Persons* was introduced and occupational therapy services dealt with any person who was 'substantially and permanently handicapped'. During the 1960s the elderly and visually impaired were incorporated into this scheme and the role of the occupational therapist began to change radically. Replanning within local government led to the amalgamation of the health and welfare departments employing occupational therapists, and this was followed by two other major changes, the Local Authority Social Services Act 1970 and the Chronically Sick and Disabled Persons Act 1970. The introduction of this legislation coincided with further widespread reorganisation within local authorities, many of whom, at that time, employed no occupational therapists. In the late 1960s and early 1970s community occupational therapists were employed by both health and welfare departments. 1971 brought about a change in this situation and thereafter the majority of community occupational therapists were employed by the newly formed social services departments. This trend has continued after the reorganisation, in 1974, of both the National Health Service and local government.

LEGISLATION

Prior to discussing the functions of the occupational therapist and her team, it is essential to consider the legislation which led to the introduction and expansion of community services and which forms the framework within which she operates.

In reviewing and summarising relevant legislation it should be emphasised that certain laws 'require' authorities to perform particular functions, which means that they must provide them, whereas others 'allow' them to do so, which means that it is left to the discretion of the local authority to perform the function. This accounts for the great variety in provision of services.

The National Health Service Acts 1946 and 1949 Section 28 stated that arrangements should be made for the prevention of illness, care and aftercare of persons suffering from disease or disability and the provision of domestic help. These services were the responsibility of the health departments of City or County Councils and were not totally mandatory.

The National Assistance Act 1948 authorised all local authorities to make arrangements for:

● promoting the welfare of 'the blind; deaf and dumb persons and others who were substantially and permanently handicapped by illness or injury or by congenital deformity' (Section 29).
● providing residential and temporary accommodation.
● making welfare arrangements in conjunction with voluntary organisations (Section 30).
● providing recreation or meals for the elderly, again in conjunction with voluntary organisations (Section 31).
● registering homes for the elderly or disabled (Section 37).
● removing to suitable premises persons in need of care and attention (Section 47).

The guiding principle for welfare services was to ensure that all persons, whatever their age or disability, be given the maximum opportunity for sharing in and contributing to the life of the community, so that their capabilities might be fully realised, their self confidence developed and their social contacts strengthened. Thus it was recognised that the provision of skilled advice and help would be the best way to achieve this in most cases.

There is an important difference between these two Acts. The National Health Service Act was concerned primarily with aiding medical treatment and the care of the sick, whereas the National Assistance Act related to the promotion of the general well-being of those permanently 'disadvantaged' by physical disability as a result of illness, injury or deformity and to the provision of assistance to enable them to overcome the limitations imposed by their disabilities.

The Disabled Persons (Employment) Acts 1944 and 1958 initiated services for disabled persons of working age and introduced the registration scheme within the then Ministry of Labour (now the Department of Employment), the Quota scheme, the services of the Disablement Resettlement Officer and others. For more detailed information the reader should refer to Chapter 12. *The Housing Act 1957* introduced both 'mobility' and 'wheelchair' housing schemes.

The Mental Health Act 1959.[1] One of the basic aims of this Act was the establishment of a comprehensive community care service to meet the needs of all types of mentally disordered persons not requiring hospital treatment. Its services include:

Support to discharged patients who are re-entering community life.

Maintenance of the elderly mentally infirm in their own homes or residential accommodation.

Training the mentally handicapped in social and work habits.

Health Services and Public Health Act 1968. In addition to the legislation mentioned above, the services to be provided within this Act include:
1. residential accommodation
2. training centres
3. prevention and after care centres (Section 12)
4. home help and laundry facilities (Section 13)
5. the promotion of the welfare of the elderly (Section 45).

Local Authority Social Services Act 1970. This Act preceded local government reorganisation in 1971 and describes the duties of social services departments in relation to all relevant legislation. Those applicable to occupational therapy services are dealt with in this text.

Chronically Sick and Disabled Persons Act 1970 and 1976 Amendment. This much needed legislation extends the provisions of the National Assistance Act 1948 in its description of the provision of specific services for the sick and disabled in the community. The major points of reference concerning the occupational therapist are mentioned below:

Each local authority is obliged to obtain information regarding the number of disabled persons within its geographical area, register them with the authority where appropriate, ascertain the need for welfare services and publicise these available services. (Section 1).

Having ascertained that needs exist the local authority would arrange:
1. practical assistance in the home.
2. provision, or assistance in obtaining, wireless, television, library or similar recreational facilities.
3. provision of lectures, games, outings or other recreational activities outside the home, or assistance in taking advantage of educational facilities.
4. assistance with transport to facilitate participation in other services.
5. assistance with adaptations to the home and

provision of additional facilities to secure greater comfort, security and convenience.
6. to facilitate the taking of holidays.
7. provision of meals.
8. provision, or assistance with obtaining, a telephone and any special equipment necessary to enable its use. (Section 2).

Housing Authorities should consider the special needs of chronically sick and disabled persons when planning, designing and building premises (Section 3).

Access to, and suitable facilities in, premises open to the public, including parking, sanitary conveniences and display signs indicating these provisions (Sections 4 and 7).

Access to, and facilities within, educational establishments (Section 8). In the amendment of 1976 places of employment were also included in this section.

Co-option to local authority committees of chronically sick and disabled persons, or others who are knowledgeable about their needs (Section 15).

Separation of younger chronically sick and disabled persons from those over 65 years of age in hospitals and residential accommodation (Sections 17 and 18).

Provision of chiropody services (Section 19).

Provision of badges for display on motor vehicles (Section 21).

Education facilities for special groups (Sections 25–27). (See also Education Act 1981[3])

The Local Government Act 1972 made provisions for the accommodation of disabled people (Section 195.2).

Housing Finance Act 1972. The provision for needs allowances for rent rebates for disabled people (Schedule 3).

Housing Act 1974 and 1975 Amendment.[4,5] Occupational therapists, whether employed by the National Health Service or Local Authority, should have a working knowledge of sections 56 and 61 to 68 of this Act. It gives details regarding grants for house improvements and adaptations and is most beneficially used in conjunction with the booklet *Housing Grants and Allowances for Disabled People.*

The Health and Safety at Work Act 1974. The guidelines set out in this Act should be familiar to all therapists, wherever they work. However, for the therapist working in the community, these guidelines are particularly important. They apply to the office, clients' homes, centres used by her and her colleagues, in fact wherever she carries out her duties. She must remember that health and safety are everyone's responsibility, that they are an important part of good management and basic-ally common sense. In her role as assessor, advisor and teacher, of clients as well as of colleagues, she therefore needs to bear the following in mind:

Good planning, whether applied to the design of a new centre or to a client's home.

Safety, by instructing in safe working methods, initiating steps to improve safety, setting a good example.

Access, should be well lit and free from un-necessary obstructions.

Flooring should be in good condition, properly maintained, easy to clean and free from any items or substances likely to cause falls.

Equipment and tools should be properly main-tained stored and used.

Lifting, moving and carrying — whether of heavy objects or a client — should be done correctly to prevent injury.

Clothing and footwear, be it essentially protec-tive or everyday wear, should be suitable for their purpose. This applies to both staff and clients.

Fire is a hazard which everyone dreads and therapists must pay particular attention to precau-tions and exits, especially in clients' homes.

General health: working and living in an en-vironment that is healthy means avoiding unneces-sary noise, physical stress and fatigue. Therapists are able to advise colleagues and clients about safe and healthy means of undertaking either simple or arduous tasks.

Above all, therapists must ensure that all special equipment is safe to use. If it is not it should be withdrawn immediately.

The Rating (Disabled Persons) Act 1978 amends the law relating to rates relief in respect of premis-es used by disabled persons.

The disabled person who is an owner occupier or tenant may be eligible for rate rebates in respect of the following:

1. A room used to meet his needs
2. An additional bathroom or lavatory required to meet his needs

3. Heating installation for two or more rooms
4. Sufficient floor space to permit wheelchair mobility
5. Garage, carport or land needed to accom-modate a vehicle used to meet the requirements of the disabled person (Section 1).

Rebates may be obtained by local authorities or other organisations who provide:

1. Training and/or occupation centres.
2. Welfare services, excluding medical and dental care and residential accommodation.
3. Facilities under Section 15 of the Disabled Persons (Employment) Act 1944, that is work-shops.
4. Workshops or other facilities under Section 3 of the Disabled Persons (Employment) Act 1958.[2]

Following increased legislation and the realisa-tion that community care was, and still is, a growing necessity, more authorities became aware of the value of the paramedical professions, espe-cially occupational therapists, in community ser-vices and the number of occupational therapists employed by local authority social services depart-ments has risen steadily and is now about 20 per cent. As occupational therapists are particularly concerned with the 'achievement of normality', be it personal independence, social skills, acceptable patterns of behaviour or preparation for work, they give a most valuable service to the ill, handicap-ped and elderly.

DOMICILIARY OCCUPATIONAL THERAPY

This is carried out in the person's own environ-ment rather than the somewhat artificial setting of a hospital or rehabilitation centre. It is not in-tended to give the impression of denigrating the latter, on the contrary, hospital departments and special centres have a vital role to play in the treatment and rehabilitation of the sick and dis-abled and very close co-operation between all concerned is essential in order to benefit the patient or client.

The role of an occupational therapist working in a particular area is much the same as that of her health service colleague, except that her primary working environment is the client's home. She does not operate in isolation but in cooperation with others, that is, doctors, nurses, health visitors, home helps, physiotherapists, social workers, housing departments and voluntary organisations, to name but a few.

She will function as a member of three teams:

1. The social work team. This covers a particular geographical area and comprises social workers and their assistants, home help organisers and the home helps, administrative staff, the therapist herself and her supportive staff, i.e. the aide, craft instructor and technician.

2. The occupational therapy team comprising her professional colleagues within the authority and all their supportive staff. The primary aim of this team is to contribute to the resettlement of the disabled person through the provision of professional advice, support, training and guidance to both colleagues of other disciplines within the authority and to clients.

3. Possibly the most important team is that concerned with a particular individual; it may comprise personnel from several departments or services and of course the client himself.

In addition to working with the disabled person in his home the therapist may also be employed, usually on a sessional basis, in any of the following:

Day centres for the elderly, physically handicapped, mentally infirm, ill and handicapped, where emphasis may be on social and recreational activities.

Special Care Units for the severely mentally handicapped, many of whom also suffer additional physical impairment. Her work in these units may include advice, guidance and the teaching of staff in personal care, social skills, means of communication and recreational activities in order that they can teach and guide the trainees.

Adult Training Centres which cater primarily for the training of mentally handicapped persons over 16 years of age in social and work skills. In addition these centres may offer places to a small number of mentally ill or physically handicapped people. Occupational therapists may be involved in assessment of abilities, both physical and mental, training in personal activities of daily living (ADL), teaching of social skills and recreation.

Sheltered workshops or work centres for sick and disabled persons of working age.

Toy libraries for mentally and/or physically handicapped children in which the therapist, with her health service and education department colleagues, advises parents about the development of their children and the services provided by the Toy Library Association.

Playgroups which either cater exclusively for handicapped children (Opportunity playgroups) or make provision for a small proportion of pre-school age children with handicaps, thus integrating them with their able-bodied peers.

Assessment Centres where sick and disabled clients may be assessed and treated, if the home environment is unsuitable.

Schools, usually 'special' or private ones, where the therapist will liaise with the teaching, medical and paramedical staff regarding the care and treatment of a child whose home is in her geographical area.

Old people's homes, including those for the elderly mentally infirm, where she may assess, advise, guide and treat the elderly person as she would in his own home. She will also be involved in advising, guiding and, in certain instances, in teaching the staff of the home the practical aspects of resident care, i.e. daily living, mobility and social and recreational pursuits.

Recreation groups, which are usually very specific to her area and may include swimming, riding, wheelchair dancing, archery or more sedentary recreational pursuits.

Intermediate treatment for young offenders, undertaken in conjunction with social work colleagues who are responsible for this form of treatment within the department.

Residential accommodation for the younger chronically sick and disabled, run either by her employing authority or by voluntary organisations, for example Cheshire Homes, in which her involvement is very much the same as with individuals in their own homes.

Self-help groups, clubs and societies within her area, in which she may have a variety of roles, for example as adviser, committee member, or helper.

This list is by no means exhaustive, for any therapist may become involved in particular aspects of community service which interest her or for which there is a specific need within her area.

Aims

The principal aim of the domiciliary occupational therapist is 'to develop, restore to, or maintain a client in his normal place within the community, enjoying the maximum independence in the physical, psychological, social and economic aspects of life'. This is obviously a very broad aim which needs much expansion and explanation. First it is necessary to consider the origins of referrals to the occupational therapy service. A client may be referred from virtually any source, for example a relative or neighbour, the hospital therapists, home help, doctor, social worker, the housing department or the Citizens Advice Bureau. Whatever the origin of the referral, the occupational therapist must ensure that she has medical support from the client's general practitioner, so that, abiding by her professional ethics, she is working under medical direction and has access to an individual's case history.

The primary role of the community occupational therapist is one of assessor, adviser and teacher in all spheres of her work.

Assessment

Assessment of the individual's needs with a view to full participation in the community will have to take his family's needs and wishes into account. The client himself will be assessed for:

1. Independence in activities of self care, mobility, communication and his ability to manage and care for his home and family. For example, a person confined to a wheelchair or able to walk only with walking aids may have difficulties in moving about the home, managing his personal toilet, cooking his meals and so on; therefore the therapist will have to ascertain his capabilities, if necessary including practical trials, and advise accordingly.

2. Psychological impairment. Occasionally this is the sole reason for a referral, as for example, in the case of a housewife who is unable to cope with the normal running of the home and caring for her family. The therapist, together with the psychiatrist, nurses and social worker, will plan a treatment programme aimed at helping the housewife to overcome her inadequacies or learn to cope

with them. On the other hand the therapist must never ignore the psychological effects of physical impairment. A client with Parkinson's syndrome may suffer from depression which will undoubtedly affect his physical ability to manage his daily life.

3. Social contacts. Sick and disabled people tend to become isolated, either because they are unable to cope with or face other people or because their impairment prevents them, physically, from doing their own shopping, attending local clubs, going to the cinema or theatre, or from going out to work. In this situation the occupational therapist may help to organise special social or self-help groups to meet social, recreational or purely practical needs. She may also encourage the individual to join community groups, such as residents' associations, the local Women's Institute and so on, initiating the introduction if she is unable to do this for herself. It is useful to include recreational activities here, for often social contacts are made through them. The therapists will be able to give advice about facilities in the community, and about groups organised by voluntary and statutory bodies.

4. Capacity to return to work. Despite high unemployment, early retirement and increasing redundancies, work is still important in the lives of most people. As well as providing an income on which to live, run a home for a family and go on holiday, it can provide the satisfaction of useful employment and some social contacts. The unemployed disabled person leads a somewhat restricted life, for he has to rely on State benefits and pensions and/or income from other members of the family. The therapist, together with the Disablement Resettlement Officer, will be able to advise the disabled person about assessment and training schemes, sheltered workshops and special employment. For additional information see Chapter 12.

The therapist must encourage the client to play as active a role as possible in any discussions or decisions relating to his lifestyle. The family will play an important part in the team effort to maintain the client in his place in society.

As a result of her initial assessment the therapist may register the client as a handicapped person — see Section 1 of the Chronically Sick and Disabled

Persons Act 1970. This may or may not entitle him to certain services provided by his local authority departments.

Follow-up

The following up of initial assessment and advice is imperative, for it is often during subsequent visits that more specific needs are realised. It is of prime importance to teach the client how to reach and maintain his highest possible level of independence, remembering that habilitation (reaching levels of function not previously attained) or rehabilitation (restoring him to previous levels) are continuous processes. Her medical knowledge will help her to make a correct assessment. This will depend on the client's age, diagnosis, prognosis and his psychological adjustment to his condition. Adequate teaching and advice will enable her client to assume a positive attitude towards life. Before considering the provision of aids the therapist should advise on and teach alternative methods. However, in certain circumstances it may be obvious that an aid is essential. She may advise rearranging certain rooms in the home, for example moving a bedroom downstairs or reorganising kitchen fitments; she may teach the family how to lift the patient safely and comfortably or she may teach the client how to manage his clothing when going to the toilet. All this will help the client to overcome frustrations, tensions and physical barriers and so raise morale.

An initial assessment and subsequent findings may entail informing other departmental personnel or local authority departments about recommendations. It is the therapist's responsibility to follow up her own suggestions; she should make sure, for example, that her aide is giving domestic independence training to a severely disabled housewife or that the environmental health department is dealing with the therapist's referral for grant aid.

Advice on remedial, leisure and social activities

Therapists, by the very nature of their role, are able to advise or, in certain circumstances, initiate appropriate remedial, leisure or social activities.

These aspects of life are particularly important to the disabled who are unable to participate in gainful employment. Leisure hours should be filled purposefully if possible, otherwise the client may reach a state where life seems totally meaningless. Careful assessment and observation of his personality and interests will enable the therapist to advise and guide him. Some disabled people who are unable to find or accept work may want to join local organisations, such as groups for the young disabled, action groups, information services or more specific organisations, for example the Spinal Injuries Association or the Multiple Sclerosis Society. Wherever possible, the occupational therapist should take an active interest in such groups. This will not only give welcome support to these organisations, it will also enable her to gain additional help and information which may assist other clients or colleagues.

The therapist as a leader

An occupational therapist has much to offer her colleagues in social services, owing to the practical nature of her training and subsequent experience. Willingness to share knowledge, apart from being a sign of maturity, is of paramount importance if one is to gain benefit from ancillary and other staff. All occupational therapy aides, technicians, craft instructors and volunteers should have an understanding of the therapist's role and one another's roles in relation to clients' and departmental requirements. The roles of ancillary occupational therapy staff are described later.

The therapist will not only have a commitment to teach the client and his family, but also other staff, both in social services and other agencies, for example:

1. Social workers and social work assistants, helping them to understand the role of the therapist within the department and informing them about the skills she has to offer in the management and treatment of the elderly, the handicapped, the mentally ill and others.

2. Home help organisers and home helps. The home helps are frequently referred to as 'front line troops' and this is a very apt description. The services they provide in the community are invaluable. Occupational therapists work in very close

cooperation with them and they should therefore make every effort to explain their role, and give practical advice in client care and support. The writer has, in the past, been involved in home help training courses in which occupational therapy was discussed at length. These sessions, albeit brief, enabled the home helps to understand the therapist's function in relation to their own and to see how both could work together to the advantage of the client. The home help sees the client far more regularly than the therapist and is able to 'keep an eye' on things, for example checking ferrules on walking aids or noticing sudden deterioration in the client's condition. Time spent explaining a situation from the therapist's point of view and informing the home help of the therapist's aims is time very well spent.

3. Care staff in residential homes often appreciate the practical advice and assistance an occupational therapist can offer. Residents may be assessed and treated in exactly the same way as those living at home and the therapist must gain the cooperation of staff to ensure that the resident reaches and maintains his maximum level of independence. The therapist may also be asked to teach ways of moving and lifting residents in a safe and comfortable manner, for often only the person in charge of the home will have had any professional training.

4. The therapist's teaching role in relation to voluntary organisations is a very broad one and mainly concerned with explaining her own function and showing how various organisations and departments may work together for the benefit of the individual client.

Remedial treatment

Specific remedial treatment will often improve the overall functional ability of a client. The domiciliary occupational therapist visits many people who are cared for wholly by community services and therefore do not receive treatment within local hospital departments. The patient with hemiplegia, for example, who has been cared for at home by his family, his general practitioner, the community nursing sister and the occupational therapist, will need treatment and advice in specific methods and activities to aid maximum recovery.

The choice of treatment will often depend on the individual's interests and house surroundings. A housewife who has suffered a cerebral vascular accident may be asked to participate in certain routine household duties, such as dusting or polishing, using specific upper limb movements to accomplish both the task and the prescribed physical activity. A retired man, after a similar episode, may be encouraged to continue with his gardening, using both upper limbs and walking as normally as possible.

The treatment of physically and/or mentally handicapped children follows a similar pattern, in that the therapist uses specific activities to aid the child's development in mobility, self care and play. By using a mobile toy she will encourage him to walk and balance whilst gaining support from the toy. By letting him play on the floor (and thus lie on his stomach), she may prevent hip flexion contractures.

Information about available help

It is important for every therapist to be aware of the variety of grants and allowances available, be they grants to assist with home alterations, rate rebates or benefits such as invalid care allowance, attendance and mobility allowance. She must know where to obtain information concerning these resources and have a working knowledge of the conditions attached to them. Obviously her information must be up to date. Financial and practical assistance may also be available from other sources, such as voluntary organisations and a working knowledge of these is important.

Assessment for aids, alterations and adaptations

It is unfortunate that therapists working in the community are primarily seen as purveyors of aids. A therapist should reach alternative techniques if possible, but inevitably aids or equipment will be necessary in some cases. Her involvement in the issue and maintenance of equipment can be complex. Apart from undertaking a comprehensive assessment for the most suitable aid the therapist will use all her expertise in advising, teaching and gaining the cooperation of the client and his family. She may undertake research for special aids and equipment if the item required is not readily available from regular suppliers. Organisations such as the Disabled Living Foundation can give invaluable advice to the therapist.

The occupational therapist has a very important function where structural alterations or adaptations are concerned. She may find, for instance, that the layout of the client's home contributes to his disability, because he cannot walk up and down stairs, or that a grabrail would help him to be independent in toilet management.

Supervision of students and ancillary staff

Therapists have not only responsibilities towards ancillary staff, but also towards occupational therapy students undertaking clinical placement in their areas. They will be involved in the daily supervision of students, the teaching of the clinical aspects of their work and in guidance towards a better understanding of 'the community'.

Preventive work

Last, but by no means least is the preventive work of the occupational therapist. Her work with the elderly and disabled will often allow them to remain in their own homes, if necessary, with support from outside services, rather than being admitted to residential accommodation or long-stay hospitals. Her work with children and young people — and their parents — is of particular importance in this respect, for the younger the child when referred the better his chances of being able to remain at home. In this way problems tend to ease rather than increase with time. For example a small child who is taught to dress, wash and brush his teeth despite his handicap is more likely to retain these practical skills with practice, making him less dependent on his parents. Should the child remain dependent despite his ability to reach a certain degree of independence, insurmountable difficulties may arise in adolescence and early adult life when personal independence may be unattainable.

Case histories

The following case histories serve to illustrate the types of problems the community therapist may have to deal with; they demonstrate the scope of work which is a constant challenge, calling on all her knowledge, skills and ingenuity.

Most mentally handicapped adults and children live in the community, either coping independently within the family and/or with support from various agencies. The occupational therapist may be involved with the family in helping a child or adult. In this respect habilitation, as opposed to rehabilitation takes place; teaching, training and advising the child or adult and family regarding development, daily living skills, communication and social and work skills.

Case No. 1: M was referred to the occupational therapist in 1974 by the health visitor with a request for advice and assistance regarding his care and future development. The therapist's initial report of M, the youngest of three children, described him as a pale, slight boy of three years and nine months, whose diagnosis was cerebral palsy with mental handicap. He was born three months prematurely and was slow to develop. His hearing was normal, but his speech limited to one or two words. He was able to sit and get up from a sitting position and he walked with a 'scissor-like' gait. His left leg showed weakness and he tended to drag it. Both Achilles tendons were shortened and he walked on his toes. He was able to crawl normally, his balance was slightly unsteady and he had difficulty running. He was able to sit at the table, feed with a spoon and drink from a cup. He could take his clothes off, but needed help in putting them on. His shoes had been built up. He was not toilet trained, but would use a potty. He had not yet tried sitting on the toilet. His hand-eye coordination was quite good for his age, he tended to use his right hand in preference to his left, his concentration span was limited. The therapist observed that M was hyper-active.

Recommendations regarding his management included:

1. Continuation of the specific exercises shown by the physiotherapist to increase stretching of his Achilles tendons and improve external rotation of his hips. He was to be encouraged to sit cross-legged on the floor to play.

2. Occupational therapy to concentrate on his dressing and toilet training.

3. Hand-eye coordination through play activities was to be encouraged at a local playgroup and toy library.

The therapist liaised with the physiotherapist, advisory teacher for pre-school age handicapped children and the speech therapist to devise a specific treatment programme for him. At this stage M's mother realised that he would have to attend a special school.

Following her initial assessment and advice the therapist introduced them to the local playgroup and toy library. M attended the former once a week and the therapist discussed his treatment with the playgroup leader. During the months spent at the group M played as any small child would, but with emphasis on his positioning. He sat cross-legged on the floor to put jigsaws together, and when he sat in a chair it was a low one so that his feet were flat on the floor.

Early in 1975 the social services department applied to the Rowntree Family Fund for financial assistance with the purchase of a car.

M's attendance at the playgroup encouraged some separation from his mother and within a month or so he started to leave her quite happily in preparation for starting school. Training in toilet use and dressing were emphasised at all times. M made slow progress and his ability to dress himself improved. Toilet training was less successful, although a routine for using the potty was established and M was not incontinent. A trainer seat was used on the toilet at home, but he rejected this. The therapist considered that this was due to his feeling of insecurity as his feet were no longer on the floor. She designed an aid to fit on top of an adult-size toilet, which would provide back, side and foot support. (Fig. 8.1). This was made by the occupational therapy technician.

M had to wear leg plasters for three months in spring 1975 to attempt to stretch his tendons and prevent inversion of his feet. The educational psychologist's report, late in 1975, stated that M was still in the oral stage of development, everything he touched going to his mouth, and that he did not relate to other children in the group. He was very active physically and assessed as being educationally subnormal (mild) and he was considered for a place at a local special school.

In 1976 the family moved house and alterations

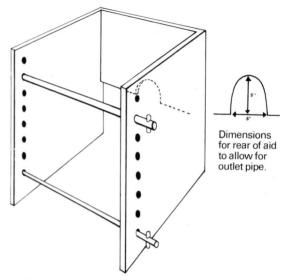

Dimensions for rear of aid to allow for outlet pipe.

Fig. 8.1 Toilet training aid for 'M'

were needed. The fence around the back garden had to be raised to prevent M from climbing over it and handrails were needed on the stairs and front steps, as M's mobility was much improved. M was still encouraged to sit on the toilet normally and was becoming accustomed to his toilet aid. By summer 1976 he was climbing stairs alone and continuing to progress in dressing and toiletting. He was still attending the playgroup and going swimming.

The paediatrician considered that M should continue all treatments and swimming and that he should be referred to an orthopaedic consultant regarding the possibility of lengthening his right Achilles tendon.

M started school in the autumn of 1976. In January 1977 he transferred to the special school nearer his home. In 1978 he was attending the toy library at school and making good progress in school work. His toilet training is almost complete, he understands simple commands and his concentration is improving.

The therapist will continue to be involved in M's treatment and development until he reaches his optimum levels and can function independently within his family. Her role with M's mother, who has always been very cooperative, is a supportive one now. Initially she gave practical advice and help, encouraging M's mother to allow her son every chance to develop his potential.

The therapist's role almost takes on social work proportions with some families when she may just listen, show empathy and give advice and help about benefits or schooling and it is virtually impossible to decide where therapy ends and social work begins and vice versa.

The physically handicapped person and his family may require much long-term advice and assistance from the community therapist, especially if the condition is progressive. Patients in this group tend to remain on the therapist's case list for the rest of their lives.

Case No. 2: Mrs B has been separated from her husband for many years; she is now 62 years old and lives alone in local authority Wheelchair Housing. She is well supported by her sons and their families who live nearby. She was a teacher. Fifteen years ago multiple sclerosis was diagnosed. Mrs B is aware of her diagnosis and the progressive nature of the disease and is a very active member of her local Multiple Sclerosis Society branch. The initial referral was for assistance with mobility and therapists have been involved since 1970. At that time Mrs B was living in a privately rented flat with her youngest son. She was able to walk with one stick and the areas of greatest difficult were mobility in the bathroom, toilet and the passage outside her bedroom. Appropriately sited hand rails were needed and the landlord's permission was sought for their installation. Mrs B was, at this time, waiting to move to more suitable accommodation and was on the local authority housing list. The therapist continued to support Mrs B in connection with mobility and social work advice was sought regarding finances for moving and furnishing a new home. Her condition remained static. Early in 1972 the question of employment was raised. Mrs B felt she was unable to cope with teaching, she was not interested in sheltered workshop employment, but agreed to contact being made with the Disablement Resettlement Officer.

During the summer of 1972 Mrs B moved into a new local authority bungalow designed for wheelchair users. Since her mobility had deteriorated further, she agreed to assessment for a wheelchair and an 8BL was supplied by the local Artificial Limb and Appliance Centre (ALAC). The possibility of an Invacar was considered, although Mrs B

had never driven, but she was very pessimistic about this. In 1974 she had a relapse, but could still stand and walk a few steps with a walking frame. She was able to deal with her personal needs and her sight and speech remained unimpaired. During 1974 her youngest son married and left home, therefore she was supplied with a telephone under the Chronically Sick and Disabled Persons Act 1970 Section 2. Because of increasing problems with mobility her ability to bath without help had to be re-assessed. The bathroom in her bungalow is designed for a wheelchair user and has ample space for manoeuvring and rails alongside the toilet, bath and shower (Fig. 8.2A and B). Those beside the bath were inappropriately positioned for her needs and it was decided that she needed a grip on the outer edge of the bath to help her to get in and out and to and from her wheelchair. By late 1975 Mrs B was dependent upon her wheelchair for all purposeful activity, but was able to manage all daily living activities. She was finding it difficult and unsafe to carry meals and hot drinks from the kitchen to the living room, because she had not been supplied with a detachable tray for her wheelchair. It was decided that Mrs B needed a detachable tray and domestic armrests, particularly for working in the kitchen (Fig 8.3A and B). By mid 1976 Mrs B's upper limb strength had deteriorated and she was finding it increasingly difficult to wheel her chair over the very small thresholds at the front door and the French windows from the living room into the back garden. The occupational therapy technician made very small ramps to enable her to negotiate both entrances. She was pleased to be able to safely manage alone. The skin on the palmar surface of her thumbs was becoming sore and callouses developed. The therapist made her a pair of wheelchair propelling gloves from very soft suede which she found invaluable. Until the end of 1976 Mrs B had managed to dress herself, but because of further deterioriation she was not able to stand for more than a few seconds and needed advice about and assistance with alterations to her clothing, particularly her trousers, to facilitate toilet use. As Mrs B's condition continues to deteriorate she will need increasing assistance from the occupational therapist. She is, however, determined to continue to live at home and manage with her home help and the support from the Multiple Sclerosis Society for as long as she is able.

Case No. 3: Mrs P is a 63 year old widow who suffers from severe generalised rheumatoid arthritis. At the time of referral she was living with her elderly parents in a two bedroomed local authority bungalow. Her condition began to place limitations on her capabilities when she was about 50

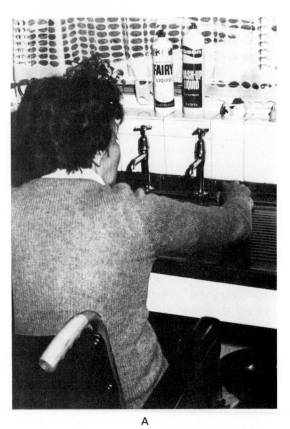

A

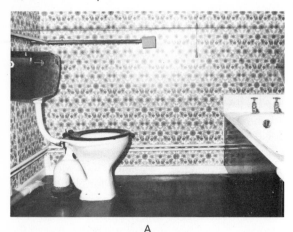

A

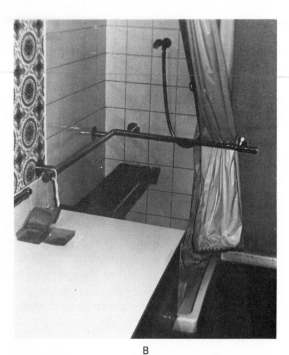

B

Fig. 8.2 A Wheelchair Housing bathroom. (A) The floor space around the toilet and alongside the bath facilitate access and manoeuvrability. (B) The plinth between the bath and shower facilitates transfers and drying after washing.

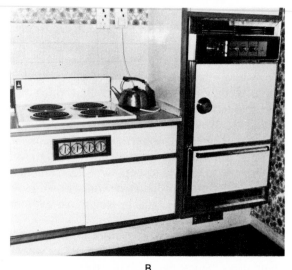

B

Fig. 8.3 A Wheelchair Housing kitchen. (A) The sink unit needs to be of an appropriate height for the wheelchair user. (B) A split-level cooker with the hob set into the worktop is ideal for Mrs B.

years old and by the time she was 56 she was quite disabled. She is in the care of a consultant outside her home district and does not have local medical contacts. The only remedial therapy she had had prior to 1975 was whilst she was in hospital. In late 1975 she was referred to the domiciliary occupational therapist for assistance in maintaining her personal independence and helping her elderly mother to cope with her father. Her particular difficulties at this time were walking outdoors, negotiating steps and stairs, managing low seats, having her hair washed and set, and bathing. Many of her personal difficulties had been solved whilst in hospital and she was, therefore able to dress herself with assistance and had special shoes made for her. She is a very resourceful woman, able to solve many of her own difficulties. After detailed assessment it was decided that the front access to her home needed ramping and a handrail, this was carried out with permission from the housing department. Both Mrs P and her mother, Mrs N who suffered from osteoarthrosis of the spine, hips and knees, were finding it difficult and painful to lower and raise themselves to and from the toilet seat. It was decided that a small grabrail beside the toilet and the loan of a raised toilet seat were needed. Although the home help service was invaluable for general household and kitchen duties, Mrs P still had some difficulties in the kitchen. Because of the impairment of her upper limbs she found it impossible to reach all but the lowest shelf in her food cupboard. The therapist suggested that an aid similar to a fish slice might be helpful and this proved very successful. The therapy technician made this special aid to the therapist's specification (Fig. 8.4). The only other items which Mrs P needed in the kitchen were a tap turner (Fig. 8.5) and an 'Unduit' (Fig. 8.6).

Early in 1976 Mrs P's mobility was further restricted by increasing pain, stiffness and deformity in her knees and she needed a walking aid. Because of the typical rheumatoid deformities of her hands (see Ch. 26) an ordinary walking stick was of little or no use; therefore she was issued with a Fischer stick (see Ch. 5) which gave her the needed support. At this time Mr N became unwell and was confined to bed for long periods. The community nurse attended to his nursing and medical needs, as neither his wife nor daughter

were able to help him to any degree. The therapist worked with the nurse, as Mr N was unable to lift himself up and down the bed and to move into a sitting position. After assessment and trials it was decided that Mr N needed a Penryn lifter, attached to the bed head. This was supplied by social services. In spring 1976 Mrs P agreed to an operation on her right knee, which had been postponed because of her father's poor health. As he was much fitter now, she felt able to leave her

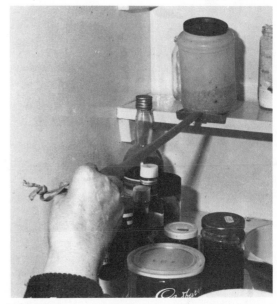

Fig. 8.4 Mrs P uses a 'slice', made by the occupational therapy technician, to help her to reach jars and packets from high shelves.

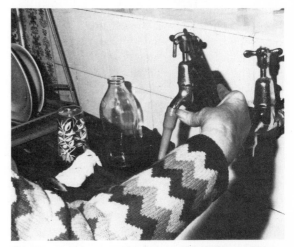

Fig. 8.5 Mrs P has a very weak grip and limited upper limb function, so she uses a tap turner to turn taps on and off.

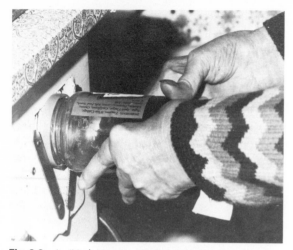

Fig. 8.6 An 'Unduit' assists Mrs P to unscrew jars and bottles.

parents. Bilateral tibial osteotomies were carried out in May and she returned home in July, walking in back slabs and with a walking frame. She received physiotherapy three times a week for six weeks to improve muscle tone and strength and joint mobility. At this time her family was very supportive. Lack of knee flexion was making it very difficult to rise from her high seat chair and bed. A forward and backward rocking movement was tried to help her gain sufficient impetus to rise and this she managed safely, until she was more mobile. Shortly after her return from hospital Mr N became seriously ill and died.

Mrs P's declining mobility made it increasingly difficult and dangerous to shower in the bath; she needed a purpose built shower unit. The housing department agreed to the removal of the bath and the installation of a shower with handrails and seat. The following year Mrs P's mother died and she was now living alone with support from a brother who lived nearby, the home help service and the occupational therapist. She is a very determined woman who will continue to live in her own home for the rest of her life if she can. She will need further surgery, i.e. bilateral knee joint replacements and correction of foot deformities, in order to retain some degree of mobility, but this she faces with optimism and cheerfulness.

This example of therapist involvement with two or more members of the same family is not unusual, because a handicapped person living with

ageing parents is not necessarily the only one needing practical assistance.

People who suffer from mental illness are a minority group in the community therapist's caseload. This is regrettable, but the position is changing slowly. There is a growing need for more therapists in this field and some authorities already employ therapists to work specifically with the mentally ill. Because of her training the therapist has much to offer to those who are trying to maintain their position in the community. She will work together with other team members, placing emphasis on coping with daily routine, building up and maintaining social and work contacts and encouraging the patient to lead as full a life as possible.

Case No. 4: Mrs G is 45 years old and lives with her husband, a quadriplegic, and one of her daughters who is an epileptic. In planning treatment for Mrs G the therapist had to consider the difficulties which this family would present to a wife and mother. Mrs G suffers from agoraphobia. She has always been a quiet woman, looking after her family. Consequently her interests and role have centred around the home. She had become unaccustomed to seeing people and social contacts became even more difficult after her husband's accident about 12 years ago. The continual stress and trauma within the family contributed to her phobia, but it was not until her condition became acute that she agreed to undergo treatment. On the recommendation of a consultant she attended the local psychiatric day hospital twice a week. Her programme included group meetings and discussions, group social and recreational activities and advice and guidance on her role as home maker.

The community therapist worked with the day hospital staff, particularly with the occupational therapists, following up their treatment on the days Mrs G was at home. Mr G attended the local Cheshire Home day-care scheme on the days his wife went to the day hospital. Mrs G knew that he was safe and being cared for and this relieved her anxieties. The community therapist supported Mrs G's interests and involvement in her husband's day care. She also encouraged her to go for walks locally, initially with others hoping that later she and her husband would go out alone. She was encouraged to make shopping trips, first to local shops and then into the town centre, instead of relying on others. She was also encouraged to take more interest in her personal appearance and to take up again the interests she had had before Mr G's accident.

As a result of an intensive period of treatment Mrs G made good progress and is now able to cope with the demands made upon her.

The elderly and infirm often suffer from a combination of medical and social problems and present a considerable challenge to the therapist. They have seen so many changes during their lifetime that upon reaching retirement they may just wish to 'sit back and be looked after'. However, for the majority of people living alone or with an elderly spouse life may not be so straightforward, as ordinary, everyday tasks which in previous years had been easy to manage, become difficult or impossible. The therapist's aim should be the patient's maximum personal independence and mobility. It is with this particular group that much of the therapist's preventive work is undertaken.

Case No. 5: Mrs S is 82 years old, widowed and lives with her two daughters. She suffers from osteoarthritis and congestive cardiac failure and has only one kidney. The health visitor had referred her to the domiciliary occupational therapist for a daily living assessment. Mrs S had impaired mobility and was walking with two sticks. She had difficulty putting garments over her lower limbs and was therefore advised about ways of dressing. She already had a 'Helping Hand'. The therapist made sure that Mrs S could manage all aspects of mobility safely, including transfers. Several months later Mrs S was admitted to the orthopaedic hospital for a total replacement of her right hip joint. After her discharge the community therapist made a re-assessment of her mobility, with emphasis on mobility and transfers, especially to the toilet. Following hip replacement she had to limit right hip flexion to a maximum of 90° and needed a raised toilet seat to help her on and off her rather low toilet. She will probably always need this because of her general physical condition. She has a commode beside her bed for night-time use and this had to be raised to assist her transfers. Mrs S has found it increasingly difficult to move up and down and in and out of bed. A variety of methods were tried to no avail and it was decided that she needed an overbed lifter with which she could lift herself using her unaffected upper limbs. Her bed was replaced by a higher one. Mrs S was finding that at times her two sticks were inadequate for safe mobility; therefore, following further assessment, she was issued with a walking frame. She enjoys going out whenever possible and because access to the house was made difficult by a sloping path the installation of a handrail was recommended.

All work involving children, whether physically or mentally handicapped, is of great importance and the therapist must have a thorough knowledge of normal child development before she can assess, treat, advise and teach the child and his family.

Case No. 6: K lives with his parents and three brothers in a council house close to the town centre. He is quiet and introverted and of average intelligence. In 1973 at the age of 13, K suffered a C5/6 lesion of his spinal cord as the result of an accident at the school swimming pool. He is now a quadriplegic, wheelchair bound, with only minimal thumb movement and some abduction and extension of his shoulder joints enabling him to propel himself short distances. K was referred to the community occupational therapist in 1976 by the National Spinal Injuries Centre at Stoke Mandeville as he and his family were moving house in order to be nearer relatives and friends. The therapist was asked to make an initial assessment of K in relation to his new home. K had been provided with a detachable table for his wheelchair, a 'pick up stick' and a transfer board. He could write with the aid of a splint and could type. He was able to feed himself and needed help with dressing. His main interests at that time were watching television, reading and playing with his younger brothers. Schooling had been arranged at the local comprehensive. Access to the house was impossible in a wheelchair and a temporary ramp was therefore provided with a view to more permanent alterations as soon as possible. K received both attendance and mobility allowances and he and his parents were given information about facilities and services for handicapped young people in the area. Shortly after initial assessments, it became obvious that the house needed altering. One of the downstairs rooms was used as K's bedroom, but as the bathroom was upstairs, provision had to be made for washing and showering facilities on the ground floor and use was made of a storage area off the kitchen. Switches were lowered so that K could reach them and access to the house was permanently ramped. K was encouraged to take part in physical activities, as he needed to lose weight. As well as going swimming he was encouraged to play table tennis using school facilities. Early in 1977 K's future needs were assessed. He was now 16 years old and plans had to be made for further treatment, advice and training. At this time little progress had been made with K's claim for compensation from the education authority. A variety of services and provisions were considered and these were environmental control systems, indoor and outdoor electric wheelchairs, an extension to the house, a hoist, a stairlift and assessment for an automatic hand control car. K was very dubious about driving at all, but after talking to a quadriplegic man who drives his own adapted car, he became more optimistic about having his own car in the future.

Other needs at this time were a sheepskin cushion for his wheelchair to prevent pressure sores, a mobile hoist to assist in transfers and fracture boards to facilitate transfer from wheelchair to bed. He also needed a holiday. A social worker was able to advise K and assist him in holiday plans, and to discuss his future with him, his parents and the therapist. It was arranged that a careers officer visit K at school as soon as possible. The careers officer suggested further education at a special college in Coventry as K had so far only received 18 months secondary education and it was considered that he should be able to obtain several CSE subjects. Early in the summer of 1977 K received intensive physiotherapy for six weeks, special attention being paid to utilising his residual muscle power for transfer to and from his wheelchair, which he and his parents were finding extremely arduous, as K was still overweight. He was reminded again to lose weight and it was pointed out to him and his family that he would probably always need to watch his diet and take sufficient exercise.

In April 1978 the therapist had to prepare the following report regarding K's capabilities for the court hearing in connection with his compensation:

K uses an Everest and Jennings self-propelled wheelchair which he can propel up gradients of 1 in 20. He is unable to transfer alone and uses a swivel overbed lifter to aid transfer from bed to wheelchair with the help of one other person. He is independent in feeding and drinking. He needs help with undressing, dressing and washing, and wears a urinary appliance. His bowels are manually evacuated. He prefers to bath but has a shower at home with which he needs assistance. His father lifts him in and out of the car. He has regular physiotherapy. He enjoys television, records, table tennis and swimming. He now attends a further education college, has settled in well and joins in most activities. He is studying English, mathematics, biology and German. His future needs include: (a) reduction in body weight to increase his efficiency in transfer techniques and dressing (b) provision of more suitable accommodation (c) provision of an environmental control system, for example Possum (d) provision of an electrically operated hoist for transfer independence between bed and wheelchair (e) provision of some form of transport in addition to his wheelchair.

Late in 1978 the occupational therapist attended the court hearing where K was awarded a considerable amount of compensation. The therapist will be involved with K and his family for some time yet, for K still needs much assistance. It was suggested at the hearing that the social services department advise and guide K and the family regarding a suitable home and financial investment for his future, i.e. training, employment and recreation, and/or continuing care should he wish to live apart from his family.

The community occupational therapist's caseload may include clients with literally any type of condition be it physical or psychological, common, such as arthritis or depression, or rare, such as Morquio-Brailsford disease or Zoophilism. In spite of the needs of the elderly, children and the physically handicapped, the therapist will often find that she is able to develop a particular interest in one area, for example assistance and treatment for the elderly mentally infirm. Whilst developing her 'speciality' she gains expertise and is often able to advise colleagues and share her knowledge to everyone's advantage.

Ancillary staff

The role of the occupational therapist is a complex one and to fulfill it single-handed would be impossible. Many authorities employ ancillary staff as members of an integrated therapy team. It is essential to review the functions of those staff in relation to the therapist.

1. The occupational therapy aide, assistant or helper assists the therapist in the care of clients in the following ways:

They will carry out remedial work under the therapist's guidance, for example dressing practice.

They may issue certain aids and teach clients and their relatives how to use, check and maintain them. Some authorities exclude aids to mobility, leaving the therapist to deal with them.

The aide will collect items no longer in use and help with the general maintenance of aids and equipment.

They will undertake follow-up visits, for example to a client with a progressive disease who may need additional advice and assistance as he becomes less able.

They may attend craft groups to help the instructor.

They may work with special groups or individuals, such as self-help, recreational or educational groups. These groups may have been initiated by the therapist who will continue to guide her staff in their organisation even though she may not attend each session. In some instances an aide may be given responsibility for one person, for example a man with multiple sclerosis who attends a weekly swimming group run by social services with the help of a voluntary organisation.

Other work may include clerical duties, follow-up of telephone and car badge requests and running a 'call-up' or check system by post.

2. Craft instructors. Many authorities have developed craft services as a natural progression from the days when community occupational therapy dealt with handicrafts. Some craft instructors or teachers work in comparative isolation, whereas others work as members of the integrated therapy team. The therapist advises the latter and supports and helps them by organising home tuition and groups for recreational, remedial and social purposes.

The guidance given by therapists is especially valuable when specific remedial work is required or when the patient's medical condition precludes him from certain activities; for example a man with severe respiratory disease may not be able to work with certain adhesives or in a particular atmosphere.

They will arrange craft classes or groups (Fig. 8.7) and be responsible for booking suitable accommodation and transport for both ambulant and non-ambulant clients.

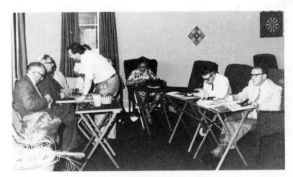

Fig. 8.7 An informal craft group for the elderly and handicapped, held in a community centre.

The instructor may recruit volunteers to assist and be trained in craft work and later to take over responsibility for the class under his/her guidance.

The instructor is responsible for the allotted budget, for the purchase and issue of suitable materials, stock records and receipts. They may arrange exhibitions and/or sales of work to increase the group's income.

They should be able to utilise the facilities for traditional crafts in the area and encouraging clients to be independent of the group.

In certain authorities craft instructors help with intermediate treatment for young offenders.

3. *The occupational therapy technician* (Fig. 8.8). His practical expertise makes him an invaluable member of the team. He usually holds certificates in one or more trades, such as joinery, tool making or ship/boat building.

He is responsible for ensuring that designs and specifications for aids and equipment submitted by a therapist are feasible and conform to specified standards.

The selection of materials used in construction is his responsibility.

He has to cost all items he makes and compare the cost of producing special equipment himself to manufacturer's prices.

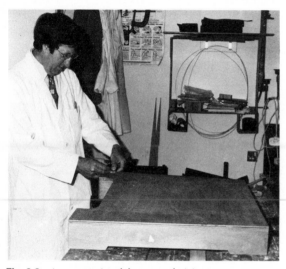

Fig. 8.8 An occupational therapy technician constructs a chair raise for an arthritic client.

In some authorities technicians are responsible for the installation of grab and stair rails. They should have some structural building knowledge to make sure that a wall will hold a stair rail *and* take the strain of the client pulling or pushing on it.

He may be involved in the maintenance of equipment used by therapists and will most certainly be responsible for his own equipment and materials.

Technicians are often able to advise therapists of the feasibility of structural alterations and may be asked for an opinion prior to involving architects and builders.

Liaison

The occupational therapist will often need to liaise with other personnel in social services, other local authority departments, district health authorities, education and employment departments and an increasing number of other organisations. She must understand that without good working relationships and liaison with appropriate personnel the person to suffer most will be the client. As this liaison is so important, the principle organisations and departments are described below.

Hospitals. Personnel such as the consultant, physiotherapist, occupational and speech therapist, appliance officer and nursing staff of a hospital will form part of the team with whom the community therapist liaises, usually regarding a patient's admission to hospital or his discharge into the community. While in hospital a patient will be treated by the consultant, his medical and nursing staff and by the rehabilitation team. If practical assistance and follow-up treatment in the home are necessary after his discharge, contact will be made with the domiciliary occupational therapist. She should visit the patient whilst he is still in hospital, if possible, and so establish a link between home and hospital. She may also visit his relatives at home to discuss local authority services, if these have not been necessary previously.

On the other hand, when a domiciliary occupational therapist's client is admitted to hospital she should liaise with her health service colleagues, providing information about the home, the client's capabilities before admission and services which had been provided, thus helping the hospital therapists to plan treatment.

Health and social services therapists may make a joint visit to the client's home, usually prior to his discharge. The client and his relatives should be present at this visit to find out whether they will be able to continue living as before or whether modifications to their lifestyle will be necessary. If there is a need for special services, the domiciliary therapist can make arrangements so that home help, meals on wheels or certain alterations are ready for the client when he arrives home.

Health care teams. These comprise general practitioners, community nurses and her assistants, health visitors and such personnel as chiropodists. They provide general medical and nursing care in a given geographical area. It is imperative that the occupational therapist knows the doctors and health care workers who provide services in her area and that they know about her and the treatment she is able to provide. It is essential that the therapist who is 'new' to a particular area make herself known to the health care teams, explaining her role in its relation to theirs. She should also do this to new staff in the health care teams, for an understanding of one another's work is important for successful client/ patient care. The general practitioner will be able to provide medical information about the client and let the therapist know if there are any contra-indications to treatment, for example chronic cardiac failure in an osteoarthritic client. The therapist should report back to the doctor, so that he can maintain an overall picture of his patient's condition. Regular liaison with health visitors and community nursing staff is essential, if treatment is to be consistent. The therapist will work very closely with health visitors in the care of pre-school children and the elderly, and with nurses in their care of all age groups. Most of this work will concern specific activities in personal care, mobility, development and nutrition.

Local authority housing departments. An occupational therapist's contacts with her local authority housing department and their technical services section are essentially practical and educational. These contacts should be maintained and developed because they will benefit not only her clients who are already in local authority housing but also those who may need it in the future. There are several aspects to her work with the housing department:

Alterations to housing department property for disabled or elderly people. The therapist must obtain permission from the housing department for the work to be undertaken and she will usually liaise with a housing inspector or technical officer regarding structural feasibility of the alteration. For example, a client may need alternative access to a downstairs bathroom which entails removing part of an existing wall. The therapist must seek professional advice regarding the possibility of this alteration. She needs to know whether the wall is load bearing and a doorway can be made through it or whether she has to consider an alternative.

At the time of writing this information was correct, but in April 1979 housing authorities became responsible for alterations in their own properties to meet the needs of chronically sick and disabled people. It was, however, anticipated that occupational therapists would assess clientele and advise housing departments regarding needs.

Rehousing to more suitable accommodation. The success of an application for rehousing depends largely on close liaison between the therapist and the housing department officer. Whenever alternative housing becomes necessary a therapist will visit the clients home (local authority or private) in order to assess his specific needs. She will then present a comprehensive case for rehousing or housing by the housing department.

Some authorities may also help local authority therapists when major alterations are needed in the privately-owned sector. In such circumstances therapists liaise with the housing inspector regarding the feasibility of her suggested plans. This service is offered primarily because of the excellent working relationships between the two departments. This type of working relationship takes time and understanding to develop and is only achieved through mutual respect, cooperation and education.

Local planners and architects. Therapists must endeavour to 'keep their eyes open' and 'their ears to the ground' regarding proposed building developments, particularly of public buildings, schools and colleges and special housing for the elderly and/or disabled. Therefore, they must know and be known by local planners and architects. The development of a sound working relationship with them will pay dividends and a therapist working in an area for any length of time should either ask them to contact her so that she may view plans, or should 'drop in' occasionally to ask whether any special accommodation or public buildings are being planned. This relationship may save time, effort and finances at a later date, for if the therapist can point out a feature which the planner and/or architect has overlooked or sited incorrectly, this may be corrected at the planning stage, thus saving expensive alterations when the building is partially constructed or complete. Planners and architects are far more aware of the needs of the elderly and disabled than they used to be and therapists must be grateful to Mr Selwyn Goldsmith, his colleagues and his book *Designing for the Disabled* for this improvement and awareness.

Environmental Health departments. These usually deal with improvement and intermediate grants for housing in the private sector and the occupational therapist should know when and why these grants are allocated and which conditions are attached to them. It is worth remembering that, since the 1974 Housing Act and its 1975 Amendment, Environmental Health departments have looked sympathetically at requests from registered disabled people.

1. Improvement grants are given 'at the discretion of the local authority for any works required for making a dwelling suitable for a disabled occupant's accommodation, welfare or employment', that is, the authority has the power to provide grants for alterations or enlargement of a dwelling.

2. Intermediate grants are given 'to aid the provision of any standard amenity even if this is additional to any existing amenity, if the existing amenity is not readily accessible to the disabled person owing to his condition' (e.g. a toilet).

At present both the property's age and rateable value will affect consideration for grant aid under the Improvement scheme, which may be subject to the individual undertaking other improvement work, for example loft insulation. The intermediate scheme does not specify such conditions.[5]

The application for a grant from the Environmental Health department has to be made by the disabled person himself. The therapist is usually responsible for his registration as disabled person under the terms of the Chronically Sick and Disabled Persons Act 1970, giving advice about the design of an addition to the home, alterations to existing facilities and/or financial assistance requested by the disabled person in addition to the permitted grant.

The Department of Education and Science. This is responsible for the provision of education and further education and therapists will work with local education authorities in respect of handicapped pre-school and school age children and young people in further education. The therapist will liaise with schools and special schools and colleges in her area and may work with the teaching and remedial therapy staff of a special school which is attended by a child whose home is in her area. They will discuss his levels of development and independence and his progress generally, so that an integrated approach to his problems can be formulated.

Therapists must also be aware of educational facilities available to the school leaver, for example further education departments of residential training colleges for the disabled, so that she can advise colleagues, the child and the family.

The Department of Employment and Productivity (DEP). The therapist must have a thorough knowledge of the provisions made for training and retraining and of the relevant legislation to enable her to advise school leavers or others of working age. She must liaise with Disablement Resettlement Officers and be able to discuss particular clients with him intelligently. She must be aware of employment prospects in her area, training opportunities, vocational guidance and how best she can relate to careers officers in connection with handicapped school leavers. All too often therapists may overlook employment potential, as they are so busy trying to help the individual meet his personal or recreational needs.

The Department of Health and Social Security. This department has overall responsibility for health services, local authority social services and financial provisions for those members of the public who require assistance because they are unemployed, unable to work, unable to provide for their family on a low fixed income or are handicapped and therefore entitled to specific benefits. A therapist's training and subsequent experience will provide her with a working knowledge of the National Health Service and local authority social services, but in addition she must inform herself about benefits available to the disabled.

Voluntary organisations. These provide invaluable services and support to innumerable individuals and groups of people and complement the work undertaken by statutory organisations such as social services. Without them much practical advice and assistance would not be available to a vast number of people. Many of these organisations receive annual grants from the Government or local authority departments to assist them in the provision of services. It is impossible to mention all the voluntary groups with which an occupational therapist may come into contact and only a few are described below.

The Joseph Rowntree Family Fund gives grants to families with handicapped children under 16 years of age. The fund liaises with social services departments and will make grants for such items as automatic washing machines, the deposit on a car, an annual holiday or the family's contribution to the cost of an alteration to the home. The fund will only provide for services which are not catered for by the local authority.

Social services provide the Women's Royal Voluntary Service (WRVS) with financial support to organise the meals on wheels service to the elderly and handicapped in their own homes.

The Multiple Sclerosis Society has branches throughout the country and each branch will provide advice, welfare support and, in some instances, financial help to its members.

The therapist should know which voluntary organisations exist in her area, so that she can provide clients with information about their aims and activities and refer them to an appropriate group, if they so wish. In addition to the examples given above the occupational therapist may well be involved with any of the following: Spinal Injuries Association, Arthritis Care, Chest and Heart Association, MENCAP, Action Group for Handicapped Children, National Toy Libraries Association, Opportunity Play Group schemes, Parkinson's Disease Society, Physically Handicapped and Able Bodied clubs, Agoraphobics' Society, the list is endless. For additional information refer to 'Directory for the Disabled' and the Royal Association for Disability and Rehabilitation.

Private agencies. Therapists liaise and work with various private agencies who provide residential accommodation, for example Cheshire Homes. They may also be involved in their recreation groups, to which clients not resident at the establishment may be invited. Many of these organisations provide day care services for severely disabled people, so that their families have support and relief from care for a few hours each week and may continue their personal commitments.

Community psychiatric nursing teams. These provide follow up, support and continuing treatment to patients discharged from hospital or a day hospital and to those whose psychological condition does not warrant admission to hospital. In many instances the therapist working in the local psychiatric or day hospital will continue to treat these patients, for this is as important as the continuity of treatment itself. However, in certain circumstances a patient may manage at home under the care of his general practitioner, a social worker and the community therapist. In these circumstances the therapist can help the client to cope with daily living, for example by advising him how to manage on a limited weekly budget or overcome agoraphobia, or by encouraging him to join social and/or recreational groups from which he will gain support.

Working in the community means more than just being an occupational therapist, it often means being a friend, listener or a shoulder to cry on. It means being involved with families, sharing their grief, joy and problems. It is essentially a job for those who like people no matter who or what they are, who can give of themselves and offer help, yet withdraw when it is necessary. The success of a therapist's work depends on her powers of persuasion, because she does not wear a uniform and has no 'authority' in clients' homes. Her expertise never ceases to grow. She uses it to elicit information, to make wise assessments and to plan treatment programmes, and experience gained in one case can often be applied to another. A job in the community is what the therapist makes it. It is never 'cut and dried' and the more thoroughly she knows the 'community', the more she will be able to offer and gain from it.

Acknowledgements

Miss M M Keily Dip COT, County Occupational Therapist, Devon County Council Social Services Department, for her invaluable and constructive criticism of the manuscript.
Devon County Council Social Services Department for their cooperation and permission to refer to case notes.

To family, colleagues and clients who listened, contributed and permitted photographs to be taken of their homes and work.

Notes on Recent Legislation

[1] The Mental Health (Amendment) Act 1982 has five main principles. First, the safeguarding of the rights of all mentally disordered people. Second, procedures for effecting compulsory admission must be carried out within the regulations stated. Third, compulsory care should be in the least restrictive conditions possible. Fourth, professionals concerned with the care and treatment are adequately trained and their competence assessed. Fifth, that quality of care and treatment should not fall below the accepted minimum. This Act has major implications for social workers as they will have to become accredited in order to effect compulsory admissions to hospital (see four above).

[2] The Disabled Persons Act 1981 amends earlier legislation, including the Chronically Sick and Disabled Persons Act 1970, to ensure that the appropriate local authority departments and others pay heed to, for example, (i) the needs of disabled and blind people regarding ramping pavements; the placing of bollards and lamp posts; (ii) parking spaces, and ensure that those reserved for disabled people are used solely by and for them. Those not eligible to use such parking spaces would be subject to a fine; (iii) public buildings, including educational premises, sanitary conveniences and places of entertainment should be planned and built so that they facilitate use by disabled people; (iv) signposting of facilities for disabled people be improved.

[3] The Education Act 1981 makes significant changes regarding the education of 'children with a special needs'. This Act was the result of the Warnock Report and recommendations include: categorisation be abolished, although it is recognised that some special educational facilities will be needed; no child be denied entry to a mainstream school solely on account of physical inaccessability to the school; opportunities for parents to have more influence in the placing and assessment of their child.

[4] The Housing Act 1979 amends the arrangements for adaptations to council dwellings. Local Authority Housing Departments are responsible for alterations to their own housing stock, although the advice of Occupational Therapists will still be sought.

[5] The Housing Act 1980 amended the rateable value limits set for grants. The limits were waived for disabled people. This means that on application for a grant to alter his property the disabled person is not restricted by the age or rateable value of that property.

REFERENCES AND FURTHER READING

Chronically Sick & Disabled Person's Act 1970. London, HMSO

Disabled Persons (Employment) Acts 1944 & 1958. London, HMSO

Disabled Persons Act 1981. London, HMSO

Education Act 1981. London, HMSO

Health & Safety at Work Act 1974. London, HMSO

Health Services & Public Health Act 1968. London, HMSO

Housing Act 1974 (Amended 1975). London, HMSO

Housing Act 1979. London, HMSO

Housing Act 1980. London, HMSO

Housing Finance Act 1972. London, HMSO

Local Authority Social Services Act 1970. London, HMSO

Local Government Act 1972. London, HMSO

Mental Health Act 1959, London, HMSO

Mental Health (Amendment) Act 1982. London, HMSO

National Assistance Act 1948. London, HMSO

National Health Service Acts 1946 & 1949. London, HMSO

Rating (Disabled Persons) Act 1978. London, HMSO

British Association of Occupational Therapists 1978 Occupational therapy service in the community. London, BAOT

Occupational therapy in the community 1978 World Federation of Occupational Therapists, London

9

Rehabilitation equipment

Machinery designed specifically for the purposes of rehabilitation has only been available for a comparatively short time. Some designs, such as the bicycle fretsaws and treadle lathes, have been well tried and tested and consequently new and improved designs are in use alongside older models. Others, such as the quadriceps switch, have been available for only a few years and for this reason their full potential may not yet have been realised. New equipment is continually being investigated and is, as yet, used in but a few departments — PIED switch is an example of this.

Because of this constant change it is difficult to be completely up to date with all the variations and innovations in rehabilitation machinery. This chapter, therefore, will describe those pieces of equipment most widely used in occupational therapy departments. The therapist will find that some machines have variations and facilities not described in the text, but the principles of their use will be the same. If the therapist understands the basic principles of treatment she will be able to apply them to similar pieces of machinery.

THE ELECTRONIC CYCLE (FIG. 9.1)

As can be seen from Figure 9.1 the electronic cycle consists of an adjustable static cycle unit to which a fretsaw (and on some models a sander) is attached. This is worked electronically by the action of the pedals. The seat is a separate unit which can be removed from the cycle for ease of transfer, it is firmly locked into position when in use.

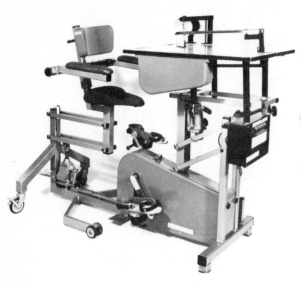

Fig. 9.1 The electronic cycle

Although models from different manufacturers vary slightly, the following adjustments are possible on the majority of them:

1. The seat unit

The seat. This is of a cycle seat design and can be adjusted in height and distance from the cycle unit. Both these adjustments can be made while the patient is sitting on the seat. The tilt of the seat can also be adjusted. The seat unit moves on braked castors and when used with the cycle it can be locked to the cycle's frame by various methods, depending on the design of the model. When the seat unit needs to be moved away from the cycle it can be wheeled freely and steered from behind by the therapist.

The backrest. On most models this is adjustable both vertically and horizontally.

The armrests. Some are hinged so that they can be raised in order to facilitate transfers. They are also adjustable sideways.

2. The cycle unit

The table. This is usually covered in formica or similar material and is adjustable for height and distance from the seat unit. Most models have hand grips onto which the patient can hold for added stability while the seat is being adjusted, during transfer or when undertaking an activity in which upper limb movement is not required.

The power driven tools. All models have a fretsaw and some also a sander or drill. Selected models have a standard 240 volt socket into which any piece of electrical equipment of the same voltage can be plugged. Switch mechanisms are available to channel the power from one tool to another.

The pedals. Pedals on the newer machines are fitted with self levelling footplates, each of which has two strap fastenings. (On some models these can be removed and replaced by toe clips.) The pedal cranks can be adjusted in length.

Resistance. As the pedal motion of the cycle is normally power assisted the unresisted movement is lightweight and therefore suitable for use by weak patients. As the action of the tools is also power assisted they will turn at a constant working speed even if the pedals are moving very slowly. Resistance can be added to this electrically assisted motion and in the later models this is done through a series of switches or by a lever, each of which is marked with the resistance it affords. In addition the power assistance can be removed thus turning the machine into one in which the tools are driven directly from the mechanical power supplied through the pedals. In this case the speed of the tools is directly related to the speed of pedalling.

Accessories. All models have a counter for the number of revolutions and some are also able to record the 'distance' travelled and the speed of pedalling. Some machines have an automatic timer which will buzz at the end of a pre-set time.

Transfer to and from the machine. For those who are able to stand the seat unit is removed and the patient stands, with feet apart, facing the machine. The seat unit, lowered to a suitable height, is then wheeled in under the patient and locked into position. As the seat is raised the patient sits on the saddle and places his feet on the pedals. The seat height and distance are then adjusted as required.

For those patients unable to stand the seat unit can be wheeled next to their chair and, with the arm rests raised, the therapist aids the patient to transfer onto the seat unit. The unit is then wheeled up to the cycle, locked into position and adjusted as required.

Adjustment and uses

Because of its wide adjustability the electronic cycle can be used to treat a variety of conditions and, since the pattern of movement involved in pedalling is similar to that of walking and running, these actions can also be stimulated. The machine is also valuable, because the patient is seated and the action therefore partially weight bearing, which means it can be used in the early stages of lower limb treatment.

A variety of lower limb movements can be obtained by adjusting the machine as described below. Note: These adjustments will give the greatest range of any specified movement.

1. Hip movement (Fig. 9.2A)
a. Flexion: seat low and forward, pedal crank long
b. Extension: seat high and forward, pedal crank long
2. Knee movement (Fig. 9.2B)
a. Flexion: seat low and forward, pedal crank long
b. Extension: seat high and back, pedal crank long
3. Ankle movement (Fig. 9.2C)
a. Plantarflexion: seat high and back, pedal crank long
b. Dorsiflexion: seat low and forward, pedal crank long.

Conditions treated

The following conditions may be treated on the cycle:

(a). Fractures and other orthopaedic conditions (such as meniscectomy) of the lower limb: To increase range of movement and strength in the affected limb once the patient is partial weight bearing.

(b). Arthritic conditions (with the exception of rheumatoid arthritis) affecting the lower limbs, e.g. osteoarthrosis, especially during maintenance treatment (see Ch. 22) and following joint replacement: To maintain and/or increase the range of movement at the joint. To increase strength in the

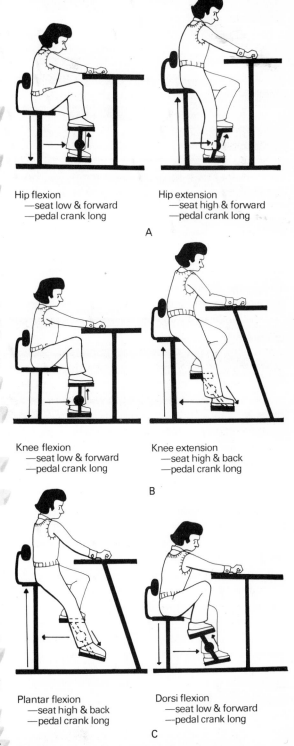

Hip flexion
—seat low & forward
—pedal crank long

Hip extension
—seat high & forward
—pedal crank long

A

Knee flexion
—seat low & forward
—pedal crank long

Knee extension
—seat high & back
—pedal crank long

B

Plantar flexion
—seat high & back
—pedal crank long

Dorsi flexion
—seat low & forward
—pedal crank long

C

Fig. 9.2 Use of the electronic cycle to increase (A) hip movement (B) knee movement (C) ankle movement

muscles controlling the joint. To stimulate a good reciprocal walking pattern.

(c). Peripheral nerve lesions affecting the lower limb, especially those of the common peroneal nerve: To maintain a full range of movement and prevent joint deformity and muscle shortening. To stimulate movement. To increase strength.

(d). Spinal injuries with partial paralysis of the trunk and lower limbs: To maintain a full range of movement in the lower limbs. To stimulate movement. To increase strength. To improve balance. To stimulate coordination and a reciprocal walking pattern. Some back injuries may be included.

(e). Amputation of the lower limbs when the pylon has been fitted. Note: the machine must not be adjusted to allow full knee extension, as this will cause the knee joint of the pylon to lock: To maintain strength and range of movement in the remaining joints of the amputated limb and to prevent joint stiffness. To stimulate coordination and a reciprocal walking pattern. To stimulate circulation.

(f). Progressive neurological conditions such as multiple sclerosis and Parkinsons disease, and other conditions in which general weakness is a problem: To maintain strength and range of movement in the lower limbs. To stimulate a reciprocal walking pattern. To maintain and where possible improve balance and coordination in lower (and upper) limbs. To increase proprioceptive input. To stimulate circulation.

(g). Head injuries and other conditions producing general weakness and incoordination: To increase strength and range of movement in the lower limbs. To improve balance and coordination in the lower (and upper) limbs. To encourage sensory return with an input of vibration to the upper limbs. To increase noise tolerance. To stimulate a reciprocal walking pattern.

(h). Soft tissue injuries, e.g. tendon injuries and burns: To increase range of movement and muscle strength following immobility. To prevent contracture. To stimulate circulation. To encourage sensory return with an input of vibration if upper limbs are affected.

Points of use

As with all moving parts on machinery the blade, sander and cycle chain must be guarded during use to comply with the Health and Safety at Work Act.

Suitable shoes should be worn during work on the machine. These should fit firmly, supply support over the instep and be low heeled. Clogs, open-toed sandles, boots or slippers are not advisable. If flare-legged trousers are worn, cycle clips should be supplied.

When putting the patient onto the machine the weaker leg should be put onto the foot rest first. The foot rest should be placed at the lowest point of the cycle for this purpose.

At the beginning of treatment the machine should be adjusted to allow the fullest range of movement at any limited joint. As movement increases the machine should be adjusted to accommodate this. The joint should never be forced beyond its possible movement.

To increase muscle strength the resistance and time spent working can be increased. An upright posture can be encouraged by adjusting the table height to mid-way between chest and shoulder.

When setting the seat high to encourage hip or knee extension or plantarflexion the therapist must ensure that the patient can reach the pedals comfortably and does not have to rock from side to side on the seat in order to move them.

Machine adjustments (i.e. seat height and distance, crank length and table height) and treatment periods should always be recorded, as well as the resistance and number of revolutions.

Patients with poor hand sensation or coordination and visual problems, or those who are confused should not use the fretsaw, drill or sanding attachment. In such a case a radio, tape recorder, slide projector or buffer may be preferable.

It is not advisable to use the machine for patients with spasm in the lower limbs as the effort involved can increase muscle tone still further.

Possible activities

Fretsaw: Jigsaws, remedial games, toys, tray and other basketry bases, cheese boards, bread boards, splints, toast and letter racks.

Sander: Any sanding activity, provided the article is big enough to handle safely (or is blocked up to be safe).

Drill: Drilling holes on bases to be used for adapted solitaire, chess, draughts, dominoes, chinese checker boards, plant tags etc.

Socket outlet: Use of sewing machine (the foot control must be taped shut), tape recorder, record player, slide projector, kettle, train set etc. These activities are especially useful if the patient's upper limbs are very weak or incoordinated.

Available:

Nottingham Medical Equipment Company, Melton Road, West Bridgford, Nottinghamshire.

Tru-Eze Creasey Co (Akron Ltd), Farthing Road, Ipswich, Suffolk.

THE LIGHTWEIGHT CYCLE SAW (FIG. 9.3)

The lightweight cycle is, in essence, similar to the electronic cycle except that there is no motor power assistance. The fretsaw is driven by the power produced from pedalling: and the speed is therefore directly related to the speed of pedalling.

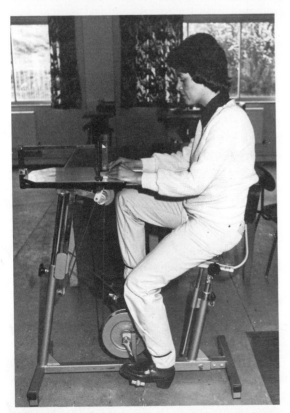

Fig. 9.3 The lightweight cycle

The machine is less adjustable and as the seat unit is not removable the cycle can only be used by those who are able to stand and climb onto it. The resistance cannot be increased on this machine and work can only be made harder by the use of harder or thicker materials.

However, the cycle is compact and because of its simplicity, reliable and easy to maintain. It is, therefore, an extremely useful piece of machinery.

1. The seat unit

The seat. The saddle is of a cycle seat design. It is adjustable in height and distance from the pedal unit. The adjustments are best made before the patient is seated on the machine.

The backrest. This is adjustable forwards and backwards but not vertically.

Armrests. There are no armrests.

2. The cycle unit

The table. This is formica topped and is adjustable for height only.

The tools. A fretsaw only is attached.

The pedals. The footrests are of the cycle pedal variety. No straps are attached and the cranks are of a fixed length.

Resistance. As already mentioned, there is no facility for adding resistance to the pedalling action.

Accessories. No revolution counter or other accessories are available.

Transfer to and from the machine. The patient must be able to climb on and off the machine as the seat unit is not removable.

Uses

As the movements and adjustments are basically the same as on the electronic cycle the points of use and activities are the same. There are, however, a few differences in addition to those already mentioned:

The lightweight cycle saw is quieter in use, compact and requires less space. It is easy to move and much cheaper and easier to maintain than the electronic cycle. It offers less support to the patient and he has to be able to balance independently.

As it is not fully adjustable it cannot be used for children. Its simplicity makes it less inhibiting to the patient. The saw works well for intricate shapes, but cuts less well in a straight line.

Available:
Nottingham Medical Equipment Company
Tru-Eze Creasy Co (Akron Ltd).

THE TREADLE FRETSAW (FIG. 9.4)

The treadle fretsaw consists of a work unit on which a fretsaw is powered by the reciprocal action of the two foot pedals. A seat unit is attached.

1. The seat unit

The seat. The saddle is of a cycle seat design and is adjustable in height. The seat unit is separate from the work unit but is not mounted on castors. On some more recent models the seat unit can be secured at a series of set distances from the work unit.

Backrest. Whether the backrest is adjustable or not depends on the model of seat used.

Armrests. There are no armrests.

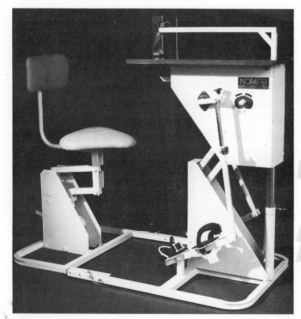

Fig. 9.4 The treadle fretsaw

2. The work unit

The table. The top is formica covered and is adjustable in height only.

The tools. A fretsaw only is attached.

The pedals. The footrests support the whole foot, which is held by two securing straps. The toe end of the footrests is attached to a pedal shaft through which the treadle action is transmitted via a crank shaft to move the fretsaw. Both pedal shaft and crank shaft are adjustable in length to obtain the required movement. On some models the length of the footrest can be altered.

Resistance. There is no facility for adding resistance to the treadle action although the use of thicker or tougher wood can make work harder.

Accessories. There are no accessories.

Transfer to and from the machine. The seat is pulled away from the work unit. The patient stands facing the unit and, disregarding any walking aids, holds onto the table top. The seat is then pushed up behind him to the correct distance from the work unit and he sits down. His weaker foot (should this apply) is put onto the pedal first. The seat height is then adjusted.

Uses

The treadle fretsaw encourages mainly dorsiflexion and plantarflexion of the ankle joint. Minimal flexion and extension of the knee joint is obtained during the reciprocal pedal action but the amount of movement is not sufficient to be used to treat the joint. The action is partial weight bearing.

Figure 9.5 shows the adjustments necessary to obtain increased movement at the ankle joints.

1. *Plantarflexion (Fig. 9.5A):* seat high and back, pedal shaft and crank shaft long.

2. *Dorsiflexion (Fig. 9.5B):* seat low and forward, pedal shaft and crankshaft short.

3. *Dorsi- and plantarflexion (Fig. 9.5C):* seat low and forward, pedal shaft short, crankshaft long.

The use of unequal adjustment. In the early stages of treatment the movement of the weak ankle can be assisted by the strong ankle by adjusting the range of movement for each foot individually. Where the strength and range of

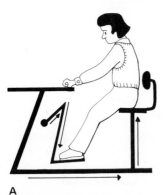

A

To increase plantarflexion
    Pedal shaft—long
    Crank shaft—long
    Seat distance—move backwards
    Seat height—high

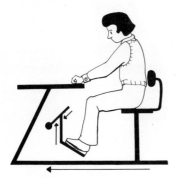

B

To increase dorsiflexion
    Pedal shaft—short
    Crank shaft—short
    Seat distance—move forwards
    Seat height—low

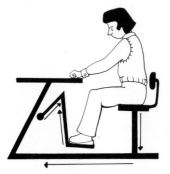

C

To increase both dorsiflexion and plantarflexion
    Pedal shaft—short
    Crank shaft—long
    Seat distance—move forwards
    Seat height—low

Fig. 9.5 Use of the treadle fretsaw

movement of the weak ankle is severely limited the strong ankle can be set to move through a full range of movement while the weak ankle is set to a range of movement within its capacity. In this way the therapist will find that the strong ankle will be able to assist the weak one by taking more of the work load.

Similarly, during the final stages of treatment, the reverse setting will require the weaker ankle to take a greater work load.

Conditions treated

The following conditions may be treated on the treadle fretsaw:

(a). Fractures involving the lower leg, ankle and foot, e.g. fractured tibia and fibula, Potts fracture, fractured calcaneum: To increase the range of movement and strength in the affected limb(s) once the patient is partial weight bearing. Dispersion of oedema.

(b). Soft tissue injuries, e.g. injury to tendo-calcaneus, burns: To maintain and increase the range of movement. To increase muscle strength which may have been lost during immobility. To prevent contracture. To stimulate circulation.

(c). Spinal conditions resulting in lower limb weakness, e.g. prolapsed intervertebral disc: To encourage balance. To increase strength in spinal and lower limb muscle groups. To encourage reciprocal walking pattern. To stimulate movement.

(d). Peripheral nerve injuries, especially those to the common peroneal nerve: To maintain a full range of movement and prevent joint deformity and muscle shortening. To stimulate movement. To increase strength.

(e). Progressive neurological disease e.g. multiple sclerosis and Parkinsons disease: To maintain and increase coordination in the lower leg in the early stages of the disease. To encourage a reciprocal walking pattern.

(f). Head injuries and other conditions causing weakness and incoordination in the lower limbs: To improve strength, range of movement and coordination in the lower leg. To encourage a reciprocal walking pattern and build up work tolerance.

Points of use and possible activities. See under electronic cycle.
    Available:
Nottingham Medical Equipment Company
Tru-Eze Creasey Co (Akron Ltd).

THE ANKLE ROTATOR (FIG. 9.6)

The ankle rotator consists of a work unit to which a fretsaw is attached. This fretsaw is operated by the rotary action of the foot pedal whose movement is transmitted to power the saw via a flywheel and drive band mechanism.
    A special seat is not supplied with the machine but an adjustable cycle seat is recommended.

The work unit

The table is made of metal and is narrower than on the cycle and treadle machines. It is not adjustable in height or distance as the whole work

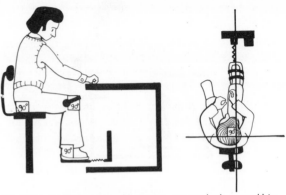

Fig. 9.7   Position at the ankle rotator. (Note: the knee and hip joints are at right angles)

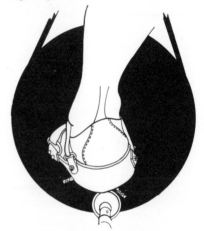

Foot plate set to encourage inversion . . .

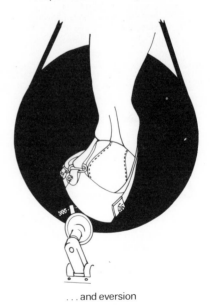

. . . and eversion

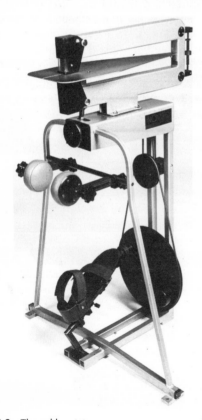

Fig. 9.6   The ankle rotator

Fig. 9.8   Use of the ankle rotator

unit is fixed to the floor. Any necessary adjustments to obtain the correct positioning and movement are made at the footplate and seat.

The tools. A fretsaw only is available.

The foot pedal. The single footplate supports the whole foot and holds it with two securing straps. The toe strap is adjustable along the length of the footplate to accommodate different foot sizes. The footplate can be tilted on its longitudinal axis either to the right or to the left in order to encourage inversion or eversion of the foot (see Fig. 9.18).

Resistance. This can be added either by an adjustable braking system or by the weight attached to the flywheel. When fixed near the centre of the flywheel the weight will add resistance to the rotary movement.

Accessories. No accessories are available.

Transfer to and from the machine. The patient stands facing the work unit and the cycle seat is pushed up behind him. He then sits down. The foot is strapped to the footplate which should be in a neutral position, so that the foot is neither dorsi- or plantarflexed nor inverted or everted.

The seat height and distance are adjusted so that the knee and hip joints are each at right angles and the hip joint is neither abducted nor adducted (Fig. 9.7). The knee is supported by two knee pads fixed against either side of the knee just behind the femoral condyles. These secure the knee, helping to reduce compensatory hip movements. The

therapist must ensure, however, that rotatory movements of the tibia are not prevented at the knee.

Uses

The ankle rotator, like the treadle fretsaw, treats the ankle joint but, because of the facility allowing inversion and eversion (Fig. 9.8), full circumduction at the ankle and foot can be obtained. The action is partial weight-bearing.

Because of the circular movement of the ankle rotator only one adjustment is necessary to obtain the required range of movement. In the early stages of treatment the toe of the footplate is set towards the centre of the flywheel so that a minimal range of movement is obtained. As movement improves the toe is moved towards the outside of the flywheel so that a greater range of movement is required (Fig. 9.9). The therapist should remember that, as the weight on the flywheel adds resistance to the movement when placed centrally, it should be fixed towards the outside of the wheel until resistance is required.

Conditions treated

The conditions treated on the ankle rotator are as those described in sections (a), (b) and (d) of the treadle fretsaw.

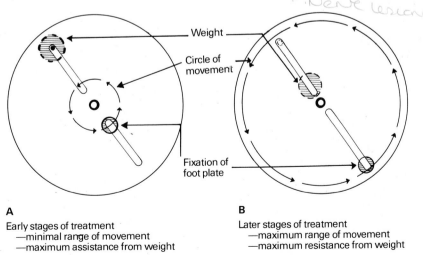

A Early stages of treatment
—minimal range of movement
—maximum assistance from weight

B Later stages of treatment
—maximum range of movement
—maximum resistance from weight

Fig. 9.9 Adjusting the flywheel

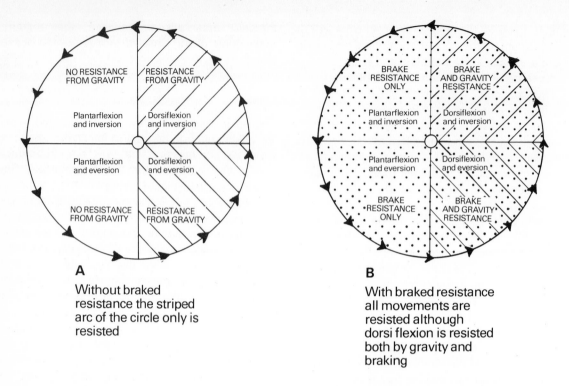

A
Without braked
resistance the striped
arc of the circle only is
resisted

B
With braked resistance
all movements are
resisted although
dorsi flexion is resisted
both by gravity and
braking

Fig. 9.10 Footplate — the diagrams show the footplate turned anticlockwise by the right foot

Points of use

See relevant points under Electronic Cycle. Additionally the therapist should note that:

Flat soled shoes are advisable to support and protect the foot during the early stages of treatment. However, as movement returns to the ankle and foot the shoe can be removed (and the foot protected by a thick sock if necessary) in order that movements within the foot are encouraged.

The ankle rotator should be well understood before being used and the therapist should be aware of exactly how much effort is involved in its use.

When no resistance is added to the rotatory movement the plantarflexion part of the cycle requires little muscle power as it is gravity assisted. Should the plantarflexors particularly need to be exercised then resistance must be added (Fig. 9.10).

Possible activities. See under Electronic Cycle.

Available:
Nottingham Medical Equipment Company.

Note: A PIED saw, designed to treat the movements of the ankle joint is now available from Tru-Eze Creasey & Co Ltd.

THE QUADRICEPS SWITCH (FIG. 9.11)

The quadriceps switch consists of a metal work unit to which an air-filled pad is attached at one end and an ankle support at the other. The user sits as shown in Figure 9.11 and when the pad is compressed by the static action of the quadriceps muscle group power is released to the socket which is positioned below the pad. In this way any electrical appliance which is plugged into the socket is activated. No special seat is supplied with the switch and any cycle seat or chair of suitable height may be used.

The work unit

The unit is made to fit under a work bench and the appliance to be powered by it is placed on the bench at a suitable working position for the pa-

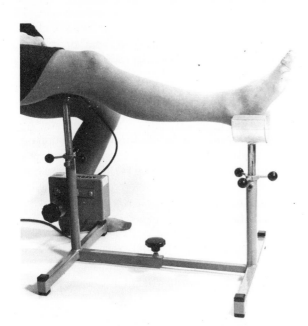

Fig. 9.11   The quadriceps switch

tient. Any suitable appliance worked from a standard 240 volt socket may be operated.

The ankle support. This consists of a metal cup padded with foam rubber. It can be raised or lowered to the required height using an adjuster. The shaft is marked in inches so that the position can be easily recorded.

The knee pad. This is an air-filled rubber pad which fits under the popliteal fossa. Adjustable in height, its shaft is marked for easy recording.

The bottom shaft. This is a metal shaft whose length can be adjusted to alter the distance between the knee pad and the ankle support.

Resistance. This can be varied by altering the air pressure in the knee pad. Three grades of pressure are available.

Transfer to and from the machine. The patient sits on a chair placed at the knee pad end of the unit and rests the ankle onto the ankle support. The unit is adjusted to a suitable length so that the ankle is supported comfortably with the knee pad under the popliteal fossa. The height of the knee pad is then adjusted so that it is compressed when the patient pushes down onto it by bracing his knee, using the static action of his quadriceps muscles. The therapist must ensure that the pad is not too low, as this would force the patient to hyperextend his knee in order to compress it.

Finally the resistance in the pad is adjusted to the required level and the appliance plugged first into the socket on the machine and then into the mains supply.

Uses

As implied by its name this machine treats the action of the quadriceps group of muscles, which is to stabilise and extend the knee. Because the machine is used in a non-weight bearing manner it can be used in the very earliest stages of treatment following injury or dysfunction.

Its particular uses are to help eliminate extension lag at the knee before mobilisation is commenced (it is vital to stabilise the knee joint before mobilisation), to maintain and increase the tone and strength in the quadriceps muscle group and to prevent flexion contractures at the knee.

Conditions treated

The following conditions may be treated by the quadriceps switch:

(a). Fractures of the lower limb where the knee joint is affected or has to be immobilised, such as fractured tibia and/or fibula or fractured patella: To maintain and increase the tone in the quadriceps group during and/or following the non-weight bearing stage. To eliminate extension lag and prevent joint deformity. To reduce oedema.

(b). Surgery or injury to the knee, including meniscectomy, patellectomy (or repair); ligamentous or other soft tissue injury around the knee and arthroplasty to the knee: To maintain and increase the tone in the quadriceps group during and/or following the non-weight bearing stage. To eliminate extension lag. To reduce oedema.

(c). Burns of the lower limb, especially those over the front of the thigh or the back of the knee: To maintain and increase the tone in the quadriceps group. To eliminate extension lag, reduce oedema and prevent contractures at the knee.

(d). Arthritic conditions affecting the knee, either during conservative treatment or following surgery: To maintain and increase the tone in the quadriceps group. To eliminate extension lag, reduce oedema (especially post-operatively) and prevent contractures at the knee.

(e). Below knee amputations: To maintain and increase the tone in the quadriceps group. To eliminate extension lag and help the patient learn to control the stump. To reduce oedema and prevent contractures.

Points of use

When setting up the machine the therapist must ensure that the knee does not fall into hyperextension in order to operate the pad, nor that the pad is set too high so that the weight of the relaxed limb operates the machine.

If using the machine to treat a below knee amputee whose stump is short it may be necessary to lengthen the ankle support in order to support the stump.

The chair on which the patient sits should be of a height that allows the machine to be operated with the hip flexed at approximately 90° for greatest comfort.

Possible activities

Any of the following electrical appliances can be operated by the quadriceps switch: Sander (firmly fixed to the bench and well guarded), drill, soldering iron (for model or splint making), small lathe (for model or splint making), sewing machine (the footplate must be taped shut), train set (this has been a great success with children), radio, tape recorder, slide projector.

Note: The appliance must be able to work in short bursts, especially in the early stages of treatment when the patient's control is weak. For this reason appliances such as record players or irons are not recommended.

Available:
Tru-Eze Creasey and Company (Akron Ltd).

THE WIRE TWISTING MACHINE (FIG. 9.12)

The wire twisting machine consists of a table mounted unit into which a double length of wire is fixed so that it is held still at one end in a tail stock and is twisted at the other end by turning a handle. A variety of handles can be fitted to the spindle. The machine should be firmly secured to the edge

of a work bench and any cycle seat, stool or chair of a suitable height placed in front of it. The machine can be used to treat most movements of the upper limb.

The work unit

The spindle and head stock. This is the end unit on which the wire is twisted. The wire is secured by a wing nut and the spindle can be turned using one of the following handles which are supplied with the machine:
(i) Spade handle
(ii) Series of disc handles
(iii) Adjustable lever handle with rigid or ball jointed hand grip
(iv) Thumb release roller handle.

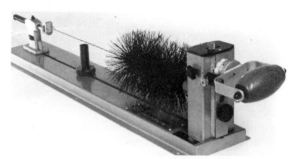

Fig. 9.12   The wire twister

The tail stock. This is the end unit over which the wire is doubled and held still, thus allowing the wire to be twisted by the rotation of the spindle. The tail stock is adjustable along the length of the work unit in order to accommodate the length of wire required.

The wire control column. This sliding column fits underneath the wire and its removable plug, when placed in position over the wire, prevents the wire beyond that point being twisted when the handle is turned. This enables bristles to be placed between the wires in short bundles and twisted sufficiently to hold them secure before the next bundle is added.

Resistance. The action of twisting and therefore shortening the wire is in itself a process of increasing resistance, for as the wire shortens it pulls against a spring in the tail stock. Further resistance can be added by the adjustment of a brake.

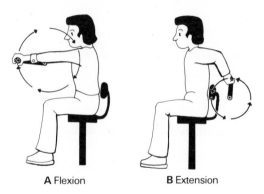

A Flexion   **B** Extension

Note: Circumduction can be obtained with a setting between the two illustrated.

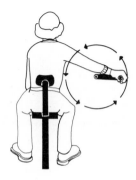

C Abduction

Fig. 9.13   Shoulder movement

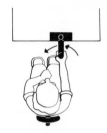

A Seating to show shoulder and forearm position

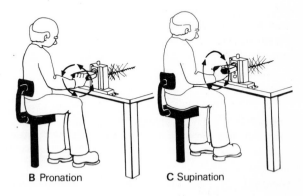

B Pronation   **C** Supination

Fig. 9.14   Forearm movement

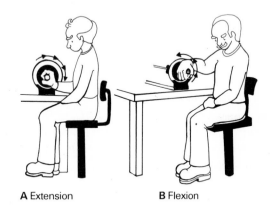

A Extension   **B** Flexion

Fig. 9.15   Wrist movement

Position at the machine

The machine should be prepared by attaching the required handle and fixing the wire. The patient sits at the end of the machine, either facing it or sideways on to it as required. The height and position of the seat are then adjusted so that the required movement is obtained. The direction of movement of the handle is set clockwise or anti-clockwise by adjusting the ratchet control.

Uses

Because of the selection of handles supplied with the machine, it is possible to treat most movements of the upper limb. Table 9.1 shows the various movements which can be obtained and the settings and positions required for each.

Conditions treated

The following conditions may be treated by the wire twister:

(a). Fractures and other orthopaedic conditions affecting the bones and joints of the upper limb: To increase the range of movement and strength and help reduce oedema.

Table 9.1 Use of the wire twisting machine

Movement	Handle	Seating	Starting Position	Action for right hand	Figure
Shoulder movement					
Flexion	Long lever – set long	Sideways on	Lever at bottom of cycle, elbow in extension	Clockwise	9.13A
Extension	Long lever – set short	Sideways on	Lever at bottom of cycle, elbow in extension	Anti-clockwise	9.13B
Abduction	Long lever – set long	Facing	Lever at bottom of cycle, elbow in extension	Anti-clockwise	9.13C
Elbow movement					
Extension	Long lever – set long	Sideways on	Lever at bottom of cycle, elbow in extension	Clockwise	As in 9.13A
Flexion	Long lever	Sideways on	Lever at bottom of cycle, elbow in extension	Anti-clockwise	As in 9.13A
Forearm movement					
Pronation	Spade or disc	Facing	Shoulder adducted, elbow at right angles and forearm horizontal and supinated	Anti-clockwise	9.14B
Supination	Spade or disc	Facing	Shoulder adducted, elbow at right angles and forearm horizontal and pronated	Clockwise	9.14C
Wrist movement					
Extension	Thumb release (thumb button omitted)	Sideways on	Shoulder adducted, elbow at right angles and forearm horizontal	Clockwise	9.15A
Flexion	Thumb release (thumb button omitted)	Sideways on	Shoulder adducted, elbow at right angles and forearm horizontal	Anti-clockwise	9.15B
Hand movement					
Cylinder grip	Thumb release or spade	Sideways on (thumb release) or Facing (spade)	As above	Clockwise	As in 9.14B or 9.15A
Span grip (and distal interphalangeal flexion)	Disc	Facing	As above	Anti-clockwise or clockwise	As in 9.14A or 9.14B
Thumb interphalangeal flexion and metacarpal phalangeal flexion and adduction	Thumb release (thumb button included)	Sideways on	As above	Clockwise	As in 9.15A

(b). Peripheral nerve lesions affecting the upper limb: To maintain a full range of movement and prevent joint deformity and muscle shortening. To stimulate movement and increase strength and coordination.

(c). Soft tissue injuries to the upper limb, especially those to the hand: To increase the range of movement and strength following immobilisation.

To prevent contracture, to reduce oedema and help skin condition. To increase coordination and dexterity.

(d). Amputation of the whole or part of a digit or digits: To reduce oedema and help skin condition. To increase the range of movement and grip strength. To increase coordination. To aid natural use of the stump.

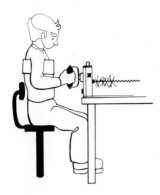

Fig. 9.16 Preventing compensatory abduction at the shoulder by holding a card between arm and chest

Points of use

1. As the wire twister is able to treat specific movements the therapist must take care that no compensatory movements occur whilst the action is being performed. For example, when treating pronation a compensatory abduction may occur at the shoulder. This can be prevented by asking the patient to maintain his shoulder in adduction by holding a piece of card or paper to his chest with his arm. (Figure 9.16).

2. When treating patients with hand injuries or those with softening of the palmar skin due to immobilisation, the therapist must take care that blisters do not develop on the hand.

3. The thumb release button on the roller handle is especially useful when treating a hand in which coordination is a problem or when treating those who must return to driving, as the action needed to release button is similar to that used on a standard floor mounted handbrake lever.

Possible activities

Wire only: Flower stakes, hanging flower baskets, children's coat hangers.

Wire and bristles: Bottle brush, clothes brush, lavatory brush, model fir trees (for cake decoration or model railways etc.), pastry brush.

Wire and other materials: Foam washing up mop, dish cloth, cotton washing up mop.

Available:

Nottingham Medical Equipment Company.

OVERHEAD SLING SUPPORT SYSTEMS (FIG. 9.17)

The OB Help Arm is described as an example. It consists of a mobile stand with a fixed overhead yoke and movable forearms. Each of these forearms holds an adjustable bar and slings which, by a series of counterweights, can be altered to support the weight of weak upper limbs. One limb or both may be treated at·a time. The OB Help Arm can be used while the patient is standing, sitting or in bed.

1. The work unit

The mobile stand. This is made of lightweight metal and stand on four castors, the back two of which can be braked. From the fixed overhead yoke two movable forearms protrude which can be adjusted for length, horizontal movement and tilt on the long axis. Each of these adjustments is measurable on the scales provided (Fig. 9.18). The stand contains a clip on which the storage box containing spare slings and cord is stored.

The slings. Each machine is supplied with slings to fit the wrist, elbow and hand. The slings are

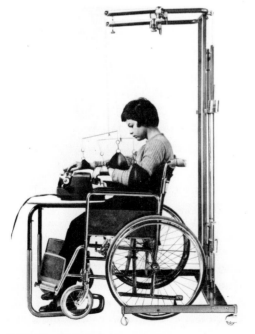

Fig. 9.17 The OB Help Arm

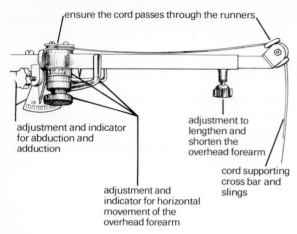

ensure the cord passes through the runners

adjustment and indicator for abduction and adduction

adjustment to lengthen and shorten the overhead forearm

cord supporting cross bar and slings

adjustment and indicator for horizontal movement of the overhead forearm

Fig. 9.18 Adjustments on the overhead gantry

attached to either end of a crossbar which, by adjusting the weight distributor, can be altered so that the patient's forearm can be correctly positioned in the slings. The crossbars are attached to a nylon cord which runs over the forearms and yoke and down to the weight basket.

The weights and weight basket. The weight of the patient's upper limbs is supported by the counterbalance of disc shaped weights which fit inside the weight basket. When the machine is not in use, or while the patient is being set up in the machine, the weight box is locked in position on the back of the stand. The weights are stored on a stand fixed to the back of the unit.

2. The seat

The Help Arm is designed to be used with any static or mobile seat. The machine can also be used for bed bound patients or those standing at a work table.

Transfer to and from the machine. It is most important that the therapist is able to set the patient up in the OB Help Arm correctly and easily. The following sequence should be used:

1. The patient is seated at a work top. For the bed bound patient a work top is placed over the bed in front of him.

2. The OB Help Arm, with the weight box and forearm bars locked and the cords looped over the forearm bars, is wheeled up behind the patient. The brakes are then secured.

3. The patient's arm is supported (by the thera-

pist, her helper, on the table top or by the patient's other hand if possible) while the slings are put around the elbow, wrist and, where necessary, the hand. They are then clipped to the crossbar.

4. The cords are unlooped and attached to the crossbar.

5. Whilst supporting the patient's arm with one hand the therapist unlocks the weight box and lowers it with her other hand. This will take up the slack on the cord, but will not yet support the patient's limbs.

6. Weights are added to the weight basket until the patient's limbs are in a good working position.

7. The forearm bars are adjusted for horizontal movement, length and tilt as required.

8. Finally the crossbar is adjusted by moving the butterfly screw along it until the forearm is correctly positioned for work.

Uses

The OB Help Arm is used to support the upper limb or limbs if weakness prevents them from being used for independent actions. Because the weight of the limb is counterbalanced by the machine any power remaining in the limbs can be used to grasp, coordinate and move during work without having to be expended on holding the limb up against gravity. In this way minimum power can be used to maximum advantage.

Additionally, because the patient is able to work bilaterally, good upper limb patterns of movement can be retained even if one limb only is affected, such as in a brachial plexus lesion or hemiplegia. Sling suspension is *not* helpful where spasticity is present as the spastic tone may be increased.

Conditions treated

The following conditions may be treated using the OB Help Arm:

(a). Fractures or other orthopaedic conditions of the upper limb: To relieve the weight of the Plaster of Paris, thus enabling the free joints of the limb to be used while the fracture is immobilised. To support the limb in the early stages of recovery from injuries affecting the shoulder joint, e.g. fractured humerus or dislocation of the shoulder.

(b). Spinal injuries resulting in upper limb

weakness: To support the limb, allowing maximum functional use of weak muscles. To aid coordination.

(c). Progressive neurological conditions such as multiple sclerosis or motor neurone disease: The purpose for treatment is the same as above.

(d). Head injuries and other conditions causing weakness and incoordination of the upper limbs: Purpose as above. Additionally to enable the limbs to help in the treatment of other affected areas such as perceptual and sensory problems.

(e). Hemiparesis: The purpose for treatment is the same as above.

(f). Peripheral nerve injuries affecting the upper limb: To support the upper limb, thus allowing maximum functional use of weak muscles. To prevent joint deformity and muscle shortening by maintaining a full range of movement. To encourage any returning strength.

(g). Other lower motor neurone conditions such as polyneuritis: The purpose for treatment is the same as above.

Points of use

Because the OB Help Arm is mobile and compact it is suitable for use in the department, on a ward or in the patient's home.

The facility to control the horizontal movement of the forearm bar allows the therapist to limit the range of shoulder abduction and adduction within the arc required.

As the strength in the upper limb returns the balancing weights are reduced so that the patient begins to support the limb against gravity using his own muscle power.

As well as the OB Help Arm, the 'Sunflower' Limb Balancer and Akron Mobile Arm support systems are available.

Possible activities

Almost any activity can be performed with the OB Help Arm. Those most commonly required include:

Personal care activities: feeding, washing and hair care.

Communication activities: writing and typing.

Activities to increase the functional use of the upper limbs: stoolseating, sanding and remedial games.

Leisure activities: painting, reading and craft work.

Available:

Both the OB Help Arm and the 'Sunflower' Limb Balancer are available from the Nottingham Medical Equipment Company.

The Akron Mobile Arm is available from Tru-Eze Creasey and Co. Ltd.

THE RUG LOOM (FIG. 9.19)

The rug loom is an upright, wooden framed loom which is adapted from the standard design to give maximum therapeutic value to the upper limb and trunk. The shed can be changed by a foot or hand mechanism and the loom is high enough to give maximum range of movement at the shoulder and shoulder girdle when using the beater.

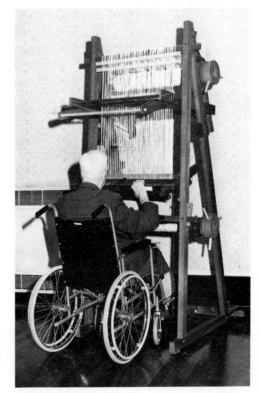

Fig. 9.19 The upright rug loom

1. The work unit

The frame. The loom frame is raised so that shoulder, shoulder girdle and spinal movement can be exercised during use.

The beater bar. When raised in its highest position the beater is held in position by two hooks. Before beating the bar is released by pushing in the release knob which is located centrally on the beater. Beating is a bilateral action.

The heddle. To change sheds the release toggle is pulled with one hand and the shed changing bar pulled or pushed with the other, depending on the previous position of the heddle. Alternatively the shed can be changed using the foot pedal mechanism.

Resistance. Resistance can be added to the 'down' beat by attachment of a weight and pulley system (Fig. 9.20A). Resistance to the 'up' beat is added by attaching the weights provided onto the screws of the beater bar (Fig. 9.20B). Resistance can also be graded according to the type of work set up on the loom.

2. The seat

Any suitable seat can be used with the rug loom.

Position at the machine. The patient sits centrally, facing the loom. The seat height is adjusted to accommodate any limitation in the range of movement of the upper or lower limbs. The patient is then taught the weaving action:

1. Pull the toggle to release the heddle catch and change the shed using the shed changing bar.

2. Throw the shuttle, pulling the thread to the correct tension.

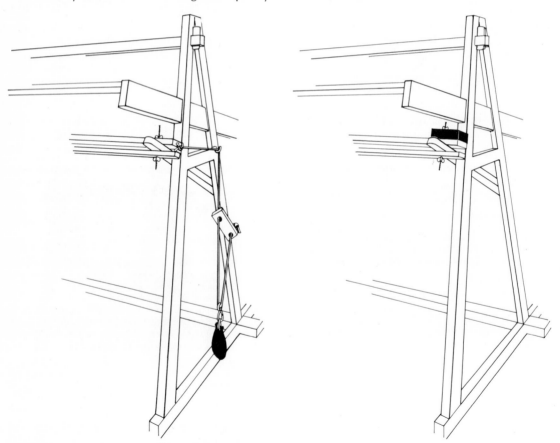

A Resistance to the 'down' beat   **B** Resistance to the 'up' beat

Fig. 9.20   Adding resistance

3. Press in the beater release knob and beat.

4. Return the beater to the 'up' position until the holding hooks lock into position.

Uses

The rug loom can be used not only to exercise the muscles of the shoulder, shoulder girdle, upper limbs and trunk, but also to improve coordination and balance owing to the wide, bilateral movement involved in the weaving action. Should the foot pedals be used to change sheds then all four limbs and trunk can be exercised, making this an excellent piece of equipment for treating conditions such as head injuries or high spinal lesions where general weakness and incoordination are a feature. Because of the physical effort involved, especially if resistance is added or long shuttles used, the loom can be used to build up the work tolerance of those in the final stages of treatment.

Table 9.2 shows the movements which may be encouraged by the rug loom.

Table 9.2 Use of the rug loom

Movement	Action	Resistance, adaptation or positioning	Figure
Spine			
Extension	Reaching for toggle or beater	Seat low	9.21A
Side flexion	Placing shuttle into shed and collecting shuttle	Long shuttle	9.21B
Shoulder girdle			
Elevation	Reaching for toggle or beater; 'up' beat of beater	Seat low, weight added to beater bar	9.21A
Depression	'Down' beat of beater	Weight added to pulley	9.21C
Shoulder joint			
Elevation	Reaching for toggle or beater; 'up' beat of beater	Seat low, weight added to beater bar	9.21A
Abduction	Placing and collecting shuttle	Long shuttle	9.21B
Adduction	Pushing shuttle through shed; 'down' beat of beater	No adjustments	9.21C & D
Elbow joint			
Extension	Reaching for toggle or beater, placing and collecting shuttle, 'up' beat of beater	Seat low, weight added to beater bar, long shuttle	9.21A & B
Flexion	'Down' beat of beater, pushing shuttle through shed	Weight added to pulley	9.21C & D
Hand			
Grip	Holding beater, holding shuttle, pulling toggle	No adjustments	9.21A, B, C & D
Lower limb, hip and knee movement.*	Using foot pedal	No adjustments	

*Note: Lower limb, hip and knee movement is only slight, the foot pedals are used more therapeutically in the treatment of incoordination and balance.

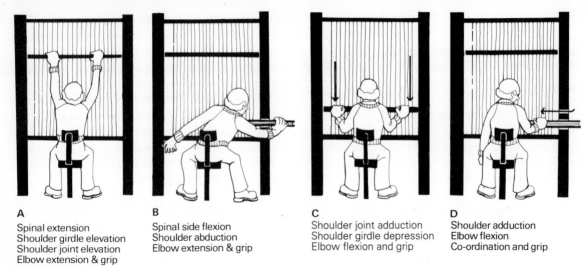

A
Spinal extension
Shoulder girdle elevation
Shoulder joint elevation
Elbow extension & grip

B
Spinal side flexion
Shoulder abduction
Elbow extension & grip

C
Shoulder joint adduction
Shoulder girdle depression
Elbow flexion and grip

D
Shoulder adduction
Elbow flexion
Co-ordination and grip

Fig. 9.21   Movements which can be treated by the use of the rug loom

Conditions treated

The following conditions may be treated using the rehabilitation rug loom:

(a). Fractures and other orthopaedic conditions affecting shoulder and upper limb movement: To increase range of movement and strength. To reduce oedema. To increase work tolerance and coordination.

(b). Soft tissue injuries such as tendon ruptures and burns or crush injuries of the upper limbs: To reduce oedema and improve skin condition. To increase range of movement and strength. To prevent joint deformity and scar contracture.

(c). Arthritic conditions such as ankylosing spondylitis, (but with the exception of R.A.) which affect the upper limbs and spine: To increase or maintain full range of movement and strength. To prevent deformity caused by poor posture or inactivity. Note: Care should be taken where cervical joints are affected.

(d). Spinal injuries, head injuries or other conditions causing general and upper limb weakness, incoordination and poor balance: To maintain and increase range of movement in all limbs. To stimulate movement. To increase strength. To improve balance and coordination.

(e). Amputations of the lower limb: To improve balance and strengthen the upper limbs.

(f). Progressive neurological conditions where general weakness is a problem: To maintain strength and range of movement in all limbs. To maintain and improve balance and coordination in all limbs. To stimulate circulation.

(g). Peripheral nerve lesions affecting the upper limb: To maintain a full range of movement and prevent joint deformity and muscle shortening. To stimulate returning movement and increase returning strength.

(h). Certain chest and heart conditions: To increase vital capacity, encourage good posture, and build up work tolerance. To stimulate circulation.

Points of use

The therapist should ensure that clothing, such as heavy jackets or neckties, is not restricting full movement.

The therapist must know exactly how much effort is needed to work the loom, as the bilateral, elevated action can be extremely tiring.

Many different materials can be used for weaving and the therapist must be aware of the differences in resistance and effort involved in using each type.

As the rug loom will be used by a number of people during the course of one piece of work the therapist must make sure that each person is capable of obtaining a reasonable standard of work, so that the effect of the piece is not spoiled by uneven weaving.

Possible activities

Scarves, head squares, rugs, floor mats, bath mats, oven gloves, shoulder bags, hand bags, place mats, dish cloths, dressing table mats, wall hangings, peg bags, work bags, cushion covers and similar items can be made on the rug loom.

Materials which can be used include cotton (fine, medium or thick), wool (fine, medium or thick, i.e. rug wool), thrums, wool mixes, nytrim, dishcloth cotton, split cane (for place mats).

Available:
Nottingham Medical Equipment Company.

FEPS (FIG. 9.22)

The FEPS apparatus was designed to aid the treatment of the forearm, wrist and hand and can be used to treat *Flexion* and *Extension* (at the wrist) and *Pronation* and *Supination* (at the forearm). The apparatus can be used for several different activities, such as weaving, printing and some remedial games. Resistance varies for each activity and can also be added to the apparatus itself by means of a screw adjustor.

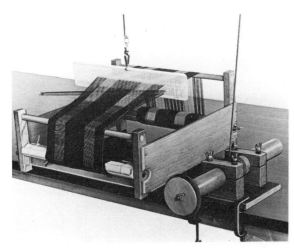

Fig. 9.22 The FEPS apparatus

1. The work unit

The frame. The wooden frame holding the roller-bar is clamped to a work top. Four screws can be adjusted to give the amount of resistance required.

The rollers. Two rollers are supplied. They can be used with three sizes of roller bar handles (for treating wrist movement). There is also an attachment for discs.

The discs. Three sizes of discs are supplied. These screw into one end of the large roller bar and are used for treating forearm movement, finger flexion and span.

The overhead bar. This is supplied with the apparatus and can be suspended by two hooks from an overhead mesh system. The cord, which is attached to the roller, passes over two pulleys to transmit the action of the FEPS to the equipment being used (see Fig. 9.23B).

Resistance. This can be adjusted by four screws on the FEPS frame or by the type of activity used with the apparatus. For example, printing offers greater resistance than weaving with a box loom.

2. The seat

The FEPS apparatus is designed to be used on a work top. The patient may need to sit either facing or sideways on to the work and therefore any seat of a suitable height for the work top can be used.

Position at the apparatus. The FEPS is secured to the work top and the cord threaded through the overhead bar (and other pulley system where necessary) and tied to the equipment being used. The patient sits facing or sideways on to the apparatus as required and the seat height is adjusted so that the adducted arm can hold the roller bar or disc with the forearm horizontal, i.e. the elbow bent to 90°.

Uses

The FEPS apparatus is not used in isolation but needs to be attached to a piece of equipment in such a way that its movement (i.e. rolling the bar or turning the disc) is transferred through a pulley system to perform the required action on the equipment in use. For example, with a box loom it can be used to raise and lower the heddle or with a hand press to depress the handle which moves the platen.

As mentioned the FEPS can be used to treat flexion and extension at the wrist, pronation and supination at the forearm and cylinder grip, interphalangeal flexion, metacarpal phalangeal extension and span grip in the hand. For specific information on the positioning for each particular movement see under 'Wire Twisting Machine'.

Conditions treated: See 'Wire Twisting Machine' points a, b, c and d.

Points of use: See 'Wire Twisting Machine' points 1 and 2.

Possible activities

The FEPS apparatus can be attached to the following: a hand printing press, a box weaving loom (note: a weight must be attached to the bottom rail of the heddle so that it will drop down far enough to create the lower shed) and remedial games. The FEPS can be adapted to move along a counting frame or other scale used with a remedial game, for example a long score board for dominoes (Fig. 9.23A). It can also be used in a 'Magnetic Fish Game' (Fig. 9.23B). In this game a magnet is attached to the end of the FEPS cord which is lowered down into a box with metal (or card and magnetic) fish. When the fish has been 'caught' the line is raised out of the box and the fish removed. The game can be played either by one person working against time or by two people using a separate apparatus each.

Available:

Nottingham Medical Equipment Company.

THE LATHE (FIG. 9.24)

The lathe is based on a treadle action, for use with either leg. It has a large footplate which can be easily altered to take an extension plate. A knee bar is available to prevent compensatory movements while working on the back of the lathe. The table can be used for wood turning or sanding. The flywheel has three gears, with the resistance wheel attached to the spindle, to allow gradual increase of resistance.

In most departments the lathe is used primarily in the treatment of lower limb injuries; fractures, menisectomies, soft tissue injuries and quadriceps lag. It plays an extremely useful part in treatment as it can be used to build up muscle bulk statically, therefore quickly.

1. Treadle. The treadle platform is 1 ft 5 in deep × 1 ft 8 in wide. There are two types of platform: a) divided foot board and b) single flat board with foot plate extension.

The platform is used as a base to increase hip and knee movement or, if the patient is working from the back, to increase ankle and sub-talar movement.

2. The pitman. The pitman is attached to the treadle and can be altered to three different heights

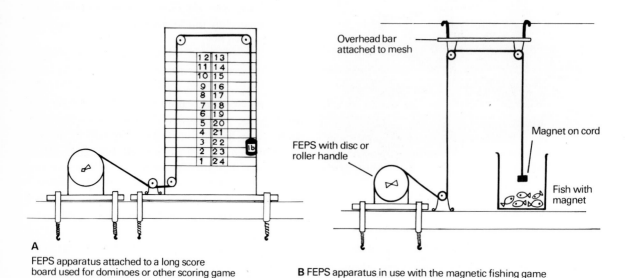

A
FEPS apparatus attached to a long score board used for dominoes or other scoring game

B FEPS apparatus in use with the magnetic fishing game

Fig. 9.23 The FEPS apparatus in use

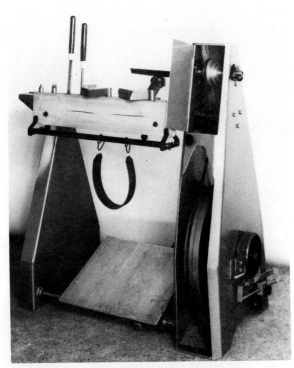

Fig. 9.24 The Larvic rehabilitation lathe

to give three different ranges of movement. This enables greater or lesser hip and knee flexion to be gained on the front of the lathe and more or less plantar and dorsiflexion on the back. In each arc, the range of movement remains the same. The treadle is secured to the pitman by a collar, thus making alterations quick and easy.

3. Footplate extension. This is 24 in long, 4½ in wide and has a safety lip at the heel end. The foot piece is 12 in long and has a non-slip surface. The extension piece is made of 1 in box section steel fitting just under the treadle platform and secured by a knurled plastic wheel. The extension foot piece can be adjusted in 11 one inch gradings. It can be slid along the platform and fixed in a wide variety of positions decided by the therapist, according to the individual needs of the patient.

4. Gears. The flywheel is on the side of the lathe and has three gears — low, middle and high. Any slack in the belt is taken up by adjusting the handwheel. The low gear is the easiest one and is the smallest pulley wheel at the base (large at the top).

5. The resistance wheel and weights. The resistance wheel is attached to the flywheel spindle. It is only effective when the wheel revolves in an anti-clockwise direction and enables the therapist to give a gradual increase in resistance more accurately. The resistance scale is graded from A—E, A being low resistance. A large metal block is pushed to the appropriate letter on the scale.

6. Tool shelf. The tool shelf is at the back of the face bed for the convenience of patients working and safe storage of tools.

7. Static quadriceps bar. This runs along the width of the face bed and is sited under the tool shelf. It is used for static quadriceps exercises — the patient is seated on a camden stool with the affected leg in a sling which is attached to the bar. The patient then treadles with the other foot. The bar is adjustable to three positions, decided by the therapist according to the needs and size of the patient.

Uses of the lathe

The lathe has a wide variety of uses, primarily in the treatment of lower limb injuries:

1. To increase the range of movement (ROM) at the hip, knee and ankle joints
2. To increase the strength of:
(i) extensors of the hip
(ii) extensors of the knee
(iii) plantarflexors
(iv) extensors of the spine
(v) grip and wrist stability
3. To increase work tolerance
4. To improve hand/eye coordination
5. To assess noise tolerance and tolerance to revolving machinery.

When planning treatment on the lathe, the therapist must always examine the patient fully *before* starting treatment. This has a two-fold purpose: (a) to assess the primary needs of the patient and (b) to make sure that there are no abnormal clinical signs and symptoms.

Before each treatment session, the patient should be asked whether there have been any additional problems since their last session.

Hip joint

The main treatment aims are to increase range of flexion and improve the power of the extensors.

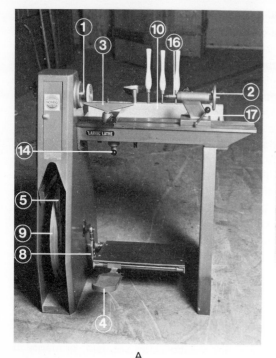

A

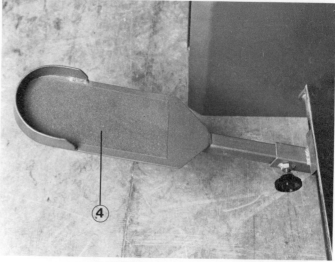

B

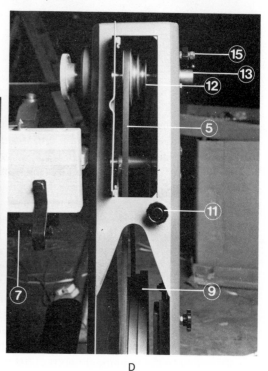

C

D

Fig. 9.25 Parts of the lathe

Key
1. Faceplate
2. Tailstock
3. Toolrest
4. Footrest extension on treadle
5. Driving belt
6. Resistance weight
7. Leg suspension bar
8. Adjustable pitman
9. 3-speed flywheel
10. Toolrack
11. Belt tension handwheel
12. Driving pulley
13. Hollow headstock spindle
14. Toolrest locking arm
15. Spindle lock
16. Tailstock barrel with central cone fitted
17. Tailstock barrel locking lever

1. Flexion. The patient stands on the unaffected leg, the height of the treadle being determined by previously taken measurements. The amount of flexion can be increased in two ways:

a). by raising the treadle by moving the notch on the pitman

b). by using the foot extension plate. The further the extension plate is pulled out, the easier it is to treadle, so this should be counteracted by increasing the resistance at the same time.

2. Extension. The patient stands on a block on his unaffected leg, with the pitman on the treadle at its lowest point and the extension plate either left off altogether or at the 'in' position. To increase resistance the drive belt should be moved to the large wheel as soon as possible and the resistance weight moved up the scale.

Knee joint

1. Full extension. The patient stands with his unaffected leg on a block and works with the affected leg on the treadle. Resistance is not usually required, but fairly long sessions are indicated.

2. Strengthening the quadriceps. This is the most vital aspect of treatment on the knee. There are two methods of achieving this. The first is used if the patient has an extension lag. The patient sits at the lathe on a camden stool seat, with the affected leg slung under the face bed and the unaffected leg treadling. In this way, muscles on the affected leg work statically by reciprocal innervation. With the second method the patient is positioned as for full extension, with the resistance weight being moved along the calibrated bar as soon as possible and the drive belt moved to the large flange of the flywheel.

The patient should be encouraged to treadle some of the time with his unaffected leg. He should then brace his affected leg well back, thus building up his quadriceps statically, as well as exercising the glutei on that side.

3. Knee flexion. When starting to treat the knee joint, flexion is not the most important aspect. Before treatment commences, it is essential that the knee is examined carefully. Effusion, pain or a hot knee are regarded as contra-indications for working towards knee flexion. However, knee flexion can be increased by adding the foot extension plate. The condition of the knee should always be checked after treatment and prior to the next session.

4. Non-weightbearing treatment. There are some conditions where weight bearing is not allowed (i.e. in the early stages of fractured shafts of femur, fractured tibia or while the leg is still in plaster of paris) but where treatment assists the venous return in an oedematous lower limb. It is also important to maintain tone in the quadriceps. In this instance, the static quadriceps exercise is given by sitting the patient on a camden stool and placing the affected leg in a long sling. This is suspended from the static quadriceps bar and the patient treadles with the unaffected leg, making sure that he does not hold on to the lathe. Thus the quadriceps and glutei have to work statically to keep the patient's balance and the muscles contract rhythmically as they stabilise the pelvis.

The therapist should always explain to the patient why she is giving him this particular type of treatment. It may help to let him feel the contractions of the quadriceps so he will have a better understanding and therefore co-operate fully.

The ankle joint

1. Plantarflexion. Powerful and well controlled plantarflexion is the key to a good walking pattern. It is therefore essential to assess the function of the ankle joint when a patient is referred, even though it may not have been the primary reason for referral. In the initial stage of treatment the patient should be treated on the back of the lathe, putting his whole foot on the footplate. While treadling with the affected foot the dorsiflexion is mainly passive, but as the plantarflexors push down there is some reciprocal innervation to the dorsiflexors.

The patient should treadle with both affected and unaffected legs. When using the toe block (see 'adaptations') and treadling with the unaffected leg, the posterior and anterior tibials work on the ankle joint, while the long flexors exert the downward pressure on the toe block. It is important to keep the knee joint braced in the 'locked' position. This is a very strenuous activity to start with and should therefore be graded carefully to avoid excess stress.

Other uses:

1. Head injuries — to assess/treat balance, hand/eye coordination, noise tolerance and reaction to revolving machinery.

2. Back injuries — general strengthening up, working in the mid-range and building up resistance, provided that the pain level is carefully watched. Equal time should be spent treadling with each leg.

3. Hand injuries — later stages of treatment, for general toughening up, to improve grip and increase stability at the wrist. It can also be used to desensitise the stumps of amputated fingers when working with the tools, as they vibrate.

4. Lower limb amputees - providing a block hollowed out is used to keep the bottom of the pylon in position. Full extension of the knee should not be attempted as the pylon will lock. This activity will help to keep the other joints mobile.

Conditions treated with the lathe

(a). Fractures and dislocations of the acetabulum, slipped epiphysis, fractured neck of femur or greater trochanter: to increase stability of the hip joint and improve ROM and strength. Fractured shaft of femur, tibia and fibula, patella, condyles and tibial plateau: to reduce oedema, remove extension lag, increase stability of the knee joint and improve ROM and strength. Fractured malleoli, calcaneum, talus, ankle (Pott's fracture) and other bones of the foot: to reduce oedema, increase plantar and dorsiflexion and in/eversion. To improve general strength, walking pattern and ROM.

Note: Remember, if the patient has been on traction or in plaster, to check the joints above and below the affected joint, or the fractured site.

(b). Other orthopaedic conditions. Meniscestomy, lateral releases, chondromalacia, osteotomies, arthrotomies, removal of loose bodies, internal derangement of the knee and ruptured tendons (quadriceps and Achilles) — aims as above.

(c). Arthritic conditions, osteoarthrosis, knee replacements, OA hip, knee. Work in the mid-range gently, building up resistance gradually. The aim is to build up muscles as far as possible,

reducing pain and maintaining adequate function for independence. To prevent joint deformity and stimulate a good reciprocal walking pattern. (In some older patients this is contra-indicated as the movement can be too jerky.)

(d). Peripheral nerve lesions, especially of the common peroneal nerve: to help promote regeneration of nerve tissue, prevent muscle wasting/contractures, maintain full ROM and increase returning strength.

(e). Amputation of the lower limb once pylon or prosthesis is fitted: to maintain and improve balance and coordination of the lower limbs and encourage a good walking pattern. To strengthen muscles of both lower limbs and prevent flexion contractures of the hip joint. To increase ROM and maintain good circulation. For work assessment.

(f). Head injuries and conditions producing general weakness and incoordination: to increase general strength and ROM in lower limb. To improve balance, hand/eye coordination, concentration and noise tolerance, as well as tolerance to moving machinery. For work assessment.

(g). Spinal injuries, if there is partial lower limb function and/or weakness in the trunk: to strengthen the muscles of the lower limbs and the back extensors. To increase ROM and improve balance. To stimulate returning movement (sanding or wood turning).

Some patients may need to sit at the lathe, especially those with an extension lag, or partial paraplegia; in such cases a camden bicycle seat can be used. This then becomes a partial weight-bearing activity.

Points of use

1. *The Health and Safety at Work Act* of 1974 demands that all moving parts of machinery are guarded. Hence the belt on the lathe has a guard on later models.

2. *Suitable clothing* should be worn when patients use the lathe, preferably shorts and a T-shirt or a tracksuit. Footwear is also important — gym shoes or training shoes are safest as they usually have a rubber non-slip sole. When patients are using the back of the lathe, the shoe should be removed from the treadling foot, as more movement is gained with less compensation, and sup-

port from the shoe is eliminated. Long hair should be tied back and ties removed or tucked out of the way.

3. *Positioning*

(a). *Front* It is important to position the patient correctly on the lathe to gain maximum benefit from treatment.

(i) When treadling, the patient should put the ball of the foot on the treadle platform to prevent the knee hitting the base of the face bed on flexion. The push down required in this position is stronger than with the whole foot on the treadle and also uses gastrocnemius in addition to the quadriceps.

(ii) When using the foot extension plate, make sure the heel is right back in the guard, to help gain the range of movement required.

(iii) When not using the extension plate, place the standing leg as near the footplate as possible without hitting it on the down movement. If using the extension plate, keep the feet as parallel as possible.

(b). *Back*

(i) Keep the heel flat down on the footplate and as near the base of the footplate as possible, to gain maximum movement.

(ii) Keep the standing leg as near the treadle plate as possible.

4. *Posture*

(a). The patient should be encouraged to stand upright and to keep the standing leg braced back when treadling.

(b). The patient should not hold on to the lathe when treadling; this is to increase his balance and strengthen the standing leg. It is also to avoid touching moving parts.

(c). The therapist should be alert to compensatory movements, especially when the patient is using the lathe from the back. The patient should then be encouraged to push the treadle with his foot and not with the whole body.

(d). When setting up the machine the therapist must make sure that the patient is quite comfortable.

5. *Range of movement (ROM).* When the patient first uses the lathe, adjust this to gain the maximum ROM at that time. As the ROM increases the machine should be adjusted accordingly. Never set the machine beyond the patient's range.

6. *Upgrading.* ROM. and resistance can be increased in the following ways:
(a). Increase time
(b). Increase weight load
(c). Alter belt drive to harder pulley
(d). Tighten belt by belt adjusting hand wheel
(e). Start sanding, then turning
(f). ROM — front: use extension plate, alter pitman
(g). ROM — back: remove heel block, alter pitman.

7. *Charts.* Adjustments in the patients' treatment programme must be recorded. The quickest and most efficient way of doing this is to keep charts with the following information near the machine:
(a). Patient's name
(b). Front or back of the lathe
(c). Time (in minutes) for each leg is appropriate
(d). Footplate number, in/evertor block, large or small block, sling if used
(e). Resistance: A — E

It has been found that the use of charts is a great help in very busy departments. It also helps therapists covering for absences, and students to alter the machine for each patient quickly.

8. *Safety precautions*

(a). Patients who are sanding or wood-turning should be closely supervised. They should also be informed that goggles and aprons are available.

(b). Patients should be told about moving parts on the lathe before they start treadling and reminded each time they attend for treatment.

(c). Patients should be told that the injured limb may swell up and ache more than usual after the first treatment session, because they are unused to the increased activity. This should be checked prior to the next treatment session.

(d). The therapist should check that long hair is tied back, ties are removed and that the patient is not wearing clothes or jewellery which may become caught in the machinery.

9. *Maintenance.* Regular maintenance of equipment is essential for good and efficient running; especially when it is in heavy use. Checks such as nuts and bolts, tightening screws and oiling should be carried out weekly. Servicing by the manufacturer or through a planned hospital maintenance scheme should be carried out at least

once a year and more often if the equipment is under heavy use.

Adaptations

We have made several useful adaptations to the lathe at Ashford Hospital to enable us to make quick alterations when the department is busy.

1. The block. We have two blocks, one 2½in and the other 2in high. When a patient has limited knee flexion, a block is placed under the sound limb. Both blocks can be used together to obtain full knee extension with the pitman in the lowest position, should this be needed.

2. In/evertor block. This is a wedge shaped block which can be attached to the back of the lathe on the treadle plate by drilling two holes in the plate and attaching dowelling to the block to correspond with the holes in the treadle.

3. Plantar/dorsiflexion block. This again is a wedge shaped block of varying angles; it is attached to the treadle plate in the same way as the in/evertor block. It is used to prevent compensation and to keep the heel down on the treadle if the patient has a short achilles tendon.

4. Numbers on foot plate extension. This enables the therapist to put the foot plate in position quickly and accurately, provided the information is recorded on the appropriate charts.

5. Toe block. A toe block is used on both the front and back of the lathe. When standing on this, the patient is on tiptoe. It is used to strengthen gastrocnemius, to improve balance and to help improve the heel-toe gait.

6. Non slip surface on treadle. We have attached a sheet of rubber to the treadle to prevent the foot from slipping.

Possible activities

Sanding: bingo pieces, draughts men, solitaire sticks, quoits, rocker bases, bag handles, towel holder ends, and any other sanding activity provided the article is large enough to be held and sanded safely.

Turning: fruit bowls, table lamp bases, egg cups, salt and pepper pots, rolling pins, mug trees, candle stick holders, handles, round boxes.

Availability:
Tru-Eze Creasey and Co Ltd (Akron); Nottingham Medical Equipment Company.

10

Remedial games

A remedial game is an activity designed to treat a specific disability or problem while, at the same time, being amusing to use. Many of the games described in this chapter are well known, but have been adapted to be played in such a way as to give very specific treatment to a particular dysfunction.

In addition to using standard commercially produced games many occupational therapy departments make their own adaptations to traditional games or, indeed, invent new games in order to treat a wide variety of disabilities and this is an admirable exercise. However, the therapist must remember that any activity presented to a patient must be well made, professionally finished and, above all, must suit the purpose for which it has been designed. A remedial game which is broken, badly made and finished or clearly designed to be played with by an infant is an insult to an adult.

Eight of the more common remedial games are described in this chapter. There are very many more in use, but the therapist who can understand the basis of adapting a traditional game to suit a specific remedial purpose can use this knowledge to widen the selection of activities she has available.

SPAN GAME (FIG. 10.1)

Construction. The span game consists of a base board into which are set three vertical dowel rods. A series of discs is available which will easily slide over the rods. The full set of discs should vary in size from approximately 1½ in in diameter to 11 in

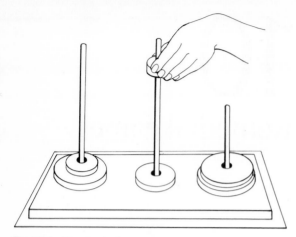

Fig. 10.1 The standard span game

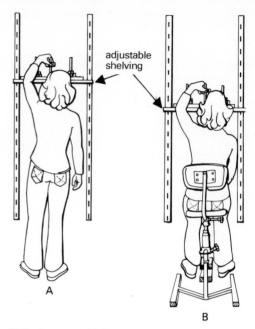

Fig. 10.2 Posture and balance. Span game set (A) to encourage good posture, back extension and standing balance (B) to encourage balance in the early stages of lower limb treatment

in diameter and in order to accommodate different span grips each disc should be approximately ½ in larger in diameter than the previous one.

Starting position. The board is placed on a table or shelf and secured by a dycem mat or clamps. The therapist chooses an appropriate series of five discs and these are placed over one of the end rods with the smallest disc at the top of the pile and the largest at the bottom. The game is for one player.

To play. The aim of the game is to transfer the discs from one end rod to the other so that they end as they start, with the largest disc at the bottom. Only one disc may be moved at a time and at no point during the game may a large disc be placed on a smaller one.

Source. A standard span game is available from 'Six to Twelve', PO Box 38, Northgates, Leicester (order: 'Tower of Brahma'). Adapted games are usually made as required.

Therapeutic value

The span game can be used to treat the following movements:

1. *Spinal extension (Fig. 10.2).* When the game is placed at eye level good posture, with back extension, is encouraged. The patient may be standing or seated. If balance is to be encouraged, for example following hip replacement or amputation of the lower limb, the patient can be seated on a bicycle stool in the early stages of treatment. Standing tolerance can be encouraged by gradually increasing the time spent standing at the acti-

vity. The therapist must take care when raising an activity such as this for use by elderly arthritic patients, as neck extension can lead to pressure on the vertebral arteries, if their cervical vertebrae are affected.

2. *Shoulder movement.* Elevation at the shoulder can be increased by raising the game relative to the position of the patient. As movement at the shoulder increases the game is raised higher. If a game is made in which the dowel rods are longer than average then a greater arc of movement is needed at the shoulder in order to remove the discs (Fig. 10.3A & B).

Abduction at the shoulder can be encouraged by placing the game to the side of the patient (Fig. 10.4).

3. *Elbow movement.* Elbow extension can be encouraged by placing the game in such a position that the elbow is extended to its maximum range when the patient lifts the disc off over the top of the rods. This can be achieved by either raising the board (see Fig. 10.2B), by using a board with extended rods (see Fig. 10.3B) or by placing the board further away from the patient when he is seated at a table.

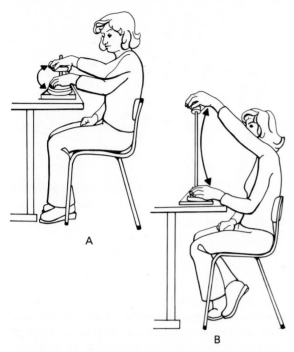

Fig. 10.3 Shoulder flexion. (A) Using a standard span game (B) Flexion is increased when the dowel rods are lengthened. (Note: the height of the board can still be altered according to the range of movement required)

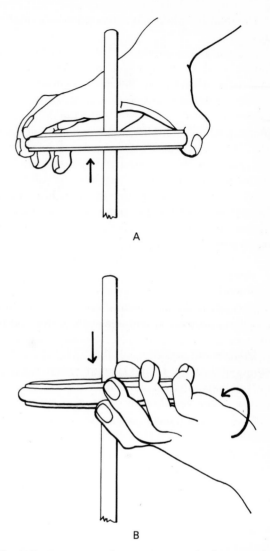

Fig. 10.5 To encourage forearm movement the disc is raised with the forearm in pronation (A) and replaced with the forearm in supination (B)

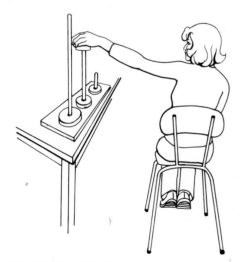

Fig. 10.4 Shoulder abduction

4. *Forearm movement.* Pronation and supination can be encouraged by asking the patient to pick up the discs with his forearm in pronation and to replace them with his arm in supination (Fig. 10.5).

5. *Wrist movement.* Wrist extension is encouraged when the game is placed on a low stool or table so that the patient must reach down to grasp the discs.

Wrist flexion is encouraged when the game is placed on a high shelf or when the game with extended rods is used. The wrist flexes as the patient grasps and raises the disc (see Fig. 10.3B).

6. *Thumb movement.* The carpometacarpal and metacarpophalangeal joints of the thumb are extended and the inter-phalangeal joint flexed when a large disc is used.

The thumb is abducted and opposed if a smaller disc is used.

7. *Finger movements.* The metacarpophalangeal and interphalangeal joints are flexed in mid-range when the smaller discs are used.

The metacarpophalangeal and proximal interphalangeal joints are extended and the distal interphalangeal joints are flexed when the larger discs are used. Span is also encouraged and the skin on the palmar surface of the hand is stretched. This particular movement is therefore useful when treating patients following an operation for a Dupuytren's contracture, burns or other injury to the palmar surface of the hand or of the injury to a distal interphalangeal joint.

Other conditions which can be treated include:

Incoordination. Upper limb coordination is encouraged during this activity as it is rhythmical and lightweight and the discs must be controlled while travelling up the rod and across from one rod to the other.

Upper limb weakness. If the game is used in conjunction with a sling support system such as the OB help arm then part of the weight of the limb can be supported thus allowing weak muscles to control its movement. Alternatively, the strong hand can be placed over the weak hand to help grasp and lift the disc. In this way bilateral upper limb movement can be encouraged. This is especially useful where extensor or release movements are to be encouraged, e.g. in patients suffering from hemiplegia.

Sensation. The appreciation of texture and pressure is encouraged while the disc is being held. The game can be played blindfold or by those with little or no sight.

SOLITAIRE (FIG. 10.6)

Construction. Solitaire consists of a square or round board on which a series of holes are made to conform with the pattern illustrated. A set of 'men' is supplied to fit into the holes. As its name implies, the game is played by one player.

Starting position. The game is usually played with the player seated at a table. However, if suitably constructed, it can be elevated either on its own stand (Fig. 10.7A) or on a wall mounted

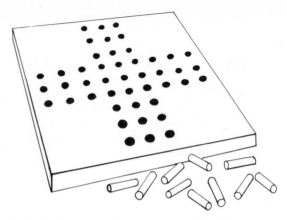

Fig. 10.6 The layout of the solitaire game. (Note: on some boards the outer line of holes is omitted)

bracket (Fig. 10.7B). A man is put into each hole except the central one.

To play. The aim of the game is to eliminate all but one of the men from the board and this final man should be left in the central hole. Men are eliminated by being jumped over as shown in Figure 10.8. A man can only jump one piece at a time and moves can be made vertically or horizontally. When a piece has been jumped it is taken off the board.

Source. The game is available commercially through sports shops or department stores. Adapted games are usually made as required in the department.

Therapeutic value

Solitaire can be used to treat the following movements:

1. *Spinal movements*

(a). *Extension.* This is achieved using a large, wall mounted game placed so that the top line of men is level with the highest point the patient can reach. The patient can stand or sit on a stool or bicycle seat. This latter method also encourages balance and partial weight bearing in the early stages of lower limb treatment.

(b). *Rotation.* The game is wall mounted at eye level with the patient standing or seated on a stool or bicycle seat. When a man has been removed from the board the patient twists and places it in a box behind him. If the hands are used alternately to remove the men the patient can be encouraged

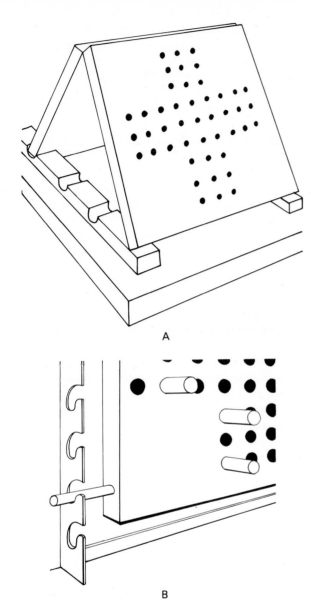

Fig. 10.7 The board adapted for (A) elevated use on table top (B) wall mounting on a slotted bracket

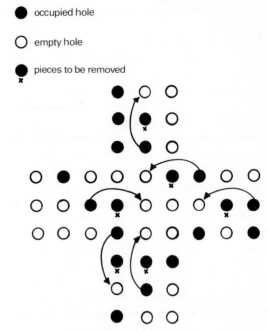

● occupied hole

○ empty hole

● pieces to be removed
✗

Fig. 10.8 To play solitaire, moves are made as indicated by the arrows. Diagonal moves are not permitted

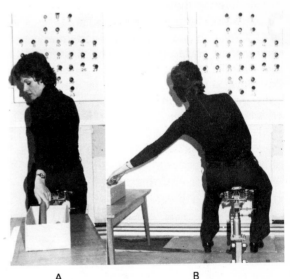

Fig. 10.9 Wall-mounted solitaire to encourage (A) spinal rotation (B) spinal side flexion

to twist first to one side and then the other (Fig. 10.9A). This can also be done with the game on a table top and the patient seated on a stool or bicycle seat.

(c). *Side flexion*. Again, the game is wall mounted at eye level with the patient standing or seated on a stool or bicycle seat. Alternatively it can be placed on a table. When a man has been removed from the board the patient leans over to the side to place it in a box beside him. As before,

if alternate hands are used then flexion to both sides can be encouraged (Fig. 10.9B).

2. *Shoulder movements*

(a). *Forward flexion*. This is achieved by placing the game on a table so that in order to reach the row of men furthest away from him, the patient must use maximal forward flexion.

(b). *Abduction*. The game is wall mounted or placed on a table and the patient is seated sideways to it so that when reaching for the men his greatest range of abduction is used (see Fig. 10.4).

(c). *Extension*. The game is wall mounted or placed on a table and the patient faces the game. When a man has been removed from the board the patient reaches behind him and – without twisting his spine – places the piece in a box behind him.

(d). *Medial and lateral rotation*. The game is wall mounted and the patient may sit or stand. When a man is removed from the board with one hand the player passes it behind his neck (lateral rotation) or behind his waist (medial rotation) to the other hand. It is then placed in a box.

(e). *Elevation*. The game is wall mounted and placed so that in order to reach the highest row of men the player is required to use his fullest range of elevation. The patient may stand or sit.

3. *Elbow movement*. The board is placed flat on the table in such a position that the furthest row of men requires the patient to extend his elbow as far as possible in order to move them.

4. *Pronation and supination*. A game in which the men are made of discs which fit over rods is required (Fig. 10.10). The men are picked up with the player's forearm in pronation and replaced with the forearm in supination — see Figure 10.5.

5. *Wrist movement*. To treat wrist extension a

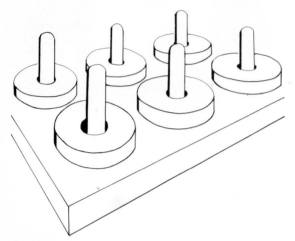

Fig. 10.10   Disc-shaped 'men' and peg design

board in which holes are drilled to take peg shaped men is required. The holes and pegs should be far enough apart to allow the hand to be placed between them. The game is played with the men held as illustrated (Fig. 10.11A).

Wrist flexion can be treated by using the board with disc-shaped men as shown in Figure 10.10, and placing it at eye level so that the patient has to reach up for the discs (see Fig. 10.2).

6. *Thumb movement*

(a). *Opposition* is treated using a board with peg-shaped men. These are held as illustrated in Figure 10.11B. Note: In the early stages of treating thumb opposition wide pegs are required. The pegs can be held between the thumb and furthest finger tip possible if the grip illustrated cannot yet be achieved.

(b). *Adduction* is treated using a board with peg-shaped men. The men are held between the straight thumb and second metacarpophalangeal joint.

(c). *Flexion* is treated using a board with peg-shaped men. The men are held as illustrated in Figure 10.11C. Again, in the early stages of treatment wider pegs can be used, progresssing to smaller ones as thumb movement improves. Note: Some people, especially those with short or large thumbs, may find this movement difficult to perform normally. Their ability should be checked by asking them to perform the movement with the unaffected thumb where appropriate.

7. *Finger movement*

(a). *Metacarpophalangeal flexion* is treated by asking the patient to hold the peg-shaped men as shown in Figure 10.11A. Again, in the early stages of treatment, wide pegs are used, progressing to thinner ones as the movement increases.

(b). *Interphalangeal flexion*. To treat this a board with men shaped as in Figure 10.12 is needed. The men can be made by gluing two discs together or, for preference, with the two discs left unjoined so that the size of the top disc can be altered to suit the size of the player's hand and the bottom disc can be changed to suit the amount of flexion he has. The discs are held as illustrated. Note: If only the distal interphalangeal joints are to be treated the disc will need to be enlarged so that these are the joints mainly concerned with grasping. The lower disc would not then be necessary.

Metacarpophalangeal and interphalangeal flexion can be treated together by using tall, peg-shaped men (see Fig. 10.11) which are held in a cylinder grip.

(c). *Adduction.* This can be treated by asking the patient to grasp the peg-shaped men between the two fingers to be treated as shown in Figure 10.11D.

(d). *Metacarpophalangeal and interphalangeal extension* can be treated by using a board and men constructed as shown in Figure 10.13.

Other conditions which can be treated include:

Incoordination. Upper limb coordination is encouraged by using this activity in most of its forms, as the limb has to be positioned and controlled while grip and release actions are performed.

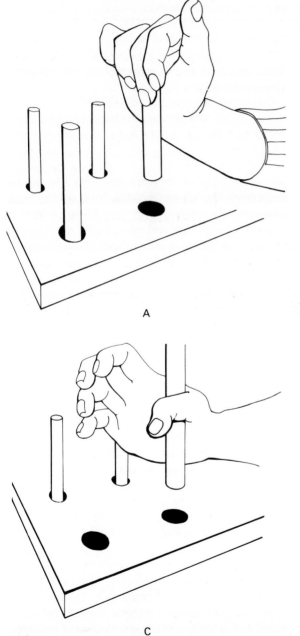

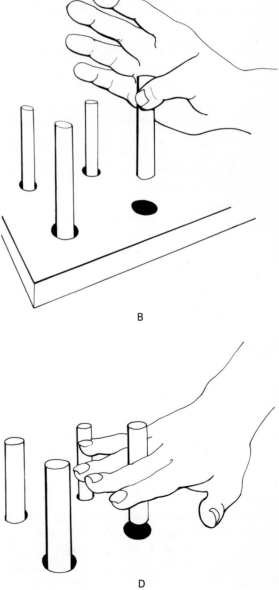

Fig. 10.11 Peg-shaped men held to treat (A) wrist extension (B) thumb opposition (C) thumb flexion (D) finger adduction

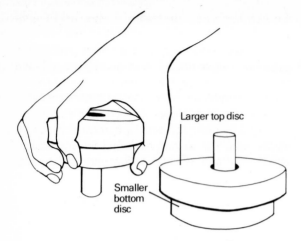

Fig. 10.12 Two disc-shaped men held to treat interphalangeal flexion

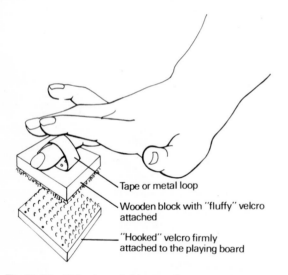

Fig. 10.13 'Velcro' men held to treat finger extension

Where coordination is poor a large board with large peg-shaped men which fit securely in position is preferable, as these will not be knocked across the board if touched accidentally. For finer finger coordination a board with small pin shaped men can be used, or one in which the men are made from dressmakers pins and the board of a material such as plastazote.

Upper limb weakness. A large table top board in conjunction with a sling support system can be employed to treat upper limb weakness. Initially, when the limb and grip are weak, the men should be large and lightweight so that they are easy to lift

handle (Balsa wood blocks or empty painted containers may be used, for example). They can be lifted bilaterally if required. For those whose strength is improving resistance can be increased in several ways. The following have been found successful:

Painted containers filled with sand, lead weights or similar heavy materials.

Wooden blocks with 'fluffy' velcro attached to the base. The 'hooked' velcro is attached to the playing positions on the board so that the player must pull against the resistance of the velcro to release the men.

Magnetic men on a metal board.

Pinch grip and opposition. These can be treated by using a board on which the men are made of clothes pegs or bulldog clips which slip onto pegs on the board secured in the playing pattern. A series of clips of different strengths should be available. The player is asked to grasp the men between the thumb and whichever finger is appropriate for his particular disability. Note: In the early stages of treatment standard peg-shaped men, which offer little resistance, can be used.

Mental processes. Concentration, perseverance and patience are encouraged with this game. If the positions are numbered and instructions written down, the therapist can also assess the patient's ability to follow instructions.

DRAUGHTS — (FIG. 10.14)

Construction. The draughts game consists of a checkered board of 64 squares and two sets of twelve men, each set of a different colour. The game is played by two people.

Starting position. The game is usually played on a table, but may be constructed to be played in elevation (see Fig. 10.7). The men are laid on the board as shown in Figure 10.14.

To play. The aim of the game is for each player to eliminate his opponent's men from the board. A piece is eliminated when it is 'jumped' by an opponent's man as illustrated in Figure 10.15. Moves and jumps can only be made diagonally, either to the right or to the left. When not jumping, moves are made diagonally, one square at a time, until a position is reached where an opponent's

for instance where the men are made deliberately large for easy handling by a weak player, the men can be painted two colours as illustrated in Fig. 10.16 so that when a king is gained, the piece is inverted) A king has the added advantage of being able to move either forwards or backwards, one square at a time unless 'jumping'. If a quicker game is needed, e.g. for children or the elderly, then a game of 'Fox and Hounds' can be played. In this, one black piece (the fox), which can move in

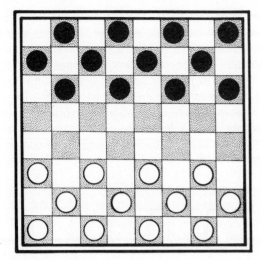

Fig. 10.14   Draughts games ready to play

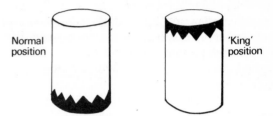

Fig. 10.16   Larger, lightweight men can be adapted to be inverted when a 'king' is claimed

any direction, attempts to escape from five white pieces (the hounds), which can only move forwards from one end (the field) to the other (the foxhole) and can be 'taken' by the fox as before.

Source. Standard draughts games can be bought from toy shops, sports and games shops or department stores. Adapted draughts games are usually made as required. An adapted set of disc draughts with a peg board is available from 'Four to Eight', PO Box 38, Northgates, Leicester.

Therapeutic value

The draughts board and men can be adapted to treat the same movements and conditions as solitaire. Additionally, because it is played by two players, the game provides:

Social interaction. This can be used to help the speech, concentration or the speed of the patient's play. For if the therapist plays as his opponent she can control the game in such a way that she demands conversation, perseverance or quick reactions from the patient.

Draughts is a universally known and socially acceptable game and this can be used to advantage. For instance, for the elderly patient who finds interaction with others difficult playing draughts may be a means to encourage communication. It

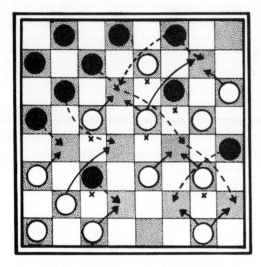

→ Moves which can be made by the white men

– – ◆ Moves which can be made by the coloured men

✗   Pieces which may be eliminated

Fig. 10.15   Possible moves. (Note: a *series* of 'jumps' can be made)

piece can be jumped and therefore eliminated. Players move alternately, one move at a time.

Should a player's man reach a square on the line at the far side of the board he can claim a king. This is usually denoted by stacking two men on top of each other. (Note: Where this is not practical,

may also help the therapist or relative to relate to the patient. Other board games as well as draughts should always be available on a ward or in a day room so that spontaneous games can be initiated by patients themselves. Adapted board games, such as draughts or solitaire, may also be given to a patient on the ward or at home so that specific treatment can be continued at times other than those spent in the department.

An element of competition. For some people a game involving competition (against another player rather than the game itself) can often help concentration. Board games such as draughts have the advantage that, provided they are not disturbed, they can be left and restarted should concentration fail.

Draughts, like solitaire, can also help to encourage concentration, perseverance and patience.

DOMINOES

Construction. The standard game consists of a set of 28 rectangular pieces each approximately 5 cm × 2 cm × 1 cm. The playing face of each piece is divided in two and marked with a number of dots as shown in Figure 10.17. The game is normally played by two, three or four players.

Starting position. The players sit round a table and each player is dealt seven dominoes face downwards. These he arranges so that the playing face is towards him.

To play. The aim of the game is for each person to play all his pieces as soon as possible so that he is left with none in front of him. Play begins with the person who has the highest 'double' piece placing it on the table (that is the double six double

five or double four). The player to the left of the starter then has to place one of his pieces next to the starting piece in such a way that the touching numbers match. Play then continues round the circle in this manner until the first person to play all his pieces is declared the winner. If a person cannot match one of his numbers to one of the end numbers in the central line, he must pass and miss a turn. An example of play in progress is shown in Figure 10.18.

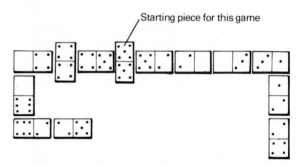

Fig. 10.18 A game in progress. The score for the last move is 3 (5+4=9; 9÷3=3). The next player must match either the 5 or the 4

Interest can be added to the game by scoring. If the sum of the two end numbers is divisible by three or five then the number of times it is divisible is counted as a score for that player.

Sources. Standard dominoes can be bought from toy, games or department stores. Adapted dominoes are available from:

1. Reeves Dryad, PO Box 38, Northgates, Leicester. Their 'Six to Twelve' catalogue includes geometric dominoes and several similar games which require skill in matching shapes and/or colour. Their 'Four to Eight' catalogue includes junior (picture) dominoes, number dominoes (the numbers are represented by pictures of groups of objects), Hexadoms (a form of six sided dominoes), Triple dominoes (a set containing picture, colour and number dominoes) and several other similar games which involve matching.

2. Large wooden dominoes, colour dominoes, picture dominoes and Domi-numbers are available from the Galt Early Stages catalogue, James Galt & Co Ltd, Brookfield Road, Cheadle, Cheshire. Galt also produces several similar games such as 'Triple Triangles', 'Connect' and 'Fizzog' which involve matching.

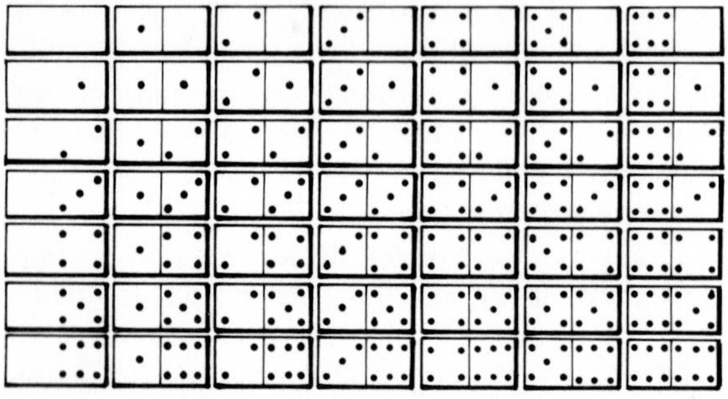

Fig. 10.17 The pieces of a dominoes set

3. Colour, picture and traditional dominoes are available from Nomeq Ltd, Melton Road, West Bridgford, Nottinghamshire.

4. Shape and picture dominoes are available from 'Learning Development Aids', Aware House, Duke Street, Wisbech, Cambs PE13 2AE.

Therapeutic value

Dominoes can be used to treat the following:

1. *Light grip and release.* Standard or slightly large dominoes are useful when treating those who have a weak grip or poor release.

2. *Incoordination.* Upper limb coordination is necessary for handling, standing and placing the dominoes. In the early stages of treatment when coordination is poor, larger dominoes will be easier to handle. A stand to hold the pieces in front of each player, as well as a backing such as felt, pimple rubber or Dycem on each piece will help prevent the dominoes from being knocked out of place. Weak limbs can be supported in a sling support system.

3. *Perception.* Depending on the design of the dominoes the game can be used to help those who have difficulty identifying the following:

Number: Dominoes with either the written number or dotted numbers on their playing face will help.

Colour: Dominoes with colour coding on the playing face are necessary.

Shape: Dominoes with various geometric shapes on the playing face can be used.

Objects: Dominoes on which the playing face denotes object outlines can be made or bought.

Picture: Picture dominoes are available commercially or can be made. They are especially useful in treating those with figure background problems.

Note: A combination of the above types may be used, for example shape and colour can be combined, as can object and colour or shape and number symbols (Fig. 10.19). For those with reading difficulties the word describing the object, picture, number, colour or shape may be added if required.

4. *Sensation.* Dominoes with different textures or raised shapes on the playing face can be bought or made. If made, these are best constructed in a

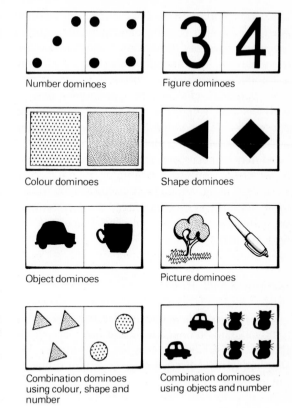

Number dominoes

Figure dominoes

Colour dominoes

Shape dominoes

Object dominoes

Picture dominoes

Combination dominoes using colour, shape and number

Combination dominoes using objects and number

Fig. 10.19 Dominoes adapted to help visual stimulus and recognition

'bridge' form so that there is no chance of visual stimulation clouding the sensory input (Fig. 10.20). If the dominoes are flat, however, then the players must be blindfold. Note: If the therapist is making her own sensation dominoes to help re-educate the patient in texture appreciation she should ensure that the various textures used have a wide *tactile* and not *visual* variation. For example, combinations of sandpaper, velvet and plastic are easier to distinguish with lowered sensation than needlecord, velvet and denim.

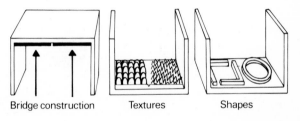

Bridge construction   Textures   Shapes

Fig. 10.20 Sensation dominoes

5. *Mental processes.* Speech can be encouraged, along with patience and perseverance, as the game involves the social contact of two or more players. If number dominoes are used simple arithmetic is required for scoring.

6. *Balance and standing or sitting tolerance.* As with any table game, balance and standing can be encouraged if the game is placed on a standing table. For those with poor balance a pelvic support band may be necessary. For those who are partially weight bearing and beginning to balance or stand again (e.g. after a back or lower limb injury) these actions can be encouraged if the patient sits on a bicycle stool with both feet placed on the floor while playing.

POST BOX (FIG. 10.21)

Construction. The game consists of a box with a removable lid, into which various holes of specific shapes are drilled. A number of counters are supplied which correspond to the shapes drilled in the lid.

Starting position. The box, with the lid in place, is positioned on a table top in front of the player. The counters are spread out around the table.

To play. The aim of the game is to 'post' the counters through the hole of a corresponding shape in the lid. The counters will not pass through a hole whose shape does not correspond to the cross-section of the counter.

Source. Post boxes of various designs are available from toy shops and department stores. The therapist must remember that a toy which looks too childish, is covered with nursery pictures or boldly states 'For 1–3 years' will be inappropriate for adults. Post boxes of painted or varnished wood are available from 'Four to Eight', PO Box 38, Northgates, Leicester. Their versions are referred to as 'Sorting Boxes Set' and 'Quantibox'. Other games involving shape recognition are also available from this and other catalogues already mentioned.

Therapeutic value

The post box can be used in a number of ways and can help with the following:

1. *Shape recognition.* The player must recognise the relationship between the holes in the lid and the cross-section of the counters. They are then matched by being posted into the box. Alternately, with the counters placed at random around

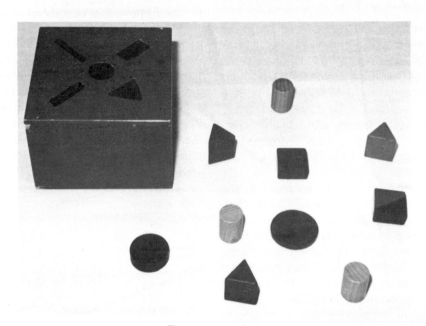

Fig. 10.21 Post box

the table, the therapist asks the patient to 'post' all the triangular counters through the appropriate hole.

2. *Colour recognition.* Using a set with differently coloured counters the player is asked to 'post' the yellow counters.

3. *Upper limb coordination.* Coordination and manual dexterity are required for, lift, manipulate and post the counters.

4. *Upper limb weakness.* As this is a lightweight activity it can be used to treat those with upper limb weakness. A sling support mechanism can be used in the early stages. The game is especially useful for treating those for whom grip and release is a particular problem. The range of movement can be controlled by placing the counters close to or far away from the patient or to his left or right. Counters placed far away from the player will encourage shoulder flexion and abduction and elbow extension. Shoulder adduction and elbow flexion movements are required for posting if the box is placed directly in front of the patient. Similarly, upper limb movement can be controlled by placing the box in a variety of positions.

5. *Figure ground discrimination.* The post box can be used to help encourage normal perceptual patterns. The box and counters should be placed against a plain, non-reflective background. In the early stages the player is asked to distinguish one shape from a small group of two or three. (Note: Ideally the shape should all be of the same colour so that this stronger visual stimulus does not cloud shape discrimination). Later he is asked to distinguish the appropriate hole from others in the lid and 'post' the counter.

6. *Hemianopia.* With the box placed centrally and the counters spread in a wide semicircle around the table the player is asked to select counters from various points in the circle (see Chapter 19).

NOUGHTS AND CROSSES (FIG. 10.22A)

Construction. Noughts and crosses is traditionally played by two players using paper and pencil. However, many sets are now available commercially or can be constructed for specific treatment.

Starting position. A grid is laid out as illustrated.

Each player is given a pen with which to draw his symbol on the paper, or is provided with a set of symbols to place within the grid.

To play. Each player adopts either the noughts or crosses symbol. The aim of the game is for each player to complete a line of three of his symbols vertically, horizontally or diagonally across the grid before being stopped by his opponent placing one of his symbols in the way. Players make alternate moves (Fig. 10.22B).

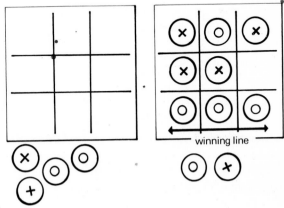

Fig. 10.22 A noughts and crosses grid and counters (left). Each player requires five counters. Game in progress (right)

Sources. Noughts and crosses can be played wherever there is a flat surface and a means of marking it. For example on a blackboard, in a sandpit, using paints on paper or chalk on the floor or drawing on an outdoor surface.

Games of noughts and crosses are available commercially from toy, games and department stores. They are also available in various forms from:

'Four to Eight', PO Box 38, Northgates, Leicester. This firm offers a wooden pegged board with wooden disc or cross-shaped counters.

Galt Early Stages, James Galt & Co Ltd, Brookfield Road, Cheadle, Cheshire. This firm produces a set of three dimensional noughts and crosses.

Therapeutic value

The various forms of noughts and crosses can be adapted to treat a wide range of disabilities:

1. *Upper limb disabilities.* For shoulder, elbow,

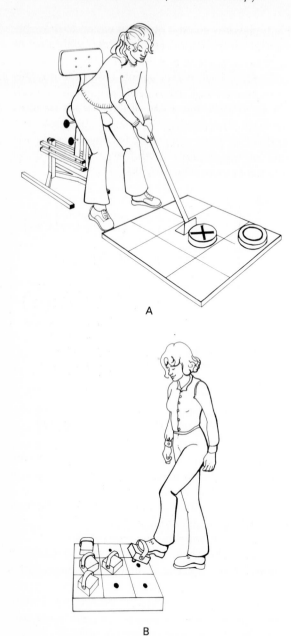

A

B

Fig. 10.23 Treating balance in (A) early stages (B) later stages

either stands supported (for example by his walking aids) or sits on a bicycle stool with some weight taken equally through both feet. The game is played using large counters which the patient pushes into position on the grid using a long-handled pusher (Fig. 10.23A). As balance improves the player stands unsupported. In the final stages of treatment the player stands unsupported and uses counters with toe loops attached which he hooks over his foot and places on the grid while balancing on one foot. (Fig. 10.23B). The game may also be played whilst kneeling or crouching.

(b). *Ankle and foot movements.* To treat inversion the player sits on a bicycle stool and picks up large, cylindrical counters between the soles of his feet and places them on the floor grid. To treat dorsiflexion the counters with toe loops can be used. As strength in the dorsiflexors improves resistance can be increased by adding weights to the counters. Note: If counters are to be used in this way they should be constructed in a box shape so that the weights can be securely placed inside (Fig. 10.24).

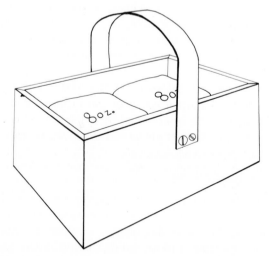

Fig. 10.24 A box-shaped counter with toe loop to take weights

forearm, wrist, hand as well as spinal disabilities the noughts and crosses game can be constructed and used in the same way as solitaire. See also Chapter 28.

2. *Lower limb disabilities.* With a large grid drawn on the floor, noughts and crosses can be used to treat the lower limb in the following ways:

(a). *Balance.* In the early stages the patient

3. *Mental processes.* This game, like the others, aids social contact because it is played by two people. Similarly, concentration can be encouraged, especially if three dimensional noughts and crosses is played, as this is a longer game and involves more possible moves.

4. *Writing.* Noughts and crosses is a useful percursor to writing practice if played with pen

and paper or on a blackboard, as the player has to hold the writing implement and draw simple figures with it.

TABLE FOOTBALL

This game is available in many forms. Two of the commoner types are described.

Puff football (Fig. 10.25)

Construction. The game consists of an edged, rectangular base board with a goal at each end, a small, lightweight ball (such as a ping pong ball) and two 'puffers'. These are circular or cylindrical containers with a nozzle through which air is forced when the puffer is pressed. Puffers can be of a variety of sizes, and slip tracers, empty detergent bottles or similar articles can be used.

Starting position. The board is put on the table and the ball is placed in the centre. The players stand one at either end of the board and each is given a 'puffer'. Note: With a large board four or six players may participate.

To play. The aim of the game is for each player or team to score a goal by puffing the ball through his goal which is at the opposite end of the board from his starting position.

Source. Puff football does not appear to be commercially available, although the base board of a blow football game can be used if required.

Therapeutic value

Puff football can be used to treat the following:

1. *Power grip and release.* As the game requires the player to continually press and release the puffer in order to move the ball it is excellent for increasing grip strength following upper limb or hand dysfunction such as a Colles fracture or nerve lesion. The therapist must remember, however, that the action is extremely tiring and therefore should initially be used for short periods only.

2. *Balance and standing tolerance.* If the game is played on a table of waist height the patient will need to stand. Initially his balance can be aided by perching on a bicycle seat or by the support of a pelvic band (Fig. 10.25B). Later he stands un-

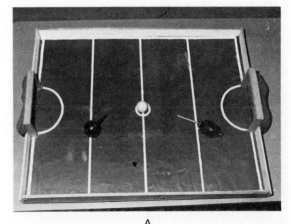

A

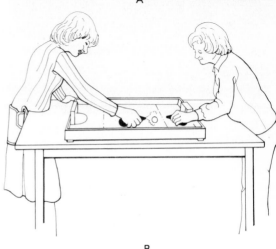

B

Fig. 10.25 (A) Puff football (B) Game being used to treat a patient with poor balance and/or weak lower limbs. A firm pelvic band supports her

aided. As his balance and mobility improve a larger board can be used which will require him to move around in order to reach the far end.

3. *Shoulder and elbow movement.* A combination of shoulder and elbow movements will be required in order to follow the ball around the board. The larger the board the more movement will be required.

Table football

Construction. A base board similar to the one described above is used. However, to move the ball several rows of players are suspended just above the table top in such a position that, when

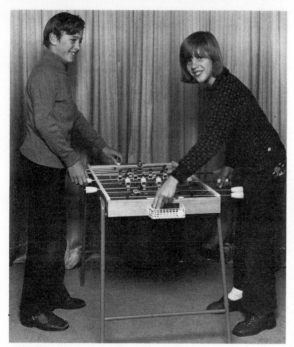

Fig. 10.26 Table football (photograph by kind permission of TP Activity Toys)

tinually grip and release with both hands in order to turn the controls and change from one control to another. Additionally, upper limb coordination is required to perform this action. If disc shaped controls are used a span grip with wrist extension and digital interphalangeal flexion is required. If cylinder shaped controls are used a power or cylinder grip is required.

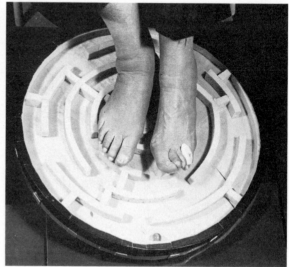

Fig. 10.27A Wobble board footmaze

swung from side to side using the controls on the side of the board, they are able to kick the ball (Fig. 10.26).

Starting position. Each player (or team of players if the board is large enough) stands along one side of the board so that he can control the handles which move his team of players.

To play. As above, the aim is to score goals by pushing the ball between the goal posts.

Sources. Table football games are available from toy, games and department stores.

Therapeutic value

1. *Shoulder movement.* Abduction and adduction at the shoulder are required to reach the controls along the side of the board.

2. *Elbow movement.* Flexion and extension of the elbow are required to reach the controls.

3. *Forearm movement.* Pronation and supination are especially treated if disc shaped controls are used. A combination of forearm and wrist movement is used if cylinder shaped controls are used.

4. *Grip and release.* The player has to con-

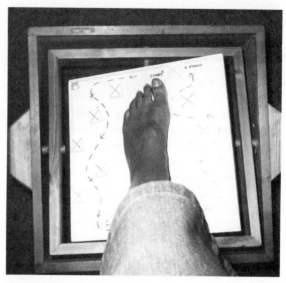

Fig. 10.27B Double-hinged footmaze

5. *Spinal movements and balance.* Spinal side flexion and balance are required when reaching sideways to the far controls.

FOOTMAZE

Construction. The game described is of a circular maze with a ball which runs between the grooves of the maze (Fig. 10.27). The maze board is mounted on a hemisphere. The maze is covered with a perspex sheet on which the player's foot or feet are placed. Different designs of the footmaze have been constructed including the double hinged variety shown in Figure 10.27B. The advantage of the design in Figure 10.27A, however, is that it will take the weight of the player, who can therefore stand on it and that both feet can be used together so that the weak foot can be assisted by the stronger one.

Starting position. The player places one or both feet on the perspex board.

To play. The aim of the game is to move the board in such a way that the ball bearing travels from its starting position in the outer ring through to the centre of the maze.

Source. The games described can both be made in an occupational therapy department.

Therapeutic value

1. *Ankle and foot movements.* A combination of dorsiflexion, plantarflexion, inversion and eversion are needed to move and control the board. In the early stages of treatment, if only one ankle or foot is affected, the player can use both feet together so that the weaker one is assisted by the stronger one. As treatment progresses the board can be controlled by the affected foot alone.

2. *Balance.* In the early stages of treatment the player can use the board with one or both feet while perching on a bicycle seat. Later he can progress to standing on one foot and moving the board with the other. In the final stages of treatment the patient stands on the board and uses the movement and balance of both lower limbs to control the board (Fig. 10.28).

As can be seen there is a wide variety of both traditional and especially created games which

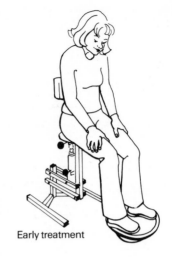

Early treatment

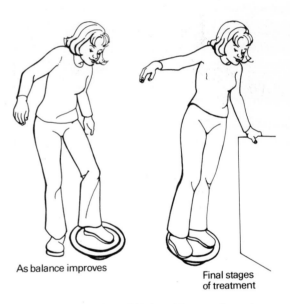

As balance improves

Final stages of treatment

Fig. 10.28 Use of the wobble board footmaze in treating balance. (Note: the player starts by standing on her strong leg and controlling with the weak leg. Later she stands on the weak leg)

can be used for specific remedial purposes. Many games are available commercially, particularly from firms specialising in activity toys for children with learning difficulties and these can be used to help patients with physical, perceptual and social problems. However, having seen how a game can be produced to suit a particular purpose the therapist should be able to adapt and construct a remedial game herself.

11

Splinting techniques

INTRODUCTION

A splint is a device supporting or increasing the function of part of the body. The term orthosis is now commonly used synonymously with the term splint, the production of orthoses being termed orthotics.

Some occupational therapists are involved daily in the production of splints, or orthoses, especially those working in specialised units, e.g. dealing with hand injuries. Opportunities to specialise in this way are certainly available but are still rare. Many more occupational therapists construct splints as part of their normal treatment process. An elderly lady, for example, with multiple problems requiring the occupational therapist's help in activities of daily living, may find lightweight purpose-made slippers temporarily helpful while her foot ulcers heal. A young male road traffic accident victim may require specific treatment for lower limb injuries in occupational therapy and a lively (dynamic) splint for his multiple hand injuries.

The reader will come across the terms 'static' or 'passive' splints, which usually have no moving parts and immobilise or rest a joint or limb; and 'dynamic' or 'lively' splints, which often have movable parts and allow controlled movement. The terms are sometimes misused, so should be used with care.

In most physical fields, the occupational therapist needs to have a knowledge of basic splinting principles, although these will continually need updating as new materials and techniques develop. Keeping up to date is difficult, but reading books, journals and medical articles, talking to manufacturers and other occupational therapists in similar units and, of course, experimentation will all help. Do not be afraid of asking around to see if someone else has solved your problem already; many occupational therapists spend hours wrestling with a tricky splintage problem only to find others have had similar problems and solved them! A special interest group of occupational therapists interested in orthotics and prosthetics (artificial limbs) meet to exchange information and report their meetings in the British Journal of Occupational Therapy.

Splinting is not just the province of an occupational therapist. She may work closely with orthotists, technicians, plaster room sisters, physiotherapists and others, all with their own knowledge of the subject and learning from each other. Some occupational therapists feel that they are in a unique position, having a specialised knowledge of function in daily living and the practical skills and facilities to manufacture splints, and in some hospitals this is indeed the case. In some hospitals the physiotherapists always manufacture the splints; if the occupational therapy department is small and demands on it are great, this may be the most practicable working policy. In other hospitals each profession specialises in a certain material, for example physiotherapists work with plaster of Paris and occupational therapists with thermoplastics. What is most important is that if a patient needs a splint, he or she is provided efficiently and speedily with one that is both functional and physiologically sound.

This chapter is intended as a very basic introduction and obviously needs to be used in conjunction with the learning of functional anatomy, and work on practical skills.

PRINCIPLES

Normal function

This chapter cannot possibly cover all the necessary aspects of functional anatomy. The reader must use knowledge gained while studying anatomy and physiology and supplement it with fur-

ther reading. For hand splinting, for example, the manuals on dynamic and static hand splinting by Malick (1972, 74), *The Hand* by Nathalie Barr (1975) and Lynn Cheshire's chapter in *An Approach to Occupational Therapy* (1977) would be useful. Observation of the hand in normal function is also invaluable. Try, for instance, observing the hands of people in a bus queue, of cyclists, a group of builders on a site, or a shopkeeper weighing goods and counting change.

When observing hand function, the following points may be noted:

Normal use of hand

Range of movement in the hand, at the wrist and through the whole arm

Types of grip

Signs of restricted function due to problems arising elsewhere

Skin condition, i.e. signs of exposure to water, chemicals or extreme heat

Shape of hand

Splint design for the hand should take into account:

1. optimum functional position (Fig. 11.1)

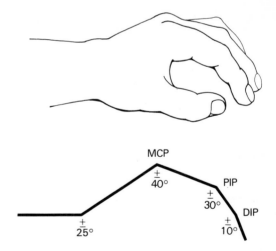

Thumb—CMC abducted and slightly opposed
MP ± 10° flexion
IP ± 5° flexion

Fig. 11.1 Functional hand position

2. hand creases
3. arches of the hand
4. axes of movement

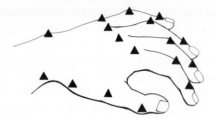

Fig. 11.2 Potential pressure points, i.e. bony prominences

5. pressure points/bony prominences (Fig. 11.2)
6. areas of increased or reduced sensation
7. any abnormality in surface anatomy, i.e. deformity
8. any undesired movement.

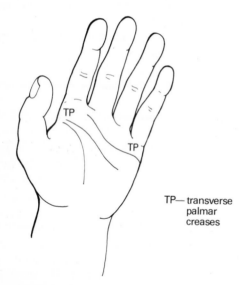

TP—transverse palmar creases

Fig. 11.3 Palmar creases

Hand creases (Fig. 11.3) show how the hand is used. The transverse palmar creases and those around the thenar eminence are particularly useful when pattern making. Try a splint that fits badly in these areas and note how your function is impaired.

The palmar arch (Fig. 11.4) has a marked curvature. Try flattening the palmar arch and note the effect on function. A 'triangle' can also be noted in the functional position; try watching the triangle in different positions, e.g. when writing and eating.

Try following each bone in turn as it moves through an arc or line of movement (Fig. 11.5).

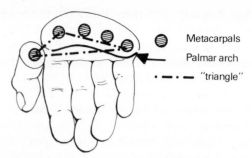

Metacarpals
Palmar arch
— · — · — "triangle"

Fig. 11.4 Diagrammatic cross-section of the hand

The resulting 'lines' of movement are very complex, especially around the thumb joint.

The same principles apply to all areas of the body which may require splintage. At the neck, for example, which is sometimes provided with a 'collar' splint, note functional positions during eating, dressing or writing, pressure points and bony prominences, directions and fulcrums of movement, any surface abnormalities and any movements to be restricted.

It can be seen, therefore, that use of anatomical knowledge, combined with accurate observation and measurement where necessary, is of considerable help in splint design where function is of prime importance.

Mechanics of splintage

Biomechanics is the application of mechanical principles to the human body. Some university

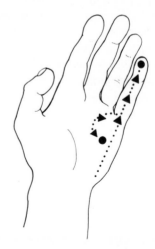

Fig. 11.5 Lines of movement

medical departments now specialise in this field, and may be able to help or advise the occupational therapist with more complex mechanical splintage problems.

Ignoring mechanical principles when producing a splint may result in a very good looking splint, but one which is not fulfilling its purpose. Some occupational therapists feel that a thorough knowledge of relevant biomechanics is necessary before lively (dynamic) splints are attempted; postgraduate courses and reading can help with this. Whilst this is particularly important for splints with moving parts, simple mechanical principles also apply to the static splint. The reader may already have some knowledge of mechanics, so it is hoped that the following may help relate its application to splint construction.

Force. Force may produce movement, for example when weak muscles are assisted by a carefully positioned spring on a lively splint; it may change or distort, for example when the elastic material of a pressure garment is placed on top of a burns scar which flattens; or it may produce strain or stretch, for example using a splint to gradually correct a deformity, regularly altering the splint to allow it to maintain a stretch on the soft tissues thus increasing joint range (serial splinting).

Pressure. This is the force applied to a certain area, often measured in pounds per square inch or kilogrammes per square centimetre. This can be critical. In a splint to correct deformity, for example, the pressure exerted by the splint has to be slightly higher than the pressure exerted by the deformity itself. If it is too high different problems may arise. Too much pressure over a body prominence, for example, may cause ischaemia or skin breakdown. Pressure throughout even a simple static splint is crucial to the success of the treatment.

Gravity. Gravity is the force by which objects tend to move towards the centre of the earth. Particular care is needed when the centre of gravity, i.e. the point about which all parts equally balance, has been altered, e.g. by amputation or severe muscle wasting. Splints need to provide correct support, particularly when the force of gravity creates a problem. If a wrist requires support because of weakness of the wrist extensors for example, the splint must be able to hold the wrist

in extension even when the arm is in pronation.

Levers. A lever is a simple device with a bar and a fulcrum (fixed point about which movement takes place). Force (or effort) is exerted to overcome the weight (or resistance). The reader will be aware of the importance of these principles in the human body. In designing a splint the balancing of forces needs to be carefully considered, e.g. where there is uneven muscle control around a joint, the positioning of the fulcrum may be crucial. A bony prominence, for example, may unintentionally act as a fulcrum, with the possibility of skin breakdown. The splint itself may incorporate a fulcrum, e.g. a spring wire coil in lively splints and this should closely approximate the body fulcrum. When using solid moulding materials, 'ventilation' holes placed over a fulcrum may severely weaken the splint.

Angle of pull. For splints using wire 'outriggers' or spring coils, the angle of pull is critical. Following tendon repair or suture, for example, incorrect pull on the tendon could result in tear or rupture of the tendon. A force is mechanically most effective when applied at right angles to a lever. For the reader about to embark on splints using spring coils, the reading of Barr (1975) is highly recommended.

Rigidity. A splint's resistance to distortion depends on the rigidity of the material and on its shape. A flat piece of material will be stronger if formed into a curve, as in a forearm gutter, and even stronger if formed into a cylinder, as in a fully enclosed wrist splint. Strengthening a splint may involve incorporating materials of different rigidity, e.g. a metal strip into a soft leather glove splint, or incorporating specially shaped sections of the original material, for example a half cylindrical strip over the dorsum of a wrist splint. The design of a splint should anticipate the points where rigidity will be needed, and thought should be given to how it can best be achieved.

It is hoped that the reader who wishes to develop her knowledge of splint design will inform herself about relevant biomechanical principles. 'Mechanics for Movement' by MacDonald (73) is a very useful reference source as a starter on mechanical principles, which are of course relevant in many other areas of physical occupational therapy.

Knowledge of disease and injury

While splinting it is important to understand the condition or injury of the patient in order to produce the correct splint physiologically, and to prevent damage to the patient while making or wearing the splint.

For a person with rheumatiod arthritis, for example, the splint should aim to prevent further deformity and may reduce existing deformity. While making the splint, the occupational therapist also needs to bear in mind pain, tenderness and skin condition of the part being splinted, as well as the careful positioning of the rest of the body to avoid pain, such as supporting the upper limb along a pillow rather than on a tender elbow joint. The rheumatiod patient must be able to fasten the splint during active and non-active phases of the disease if possible. For such patients, therefore, the occupational therapist must know exactly how each joint has been affected internally, and understand the progression of the disease.

To give another example of a thorough knowledge of diseases and injuries, some occupational therapists have been bracing femoral and other fractures of limbs ready for early mobilisation. Their knowledge of the precise anatomy and the pathological changes occurring during fracture healing is crucial to the correct application of the orthoses.

Splinting a patient with a hand injury is another example. The occupational therapist will need to know:

- what operative procedures have been undertaken, or will be necessary and what do they involve
- whether there is temporary or permanent oedema
- whether no-touch techniques are necessary for prevention of infection
- whether there are restrictions on movement, and if so what these are
- when any stitches will be removed
- whether pressure is required or contra indicated over the injured area
- whether immobilisation in a splint will render the hand permanently stiff
- the maximum skin area (especially palmar) that can be kept free for sensation/prehension
- whether later adjustments will be necessary during healing
- whether the injury has caused sensation impairment that will necessitate extra visual care when wearing a splint.

It can be seen from the above examples that the occupational therapist must use her knowledge of each condition wisely, finding out more about the disease or injury if it is new to her, before splinting.

The occupational therapist must always add to this knowledge the needs of the individual patient. No two patients are identical. A hand splint may be needed for identical medical reasons for a foundry worker and an elderly lady living in an old people's home. The foundry worker may need qualities of rigidity and heat tolerance in his splint not required by the elderly lady, while her need for a cosmetically acceptable splint may be greater, The foundry worker may indeed need two splints, one for work and one which is less bulky and conspicuous for social occasions.

THE PATIENT

The following points may help the occupational therapist who is new to splinting to approach her patient confidently:

Relax. The patient is probably more nervous than you are. If you are tense, try not to show it, as it will certainly lessen the patient's confidence in you.

Be methodical. Rushing will make you and the patient more tense; time does cost money and cannot be wasted, but rushing may lead to spoilt materials, mistakes and maybe even injury to the patient.

Talk and listen. Silence can be nerve-racking for the patient. Even if mentally you are conversing with yourself on your progress with the splint, do not forget to talk to your patient; use your knowledge of psychology appropriately and you should get a more relaxed, cooperative patient.

Involve the patient. If appropriate, give a brief explanation of what you are doing and why. The technically minded patient may be able to offer ideas for splint design, while simple involvement such as holding the wrapping bandage helps a patient feel useful. If a patient has helped in the production, he will be more likely to use his splint fully.

Comfort. Check the patient is in as comfortable a position as possible. If he has to maintain an awkward pose, try to be as quick as possible. Comfortable chairs, cushions/pillows and adjustable tables, plinths and footstools can all help. Check the room temperature; a patient and an occupational therapist with stuffy headaches are liable to be irritable. Privacy may be important if clothing has to be removed; check that all staff use procedures which ensure privacy.

Voice and manner. It may seem pedantic to mention this, but a professional yet friendly manner and being ready to respond to the patient, can help both him and the therapist. A confident and quiet tone can help calm a patient, especially if there is pain in the limb, or fear of burning from a hot splint material.

Fun. If a child is to be provided with a splint, small toys may keep tempers cool, as may having mum or a helper nearby. Children often prefer a big bandage to a discreet fastening and for toddlers this may also be more secure. Stickers, drawings or transfers on splints may also encourage their use. Check that those in charge of the children have copies of instruction sheets; children's copies tend to become drawing paper or paper darts!

Instructions for use. These need to be concise and clear. Verbal instructions, though important should not be relied upon. The patient is your legal responsibility and misuse of the splint could cause damage. Handouts are used in some hospitals, giving such information as:

Patient's name, address, telephone number
Next occupational therapy appointment
Next clinic appointment
Time to wear the splint, e.g. night time only
Care of the splint, e.g. cleaning
NB Do not adjust the splint unless you have been shown how to do so. If any problems arise, e.g. broken or irritated skin, red patches, numbed areas, broken/distorted splint, please contact (Name and telephone number of department).

MATERIALS

The choice of materials for splinting can seem bewildering and the reader needs to make him/herself familiar with the properties of each of them and keep up to date with new ones. Inevitably most occupational therapists acquire 'favourites'. Bearing in mind the patient's condition, the following points should be considered when selecting the appropriate material for his splint:

1. Rigidity/flexibility
2. Bulkiness
3. Ease of cleaning
4. Cosmetic appearance
5. Heat tolerance
6. Economy
7. Adjustability
8. Comfort
9. Need for lining or padding
10. Ease of use in production of splint
11. Suitability for the patient's lifestyle (job, sports etc).

Do not forget the possibility of mixing materials, and that scraps can sometimes be utilised for aids and adaptations.

High temperature thermoplastics

Plastazote

This is a lightweight expanded cross-linked polythene in white or pink perforated sheets of varying thicknesses. Its *advantages* are:

Light weight and comfort
Ease of cutting and handling
Direct application, though many occupational therapists prefer protection for the patient
It can be scrubbed clean, using solvents and sterilising agents if required
Auto-adhesion. This means that it can be layered and joins can be made.

Its *disadvantages* are:
Bulkiness which can hamper activities.
Limited elasticity. This makes it unsuitable for fine detail. Joints are necessary at great angles.
Limited strength. It can tear if subjected to excessive stretch or twisting.
Lack of rigidity. It requires reinforcement for

some splints, though this is easily achieved with Vitrathene.

Despite its perforations, many patients complain of excessive sweating.

Equipment. Plastazote oven, thermostatically controlled; stockinette; sharp knife; ballpoint pen or chinagraph pencil; plastic rivets; cotton gloves; soldering iron; crêpe bandages; sanding disc or glass paper; Vitrathene for reinforcement; scissors.

Patient preparation. The patient should be seated comfortably and be able to watch the preparation of materials. A layer of stockinette should be placed over the areas to be splinted. When using Vitrathene reinforcement, some occupational therapists prefer to give added protection, for example by using several stockinette layers or smooth crêpe bandage.

Choice of thickness. Thinner material is lighter and easier to mould, but does not give firm support, whereas thicker material is bulkier but gives greater support. Vitrathene reinforcement strips can be 'sandwiched' between two thin layers of Plastazote; at 140C both materials will fuse. (Remember, extra patient protection is necessary. The operator must wear thick gloves.)

Cutting. Mark the material with ballpoint pen or chinagraph pencil and remember to allow extra material for the thickness. Using 3 mm material, for example, a wrist support would need to be at least 6 mm more than the wrist measurement. For collars this is particularly important, especially if Vitrathene 'sandwich' reinforcing is used. Cut with sharp scissors, knife or bandsaw.

Heating Use the Plastazote oven at 140C. Lay the paper provided in cartons underneath the material to prevent sticking. Some occupational therapists use other dry air methods, such as hot airguns, but this needs considerable experience. If reinforcing with Vitrathene, place all the material on a layer of stockinette for easier removal from the oven. Always use gloves when using the oven. Reheating is possible, but Plastazote becomes brittle after repeated reheating. (A well-fitted Plastazote shape can be flattened to provide a useful pattern for other materials.) Place in the oven for approximately three to four minutes, depending on the thickness. The material should then be 'floppy'.

Application. Check the heat of the material on your own skin and let the patient see this. Apply it quickly and firmly, bandaging over with a crêpe bandage if possible. The material cools in approximately 20 to 30 seconds, so work fairly quickly, but remember that it can be reheated. Two therapists are often preferable, especially for well-fitted collars. Hold the material firmly in position, checking concave areas carefully, for example popliteal fossa or palmar arch.

Finishing. The edges can be angled and sanded for comfort. Lining is not usually needed, although some patients find stockinette tubing covering the splint easier to remove and wash. This also provides a little relief from the heat of wearing the splint, which many patients find uncomfortable. Joins can be riveted (see below) or touch soldered. Touch both sides for a few seconds with the soldering iron and quickly press them together. This is quite tricky, so practise before using with a patient.

If there is any rubbing or irritation the offending areas can be:

1. cut out if small and not at a leverage point. This is useful over ulcerated areas, e.g. in slippers.

2. carefully heated with airgun and pushed away from inner surface, but be careful not to tear.

3. padded *around* the rubbing area, not on top which merely increases pressure (Fig. 11.6).

4. 'slashed' in a cross-hatched fashion to reduce surface pressure. The closer the hatching, the greater the reduction in direct pressure (Fig. 11.7). This is useful over the clavicles on collars, but be

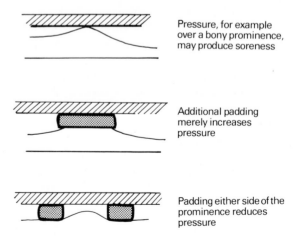

Pressure, for example over a bony prominence, may produce soreness

Additional padding merely increases pressure

Padding either side of the prominence reduces pressure

Fig. 11.6   Reducing pressure under a splint

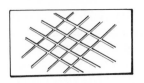

In cross section the cuts are seen to be no more than half way through the material

Fig. 11.7 Cross-hatching

careful to cut no more than half thickness and avoid weakening over fulcrums.

The material can be held together with plastic rivets at joins or where straps are required. Insert the rivet and cut off the protruding end two notches above the level of the material, touching lightly with a soldering iron to melt it into a permanent position.

Encourage patients to wash their splints frequently. Webbing and velcro straps, sometimes with metal loops, are the commonest fastenings for Plastazote.

Vitrathene

This is a lightweight, semi-transparent polythene in two thicknesses, Its *advantages* are:

Light weight and minimal thickness

Semi-rigidity. It can be reinforced with extra strips

Ease of moulding to small detail

Resistance to most chemicals and scrubbing.

Its *disadvantages* are:

For a splint of Vitrathene only a plaster of Paris cast is essential. The material is very hot to handle and two or more pairs of gloves are needed.

It can be used with Plastazote acting as a lining. This procedure should only be tried after considerable practice on a plaster of Paris cast.

It is malleable at 100C, which may be reached in some industrial jobs or when placed directly on a heat source.

Excessive stretching when hot.

Patient preparation. Take a plaster of Paris cast if using Vitrathene alone. Once experience has been gained the material may be used with Plastazote as a lining. Where good patient protection is needed a crêpe bandage wrap, or thicker protection, should be used.

Cutting. The thin material can be cut with sharp scissors or scored with a knife and cracked. Thick-

er material, especially with small details, needs to be marked, then cut on a bandsaw. (Clear the inside of the machine after each splint to prevent 'clogging' and subsequent band slipping.) If using the material with a Plastazote lining, cut the Vitrathene slightly smaller all round.

Heating. Use thick gloves at all times. Place the Vitrathene on stockinette before placing it in the Plastazote oven on paper provided in the Plastazote packs. Heat at 140C for approximately four to six minutes. The material becomes transparent.

Moulding. Using gloves, remove the material, still on the gauze or stockinette and place it into position around the cast, bandaging if possible. As the material stretches easily be careful it does not slip down the cast while moulding. Well placed key marks can help avoid this. With experience gained on a plaster of Paris cast, Vitrathene with a Plastazote lining can be placed onto a very well protected patient, though many occupational therapists still prefer to do this onto a plaster of Paris cast.

Finishing. The edges can be filed or lightly sanded. Metal rivets with webbing or Velcro straps and double sided sticky tape, are common fastenings. Wire attachments can be added using metal rivets. If considerable strain is expected, bond an extra square of material onto the outside at the point of attachment of the rivets.

Formasplint or Darvic

This is a rigid thermoplastic material, white or transparent. Its *advantages* are:

Rigidity and light weight

Spot-heating and readjustments are easy

It can be drilled and attached to metal, for example wire or special aids

Ease of care, resistance to scrubbing and most chemicals

Its *disadvantages* are:

Moulding of minute detail is impossible

Very short setting time, therefore quick work is essential

Lining is necessary in most cases and its rigidity means extra care is needed at pressure points

Lengthy preparation and particular care to prevent burning the patient.

Equipment. Electric hot plate and funnel or

thermostatically controlled oven; fretsaw or band-saw; sanding files/discs; chinagraph pencil; rubber solution; polystyrene insulation; impact adhesive; metal rivets; stockinette; crêpe bandaging or elastic bandages; gauze or thin cotton material.

Patient preparation. The area to be splinted should be covered with at least two layers of stockinette, although some occupational therapists prefer smoothly applied crêpe bandaging. The insulating material is such that, once practise has been gained, the splint can be applied directly, as long as the lining is firmly positioned and extreme care is taken. Check that the patient knows he must not touch the material.

Cutting. Mark with a chinagraph pencil and cut with a fretsaw or bandsaw. (Clear the inside of the bandsaw frequently to prevent 'clogging'.) Try not to produce jagged edges and use curves in preference to right-angles which are difficult to smooth later. If the material is warm, scissors can be used with care.

Insulation. This is very important. Cut a piece of polystyrene sheeting to pattern with scissors and glue with rubber solution onto the inner surface of the splint. Take particular care that this reaches *all* edges, especially round the thumb on hand splints.

Heating. Use thick cotton gloves at all times. Hold the material over the electric plate until pliable. If only making a small splint or spot heating a funnel may be useful. Held about eight centimetres from the plate, this should take approximately three to four minutes. Once experience has been gained a thermostatically controlled oven can be used. If this is a Plastazote oven, heat to 100C, place the formasplint on gauze or cotton (cut to pattern shape to make moulding easier) and then on a paper sheet in the oven. Spot heating can be done with an airgun or over the funnel. It can be reheated many times.

Moulding. Apply quickly. The material will be rigid in approximately one minute, often sooner. Using thick gloves, place the material quickly on the patient, with the insulated side nearest the skin. Two therapists may be necessary for a large or difficult splint. Wrap it on firmly with elastic bandaging and check the concave areas. Heated material must *not* touch the patient.

Reinforcing. This is rarely necessary. If it is, the moulded pieces require fixing with impact adhesive, as this material is not auto-adhesive.

Finishing. Remove the polystyrene lining and any blobs of glue. Smoothing the edges is important; file with sanding discs or hand files. If using a disc follow the safety procedures. Moleskin or similar material can be placed over some edges, such as the edges distal to the metacarpophalangeal crease or the popliteal fossa. Line the splint, if necessary, with moleskin, foam lining or felt. Remember, foams easily become distorted with continual wear and need constant checking. Some occupational therapists recommend a crêpe bandaging or tubinette under the splint for added comfort. Fastenings may be webbing or leather straps together with Velcro or buckles and attached with metal rivets or sometimes double sided sticky tape or impact adhesive.

Medium and low temperature thermoplastics

These include Orthoplast, Polyform, Sansplint, Hexcelite & Aquaplast, all of which are plastics which become malleable at fairly low temperatures. Several new plastics are being developed for splinting at the time of writing and it is not possible to give instructions for them all. The instructions below are for Orthoplast, but the general method of working is similar for most of these types of materials.

Orthoplast

This is a thermoplastic material obtainable in perforated/unperforated sheets. Its *advantages* are:

Versatility. It can be moulded by wet or dry methods and so can be used on wards or in the home, as well as in the department.

Ease of use. It moulds quickly and cools slowly.

Smooth edges if cut while warm. Often no lining is needed.

Auto-adhesion gives scope for additional parts and strengthening.

Light weight and comfort.

Moulding into small details is easy as it stretches while warm.

Adjustment is easily achieved by spot heating.

Its *disadvantages* are:

Sensitivity to light and air, so storage in closed containers is necessary.

Even at temperatures which may be reached in domestic use such as warm water it becomes malleable, so careful instructions to the patient are essential.

Auto-adhesion may occur at unwanted points when forming complicated shapes.

Limited strength, although reinforcement is possible.

Cleansing is not possible in warm water; a damp sponge is preferable.

Equipment. Oven: dry heat of 65C; if using a Plastazote oven it must be adjusted. Water: 65C (150F), do not allow the water to boil, as this may affect the adhesive properties. Scissors; chinagraph pencil/biro; elastic bandaging; leather punch; cold or iced water; small pointed paintbrush; drinking straws or thin wire; sharp knife; spot heater (e.g. upturned hair dryer with blow drying nozzle).

Cutting. This is best done while the material is warm, using firm, even strokes. Press uneven edges between fingers while warm for a neat edge. Use dry heat whenever possible, especially if the auto-adhesive qualities are to be retained.

Heating. Dry heat or water of 65C should be used. Do not allow the water to boil. If using dry heat, place the material on carrier sheets, e.g. those from Plastazote cases. With either method be sure the material does not fold or crease on removal or it will adhere firmly; also take care not to pull or it will stretch.

Application. Apply directly onto the skin or over a stockinette protection layer after testing on your own skin. Mould carefully, aligning the areas to be joined before bringing them together. Apply an elastic bandage to hold the splint firmly. An iced bandage will accelerate setting, as will an ice-pack (as used in picnic boxes).

Setting. This will occur in eight to ten minutes. Cold bandages or packs (as described above) will accelerate the process but ensure there are no contraindications, such as vascular insufficiency.

Bonding. This may be done during moulding or later, using spot heating. Use dry heat if possible, prior to bonding. Check that the surfaces are clean and free from grease by using a solvent such as non-flammable spot remover.

Reinforcement. Remember a curved surface is much stronger than a flat one. Clean the material thoroughly using a pointed brush over small areas. A straw, wire or similar material covered in Orthoplast will give added strength if necessary. Bonding occurs most easily when both surfaces are warm. (Some thermoplastics require adhesives; check the manufacturer's instructions.) Curling the edge over can strengthen it considerably, for example at the palmar edge of a wrist cock-up splint. Try to anticipate strengthening points and allow for an extra piece to fold or curl.

Hinge joints. These can be made with a sharp knife while the material is still warm or with a heated paring knife. To crease, the splint needs reducing in thickness by approximately one half. A cylinder splint may be hinged to allow easy application.

Fastening. Webbing, Velcro or 'D' rings, using double sided adhesive tape, are easiest. Metal rivets can be used if strengthening tabs of Orthoplast are first added to the splint.

Ventilation. If using perforated sheets, be careful to check that the pattern does not include perforations on its edges. If using unperforated sheets, check the position for ventilation carefully, then punch holes using a fine leather punch, heated skewers or a very fine soldering iron.

Finishing. No special finishing is usually required.

Plaster of Paris

This is available either in powder form or as impregnated bandages of varying widths. Its *advantages* are:

A cast of the limb can be retained in the department, even if the patient has to return home or to the ward. A complex splint can then be moulded from the cast with the minimum of fuss to the patient.

A positive cast can be used for the moulding of difficult materials such as those with a high heat retaining capacity or for experiments in design.

Extremely detailed copying is possible.

Casting is sometimes used for the production of specialised aids, such as contoured handles or switches for electrical aids. The cast can also be sent elsewhere, for instance to the orthotic workshop, when specialised appliances are required.

It can be reinforced with fibre glass if necessary.

Its *disadvantages* are:

It is messy compared with plastic materials. The working area, patient and therapist all need protection.

It is fragile and heavy. Any cast should be stored with care. For most occupational therapy purposes, plaster of Paris splints are not practical working splints, although some occupational therapists use them for resting or serial splints. It is not usually feasible to use it where there are open wounds or skin problems until sufficient experience with this material has been gained.

Some therapists feel plaster of Paris is time-consuming to use. For most simple designs this is probably true. If more advanced splinting, however, is undertaken regularly, time can be saved.

Disposal of waste can be a problem. Once the powder has been mixed with water it must not be thrown down a sink without a special plaster of Paris catch. Waste must be placed in plastic disposal sacks. If allowed to dry it can often be crumbled easily.

Equipment. Plaster of Paris powder; plaster of Paris bandages; scissors, pointed and blunt end; small wooden tool, e.g. orange stick; plastic disposal sack; plastic bowl of tepid water; towels/soap or access to sink; bowl of sand; lubricant (white petroleum jelly); paper towelling; plastic sheeting; waste bin; plastic apron; chinagraph pencil; plastic or pyrex jug; wooden rod 15 to 30 cm long.

Patient preparation. Mark the area to be covered with a chinagraph pencil directly on the skin. Protect the patient with polythene sheeting. Check the limb is in the correct position, using support rolls (foam or rolled bandages) or plasticine if needed. Lubricate area with white petroleum jelly.

Dry cutting. Cut the bandages to the lengths required. Approximately 6 to 8 lengths are needed for the leg/forearm/wrist sections (half shell) and 12 to 16 for a full cast. Experience will show the widths required, but as a guide 150 mm should be used on the leg, 100 mm on the wrist and forearm and 75 mm on the hand. For intricate moulding, such as around the fingers, cut a 150 mm width bandage into squares of approximately 75 mm and 37 mm in size. Cut the squares *on the cross* of the bandage. Boxes of these can be prepared in ad-

vance and labelled. With experience, lightweight casts can be prepared using fewer bandages.

Moulding with squares. Dip the square into tepid water and apply, placing the diagonal of the square over any rounded areas and pressing it gently into place. Apply the squares in sequence, overlapping them slightly and pressing into crevices using a tool. Try to ensure this layer is as smooth as possible. Fold back any uneven edges along the chinagraph lines and smooth them into place thus giving a strong edge. Apply several layers, usually four to six, then proceed with the rest of the cast using strips.

Moulding with strips. Check that the dry lengths have been cut accurately and that enough have been prepared. Fold one length concertina-like and dip it into a bowl of tepid water until no more bubbles rise. This time varies according to the size of the bandage, but as a rough guide a 75 mm × 300 mm length requires no more than a few seconds and a 100 mm × 600 mm length may need eight to ten seconds. Remove and gently squeeze the bandage and apply it along the length of the limb, pressing gently around protruberances. Repeat with the next length slightly overlapping the central pieces already applied and fold back the edge of the bandage where it meets the chinagraph mark to give a strengthened edge. Repeat this until the whole area is covered. When the first layer is complete, apply the next in the same sequence until four to six layers have been completed.

To mould a full cast enclosing the limb (i.e. a negative cast). Complete a half shell first, turning back the edges in the usual way. Allow the surface to dry slightly, then lightly grease the edge of the shell and its outer surface for approximately 50 mm. Now proceed with the other half of the cast, pressing up to the edges of the completed shell. Mark *across* the join in several places then prise them gently apart.

To mould a positive cast. A negative cast needs to be made first (see above). Grease the inside and edges of both shells. Place them together, matching the marks and hold together with a standard bandage. Close one open end (usually the distal end) with three to four layers of plaster of Paris bandage and allow it to set. If possible, grease the inside of the newly enclosed end. Have ready a bowl of sand in which to support the mould. Fill the cast with tepid water to within 10 mm of the top and then pour this water *quickly* into the jug. Sprinkle plaster of Paris powder onto the surface until no more will be absorbed — again work quite quickly. Leave this to become creamy (approximately 10 seconds for small quantities and 20 seconds for larger ones). Pour this cream into the negative cast and place it in the support bowl. Leave it to harden (at least one and a half hours) then gently prise off the shell. Leave it to dry out, preferably overnight. The result is a *positive* cast, that is, it is the same shape as that originally moulded. A rod can be inserted before setting, protruding approximately 100 mm. The cast can then be put into a vice, leaving the operator with both hands free. A little cream of plaster of Paris can be rubbed into any small air holes in the cast and also over any uneven surfaces, as these are likely to be reproduced on the splinting material. Alternatively, the surface can, with great care, be very lightly sanded.

Further help. If the reader has little practice in plaster of Paris techniques physiotherapists, plaster room technicians or sisters in casualty departments may be able to help. If casts are needed for the moulding of electrical switch devices dental departments (orthodontics) can often give invaluable help.

Other materials

It is not possible to cover all the materials used by occupational therapists in one chapter. The reader may come across some of the following and be able to learn from trade leaflets, reading, observing occupational therapists and most of all by experimentation.

Pressure garments

These are manufactured by various companies. They are elastic garments which apply specific pressure to help control hypertrophic scarring, e.g. after burns injuries. A special measuring technique involving purpose-made tapes and charts is required and many occupational therapists now assess the need for these garments, measure and supply them and occasionally incorporate added splintage. They also provide follow up. Companies provide explanatory leaflets and can sometimes arrange training sessions. Such garments are supplied in Britain by Jobst Inc., Pan-Med and Seton.

Some occupational therapists are designing and making pressure garments in their own departments. This needs care and skill, especially in the measurement and production of the garment, i.e. in design, seaming and fastening (Nelson 78).

Leather

Specially processed moulding leather is used primarily by orthotic technicians. Leather or synthetic leather may, however, be found useful for the following purposes:

Strappings and fastenings, especially for long-term splints with buckles

Padding under awkward fastenings, for example around the ankle

As a base for lively splints, for example gloves holding spring wire such as those used for Dupuytrens contractures, or soft opposition splints

As a cover for some splints for cosmetic reasons or to make them more hardwearing.

Leather can be handsewn using waxed or other strong thread. Use two needles to produce a gloving stitch. It can also be machine stitched using strong linen or buttonhole thread on a heavy duty machine. (Check on a sample before using modern machines.)

Sheepskin

This may be synthetic or natural — and can be used for the following purposes:

Padding. It is bulky, however, and needs care in its use.

Protection over the edge of some orthoses, especially if the patient is prone to pressure sores, or has friable or anaesthetised skin.

Padding under straps and buckles.

Protective heel or elbow muffs. These are sometimes made by occupational therapists, although also available commercially.

Sheepskin can be sewn by hand or on a heavy duty machine with adjusted tension; clean below the plate on the machine frequently.

Spring wire

This is used for lively splints in some departments, although these splints are now often made by orthotic technicians. With practice, it can be very efficient. Wire may be used on its own with padding and fastening, but is more frequently attached to other materials such as formasplint. Covering the wire, for example with catheter tubing, may give a practical finish. Jigs for producing coils are often used and the mechanics involved are complicated. Nathalie Barr (75) gives an excellent and well-illustrated account of these.

Metals

Sheet aluminium, cut carefully with tin snips and well covered, for example with foam and moleskin or leather, can be useful for heavyduty working splints. Aluminium rods are used frequently by orthotists, and some occupational therapists use them for specialised work such as bracing. Tin plate is an easier material to work with for the beginner, being easy to soft solder.

Rubber

This may be used occasionally. Examples include:
  Lightweight rubber soles for footwear.
  Thin sheeting for some hand splints, for example opposition splints for median nerve lesions.
  Pimpled sheeting for non-slip outer surfaces, for example on pushing gloves used by wheelchair users, or splints to be used in lifting jobs.

Linings

There is now a wide variety of these and only experience will show advantages and disadvantages. Jones (77) gives comparative lists. Some thick linings provide additional padding and must therefore be chosen at the fitting stage, while thin linings merely provide additional comfort. They include: moleskin, synthetic leather, stockinette, plastic foams, chiropody felt, adhesive solid foams suede/leather, non-adhesive open cell foams and tubinette.

The life expectancy of these materials has to be considered. Some may look ideal, but last only a short time, causing additional discomfort.

Fastenings

Ingenuity is often needed, Common fastenings include: webbing straps, leather or plastic straps, Velcro touch-and-close fastenings on straps or used alone, metal 'D' rings or loops used with Velcro and straps (a common fastening is made with the strap passing through the D ring, then back on itself to fasten with Velcro), double sided sticky tape (this is invaluable for all round closures, for example around the forearm, and for attaching webbing/Velcro), plastic rivets (see Plastazote) and metal rivets, bandaging/netalast, adhesives (check their compatibility, especially with Plastazote).

The ease of fastening and the appearance are often crucial factors in a patient's decision as to whether to wear or discard a splint. A well designed splint needs a well constructed fastening.

PATTERN CONSTRUCTION

Many books give excellent guidelines to pattern making, especially for the hand — see Malick (1972, 1974), Barr (1975) and Jones (1977). Plenty of experimentation is needed, preferably initially with an understanding colleague. There is no 'correct' method and the reader will see many different techniques. The following are general guidelines only. The reader will no doubt discover other factors influencing pattern construction.

1. Generally, choose the material before designing the pattern, bearing in mind the purpose of the splint.

2. Take measurements or outline with the patient in *a normal functional* position wherever possible, for example with the forearm pronated for hand splints, or with the patient standing for lower limb splints in which the patient will be mobile. To show the importance of this try Nathalie Barr's (1975) experiment (p. 110), or draw round the foot, marking key points first in raised

position, then in weightbearing and note the changes.

3. If a splint is to hold the body in a corrected position, for example following surgery or in rheumatoid arthritis, position the limb before pattern taking. Use round foam wedges for example or place the limb on a plasticine or aloplast 'mound'.

4. Common methods for pattern design/construction include:

Flat paper silhouette (e.g. draw hand flat on paper).

Block (e.g. balsawood) covered in paper, folded if necessary. The hand is positioned correctly over the block and traced. The outline is then transferred onto paper.

Paper strips stuck into position around the limb then flattened.

Cotton material stuck into position then flattened.

Aloplast. This is similar to plasticine. Roll it out like pastry and mould it round the limb, cutting out unwanted areas before flattening it to obtain the pattern, which can then be cut in paper.

Plaster of Paris mould. This is made and then the splint is moulded over it using one of the above methods, especially if a complex shape is required.

Vacuum bags filled with silica sand, placed round the limb. The air is then sucked from the bag, leaving a rigid mould which can form the basis for a plaster of Paris mould. This is mainly suitable for large areas requiring no detail, such as a knee extension slab or spinal support.

Simple tape measurements. This may be the only way, for example, across open wounds (when the tape should be sterilised) or collars when the patient is lying flat and unable to sit until the collar is fitted. Flexicurves (available from mathematical suppliers) or electrical cable wire are useful for awkward measurement of lengths or angles.

Pattern material should resemble chosen splint material, for example paper should be used for materials which do not stretch, e.g. Formasplint, and cotton material or aloplast for those that do, e.g. Polyform.

5. Remember normal functional anatomy wherever possible. For example if thumb opposi-

tion is required there should be no restriction over the thenar eminence, therefore hand splints allowing this movement must be cut well away around this point. Similarly, flexion at the metacarpophalangeal joints requires an unimpeded area to just proximal to the palmar crease. Similar observations can be made for all areas requiring splintage.

6. Place key marks, for example at the centre of anatomical joints, over skin creases and bony prominences, clearly onto the pattern. These give guidelines for allowing or preventing movement, especially for lively splints. Selected key marks can also be placed on splint material to ensure accurate positioning. Corresponding marks may also be made on the patient.

7. Remember to allow for bulk of the material; for example, for 10 mm material allow 20 mm extra for wrap around.

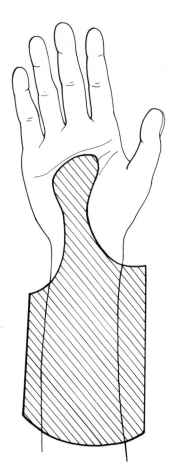

Fig. 11.8 Basic wrist cock-up splint

8. Refer to pattern books or journals. Many departments keep stocks of useful pattern designs. If the case is unusual, use an adapted pattern or develop a suitable design and keep it for reference.

The following patterns are suggestions for experiments; remember to use such patterns as guidelines only, making individual patterns dependent on the individual's anatomy, the condition, functional anatomy and mechanical principles.

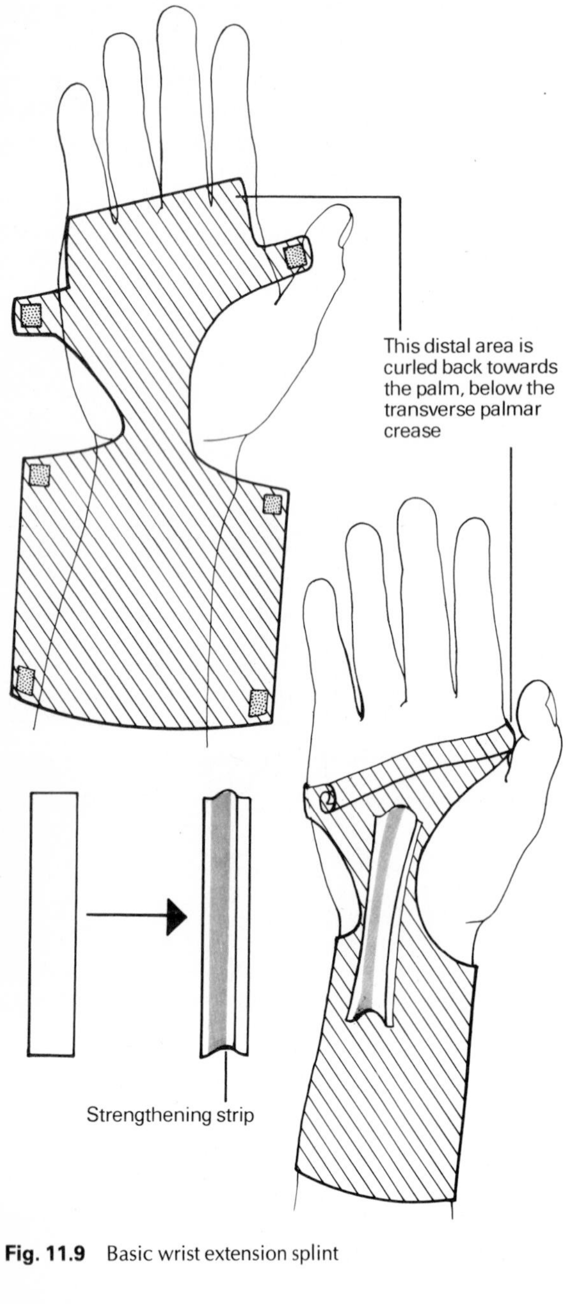

BASIC SPLINTS

Basic wrist cock-up splint (Fig. 11.8)

Material: High temperature Formasplint/Darvic (try reinforced medium temperature thermoplastics once experience has been gained).

Examples of use: Tetraplegia (quadriplegia), tenosynivitis.

'Stock' supplies are sometimes kept in three sizes.

Moulding. Mould on a polystyrene lining cut to shape and stuck. The wrist is usually placed in 20–25° of extension. Curve carefully into the palmar arch.

Fastening. Webbing/Velcro and double sided tape or firm bandaging, especially for night-time use.

Basic wrist extension splint (Fig. 11.9)

Material: Low temperature plastics, such as Orthoplast or Polyform. (Try medium temperature plastics once experience has been gained.)

Examples of use: Wrist injuries, Rheumatoid arthritis, tetraplegia.

Moulding. Heat both pieces and mould the reinforcement over its 'support' (e.g. drinking straw or wire). Join to main piece while still warm. (Use adhesive if material is not auto-adhesive.) Reheat and mould onto hand, fitting well into the palmar arch. The distal area should be curled towards the palm to a level below the transverse palmar crease.

Fastening. Webbing/Velcro and double sided tape or metal rivets.

Basic paddle splint (Fig. 11.10)

Material: High temperature plastics, e.g. Formasplint/Darvic. (Try medium temperature plastics with reinforcement when experience has been gained.)

Examples of use: Night resting only (e.g. rheumatoid arthritis); hand injuries, nerve injuries and burns (with adjustments according to condition).

This distal area is curled back towards the palm, below the transverse palmar crease

Strengthening strip

Fig. 11.9 Basic wrist extension splint

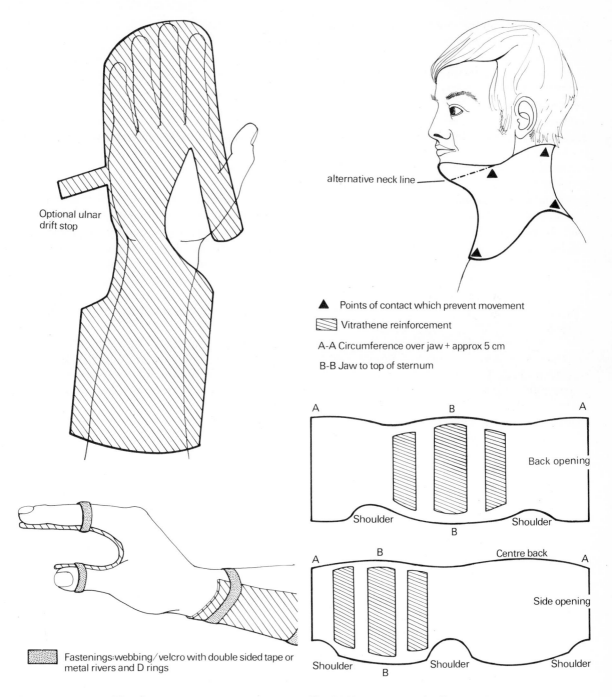

Optional ulnar drift stop

Fastenings: webbing/velcro with double sided tape or metal rivers and D rings

Fig. 11.10 Basic paddle splint

alternative neck line

▲ Points of contact which prevent movement

▨ Vitrathene reinforcement

A-A Circumference over jaw + approx 5 cm

B-B Jaw to top of sternum

Back opening

Shoulder   Shoulder

Centre back

Side opening

Shoulder   Shoulder   Shoulder

Fig. 11.11 Basic cervical collar — medium support

Moulding. Over a polystyrene lining cut to shape and stuck.

For short-term use the hand should be in a functional position. For long-term use the inter-phalangeal joints should be in extension. Fit well into the curved palmar arch.

Fastening. Webbing/Velcro with double sided tape or metal rivets and D-rings.

Basic cervical collar – medium support (Fig. 11.11)

Material: Plastazote and Vitrathene. (Low temperature plastics can be used once experience has been gained.)

Examples of use: Medium strength support for neck injuries, instability or nerve involvement. Postoperative medium strength support.

Moulding. 'Sandwich' Vitrathene reinforcement between thin sheets of Plastazote or place it on the outer surface of one thick sheet once experience has been gained. Mould quickly and firmly, fitting well. Trim and chamfer the edges. Minimal crosshatching if necessary, e.g. over the clavicle.

Fastening. Webbing/Velcro and D rings attached with plastic rivets (usually at the top, middle and bottom of the opening).

Basic temporary slippers (Fig. 11.12)

Material: Plastazote rubber soling (sheet or ready cut soles).

Examples of use: Ulcerated or gangrenous areas on the feet (cut out areas where necessary), oedematous feet, foot injuries or surgery.

Moulding. While weight bearing where possible over all Plastazote pieces, which will then bond. Wrap round firmly. Spot solder or insert plastic rivets at the heel to close the slipper.

Fastening. Velcro tabs or strips with plastic rivets. Check the fit carefully.

These slippers are not particularly pleasing aesthetically, but are substantial for temporary use, especially where the foot is swollen. Cut out areas are easily achieved. Simpler sandal types may be used — see Jones (1977). Ready made shoes which can be similarly adapted are commercially available.

Mass-produced shapes

Some departments have great demands for certain simple splints, for instance cervical collars or small wrist supports, and keep several sizes ready cut out. These require only moulding onto the patient and adjustments for the individual can be made at this point. This is usually only satisfactory for simple splints or those which can be easily adjusted.

Time taken experimenting with patterns and materials is invaluable. Even if a particular splint is never made for a patient, the reader will have gained experience in developing patterns and using tools, equipment and materials.

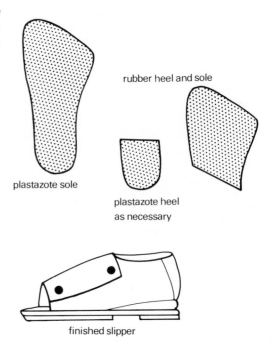

rubber heel and sole

plastazote sole

plastazote heel as necessary

finished slipper

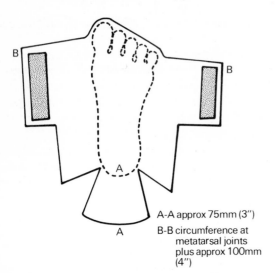

A-A approx 75mm (3")

B-B circumference at metatarsal joints plus approx 100mm (4")

Fig. 11.12 Basic temporary slipper

SAFETY

Workshop safety is vital and the following points should be borne in mind:

Health and Safety at Work Act. Check that regulations which cover the use of equipment and material are implemented within the school, department and hospital, for example wearing goggles when using sanding discs.

Storage of equipment. Storage of knives and inflammable liquids, for example, should be safe. Peg boards, labelled drawers and locked cabinets may help. Check the storage of inflammable materials with the fire safety officer.

Electrical equipment. Again check with the safety officer. The position of sockets, trailing wires, worn flexes, safety cut outs for disc sanders, goggles, adequate guards for cutting machinery and stands for soldering irons should all be checked.

Water. If boiling water is used, make sure that it is away from table edges and electrical equipment.

Materials. Storage should be in accordance with the manufacturer's instructions. Also check inflammability and chemical reactions. All materials should be stored safely out of the way.

Allergies. Some patients may be allergic to certain materials although this is rare. Ask the patient if he has any known allergies. Those with reactions to nylon are sometimes susceptible. If there is time, use a full allergy test, with small samples of the materials to be used firmly attached to the inside of the forearm for 24 hours. As this is rarely practicable, always check that the patient knows where to contact you. Keep a careful record of any minor allergic reactions.

Handling materials. Hot materials should obviously be handled according to the manufacturer's instructions. As a rule, thick gloves should be worn for materials requiring high temperature moulding and thin gloves for low and medium temperature materials. The latter may also be handled without gloves once experience has been gained. But if removing material from ovens or hot water it is obviously sensible to use thick gloves or a heat resistant implement such as wooden tongs or spatulas.

Patient care. The patient should avoid touching anything within the splint area. A supply of magazines may be appropriate if moulding will take time. Protection of the patient will depend on the material being used.

Room ventilation. If using inflammable or noxious materials, this is particularly important, especially if splinting takes place in a small room.

Accident procedure. Be sure you know where the first aid box is kept and how to alert medical staff. Do not forget to record on the appropriate form even the most minor of accidents, in case of later complications.

RECORDS AND FOLLOW UP

Referrals

These usually come from consultants, but may come from other medical staff or from general practitioners. Their request may be made by letter, on an occupational therapy referral form, or on a specific splint request form.

The consultant may be very exact in his request. Besides giving medical details, he may also state, for example: 'MCPs 80° flexion, PIPs maximum passive extension within limit of pain'. Some consultants with a good working knowledge of orthotics may even specify the materials to be used. Most will state the length of time they wish the splint to be worn and when they next wish to see the patient.

The reader will no doubt meet occupational therapists with considerable experience who are left to make their own decisions about the design of the splint, as well as materials and fastenings to be used. A consultant should be able to trust an occupational therapist's specialised knowledge, especially when backed by experience. Referrals ensure medical supervision of the patient's progress; the consultant after all has overall responsibility for the patient's medical and surgical care. Requests should be carefully kept in the patient's records.

Records

Systems vary considerably. Departments using splints regularly have special systems, while those who splint infrequently may simply use normal occupational therapy records. In either case, accuracy is essential for correct treatment, in case of future complications, to provide accurate information for statistics (for example for research), and to help build up knowledge.

Notes. Simple and clear notes are most effective. A lengthy past medical history is not needed unless it is relevant. For example, it is not necessary to know that a patient with a hand injury had a hysterectomy 15 years ago, whereas it would be important to know whether there is a history of rheumatoid arthritis, as this would indicate care with the design of the splint, especially the fastening. Where progressive diseases are involved, a short note on these could help ensure that no unfortunate statements are made to patients or relatives and that the splint design is appropriate. Current medical details do need to be noted clearly for accurate splint production, especially in surgical cases. The art of taking these quickly is invaluable.

Splint instructions. These should be given as described earlier in this chapter. They should be clear and concise and preferably in writing.

Reports. Copies of reports written for clinics, letters and short notes on telephone calls should all be retained.

Photographs: Some occupational therapists find black and white or colour photographs or slides useful as a:

Visual note of progress.

Reminder of an unusual splint design.

Teaching material, for example for new occupational therapy staff, students and technicians and for lectures to medical or nursing staff. The patient's permission should be obtained if the face is visible.

System of storage or display. This should be constructed to avoid damage and encourage use. Most occupational therapists do not mind students taking photographs as long as the patient gives permission (and obviously as long as the photograph taking does not impede treatment!).

Follow up

This may be arranged by the occupational therapist and/or the consultant. Dates should be given in writing. Where the consultant is following up, a short report may be sent to him regarding splint instructions. In some hand clinics the occupational therapist routinely sees the patient prior to the consultant to note function, ranges of movement, oedema, or power. If the splint is long term, a follow up letter can be sent to check the splint's use and condition, for example three months later. This often takes the form of a questionnaire which can help in evaluation of the splinting programmes.

Acknowledgements

Many thanks to all who helped in the preparation of this chapter, especially Lynn Cheshire, Carolyn Rutland and Diana Wharton.

REFERENCES AND FURTHER READING

Barr N 1975 The Hand. London, Butterworths
Broadley H 1974 Management of the foot in rheumatoid arthritis. British Journal Occupational Therapy 37:4
Jones M 1977 An Approach to occupational therapy, 3rd edn. London, Butterworths
Lawton D S 1974 Hand Splinting in rheumatoid arthritis. British Journal Occupational Therapy 37:219
Macdonald F 1973 Mechanics for movement. London, Bell
Malick M 1972 Manual on static hand splinting. Pittsburgh (U.S.A.), Harmaville Rehabilitation Centre
Malick M 1974 Manual on dynamic hand splinting with thermoplastic materials. Pittsburgh (U.S.A.), Harmaville Rehabilitation Centre
Malick M 1975 Management of the severely burned patient. British Journal Occupational Therapy 38:76
Nelson J 1978 The prevention and treatment of hypertrophic scars. British Journal Occupational Therapy 41:159
Rodocanachi C 1978 The disappearing neck. British Journal Occupational Therapy 41:107
Unsworth H 1977 Why don't people wear splints?. British Journal Occupational Therapy 40:241
Wynn Parry, C B 1973 Rehabilitation of the hand, 3rd edn. London, Butterworths

12
Work resettlement

Rehabilitation, it has been said, should start in the ambulance on the way to hospital and not finish until the person returns to open employment and pays his next income tax contribution! However true or untrue this statement may be, it certainly seems fair to say that in the majority of cases a patient is not considered to be fully rehabilitated until he can return to work, be it his former job, a new one for which he has been assessed and retrained or, in the case of a housewife, back to the role of homemaker which she fulfilled before.

This assumption, therefore, seems to point to the fact that the majority of people expect to work and that there are only certain groups (such as mothers with young children, the elderly or the 'sick') whom society accepts as being unable to do so. One may ask, therefore, why do we want to work? Certainly, in these times of high unemployment and apparent ease of 'social security living' it may seem rather strange to find that the majority of patients certainly do what to return to employment and also that members of the medical and para-medical professions still feel that they have 'failed' if they cannot resettle their patient at work. Unless there is an obvious reason for not working, it appears that most people still feel slightly guilty about being unemployed and statements that a woman is 'just a housewife' or that a man was 'made redundant' or is 'under the doctor' seem to reflect this guilt and try to justify a probably quite acceptable reason for not being at work.

Clearly, there will invariably be a percentage of people who are quite content with their unemployed state, but for the majority the strong desire to be at work would seem to stem from more than just a wish or a need to earn money. It appears, therefore, that we wish to work for a variety of reasons and these may be thought of as:

The desire to be part of a group. Man is a naturally gregarious animal and his need to gain status within a group and have a definite role within society is a constant pull. People gain support and social contact from those with whom they work and many will claim that they do not work 'for the money' (as if, perhaps, this is an undesirable reason!) but to get out of the house, to meet others, to be a 'useful' member of society or to be part of a social and/or employment circle.

The ability to be self supporting. In societies where self sufficiency or subsistence farming provides for physical needs such as food, clothing and shelter and where bartering brings comforts or satisfied desires the individual is unable to fulfil for himself, his own labour will directly meet his physical needs. Little has basically changed in our complex society, although our reward is now provided in the form of money with which to buy the goods we require.

The need for self esteem. Regardless of the changes in society, our lives are still dictated by our work and the majority of those who cannot or do not work feel inadequate unless they can show some positive reason for not doing so. Some jobs carry with them self esteem, interest and status and the jobs which we hold certainly shape our lifestyle for, apart from occupying more than half of the daylight hours for most people, the work we do determines the type of house we live in, the people we meet, the items we can afford to buy and, in some instances, the area in which we live and the opinions we hold. Those who can find little satisfaction in their work often compensate by fulfilling their need for self esteem in more rewarding leisure time pursuits, e.g. by captaining a local sports team or growing their own vegetables.

To gain security. Work provides not only financial security but also a routine and familiar environment from which the worker can gain a sense of belonging and a feeling of being needed.

Unemployment and its problems

When a person is unemployed over a long period

of time certain problems may arise because of his inability to fulfil these needs. These problems can particularly affect those who are unable to work because of sickness and, although obviously interrelated, they can be seen as:

Financial Although our welfare state provides financial benefits for the sick, these are comparatively small and do not allow for 'extras' such as holidays, personal transport or home ownership, which are now often considered as a right by those in open employment. Additionally many illnesses can carry hidden expense as, for example, the special diet required by the diabetic person or the extra heating needed to keep an inactive disabled person warm and this can easily strain an already low income.

Emotional. As previously mentioned, many people who cannot work feel a 'burden on society'. Some lose their self respect, for they feel that they do not contribute to the society in which they live. Some still think of themselves as living on charity when receiving benefits or other services to which they are entitled and for this reason (as well as others) may not apply for the help available to them.

Social. In spite of the additional leisure time available to the unemployed, the opportunity for social outlets and contacts is often greatly reduced. Many people find at least part of their social needs are fulfilled at work and a source of contact and feeling of belonging to a social group may become very limited if such outlets are not available.

Physical. A routine job, however sedentary, does provide a certain degree of physical exercise even if only walking around the office or upstairs to the canteen, and those who do not exercise regularly find that they easily become unfit and possibly overweight.

For those who have been out of work for any length of time or those who have never been able to work, the process of finding a suitable job and returning to employment can be extremely demanding, and some may well fail to retain their job simply because they have not been adequately prepared for the extra stresses and demands which employment brings. Physically, employment demands extra effort and in some cases a sustained level of physical activity is needed during the working day. By contrast some work, such as typing or electrical assembly, demands a high degree of coordination and dexterity and where skills are unpractised or illness has left a residual manual disability, these demands may prove too great. Psychologically any work demands a degree of concentration and adherence to a routine. Certain rules and regulations must be followed and acceptable levels of dress, language, social habits, time keeping and personal hygiene must also be displayed. Work tolerance, which may also include the ability to tolerate noise, heat, cold, heights, dust, outdoor work and long hours, may therefore actively need improving in some people whose physical and psychological fitness have been seriously impaired. Similarly, people who have been unemployed for a substantial period of time may need help in achieving the correct level of 'adult' skills such as budgeting, the adjustment of personal life around a work routine, the ability to use public transport, to work unsupervised or to a high level of accuracy, to relate adequately to their workmates and employers and to be personally independent in all activities of daily living, all of which may be necessary when working.

Clearly, many people will not lack in all the above mentioned skills but, equally, many will need help in regaining, improving or learning such skills following a period of physical impairment. For this reason a variety of services are available to the disabled in order to help them become fit for work, to train for suitable employment if they cannot continue with their previous work and also to help them find work once fit and ready to do so. Such services are available both in hospital and in the community and each has its own role to play in helping the disabled person return to work (Fig. 12.1). These services are either medically based, such as those available in hospitals, rehabilitation centres or by contact with the patient's general practitioner, or they are the responsibility of the Manpower Services Commission. The MSC, operating via the Employment Service Agency (responsible for the training of Disablement Resettlement Officers and the running of Employment Rehabilitation centres etc) and the Training Services Agency (responsible for the running of Skills Centres, the Training Opportunities Scheme — TOPS — residential training centres and similar schemes) is responsible for providing employment and training services for disabled people under the Disabled Persons (Employment) Acts of 1944 and 1958.

A disabled person may first come into contact with the available services whilst in hospital, through community services which he has approached (such as his general practitioner or Social Services department) or via his local Job Centre where he has gone to find employment. Young disabled people will usually find help through their school or special school. The role and method of referral of each service is described below. The therapist must remember, however, that some of the lines of communication and referral may vary from area to area and also that some services are more readily available than others in certain parts of the country.

THE ROLE OF THE OCCUPATIONAL THERAPIST

The occupational therapist working in a hospital may first come into contact with a patient during the early stages of his illness, when it is felt that work resettlement may pose a problem to him later on, for example following a spinal injury, head injury or cerebral vascular accident in a younger person. He may, however, be referred specifically for work assessment as, for example, following a cornonary thrombosis, back injury or burns accident in which residual disability has inhibited a full return of function. In all such cases the role of the occupational therapist is a wide one and may involve all or some of the following aims:

Teaching independence in the activities of daily living. Where personal independence has been lost, the therapist must help to restore this before full resettlement can be achieved. Where the person is severely disabled and/or may need to attend an assessment or training centre, it will be necessary for him to become independent in all personal activities before he will be accepted for such a scheme.

Improving physical ability. Where physical function has been lost or impaired, the occupational therapist will be concerned with the restoration of the range of movement, strength, dexterity, coordination and balance which he will need in order to function adequately at work.

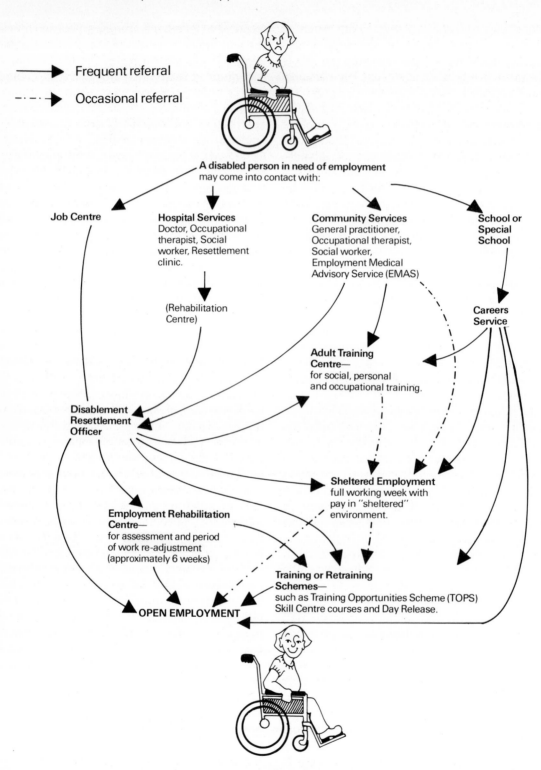

Fig. 12.1 Services available to help the disabled person with employment

Improving psychological skills. If concentration, perception or other mental processes have been affected, the therapist will help improve these. Similarly, if the functions of speech are affected the occupational therapist will help to complement the work of the speech therapist in order to improve the patient's communication skills.

Teaching or improving basic skills. Where confidence or ability have been lost in the performance of basic skills such as the use of public transport, handling money, relating to workmates or driving a car, the therapist, along with other members of the rehabiliation team, will be concerned with improving the patient's level of function in these fields.

Initiating or improving work tolerance. Following illness and a long period away from work, many people may find difficulty in regaining a work habit or sufficient stamina to cope with a full working day. In such a case the occupational therapist can begin to build up the patient's work tolerance by gradually increasing the amount of time, effort and concentration required in the activities he is performing. Similarly, it may be necessary to accustom the person to specific working conditions such as noise, dirt, outdoor work or benchwork where this is felt appropriate. It is frequently difficult for the therapist to simulate the demands imposed by a full day's work in industry or commerce but, where work tolerance is lacking, improvement in this area can certainly be initiated whilst the patient is still attending the hospital for treatment.

Assessing the patient's potential for return to work. Often the occupational therapist may be asked to assess a patient specifically to see if he will be able to return to his former occupation or, where this is not felt feasible, to discover his ability to undertake assessment and training for a new job. The activities performed in a 'work assessment' are extremely varied. Certainly many of the skills and abilities described above should be assessed and improved, for no person will be accepted for open employment if he is not personally independent or cannot make his own way to work. In addition, certain specific assessments may be appropriate. For example, it may be necessary to note the ability of a storekeeper to climb ladders and lift weights or of a clerk to write

clearly, sit for long periods and use a typewriter. In some hospitals the occupational therapist may arrange for the patient to work within a hospital department performing jobs related to those to which he will return. Such an arrangement is obviously useful to both the patient and therapist as it will give a more realistic setting in which both can see the patient's ability, but clearly such arrangements must be made only with the full consent of all departments involved. When assessing a patient's ability to return to work the therapist should ensure that she is well aware of the demands imposed on her patient by his work. This can usually be done by asking the patient himself what his job entails, but where this is not possible the therapist should ensure that she receives accurate information by either contacting the patient's employers or another reliable source.

Many occupational therapy departments devise their own work assessment and report forms for use with patients undergoing this type of assessment. An example of a work assessment is shown in Figure 12.2, but the therapist will find that invariably it is necessary to compile her own form, as the circumstances, facilities are requests she receives will be different in each department.

Giving information and guidance. Frequently people whose employment prospects are doubtful have little idea of the type of help available to them in order to get them fit enough to return to work or to retrain them should they be unable to retain their previous job. It is often a source of great concern to the patient that his future employment prospects seem poor and therefore the occupational therapist should be able to supply accurate and appropriate information and reassure the patient that he can receive help. The therapist may also be the member of the rehabilitation team who makes initial contact with people such as the Disablement Resettlement Officer or with the local Employment Rehabilitation Centre in order to further the patient's return to work.

THE PHYSIOTHERAPIST

While the patient is still in hospital the physiotherapist will be concerned with restoring the patient to the highest level of physical function.

M.R.C. ASSESSMENT REPORT

Name .... Age .... Date ....

Diagnosis .... Consultant

Former Employment ....

Period of Assessment ....

Regularity of Attendance ....

PERSONAL – SOCIAL ADJUSTMENT

1. **Personal appearance**
   (a) Grooming
   (b) Does disability distract from appearance?
2. **Relationship with fellow workers**
   (a) Can he work with others?
   (b) What is his attitude to workmates?
3. **Relationship with supervisor**
   (a) Can he accept criticism and correction?
   (b) Does he depend on supervision?
   (c) What is his reaction to pressure?
4. **Attitude towards work**
   (a) Does he like to get down to work?
   (b) Has he good judgment?
   (c) Is he able to make decisions?
   (d) Is he responsible and honest?
   (e) Does he show initiative?
   (f) Is he able to budget time effectively?
   (g) Can he concentrate?
5. **Adjustment to disability**
6. **Self Confidence**

PHYSICAL CAPACITY FOR WORK

1. **Extent to which disability is a handicap**
2. **Physical tolerance and ability:**

   (a) Standing   (f) Stooping
   (b) Sitting   (g) Climbing
   (c) Carrying   (h) Co-ordination
   (d) Balance   (i) Manual dexterity
   (e) Lifting   (j) Public transport

WORK TESTED – WORK PERFORMANCE

1. **Results of the work patient has been tested on**

   Areas of   (a) Clerical – Educational
   work   (b) Service, e.g. Kitchen, Janitor, etc.
   assessment   (c) Mechanical
                     (d) Manual
2. **What type of work does he produce?**
3. **Does he learn a skill easily and how much practice does he need to develop it?**
4. **Can he retain and follow instructions?**
   (a) Written
   (b) Verbal
   (c) Diagrammatic
5. **Has he special vocational interests?**

CONCLUSION

1. **Employable** – type of work.
2. **Trainable** – what sphere?
3. **Unemployable** – why?

Fig. 12.2 (A) Work assessment report guidelines (B) & (C)   A
Work assessment reports using form (a) as a guideline.

OCCUPATIONAL THERAPY REPORT

Name Mr A. S.　　　　　　　　　　　　　**Age** 23yrs

Consultant Dr S. G.　　　　　　　　　　**Case No.** X 99988

Diagnosis: Gilles de la Tourette Syndrome　　　　**Date** 14th July

Period of assessment: 3 weeks　　　　　**Regularity of attendance:** Daily

Former employment: (1) Newspaper staking, operating compressor in a scrap yard.
(2) Loading lorries for inter-country express. Was unable to continue with this as he could not use public transport.
(3) Honorary assistant play group leader for children between the ages of 3 and 5 years.

PERSONAL – SOCIAL ADJUSTMENT

Mr S. is a tall, dark, slightly built young man of 23yrs. He displays obvious involuntary facial and tongue grimaces together with rather bizarre noises and inappropriate speech in a repetitive fashion. Initially this is threatening and off-putting. Mr S. finds first encounters difficult, which tends to exacerbate these problems.

During Mr S.'s assessment period he gradually settled down and demonstrated that he is a very sensitive and aware person. Once he had gained confidence he was a keen and willing worker with a great sense of humour and a natural ability and wish to help others. He has also shown that when he is interested in what he is doing the involuntary gestures and vocalisations are greatly reduced. They are, however, increased with tiredness, anxiety and boredom.

Mr S. is obviously very apprehensive about the future with regard to his work, finding it at times extremely difficult to accept and adjust to his particular disability and is occasionally resentful of the sheltered and somewhat isolated life that this disability has forced him to lead.

PHYSICAL CAPACITY FOR WORK

Mr S. has carried out various practical tests and shown no physical limitations. He has a good standard of dexterity and co-ordination. In the past he has found relaxation techniques beneficial, so these were incorporated into his programme. He also gains great pleasure from music, dancing and sport. Physically he is perfectly capable of using public transport but finds it psychologically and socially very stressful.

WORK TESTED-WORK PERFORMANCE

Mr S. has a rather immature letter formation, no mis-spellings and minimal punctuation errors. However, he took 40 minutes to complete a 20 minute passage, saying that he finds difficulty in concentrating when he is not allowed to smoke.

Reading He is quite able to carry out written instructions provided they are simple and clear.

Time/Money He is independent in basic everyday calculations.

Light woodwork When sanding down and revarnishing a stool he carried out the work methodically and thoroughly once the instructions had been given slowly and clearly. He worked at a slow, steady pace.

Repetitive assembly work (C.S.S.D. sorting theatre dressings) Mr S. followed verbal instructions and carried out the work correctly but soon became disinterested saying that he found the task extremely boring. He became restless and showed signs of increased involuntary vocal and physical activity.

Gardening Mr S. expressed a keen interest in this. He went to the library on two occasions to borrow books on the subject. During his time of assessment he prepared the earth for planting and pricked out various herbs, vegetables and bedding plants. Although a little slow, he worked quietly and methodically under limited supervision.

Cooking Mr S. lives with his parents and his mother carries out most domestic duties. However, when his parents are out or away Mr S. is quite capable of cooking himself a meal and has occasionally done some baking, which he says he enjoys. During his assessment he carried out written instructions correctly, weighed out ingredients and followed the cooking method step by step to gain a successful result. Again he worked quietly.

Specific interests Mr S. has shown that he has an artistic and creative talent which he regrets not being able to develop further in the past. It was also interesting to note that while he is doing artwork he is often completely quiet with minimal involuntary activity.

CONCLUSION

A government training course at a Skillcentre would be suitable for Mr S. provided the work was of a practical/creative nature and he was accepted by other members. In the future he may have to accept sheltered employment because of the nature of this particular disability.

B. Hawkins
Occupational Therapist

OCCUPATIONAL THERAPY REPORT
Work Assessment

Name Miss B. H.   Age 44yrs

Consultant Mr E. W.   Case No. 11122

Diagnosis: Cerebellar tumour removed   **Date** 21st March
at the age of 7yrs

Period of assessment: 2 weeks   **Regularity of attendance:** Twice daily

Former employment: Electrical sub-assembly

PERSONAL – SOCIAL ADJUSTMENT

Miss H. is a neat, bespectacled lady of average height who has a rather unco-ordinated walking pattern. I have found her to be quiet, friendly, with a pleasant manner. She is extremely willing to please and will try her hand at most things. She is very aware of her limitations but is most anxious to be treated normally and to be given the opportunity to work and contribute to society. She does have a tendency to initially appear more capable than she really is.

Miss H. left school at the age of 16 years. Since then she has worked for several firms carrying out repetitive assembly type jobs. Unfortunately her last firm closed down a year ago. Since then she worked briefly (two weeks) for County Electrics doing electrical sub assembly but was found to be too slow to continue.

At the moment she assists her mother with the domestic duties, goes to swimming classes and belongs to several community clubs, but she is extremely anxious to have a job again.

PHYSICAL CAPACITY FOR WORK

Miss H. has a tendency to be rather slow and unco-ordinated in her movements, but is quite capable of standing, sitting, carrying, stooping and climbing. She is also able to use public transport provided she is familiar with the route.

WORK TESTED – WORK PERFORMANCE

Miss H. has a tendency to become rather nervous under formal test conditions and I have therefore taken this into account.
Reading Slow but good.
Writing Rather slow, immature writing with a tendency to miss out words. Spelling poor.
English Once again very slow, taking three times the average to complete the task. Poor punctuation and limited grammar and vocabulary.
Arithmetic Only capable of very limited addition, subtraction and multiplication.
Repetitive assembly work (C.S.S.D. – assembly of dressings. Clerical work stamping forms)
Miss H. initially required repeated verbal instructions to complete these tests correctly. She produced a good standard of work but was extremely slow. She tends to be easily distracted and her short-term memory is poor. Miss H. is only capable of following very simple written or diagrammatic instructions and she does not work well under pressure.

CONCLUSION

Training Miss H. does not have the academic ability to cope with any of the government training courses that are offered at a Skillcentre.
Employment Miss H. has tried hard during her asseesment but she does not apear to be up to the reuirements of open employment because of her slowness, poor concentration and her need for careful supervision. However, as she is so keen to work I feel she should be given the opportunity to try Section 11 employment (Sheltered). She is quite capable of simple, repetitive work provided she is supervised and not pressurised.

S. J. Jenkins (Mrs)
Senior Occupational Therapist

Fig. 12.2 (contd)   C

THE SOCIAL WORKER

It is important that the social worker has a knowledge of the patient's background so that any financial or social problems can be dealt with. In some areas the social worker may have direct contact with the patient's employers about the possibility of him retaining his former job.

THE RESETTLEMENT CLINIC

In some hospitals and centres, especially those with specialist units, a resettlement clinic may meet regularly to decide on the future work prospects of patients within the hospital. Such clinics are usually run by the doctor in charge of the unit or the consultant responsible for rehabilitation services and are attended by an occupational therapist, physiotherapist, senior nurse of the unit (where appropriate) and a social worker. Often the local Disablement Resettlement Officer (or hospital disablement resettlement officer) will attend and any other people, such as the psychologist or patient's relatives, as appropriate. In the clinic the patient's case will be presented, his progress charted and his future work prospects discussed. Should any further information be required, such as an additional assessment or the availability of a training scheme, this can be requested.

THE MEDICAL REHABILITATION CENTRE

The aim of a medical rehabilitation centre is to provide an intensive programme of rehabilitation following serious illness or injury. Patients may be referred to such a centre after initial assessment and treatment in hospital. Most rehabilitation centres are run under the auspices of the National Health Service and provide facilities to build up physical fitness and work tolerance to a higher degree than would be possible in most hospital departments. Close liaison is kept with the Disablement Resettlement Officer and regular staff meetings aim to discuss the patient's progress and work prospects. Many rehabilitation centres are residential and each patient is given an individual treatment timetable to which he is encouraged to adhere. The treatment, given under medical supervision, frequently includes physiotherapy (often with hydrotherapy and gymnasium work), occupational therapy and speech therapy, but the centres offer a 'non hospital' atmosphere and patients are encouraged to be personally independent and make their own travel arrangements and social entertainment during their stay.

THE DISABLEMENT RESETTLEMENT OFFICER

The Disablement Resettlement Officer (DRO) works for the Department of Employment and is usually based in the local Job Centre, although some hospitals now employ their own DRO. His work (for which he has undergone specific training) involves advising and introducing people to open employment, vocational or professional training schemes, assessment centres and sheltered or alternative work. The DRO will keep the patient informed of any suitable jobs available for him in the area and will contact local employers on his behalf.

Where medical information may be required in order to alert the employment services of any limitations imposed upon the patient by his disability, the DRO may ask for a confidential report to be completed by the patient's doctor. This confidential information is usually supplied on the Department of Employment's blue form D.P.1. Frequently the occupational therapist may be asked to supply the results of her work assessment in order to complete the required information on questions concerning the patient's upper and lower limb function, his ability to work at heights, out of doors and so on.

Where it is felt appropriate, the DRO may help the patient to enlist on the Disabled Persons Register which is held by the Department of Employment. This is a voluntary register for people over 18 years old and is designed to help disabled people obtain and keep a suitable job as determined by the Disabled Persons (Employment) Act of 1944 when the following points were established:

1. Every employer with 20 or more workers has a duty to employ a proportion (about three per cent) of registered disabled people.

2. Vacancies arising for car park attendants and passenger electric lift attendants are reserved for registered disabled people.

3. Employment in sheltered workshops such as those run by Remploy, some local authorities and voluntary bodies is generally reserved for registered disabled persons.

It is not necessary for a person to register as disabled in order to benefit from the services of the DRO, but if wishing to do so the patient must satisfy him that the disability will last for at least 12 months, that he is available and willing to work and that he has a reasonable chance of keeping work once it is obtained. Once the person's application has been accepted he will be given a certificate of registration (a 'Green Card') which he should show to his current or prospective employer. A disabled person can also apply for his name to be withdrawn from the register at any time.

The DRO may meet his clients either through his local hospital when a doctor or therapist has felt it appropriate to contact him about a particular patient, or through the Job Centre where the disabled person has gone to find work.

EMPLOYMENT REHABILITATION CENTRES

A network of employment rehabilitation centres (ERCs) has been set up by the Employment Service Agency to provide opportunities for people who, following illness, injury or a long period of unemployment, need a chance to adapt themselves gradually to normal working conditions. The ERC will also assess the client's employment capabilities. Courses vary according to the individual's need but the average length of stay is about six weeks and the facilities offered can include woodwork, machine operation, clerical work, bench engineering and assembly work. The ERC aims to work along the lines of a factory so that a realistic work atmosphere is achieved.

During their stay at the centre clients are paid a tax free maintenance allowance which is at a higher rate than basic unemployment or sickness benefit. Each person's programme is regularly discussed and reviewed at a case conference which is attended by the manager of the centre, an employment medical adviser, an occupational psychologist, a social worker, an occupational supervisor and a disablement resettlement officer.

A variety of training and work facilities are available which are designed either specifically to help disabled people or which can be used by both disabled and able bodied. These facilities include:

THE TRAINING OPPORTUNITIES SCHEME (TOPS)

This is a scheme run by the Training Services Agency which provides a wide variety of courses in skilled and semi-skilled occupations. TOPS courses can be followed in a wide range of places including Skillcentres, educational centres of all types (such as technical or commercial colleges), residential colleges for the disabled or on the job itself with training from the employer. Most courses last six months or longer and training for professional occupations can be given where appropriate. All TOPS courses are free and the trainee additionally receives a weekly, tax free allowance, free National Insurance benefits, mid-day meal, accommodation and fares. Applications for TOPS courses should be made through the DRO.

RESIDENTIAL COLLEGES

At present the four residential colleges in this country are run through the Training Services Agency and their aim is to provide residential training courses for disabled people. The colleges offer a variety of courses, each of about six months duration, and areas covered include commercial studies such as typing, book keeping, office skills, hotel and reception work and telephony; bench carpentry and joinery; engineering skills such as draughtsmanship, electronic wiring, machine operating and mechanical servicing as well as other courses such as TV and electronic servicing, typewriter repairing and watch and clock repairing (Fig. 12.3A & B).

The four colleges offering such training are:

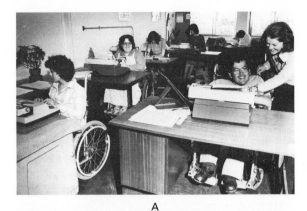

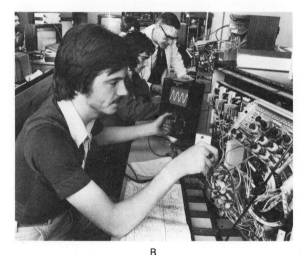

Fig. 12.3 Trainees at St Loyes College for the training of the Disabled for Commerce and Industry, Exeter. (a) Shorthand-typing course (b) Radio & television workshop.

Finchale Training College, Durham

Portland Training College, Near Mansfield, Nottinghamshire

Queen Elizabeth's Training College, Leatherhead, Surrey

St Loyes College, Exeter, Devon.

Trainees receive a training allowance whilst on the course and all applications should be through the patient's local disablement resettlement officer.

SHELTERED EMPLOYMENT

Where the disabled person is unable to work in open employment sheltered work provides an opportunity for him to offer a productive day's work under realistic conditions. Sheltered employment — established under the Disabled Persons (Employment) Act of 1944 — can be provided either through Remploy Ltd, local authority workshops or schemes offered by voluntary organisations.

The Remploy organisation runs over 80 factories in Great Britain and provides jobs for severely disabled people under sheltered yet realistic commercial conditions. Products include furniture, leather goods, textiles and other goods and employees are paid a wage while working. Local authority workshops and those run by voluntary organisations such as the Royal British Legion and the Spastics Society also provide work (usually under contract from local firms) in a realistic setting for disabled people. In most workshops those who attend must be capable of working a standard working week even if their rate of work is slow. Application for Remploy work should come through the local DRO, those for local authority and voluntary workshops will vary and the therapist should be aware of requirements in her area.

SKILLCENTRES

Organised by the Training Services Agency, Skillcentres run courses aimed at offering an intensive period of training in skilled or semi-skilled occupations to men and women who wish to improve their job prospects. Although not organised specifically for disabled people Skillcentre courses are open to them. At present there are over 60 Skillcentres through Great Britain offering a wide variety of courses ranging from bricklaying and plumbing to men's hairdressing and tailoring. Applications for Skillcentre courses should come from people of 19 years of age and over and are normally made through the local Job Centre. Courses provide a thorough grounding in the basic skills required for the job which enables the person to go either into open employment where, following a period of experience, he will be able to compete on equal terms with other trained workers, or on to further training provided on the job by the employer.

Trainees are paid an allowance during training.

ADULT TRAINING CENTRES (ATC)

For those unable to cope with either open or sheltered employment, adult training centres (which are run by local authorities) offer social and occupational training. As well as simple work tasks which are performed in a realistic work atmosphere usually under contract from local firms, ATCs provide training in basic social and domestic skills such as cookery, shopping and self care. Where necessary some educational instruction may be given and centres will often organise outings, dances and activities in order to widen the person's social, personal and work skills to their greatest potential. Trainees receive standard state benefits whilst attending the centre and small remuneration for the work they produce. Some trainees may progress to further training after a period at the centre. The method of application for a place in an ATC may vary from area to area but should come through the system agreed by the local authority in each area.

Other schemes

Other help which may be available to disabled people can include:

1. The provision of adaptations and equipment at his place of work in order to help the physically disabled person in his employment. Such help may take the form of adapting existing machinery or the provision of a special seat or bench to enable the person to cope more easily. This help is available through the DRO.

2. Help with moving expenses in order that a person can take up a job which he has trained if there is a vacancy in another area. This scheme, called the Employment Transfer Scheme, particularly applies to people who have completed a TOPS course and is run by the Employment Service Agency. Information should be obtained through the local Job Centre.

3. 'Enclave' work. These schemes, often run by Local Authorities, involve the employment of groups of severely disabled people who work under special supervision in an otherwise normal working environment. The group work in areas such as municipal parks and gardens and are paid a wage for the work they do.

4. Job Introduction Scheme. If an employer is uncertain about the suitability of a disabled person the NSC will make a contribution towards the wages of that employee for a six-week trial period.

WHY DISABLED PEOPLE CANNOT FIND WORK

It would seem that with all the help which is available to disabled people by way of assessment and training and through other assistance, such as mobility allowances, parking stickers and adaptations to cars, most disabled people should be able to find work. Sadly, however, this does not appear to be so, for many disabled people still have difficulty in finding and keeping work. Although no one factor would seem to account for this, the reason may lie in a combination of the following:

(a). Ignorance of the help available. Many disabled people have no clear idea of the type of help they can get or where they can obtain information about the assistance available.

(b). Inability to get to work and get around once there. This seems to be a common problem for, although a mobility allowance is payable to most people of working age at present it is often not enough to cover the hire of transport to and from work, nor to run a car, and the disabled person may not be able to use public transport. Coupled with this problem of transport may be the person's inability to cope with stairs, steps, slopes, awkwardly placed WCs or other facilities once at work. Similarly, although help is available to adapt machinery for the disabled person, many employers are not aware of this scheme or may be reluctant to have their machinery altered.

(c). Circumspection of employers and workmates. It may happen that, because of ignorance, prejudice or simply fear of the unknown, employers or workmates find difficulty accepting a new disabled person into their workforce. Fears that they may slow down production, that their illness may cause problems with which the establishment is unable to cope or that the condition may in some way be embarrassing, can all account to some degree for this reluctance.

(d). Loss of work habit. If, after a prolonged absence from work, the disabled person tries to return without a period of adjustment, he may find

that the work is more demanding than he anticipated and that he cannot cope. Similarly, it may
happen that the stresses of work may exacerbate
his condition and result in frequent periods of
sickness which make his employers reluctant to
employ other disabled workers.

(e). Stigma. Although the disabled persons register is designed to help those who have difficulty
in finding or maintaining employment, some disabled people feel that there is a stigma attached to
being labelled as disabled and are, therefore,
reluctant to register as a 'green card man'.

Clearly, the process of work resettlement can be
a long and complex one and it is important for the
occupational therapist, who often meets the person in the early days of his rehabilitation into
work, to understand the role she plays in her
patient's programme and be able to give accurate
and realistic information as to the type of services
available to him.

REFERENCES AND FURTHER READING

Employment Services Agency and the Central Office of
Information Monthly publication: Outlook – The
Rehabilitation and Resettlement Service magazine. HMSO,
London

Employment Services Agency and the Central Office of
Information 1976 Rehabilitation, retraining, resettlement –
Employment services for handicapped people. HMSO,
London

Jones M, Jay P 1977 An approach to occupational therapy, 3rd
edn. Butterworths, London

MacDonald E M 1976 Occupational therapy in rehabilitation,
4th edn. Balliere Tindall, London

Manpower Services Commission and the Central Office of
Information 1978 Employing disabled people. HMSO,
London

Training Services Agency and the Central Office of Information
1974 Training services – for industry and commerce. HMSO,
London

Training Services Agency and the Central Office of Information
1975 Recruiting Skillcentre trainees. HMSO, London

13
Departmental management

Departmental management is an important aspect of all occupational therapists' work. This chapter describes the basic principles of management in occupational therapy and relates this to the overall structure and organisation of the Health Service.

ORGANISATION OF THE HEALTH SERVICE

There was a major re-organisation of the National Health Service in 1974, and on 1st April 1983, further changes were made to streamline the service.

The new structure is as follows:

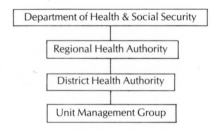

Department of Health and Social Security (DHSS)

This is the governing body at national level which has ultimate responsibility for the Health Service and is responsible for disseminating information to Regions and Districts.

Regional Health Authority (RHA)

This monitors the work of the District Health Authority, in particular planning, allocation of resources, and major building projects. It may also provide special regional services e.g. a computer centre.

District Health Authority (DHA)

The employing authority for National Health Service staff. A District Health Authority usually consists of the catchment area around a District General Hospital, plus mental illness and mental handicap units, and their associated community services. The Health Authority is managed by a team of 16 people from a wide variety of backgrounds, who are responsible for policy and decision making.

The operational unit of the DHA is the District Management Team (DMT), comprising the District Medical Officer, District Finance Officer, District Administrator, District Nursing Officer, a consultant and a G.P.

The DMT delegates the day-to-day running of the service to Unit Management Groups, who are responsible for a large hospital or group of hospitals. The 1983 re-organisation was aimed at enabling more decisions to be made at Unit level, thus making the service more effective.

ORGANISATION OF OCCUPATIONAL THERAPY

Occupational therapists may work either in the Health Service or for the Local Authority Social Services Department.

Occupational therapy in Social Services

Since the Chronically Sick and Disabled Persons Act was introduced in 1970, Local Authority Social Services departments have employed more occupational therapists to help implement the act. They are usually attached to social work teams and work in a particular Social Services Division, but are professionally responsible to a head occupational therapist based centrally. Most Social Services occupational therapists work in the community, visiting clients in their own homes, but they may also work in centres for the disabled or in residential homes.

Occupational therapy in the Health Service

Occupational therapists working in the Health Service are employed by and work in a particular District Health Authority. They are mostly hospital based, although a few Districts also employ community occupational therapists who provide a service for the general practitioner and his team and liaise with the Social Services Department under the obligations of the Chronically Sick and Disabled Persons Act.

MANAGEMENT STRUCTURE WITHIN THE NATIONAL HEALTH SERVICE

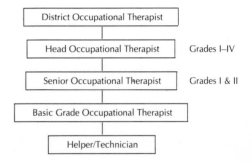

District Occupational Therapists are now being appointed to manage their own service. They may still be attached to a particular hospital or unit and have a clinical committment within that unit, but their primary function is to coordinate and develop the whole of the occupational therapy service within the District. The District Occupational Therapist has a direct link with the DMT via the District Medical Officer or the District Administrator.

Head Occupational Therapists are responsible for all the occupational therapy staff in a particular working area. There are four grades (I to IV) depending on the number of staff for whom she is responsible.

Senior Occupational Therapists are either Grade I or Grade II, depending on whether they work single-handed, are responsible for another member of staff or work in a specialised field.

Basic grade occupational therapists work under the supervision of a Head Occupational Therapist or Senior Occupational Therapist.

There may also be unqualified staff working in the Occupational Therapy Department, for example:

Occupational therapy helpers. They undertake certain duties delegated by occupational therapists, such as diversional craft activities or dressing practices. They must always work under the supervision of a qualified Senior Occupational Therapist.

Occupational therapy technicians. These are people with a specific skill such as wood work who run the technical side of a workshop. They must only treat patients under the direction of a qualified occupational therapist. They may also be employed in the Community to make aids and install them in the clients' homes.

Clerical staff. They help with clerical and administrative duties not requiring the professional skills of an occupational therapist; for example, ordering and control of stock, patients' transport, departmental statistics. They may also provide secretarial help.

Volunteers. These are not hospital staff, but may help in occupational therapy departments by arrangement with the Voluntary Services organiser. While in the department they are responsible to a qualified occupational therapist and may assist by making tea for the patients, adapting patients' clothing or helping to run a social activity.

THE MANAGEMENT ROLE OF OCCUPATIONAL THERAPISTS

All occupational therapists, even those at basic grade level, are involved in some sort of management. It has now been recognised, by the appointment of District Occupational Therapists, that occupational therapists are able to manage their own service, instead of being managed by doctors or administrators, and the development of management skills is emphasised at all levels. A well managed department runs efficiently, uses staff time and resources to the full and therefore, ultimately, gives the best possible service to the patient.

Management at all levels covers several aspects:
1. Personnel
2. Professional/clinical
3. Administration
4. Communication.

Personnel

Staffing establishments

There is a funded establishment for every department agreed by the Head or District Occupational Therapist, District Personnel Department and District Finance Department.

Establishment figures are usually considered in whole time equivalents, although a department may employ several part-time staff whose aggregate hours equate to full-time posts. The number and grade of staff required for an occupational therapy department depends on the following factors:

Type of hospital, number of beds, categories and numbers of patients likely to be referred

Type of treatments carried out and treatment time available

Siting of treatment areas and their facilities and space

Availability of support staff

The department's other committments, e.g. teaching, research.

Orientation of staff

Proper orientation of new staff is important to help them settle down quickly and enable them to contribute to the department as soon as possible. It is often very confusing for new staff to be bombarded with facts on their first day, so it is better to let orientation take place gradually. A written hand-out, giving basic information about the department, can be very useful for new staff. The Head Occupational Therapist usually sees new staff on their first day and deals with the necessary administrative procedures, but may delegate to a senior member of staff the responsibility of introducing the new occupational therapist to her particular work area.

A full orientation should include the following:
● information about the occupational therapy department and a staff timetable showing where and when they work.
● introduction to all members of the occupational therapy staff.
● explanation of the lay-out of the department, including storage of tools, materials, stationery and patients' cards.
● explanation of administrative procedures within the department, such as booking out of stock and time sheets.
● familiarisation with referral systems, patients' notes, statistics, methods of recording and reporting treatment and any other patient-related activities.
● location of the first-aid box and fire appliances and knowledge of emergency procedures such as fire drills and crash call systems.
● information about current legislation which may affect her work, e.g. the Health and Safety at Work Act, and about local codes of practice such as grievance and dismissal procedures.
● introduction to the union representative and information about unions.
● staff catering and cloak room facilities and the availability of social facilities.
● lay-out of the hospital and introduction to relevant departments.
● introduction to other members of the treatment team, for example, ward sister, medical staff, health visitor, district nurse.
● information about outside agencies with whom the department liaises, such as the Social Services departments.

In addition to departmental orientation, multi-disciplinary induction courses are sometimes organised by the hospital administrator. These may include some background history of the hospital, a comprehensive tour of all departments, information about the structure of the Health Service and useful local information. This is often a good opportunity for the occupational therapist to meet new members of staff from other departments.

Deployment of staff

In most areas there is a shortage of qualified occupational therapists, so staff deployment should be kept under constant review in order that scarce professional skills are used to the best advantage.

In most departments each post within the establishment has a job description, defining specific areas of responsibility and staff are appointed to work in those areas. However, the needs of different units can change, so regular reassessments of the areas to be covered and staff available are essential. When deploying staff the following points should be considered:

● the number of patients, number of beds on the unit and number of referrals.
● the type of treatment required and whether it is group or individual.
● the need for specialist skills (e.g. splint making).
● personal qualities required, for example a therapist with a quiet, or outgoing approach.
● units which are building up an occupational therapy service.

Additionally, the availability of staff, including their grade, career development, experience, personal qualities, whether full- or part-time and their needs for training should also be considered.

For example, part-time staff can often be used economically when the biggest demand is at certain times of the day, for example in a Day Hospital where patients attend between 10.00 am and 3.00 pm, or on geriatric wards where patients have dressing practice in the morning.

Staff development and job satisfaction

The career development of an occupational therapist depends to a large extent on her ambition, motivation and needs. However, staff should be encouraged to develop their potential to the full, so that they achieve job satisfaction and contribute their maximum to the department in which they work.

Within the occupational therapy department, staff development can be helped by:

A rotation system for staff to broaden their experience.

Provision of adequate reference, training and research facilities, which staff are encouraged to use.

A flexible career structure to give opportunities for promotion within the department.

Regular staff appraisal, so that deficiences can be overcome and future needs identified.

Ensuring that all staff have some kind of administrative or managerial responsibility within the department, to encourage the development of management skills.

Encouragement of new ideas and techniques and help with the implementation of these.

Professional/clinical function

Code of professional conduct

Upon qualification occupational therapists agree to uphold a code of professional practice. In broad terms this states:

1. That they will only treat patients under medical direction. Although the actual system of referral may vary greatly, occupational therapists in hospitals should only treat patients if requested to do so by a doctor. In the community, referral systems are often much less rigid, but the community occupational therapist has a responsibility to inform the general practitioner that his patient is being treated.

2. That they will maintain confidentiality about all aspects of their work with patients. All patients' notes and records should be kept in a safe place, so that they are only accessible to staff. Staff should take care not to discuss a patient in front of other patients or non-professional staff in the hospital or outside the hospital. If case histories are

presented by students or staff for teaching purposes outside the hospital, the patient's real name should not be disclosed. Staff should be aware that there could be certain facts about a patient, for instance, aspects of his personal behaviour or social background, which should not be written down. They should establish how much the patient has been told about his illness before discussing it with him.

3. That they will conduct themselves in a professional manner. Staff should have no personal involvement with patients still undergoing treatment or use any knowledge about the patient for personal gain. Patients should always be respected as individuals, and should not be made fun of or abused in any way.

A professional approach is often difficult to define and may only develop with experience. Senior staff, therefore, have a responsibility to show an example to their junior staff, especially unqualified members such as occupational therapy helpers, and they should set the standard of behaviour in their department. Inexperienced staff should ask for help if they find themselves in a difficult relationship with a patient.

Patients' records

Every department should keep accurate records of the patients they are treating. Apart from being useful for reference purposes, they may be important from a legal point of view, for instance if a patient brings an action for damages against the hospital. The type and detail of patients' records varies enormously from department to department, but they should include:

Statistical information. Certain information is required by the Department of Health and Social Security for statistical purposes. This will vary according to the type of hospital. A register should be kept of the numbers and names of patients, the frequency of attendance and amount of treatment given. In-and out-patients are usually recorded separately and the number of new patients and discharges is also shown. This information is usually collected at the end of every month and sent to the hospital records department who forwards it to the DHSS. Treatment figures are often useful for assessing the changing demands on a particular service or the need for additional staff.

Many departments may keep additional records for specific purposes, for example to evaluate the treatment of a particular patient group, or to assess how therapists are using the treatment time.

Patients' referral cards. All patients treated by the occupational therapist should have some kind of referral card. This should give:

Name of patient
Marital status
Social circumstances, e.g. if patient is living alone
Address or hospital ward
Date of birth
Primary diagnosis
Other medical conditions
Precautions and contra-indications
Reason for treatment
Occupation
Name of referring doctor
Name of patient's general practitioner.

If necessary, the occupational therapist should have access to the patient's notes and be able to supplement this basic information with relevant information, such as past history, current drug regime, social history and previous hospital admissions. It is also useful to file old referral cards centrally, so that reference to them can be made if the patient is re-admitted.

Recording progress: Patients' treatment cards are only of value if they are kept up to date. It is particularly important to record changes in the patient's condition and his response to treatment, as well as the type of treatment given. There should be sufficient information on the card to enable another therapist to carry on treatment if required. Regular recording also helps the therapist to monitor and evaluate the treatment and change it if necessary.

Many departments use forms or charts to record progress. These have the advantage of being quick and easy to fill in and often make more impact than a long written report. However, care must be taken to explain any grading system used, so that the form is correctly interpreted by other staff. It is also important to allow space for additional comments, otherwise these records may become too impersonal.

Reporting. It is essential for therapists to have some kind of feed-back to the referring agency, so that progress can be discussed and treatment modified where appropriate.

Written reports should be clear and concise, be typewritten if possible and only contain relevant information. A copy of the report should be included in the patient's notes and copies may be sent to others who may be involved, such as the general practitioner or social worker.

Verbal reporting usually takes place in ward rounds, clinics or case conferences. Discussion is the most useful form of communication, but this may need to be followed by a written report at a later date. Short written records should also be made of telephone conversations and informal talks about the patient, as these are easily forgotten or misinterpreted.

Planning patient treatment

It is important to make the best possible use of the time a patient spends with the occupational therapist. The patient should feel that he has achieved something during the treatment session and be motivated to continue treatment. The occupational therapist should feel that a good relationship has been formed with the patient, that some of the treatment aims have been fulfilled, and that there has been a definite response from the patient, enabling future treatment to be planned.

The following factors are important in planning treatment:

1. *Preparation.* Look up the treatment cards of the patients about to attend and collect all relevant information about them. If a patient is new, try to read the case notes as well. If more than one member of staff is involved in the treatment meet before the patients arrive to discuss work and allocate specific tasks. Make sure that all the equipment which may be used is accessible and in good working order. Check that there are enough chairs and tables of the correct height and plan where patients are going to sit, for instance ensure that a heavily disabled patient in a wheelchair is not blocking an exit. Decide on the activities to be used, but have alternatives if necessary.

2. *Programming.* Careful programming will ensure that the patient receives the maximum benefit from each treatment session, and does not waste time waiting for treatment to start. Consider:

Any other treatments the patient may be having, such as physiotherapy, and liaise with the appropriate department

Other demands on the patient's time, for example ward rounds, meal breaks

Constraints of transport

Other patients being treated at the time

The stage of the patient's illness, his ability to concentrate and his stamina.

Ideally, each patient should have an individual programme, copies of which should be sent to relevant departments.

3. *Treatment plans.* All patients should have some kind of plan for their treatment. This needs to be flexible enough to allow for change and should be regularly reviewed and modified according to the patient's progress.

The format of the treatment plan will vary enormously depending on the type of treatment. A useful framework could be:

(a). *Interview and assessment of patient.* Some information about the patient will be available from the referral card or the patient's notes, but an additional assessment by the occupational therapist is essential in order to plan effective treatment. Specific assessment forms may be used (for example to measure hand function or list problems in the activities of daily living) or the therapist may make a more informal assessment of the patient's condition. Findings and impressions should be recorded on the patient's treatment card.

(b). *Aims of treatment.* These should be decided once the patient has been assessed. Although for most patients the overall treatment aims are interrelated, it is often useful for the therapist to break these down into single components in order to get a clearer picture of what is required, for example: Improve extension of wrist, build up concentration, teach independence in putting on stockings.

(c). *Planning activities.* These should always relate to the aims of treatment, for example — coil pottery to improve extension of wrist, copy typing to build up concentration and dressing practice to teach independence with stocking aid. The activities selected should also reflect the patient's interests and be as relevant as possible to his normal life.

(d). *Patient's response to treatment.* This should be carefully noted, even if the response is negative. A formal reassessment after treatment may be necessary, such as a repeat of joint measurements. Observations by other staff should also be noted.

(e). *Plan of future treatment.* This will depend on the patient's response to treatment, but it should involve some change or modification; a new activity might be suggested, the length of treatment time increased or discharge considered. Future plans, for example planning a home visit or making arrangements regarding employment, should also be made.

Administration

A number of administrative duties are necessary for the smooth running of an occupational therapy department. In some departments these duties are delegated to clerical staff.

Ordering materials and equipment

Many departments have an annual budget for materials and equipment. It is therefore important to be as economical as possible and compare prices and discounts of different firms before ordering, although it must be borne in mind that the cheapest goods are not always the best value. The Supplies Department through which the goods are usually ordered, often have contracts with certain firms, and it is best to use these firms if possible.

Each Health Authority has its own system for ordering, but individual departments can usually order single items up to a fixed amount. Requests for more expensive items usually have to be approved by the District Management Team.

The following information is required when ordering:

Name and address of supplier

Name and address of department requesting goods or service and appropriate costing code if used

Address to which goods should be delivered

Address to which invoice should be sent

Full description of goods — quantity required, description, catalogue number, unit price, total price.

Authorised signature.

Orders are usually made out with several copies, one each for example, being sent to the

Requisitioning department
Supplier
Unit Finance Department
Delivery point
District Finance Department.

Receipt of goods

It is important that goods are checked as soon as possible after delivery. Many firms will not accept responsibility for shortages or damages after six days.

Make sure that the goods received are the same as those ordered, as far as quantity and description are concerned. Ensure there are no faults or breakages. There is usually a packing note enclosed; check this against what was ordered and what has been received. A 'goods received' note should then be made out and sent to the Finance Department, who will usually not pay the invoice until the order is complete.

Booking in stock

Once goods have arrived, they need to be booked into the department. A variety of systems can be used, of which the stock card system is the easiest.
The stock card should show:

Name of commodity
Where ordered from and order number
Unit price
Quantity booked in
Balance in stock.

Booking out stock

If several staff are taking goods from the stock room, the booking out system needs to be simple and effective. A note book giving the description and quantity of goods taken, the unit for which they are taken and the initials of the staff is useful and should be kept in the stock room. The information can then be transferred to the stock card at a later date and the balance adjusted accordingly.

Stock sent to other hospitals may be booked out on a similar basis, except that there needs to be an inter-hospital debit system, so that the receiving hospital is charged for the goods it requests.

Pricing materials

In Districts where there are occupational therapy budget holders, invoices are checked, coded and authorised by the District or Head occupational therapist. The occupational therapy department needs a copy of the final invoice from the firm to enable them to price goods accurately. Many departments add a small percentage to the cost of materials when pricing finished articles, to cover carriage charges and wastage. There should be a comprehensive list in the department of the prices of most finished articles, and non-standard articles can always be priced from the information on the stock card.

Selling finished articles

Departments should, if possible, avoid accumulating large stocks of unwanted finished articles. Patients not wishing to buy their articles could be encouraged to produce items which have been ordered by staff in other departments and should not be allowed to produce work of such low standard that it cannot be sold. Patients who are only capable of simple tasks should work with cheap or scrap materials, as it is very demoralising to make an article which remains on the shelf for months. A display cabinet is often useful for selling surplus finished articles, or the department may organise a sale of work, which could be run by volunteers.

Stocktaking

Stocktaking takes place at the end of the financial year in order to compare the actual stock with the amount shown on the stock cards. All materials in the stock room or store need to be counted, plus finished articles, work in progress and stock in ward cupboards. It is also useful to take an inventory of tools and equipment, although these do not usually appear on the stock returns. The final figure should enable the department to compare what has been ordered with cash receipted and items still in stock, and ensure that there is a movement of stock. Items that have not been used for a long time can sometimes be transferred to another hospital or small amounts may be written off.

Storage and care of equipment and materials:

Equipment. All equipment, especially that used for treatment, should be regularly serviced and maintained. This should be carried out by the hospital maintenance department or the occupational therapy technician, if this is part of the job description. Any suspected defect in a piece of equipment or machinery should be reported immediately and the equipment not used until it has been checked by a suitably qualified person. Basic procedures, such as changing saw blades on a fretsaw or oiling a sewing machine, should be able to be undertaken by all staff using that particular piece of equipment. Occupational therapists working with machinery or equipment should familiarise themselves thoroughly with the particular model before using it to treat patients.

Tools. These should be sharpened regularly and stored properly. A shadow board is useful for keeping a check on tools, especially items such as sharp scissors which may be a hazard to patients. Occupational therapists should ensure that they always use the correct tools for the job, so as to set a good example to the patients and help prevent accidents.

Materials. Every department should have adequate space for the proper storage of materials, so that they are easily accessible to all staff and do not deteriorate in storage. Certain materials need special attention, for example:

Timber should not be allowed to become damp

Cane should not be allowed to become too dry and should be hung or stored flat (never in coils)

Glues, varnishes, turpentine and any other inflammable substance should be stored in a metal cupboard, away from direct heat

Seating cord, wool, or any item containing dye should be stored away from direct sunlight.

General care of department

The department as a whole should be kept clean and tidy. The Health and Safety at Work Act made all staff responsible for identifying and avoiding hazards and establishing safe methods of use for equipment and machinery.

In the occupational therapy department attention needs to be given to the following areas of concern:

Fire precautions
First aid facilities
Hazards in the kitchen
Storage facilities
Adequate safety guards on machinery
Protective clothing, including goggles
Ventilation
Lighting
Heating
Handling of toxic substances
Floor covering
Staff facilities
Hygiene and decoration.

Communication

An occupational therapy department needs to have links with many other agencies and departments, to enable the many facets of patient treatment and departmental administration to be carried out smoothly.

Communication within the occupational therapy department

This is especially important if the department is scattered or if there is a large number of staff. Communication is necessary in order to pass on basic information, exchange professional knowledge and skills, integrate staff into the department, promote good staff relationships, encourage democratic decision making and discuss problems.

Methods of achieving good communication include regular staff meetings, at which all staff can bring up topics for discussion; meetings between senior staff or unit heads to discuss problems; informal meetings for coffee, lunch or tea breaks; department information sheet or newsletter, which could include Minutes of staff meetings; case presentations or lectures and social events.

Communication within the hospital

Informal communication exists between occupational therapists and:

(a). Medical, nursing and other professional staff, usually to convey or exchange information about patients. This may take the form of ward rounds or case conferences, informal ward meetings, patients' programme planning meetings, written reports, verbal reports or informal discussions.

In the hospital the professional team may include the consultant, nursing staff, physiotherapists, speech therapist or psychologist as well as the occupational therapist.

In the community the team could be the general practitioner, health visitor or district nurse and the occupational therapist.

(b). Administrative and clerical staff who act as coordinators for all groups of staff in the hospital or unit. The occupational therapy department may need to communicate with the Salaries and Wages department, Supplies department, Personnel department (especially for legislative and employment procedures), Unit Administrator and the Finance department.

(c). Ancillary staff, such as porters, domestics, engineers, and caterers, whose co-operation is invaluable for such jobs as cleaning the department, maintaining equipment, repairs and decoration, the transport of patients, supplying catering requisites and laundry.

Formal communication in the hospital is via interdisciplinary meetings such as:

(i) Heads of Department Meetings chaired by the Unit Administrator to pass on general information and discuss common problems.

(ii) Representative Committees of particular professional groups. For example, occupational therapists may sit on Therapeutic Professions Committees, which may also include chiropodists, dietitians, orthoptists, physiotherapists, radiographers, remedial gymnasts and speech therapists.

Their function is an advisory one. They are, for instance, asked for comments on reports and circulars affecting their professions, but the committee can also ensure that its members are involved in new building projects and the re-organisation of wards, by making representation to the District Management Team or District Health Authority.

(iii) The Staff Consultative Committee is the official meeting point between management and staff organisations. It discusses policies and plans made by the District or any problems raised by its members, such as grievance procedures, travelling expenses or the provision of creche facilities.

Communication with other occupational therapists in the area

It is important to be aware of other occupational therapy facilities within the area, for exchange of information, use of specialist facilities or transfer of patients. Communication between hospital and community occupational therapists is especially important to ensure continuity of treatment and prevent duplication of work. Hospital occupational therapists should check with the community occupational therapists before planning a home visit and a joint home visit is often valuable. Community occupational therapists may be able to use some of the hospital facilities to assess their patients or may like to make use of the library or teaching facilities in the hospital.

Communication with outside agencies and services in the area

A number of outside agencies could be involved with the patient, for instance:

Social Services: Meals on Wheels, Home Help and old people's homes.

Local organisations, both voluntary and official: Red Cross, Age Concern, Multiple Sclerosis Society, Local Artificial Limb and Appliance Centre (ALAC), Local Housing Department.

Disablement Resettlement Officer (DRO) and Local Employment Office for patients returning to work.

Up-to-date information needs to be kept in the occupational therapy department about the role of these agencies, and how they can be contacted.

In some areas useful links also exist between occupational therapy departments and local educational establishments, who may help with research projects, loan specialist equipment or library facilities. Occupational therapists may be involved in careers talks to schools, or pupils may be seconded to the department for voluntary work or work experience projects.

Communication with national bodies

The British Association of Occupational Therapists is the trade union or representative body at national level, with negotiating rights on the Whitley Council. It maintains links with its members via the Council Representatives which represent each Region. The College of Occupational Therapists is the professional body which awards the professional diploma and organises study days, teaching courses and other related professional schemes. There is now also an occupational therapist at the Department of Health and Social Security to advise and collect information about occupational therapy.

REFERENCES AND FURTHER READING

British Association of Occupational Therapists 1975 Code of professional conduct for occupational therapists. B.A.O.T., London.
Harding L 1973 The reorganisation of the National Health Service. N.E. Metropolitan Regional Hospital Board, London.
The Health and Safety at Work Act 1974. H.M.S.O., London.

SECTION | **TWO**

Occupational therapy related to specific physical disabilities

The cure for this ill is not to sit still
Or frowst with a book by the fire
But to take a large hoe and shovel also
And dig till you gently perspire

RUDYARD KIPLING
1865 — 1936

14

Amputation

Amputation, that is the loss of whole or part of a limb or projecting part of the body, is not a new phenomenon. Records written nearly 500 years BC tell of a Persian soldier, Hegistratus, who escaped from the stocks by cutting off his foot and later replacing it with a wooden one; early pictorial evidence on walls and vessels show lower limb pylons in use, and who has not heard of Douglas Bader and Long John Silver!

Many old prostheses still exist in museums throughout the world showing that amputation is and always has been a universal problem. Much advance has been made in recent years in the fitting and powering of artificial limbs, possibly spurred on by events such as the World Wars and the Thalidomide tragedy, both of which excited public interest and sympathy for those left with deformed or missing limbs. Today, the routine care of the amputee continues and the occupational therapist plays an important role in helping the patient attain his highest level of function.

AMPUTATIONS OF THE LOWER LIMB

Causes

Peripheral vascular insufficiency. This is the cause of by far the greatest number of amputations and can be the result of:

(a). *Arteriosclerosis.* The arteries become hardened and the lumen narrowed due to deposits on the arterial walls. This diminishes blood supply and raises the possibility of blockage or gangrene following slight trauma.

(b). *Diabetic gangrene.* This occurs most frequently in patients over the age of 50. Frequently these patients suffer from peripheral neuritis as a long-term result of their diabetes and this interferes with the sensory input to the limb. Therefore, any minor trauma such as banging the toes or rubbing of sores by badly fitting shoes can lead to tissue breakdown. Because of the lack of sensation and possibly poor circulation, the wound may remain untreated. Healing is slow or may not occur and gangrenous changes appear.

(c). *Embolism or thrombosis.* Thrombosis occuring in the limb will wholly or partly block the blood supply distal to its site.

The conditions above are seen most commonly in older patients. Over 70 per cent of amputations are performed on those of 70 years or older. In most cases healing is slower than normal as blood supply is poor.

Malignant neoplasms. Primary growths in bone (osteosarcoma) usually occur in younger patients. Amputation may also be necessary for metastatic invasion of a limb arising from a primary focus such as the breast.

Infection. For instance gas gangrene (death of tissue caused by a gas-producing bacillus), leprosy and scleroderma.

Trauma. If limbs are irreparably damaged, amputation may be indicated. Trauma is more commonly seen in younger patients. Amputation may also be considered if there is gross nerve damage, e.g. at the brachial plexus, which leaves a flaccid and anaesthetic limb. The stump usually heals well as blood supply is good.

Congenital. Infants can be born with absent, deformed or partly formed limbs.

Other tissue damage. For instance burns and frostbite.

Treatment

This can be divided into four stages.

1. *Preoperative.* The period before anticipated surgery is important and the patient should be prepared physically and mentally for the operation and subsequent rehabilitation.

(a). Exercises. These should aim at maintaining the patient at his highest level of function. All uninvolved joints should be exercised to maintain or increase strength and mobility. If lower limb amputation is to be undertaken, it is especially important that the upper limbs are exercised as they will have to support much of the body weight after operation when the patient is transferring, walking and learning to balance again. It is equally important that trunk mobility is encouraged, as good trunk control is also essential for the above activities.

(b). Explanation. The patient should be told exactly what will happen to him and what level of functional recovery he may expect.

(c). The institution of services. In preparation for the postoperative period the limb suppliers should be contacted (this is not usually the job of the therapist). A home visit may be appropriate and a wheelchair can be ordered, should this be considered necessary.

2. *Surgery.* Amputation should produce a stump of optimum length to afford the best leverage and mechanical advantage for the prosthesis. For example, a very short femoral stump offers little leverage for the prosthesis, whereas one which is too long may interfere with fitting the mechanism of the knee joint. It should be shaped so that the prosthesis fits well and the scar should be positioned either slightly anteriorly or posteriorly to the end of the stump (Fig. 14.1). This is especially important in stumps which will be weight-bearing, such as in through-knee and Syme's amputations, so that weight is not taken through the hard scar tissue.

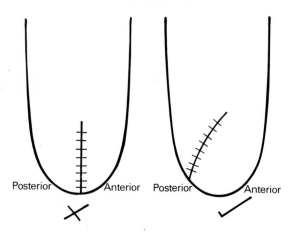

Fig. 14.1 Scar position on the amputated stump — the well-positioned scar is on the right

Encourage . . .

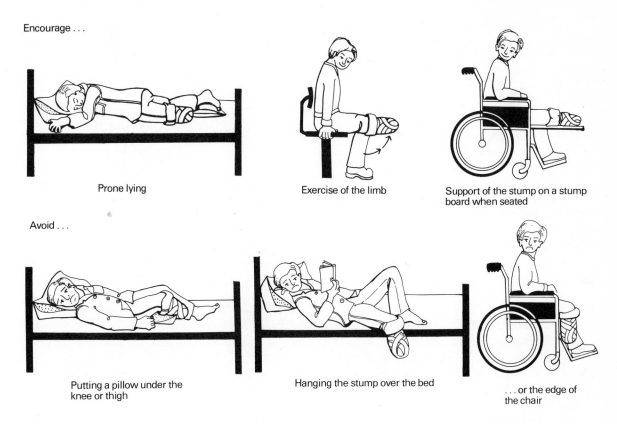

Prone lying

Exercise of the limb

Support of the stump on a stump board when seated

Avoid . . .

Putting a pillow under the knee or thigh

Hanging the stump over the bed

. . . or the edge of the chair

Fig. 14.2 Avoiding contractures

Amputations are usually classified according to the level at which they are performed, for example above-knee or hind-quarter amputations. Some specific operations are referred to by name, such as the Syme's amputation, performed at the ankle, and the Gritti-Stokes amputation, performed at the knee.

3. *Preprosthetic.* Patients who have undergone traumatic (emergency) amputation will need help to adjust to the loss of their limb at this stage whilst those who have undergone 'cold' surgery will be partly prepared. Complications which may arise after amputation include medical problems such as infection, haemorrhage or neuroma and psychological problems such as anxiety, depression and occasionally psychotic states. These are more common in the elderly.

Some degree of 'phantom limb syndrome' invariably occurs postoperatively. The patient feels that the amputated part of his limb is still present and may complain of pain in it. He should be reassured that this is quite a normal sensation which should diminish in time.

Correct care of the stump is important, especially in the early, preprosthetic days, as neglect in this period can lead to a poorly shaped stump making it difficult to fit a prosthesis.

(a). Avoid contractures, especially at the hip and knee joints. This can be done by putting the remaining joints of the affected limb through a full range of active and passive movement at regular intervals. The patient should avoid sitting with his knee flexed or hanging over the edge of a bed or chair and putting a pillow under his knee or thigh, as this will encourage flexion. Prone lying several times a day should be encouraged to promote hip and knee extension (Fig. 14.2).

(b). Condition and shape the stump. The most widely used method is to apply elastic bandages over the stump as shown in Figure 14.3 to condition the stump to constant pressure and maintain its shape by preventing oedema.

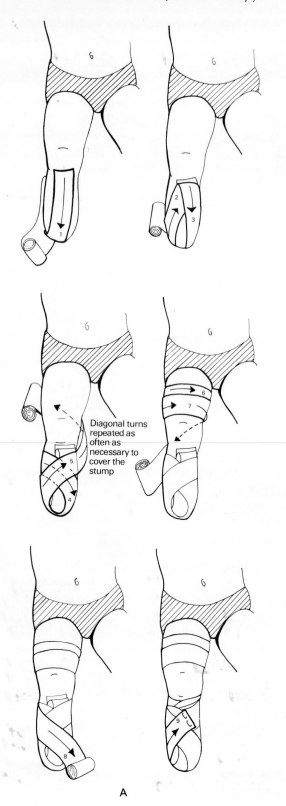

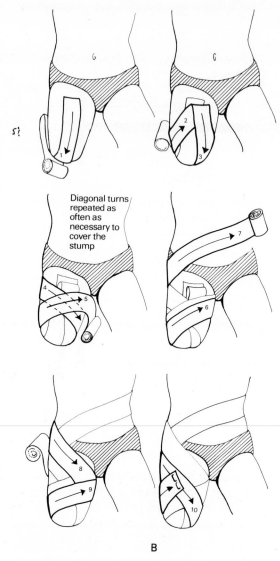

Fig. 14.3 Stump bandaging for A. Below-knee amputation B. Above-knee amputation

(c). Help the patient get to know his stump. The patient must be taught to accept his new body image. He should be encouraged to handle and look at his stump. He is likely to be very protective towards it so that there is little danger of injury at this stage.

(d). Encourage mobility and personal independence. As soon as his general condition allows, the patient should get up. Independent mobility and balance are encouraged, as this not only aids circulation and thus promotes healing, but also means that basic independence activities can begin. The unilateral lower limb amputee may begin mobility training by learning to balance and move on his remaining limb while supported between parallel bars. For those who are able to handle them axillar crutches may be issued. Wheelchair mobility is encouraged for both unilateral and bilateral amputees, especially the elderly.

(e). Encourage good skin care and personal hygiene. This is important as a preparation for fitting the prosthesis.

4. *Prosthetic.* In the United kingdom prostheses are measured for and supplied by the patient's local Artificial Limb Centre.

(a). Early walking aids. In some centres an early walking aid is fitted for lower limb amputees about eight to ten days postoperatively, in order to encourage early bilateral mobility. These early aids are made of a variety of materials and some, such as the Pneumatic Post Amputation Mobility Aid (PPMA), are commercially available. They are, however, by no means universally used.

(b). Temporary prostheses. The design depends on type and level of amputation. For unilateral amputees the initial prosthesis is usually a pylon (Fig. 14.4). This commonly consists of a socket which holds the stump and a pelvic band which fastens round the patient's trunk between the iliac crest and waist. The foot is a wooden rocker with a rubber sole and the hinged knee joint can be manually operated.

Bilateral pylons are usually of the same basic design as unilateral ones but shorter, as this makes it easier for the patient to regain balance soon after operation. Later they can be exchanged for those of normal length. They may have no knee joint (Fig. 14.5).

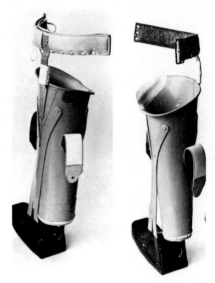

Fig. 14.5 Short 'rocker' pylons for a bilateral lower limb amputee (photograph by kind permission of Robert Kellie and Son Ltd)

The therapist must be aware that especially elderly amputees with vascular complications will not be likely to use their prostheses all the time. A wheelchair will most probably still be necessary.

Once the prosthesis has been fitted the patient, with help from the staff, must work towards the following aims:

an even and steady gait

strengthening of the stump and other limbs and coordination of the new limb

full independence in the activities of daily living

proper care of the stump, prosthesis and remaining limbs

resettling at home and in the community, and at work where applicable.

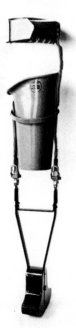

Fig. 14.4 Temporary above-knee pylon for the unilateral amputee (photograph by kind permission of Robert Kellie and Son Ltd)

(c). Definitive limbs. These are supplied once the patient has gained a reasonable level of proficiency with his temporary limb. They cannot be fitted before the stump is fully shrunk and shaped and the wound is completely healed. A definitive limb may sometimes not be supplied for six months or more after amputation.

Many types of definitive limbs are available and the choice will depend on the age of the patient, the level of amputation and the proficiency of control the patient attains. Definitive limbs are controlled by muscular power of the patient and by leverage of the stump. Some common types of definitive limbs are illustrated in Figure 14.6 A, B and C.

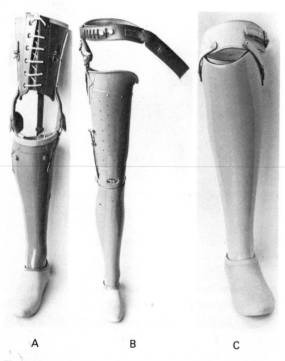

Fig. 14.6 Definitive lower limb prostheses. A. Below-knee prosthesis B. Above-knee prosthesis C. Patellar tendon-bearing prosthesis (photograph by kind permission of Robert Kellie and Son Ltd)

Patients who are not fitted with definitive limbs are usually in the older age group. Because of diminished adaptability and often multiple pathology, many elderly patients achieve independent mobility only through a combination of pylon, walking aid and wheelchair. Only very few pa-tients lose complete walking mobility and become fully dependent on a wheelchair.

The role of the occupational therapist

Whenever possible the occupational therapist should see the patient before, as well as after, the operation. Her role is important to his rehabilitation and should be explained both to him and his relatives.

Preoperative stage

If possible the therapist should get to know the patient and his family before operation. It must be remembered that the patient is likely to be in considerable pain and may therefore not remember all that is said to him. Nonetheless, the therapist can already make arrangements for suitable clothing to be brought in so that practice in the activities of daily living can commence as soon as possible after operation.

A home visit. If the patient is elderly or lives alone or with an elderly partner, it is advisable to carry out a preliminary home visit so that if any alterations or aids are likely to be needed, the wheels can be set in motion for their supply, as the patient is likely to be in hospital for only a relatively short period after operation. Even though a completely accurate assessment of the patient's eventual level of mobility can obviously not be made at this stage, the therapist should be able to make a reasonable estimate of his level of function on discharge by taking into consideration his age, general health and level of amputation.

Strengthening upper limbs and trunk. It is likely that the patient has been relatively immobile for some time before his admission to hospital and as strength in his upper limbs will be needed for activities such as transfers and manoeuvring a wheelchair or walking aids, it is important that this be increased as far as possible. Suitable activities include stoolseating, benchwork, cookery or macrame.

Education. A clear explanation of what is likely to happen after the operation will help to dispel fears of what is to come. Some patients will be interested in and helped by a simple medical explanation of their condition and operation and

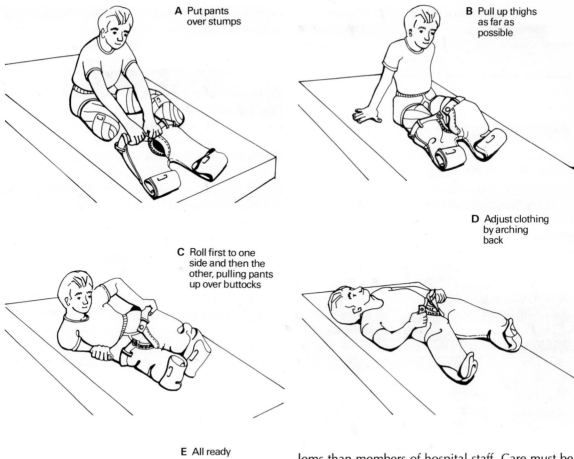

A Put pants over stumps

B Pull up thighs as far as possible

C Roll first to one side and then the other, pulling pants up over buttocks

D Adjust clothing by arching back

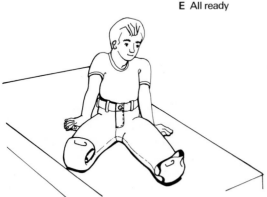

E All ready

Fig. 14.7 Dressing method for lower limb garments for the bilateral amputee

the therapist should be able to give this. It is often helpful to introduce the patient to another amputee who is undergoing, or has undergone, rehabilitation, as he will frequently feel freer to ask a fellow sufferer about future treatment and prob-

lems than members of hospital staff. Care must be taken, however, that the patients are of similar age, amputation level and physical capability so that the patient awaiting amputation will not be misled by seeing an amputee with a much higher or lower level of independence than he can expect to achieve himself.

Ordering a wheelchair. If in view of the patient's age and general health it seems likely that he will spend at least part of his day in a wheelchair, this should be ordered as early as possible, so that he can use it as soon as he is allowed out of bed after the operation. For elderly amputees a wheelchair is ordered almost routinely. A suitable wheelchair is especially important for the bilateral above-knee amputee who because of his altered centre of gravity must use a modified chair with the large wheels either set back three inches or fitted at the front with the castors at the back. These alterations compensate for the weight lost by amputation of the lower limbs and therefore make the chair more stable. The first method of adaption is preferable, as it encourages good posture and the large wheels do not hinder transfers. Because these chairs are not always held in stock at the Limb Centre, it is advisable to order them as soon as it is apparent that one will be necessary.

Preprosthetic stage

This stage may last up to several weeks depending on the delay in providing the prosthesis and the state of the stump.

Encouraging personal independence. The lower limb amputee should be encouraged to be up and dressed as soon as he is allowed and should be mobile with walking aids such as axilla crutches and/or a wheelchair. Dressing should present little problem to the unilateral amputee if performed sitting on the side of the bed with the remaining foot touching the floor or on a chair by the side of the bed. As with all lower limb disabilities, the affected leg should be put into the garment first. The patient should sit with his thighs apart to form a wide base, if balance is a problem. For the bilateral lower limb amputee it is easier to dress sitting on the bed. Upper garments should pose little problem, but lower limb garments are often most easily put on whilst lying flat on the back. Pants and trousers are put on and pulled up by rolling from side to side and are finally arranged by arching the back (Fig. 14.7). A monkey handle is often helpful for sitting up. If this early rolling action causes a problem the occupational therapist should ask the physiotherapist to let the patient practise this movement during treatment sessions in the gym as it is often more easily learnt on a firm floor than on the bed. The patient will be bed-bathed until the wound has healed, but he may wish to use the bath later on. This should not pose any problems for the unilateral amputee with adequate balance. He should be taught to sit on the side of the bath and swing the remaining limb over the side. However, for those slow in relearning to balance and for bilateral amputees a wash down or a shower taken whilst seated (which is now possible in many hospitals) will be easier until balance has improved. The patient should be encouraged to use the toilet rather than a bedpan or urinal.

Encouraging balancing, standing, mobility and strength in the upper limbs. The patient should be both up in a wheelchair and also start walking as early as possible and the occupational therapist should encourage a correct walking pattern during treatment sessions. Transfers should be taught as early as possible so that activities of daily living can be carried out independently.

The unilateral lower limb amputee should be taught to stand by first sitting well forward in his seat with his remaining leg back and the foot firmly on the floor. He should and then push up from the seat, or pull up on a firm support, whichever is easier or more convenient (Fig. 14.8). The walking

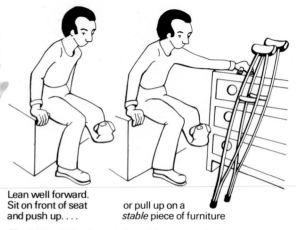

Lean well forward.
Sit on front of seat
and push up. . . .   or pull up on a
                                 stable piece of furniture

Fig. 14.8 Rising from sitting without a prosthesis

aid should be collected once standing balance is attained. With practice this should present little problem although care must be taken that the patient with phantom limb sensation does not try to put weight through his amputated limb.

For sitting down this sequence is reversed. The patient balances firmly on the sound leg and, putting the walking aid aside, holds on to a firm support and lowers himself slowly onto the seat. As soon as the unilateral amputee is sufficiently steady when walking, activities to encourage balance, mobility and independent transfer can begin. These can include any activity of interest that will help the patient to move around, stand and sit with ease, for example printing, gardening, stoolseating or cookery. All these activities will also improve strength in the upper limbs. The use of a Camden stool and standing table will help the patient to regain balance.

The bilateral lower limb amputee can be taught side and/or forward transfers (Figs. 14.9 and 10). It is important to ensure that initially the patient's wheelchair and bed are at the same height. If the bed height has been altered for any reason, for example for nursing purposes, it is essential that is is returned to the required height afterwards. A transfer board and monkey pole may help the patient's independent mobility. The therapist should encourage the patient to be as active as possible in his wheelchair, not only to increase his proficiency in manoeuvring it, but also to strengthen his upper limbs. Activities to extend his use of the wheelchair and to improve balance can include skittles, bowls, benchwork, cookery, gardening and printing, all of which can be done sitting in the wheelchair. When balance has improved the arms of the chair can be removed to allow greater trunk mobility.

Encouraging social contact. If the patient is

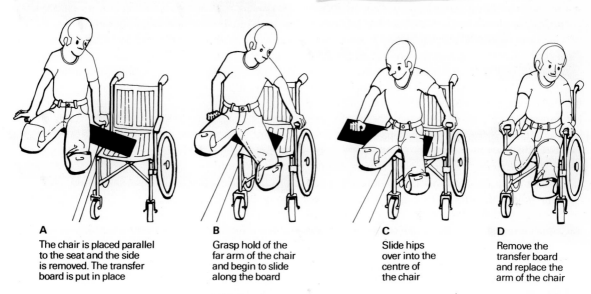

A
The chair is placed parallel to the seat and the side is removed. The transfer board is put in place

B
Grasp hold of the far arm of the chair and begin to slide along the board

C
Slide hips over into the centre of the chair

D
Remove the transfer board and replace the arm of the chair

Fig. 14.9 Side transfer using a sliding board

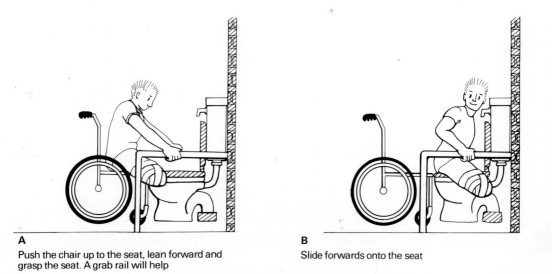

A
Push the chair up to the seat, lean forward and grasp the seat. A grab rail will help

B
Slide forwards onto the seat

Fig. 14.10 Forward transfer

treated in a unit with other amputees, social acceptance of his new body image is perhaps easier. However, whatever the circumstances, the patient should be encouraged to lead as full a life as possible during this period. He should be encouraged to take his meals in the ward dining room rather than by his bed and to go out and about around the hospital and grounds. Occupational therapy sessions should take place in the department rather than on the ward and if the patient is reluctant or embarrassed to leave the ward, the therapist should use the treatment periods to gradually wean him from the protection of the ward. Activities carried out in groups rather than individually will help the patient to get used to meeting others. Hobbies which may be continued after his discharge, such as chess, wheelchair dancing and whist, will show the patient that he can still take part in an active social life (Fig. 14.11). The occupational therapist should be aware of local clubs and associations with which the patient can be put in touch before leaving hospital and should remember that there are many 'normal' clubs and groups that the patient can join in addition to those for the handicapped. For the younger patient the Sports Association for the Disabled may be of interest and, if so, he should be put in touch with his local branch.

Preventing contractures and strengthening the stump. This is most important before the prosthesis is supplied, as contractures will make the artificial limb difficult, if not impossible, to wear. Sessions of prone lying are necessary and the therapist should ensure that treatment times do not conflict with times set aside for this. The precautions illustrated in Figure 14.2 should also be taken.

For above-knee amputees activities adapted for hip extension such as weaving and for below-knee amputees static quadriceps activities (Fig. 14.12) or work on the quadriceps switch can be used. However, in the elderly amputee the effort involved in learning to be mobile and independent leaves little energy for these activities.

Encouraging good care of the stump. Apart from regular bandaging of the stump to shape it, the patient has to learn to care for the skin of the amputated leg. Hygiene is important and the stump should be washed, well dried and dusted with talcum powder morning and evening. The patient should take special care to ensure that he is dry after visiting the toilet as the prosthesis will reach high into the groin and if this area is not well

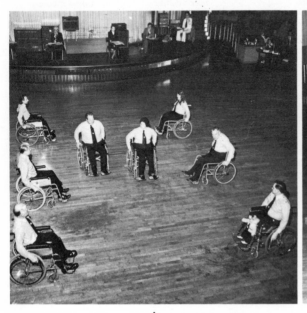
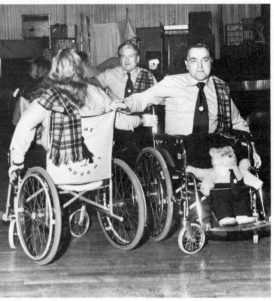

A   B

Fig. 14.11   Wheelchair dancing. A. Swinging in the Oggie Dance B. Stripping the Willow (The Choughs participating in the International Festival 1976)

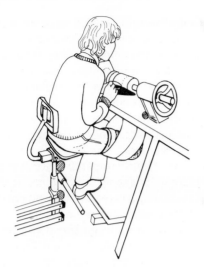

Fig. 14.12 Using the lathe to encourage static work of the quadriceps in the slung limb

dried, rubbing can lead to soreness and skin breakdown. He should check daily for signs of rubbing or bruising at this stage and report them immediately should they occur. Often the stump is hypersensitive to pressure and as some definitive limbs require weight to be taken through the stump, desensitisation should be started. This can be done by asking the patient to percuss the stump regularly with his fingers to get it used to touch and pressure. Once initial healing has taken place he can also be encouraged to rub and massage the stump in the bath or shower. He should be encouraged to bandage his own stump and use a new or freshly-laundered bandage each time, as a bandage that has been used will have lost its 'spring'.

Prosthetic stage

A temporary prosthesis is supplied first and along with this lower limb pylon the patient should also receive several stump socks which are worn under the pylon to act as a cushion between it and the leg. In Britain the handbook *Hints on the use of an Artificial Limb* is also supplied by the Limb Centre.

Once the limb has been supplied the emphasis of treatment will change.

Increasing independence in activities of daily living. The lower limb amputee must now learn to put his limb on, take it off and to perform the basic tasks of everyday living.

Dressing. The order of dressing is important and some elderly amputees find difficulty in remembering that the artificial limb must be put on before most other clothes and not after it. Dressing for the unilateral amputee is best done sitting on the side of the bed and for the bilateral amputee sitting on top of the bed. Dressing should be done in the following order (Fig. 14.13).

Bra. (if worn)

Vest. Most elderly patients wear a vest and a long cotton or lightweight woollen one will help to

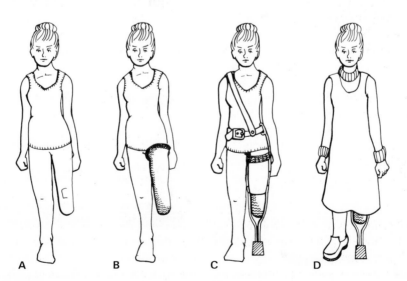

Fig. 14.13 Dressing order with a pylon (A) Vest (B) Stump sock (C) Pylon (D) Rest of clothing

prevent the pelvic band from rubbing. If this is explained, those who do not usually wear a vest may be persuaded to do so. A lightweight T-shirt may prove more acceptable to younger patients.

Stump sock. This should be pulled up over the end of the stump so that there are no wrinkles or flaps that can rub and cause soreness. The therapist should ensure that the sock comes up high enough into the groin to allow sufficient overlap for folding over the top of the socket, especially in the pubic and ischial areas.

Pylon. This is most easily put on if the knee joint is locked and the pelvic band hinged forwards. The stump is put into the socket which is then pulled up as far as possible. If there are any fastenings on the socket they should be secured at this point. Balancing on the sound leg, the patient stands and slowly puts weight through the prosthesis to allow the stump to settle into the socket. The pelvic band and shoulder strap are then fastened and the stump sock pulled up and rolled over the top of the socket to act as a cushion. The patient then sits down.

Remaining clothes. These are put on in a normal manner. Many patients prefer to 'dress the prosthesis, i.e. put the pants and trousers over the rocker, before putting it on, as this saves bending right down to reach over the foot. For women a self-support stocking or one-legged tights can be recommended for the sound leg. If trousers are worn those with wide legs are obviously better for disguising the prosthesis and pleats at the waist give a more comfortable fit at the hips. Dresses, especially those with no definite waistline, may be preferred to skirts and tops and the 'with it' octagenarian may be persuaded to wear slacks if she is embarrassed by her pylon.

For the bilateral lower limb amputee the order of dressing is the same, although much more practice is needed before the patient can become fully independent, as it is often more difficult to roll in order to pull the prosthesis up high enough to fasten the band.

Toilet. Provided the patient has dressed correctly, using the toilet should pose little problem to the unilateral amputee once he can transfer efficiently. The bilateral lower limb amputee may use a forward transfer if there is sufficient room at the side and back of the toilet. Alternatively a side transfer may be appropriate, depending on the layout of the patient's bathroom at home. A third method is to use the toilet routinely in the morning before dressing, at lunchtime rest periods and again in the evening when the patient is without prostheses, as especially in the early days he may not be able to tolerate them for more than a few hours in the morning. Once he is more tolerant of them and more agile, transfers can be practised with them on. Front-flap pants for both male and female bilateral amputees may be easier to manage than normal underwear, as they do not need to be pulled down when using the toilet.

Bath. The more agile unilateral amputee will probably manage without any aid other than a non-slip mat, provided he can hold on to a firm support or rail whilst sitting and swinging the leg over the bath. The elderly person may need a bath board and seat, and possibly a grab rail on the wall by the bath. Unless extremely agile and strong in the upper limbs the bilateral amputee is unlikely to be able to use a bath, and a shower taken on a wooden or plastic seat, or a wash down, should provide the answer.

Housework. For the lower limb amputee balance will be a major problem and the housewife should be shown how to arrange her tasks so that walking is reduced to a minimum. If she is unsteady on her feet or has a long way to carry utensils a trolley will help with both balancing and carrying. Activities needing short preparation and little movement (such as making a mid-morning snack) should lead to those requiring greater mobility and balance and longer preparation. Remember that the patient only needs to reach the level of competence required at home.

Care of the prosthesis. The pylon must be cared for regularly if it is to work efficiently and the patient should be taught to:

wipe it with a damp cloth each evening after removing it

lock the knee joint when the prosthesis is not in use

keep it free from dirt, dust and damp

A clean stump sock should be used every day and dirty ones washed as soon as possible, preferably in soap flakes. Fabric softener not only keeps the sock soft but also helps to prevent the accumulation of static electricity.

Teaching transfers. The unilateral amputee will now need practice in getting up and down from a seat (Fig. 14.14). He should be taught to:

● sit well forward on the seat with the remaining foot well back
● lock the knee of the prosthesis (where applicable)
● stand by balancing on the sound leg and pushing on a firm support such as the chair arms, grab rail or nearby sturdy furniture.

Once the patient is up the pylon should be brought level with the sound foot by hitching the pelvis up on the amputated side. Weight can now be taken through it.

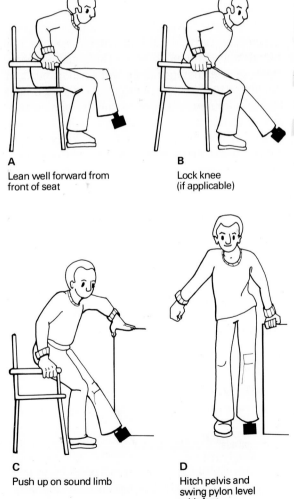

A Lean well forward from front of seat

B Lock knee (if applicable)

C Push up on sound limb

D Hitch pelvis and swing pylon level with foot

Fig. 14.14 Rising from sitting with a pylon

Note: although it is possible to stand with the knee unlocked and lock it when standing, it is safer to start by using the method described so that there is no danger of the patient trying to put weight through the unlocked prosthesis.

Sitting down is the reverse of this process so that while balancing on the sound limb the prothesis is hitched forward and the patient then slowly lowers himself onto the seat holding on to a firm support.

Transfers for the bilateral lower limb amputee can prove more difficult. Side and forward transfers can continue as before, but as there is no knee lock and the limbs are short standing and sitting are controlled from the hips and the patient must learn to lever himself in and out of a chair. This is most easily done by shuffling forward on the seat and then pushing up on the arms of the chair until the rockers reach the floor and the patient can gain his balance (Fig. 14.15).

Teaching tolerance and coordination of the prosthesis. The lower limb amputee, whether unilateral or bilateral, will need to learn to tolerate his new limb and the period it is worn should be increased each day. Initally a few hours may be all he can manage, as learning to put the prosthesis on and to control the knee lock, transferring and learning to walk will probably take up most of his energy. Later, activities can be included that encourage the patient to make full use of his new limb. This applies mainly to younger patients whose general health and limb tolerance are good.

Activities such as gardening, work on the electronic or lightweight bicycle fretsaw, lathe work, golf, darts, bowls and benchwork will encourage a

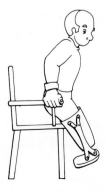

Fig. 14.15 Rising from sitting with a bilateral 'rocker' pylon

wide range of mobility and limb tolerance in unilateral amputees. For the bilateral amputee the therapist must ensure that work heights are correct for standing activities and a hydraulically operated workbench (supplied by some manufacturers of remedial equipment) can prove extremely useful. The elderly amputee will also have to learn to be as proficient as possible in his wheelchair, as he will undoubtedly use it at some time.

Making a home visit. Any aids or equipment the patient has found necessary for independence in hospital should also be supplied to him for use at home. The therapist should check the patient's mobility within the house, as well as outside. He may need a grab rail or additional banister to cope with steps and stairs. Height and position of grab rails should be determined, and the height and stability of the bed, as well as the firmness of the mattress, should be checked to ensure that they are suitable for easy transfer. If the mattress is too soft, fracture boards may be placed between it and the bed frame to form a firm base for transfer. The height and stability of the toilet and favourite easy chair should also be noted.

If a wheelchair has been supplied the width of corridors and doors and the negotiability of steps should be checked. Floor coverings and outdoor surfaces should be noted, remembering that wheelchairs fare badly on gravel paths! The height of locks and catches which will be used from the wheelchair should not be forgotten. The patient's relatives who should have been taught how and when to help, should be asked to demonstrate their ability to assist at home. Helping a patient on to a firm hospital bed in a roomy ward is different from doing so in a small bedroom.

The local authority occupational therapist should be involved at this stage and both therapists should satisfy themselves that the patient can cope safely at home to the level required of him.

Once the lower limb amputee reaches the level of proficiency at which a definitive limb can be fitted, it is rare that the therapist will still be treating him. The Limb Centre will explain how the prosthesis works and how it should be worn and most patients will adapt well to their new limb.

For all amputees of working age a work assessment should be performed (see Ch. 12).

AMPUTATIONS OF THE UPPER LIMB

Occupational therapists may be asked to treat patients either awaiting amputation or after amputation and it is important that they are able to give immediate help and support in addition to remedial therapy.

Upper limb amputations are performed most often in young to middle-aged patients who present very different problems to other amputees, often elderly patients with lower limb amputations whose problems are familiar to most therapists. Patients with upper limb amputations need a great deal of time, patience and understanding and may sometimes be uncooperative, resentful and even aggressive. They should be allowed to express these emotions.

Patients who have had amputations of the hand, forearm or wrist should be encouraged to use gauntlets as early as possible. These can easily be made by the therapist from soft leather, cut and stitched to fit the shape of the stump. If the gauntlet fits well, implements such as cutlery, pen or tools can be attached. This ensures that there is no delay in getting the patient used to a prosthetic aid. Patients have been known to reject a prosthesis simply because they never realised its potential function.

As upper limb prostheses vary considerably and have already been described in detail in other publications, this is only a general outline of conditions and treatments. The help and advice of the Area Artificial Limb and Appliance Centre of the Department of Health and Social Security is invaluable and close cooperation is particularly important when treating patients with upper limb amputations.

Causes

Trauma. The most common injuries result from:

(a). road traffic accidents, especially motor cycle accidents

(b). accidents at work, involving machinery and equipment.

These patients are commonly seen in general hospitals as emergency admissions. In the early stages they are therefore likely to be treated by hospital therapists.

As primary amputation may not be at the desired level and may leave a stump which is impossible to fit with a prosthesis, further operation may be necessary. Even if re-amputation can be avoided, some trimming or other surgery will be required. Other damage caused at the time of the accident, such as tendon, nerve or bone damage, has considerable bearing on the future treatment and may affect the later use of a prosthesis. For example, a fisherman who had lost his arm by catching it in the winch on his ship was fitted with an above-elbow prosthesis. Even though he became quite proficient, the result was not as good as it might have been, because of additional damage to the shoulder joint with consequent stiffness and weakness. On the other hand, a forestry worker who severed his arm with a saw, without any other damage to the limb, regained excellent function when fitted with a prosthesis.

Through-wrist and hand mutilations are most often the result of accidents with machinery in factories or at home, although more serious injuries may occur with, for example, conveyor belts in operation. Clean amputations of hand or fingers, however, are far more common.

(c). brachial plexus lesions which have been diagnosed as irrecoverable may be treated by amputation of the limb and arthrodesis of the shoulder joint. A fairly good result can be expected from this procedure. Scapular movements give adequate compensation when the shoulder is arthrodesed and an above-elbow prosthesis gives a reasonably functional arm. At the present time this is the best available treatment for these patients.

Disease

1. Malignant disease in the upper limb may necessitate amputation. This may be at any level from the hand to the shoulder. Lesions at or above the elbow will usually result in a through-shoulder or forequarter amputation.

2. Scleroderma, which is not a common condition, causes tissue necrosis and may necessitate total or partial amputation of the fingers or hand. Further surgery is often indicated as the disease progresses. Usually both hands are affected.

3. Gangrene is sometimes seen as a complication of injury or disease. It may necessitate amputation or secondary amputation at a higher level than the original injury.

4. Severe post-operative or post-traumatic infection or thrombosis may be the cause of amputation.

Peripheral circulatory failure. This is relatively uncommon in the upper limb. However, Raynaud's disease, a circulatory disease affecting the extremities, may result in amputation of the fingers or hand in severe cases. This may be bilateral.

Congenital abnormalities. These are perhaps the most common reason for the treatment of upper limb absence by the occupational therapist.

Treatment

Traumatic amputation

Patients who have suffered trauma resulting in amputation are at first usually seen in a general hospital and only later in special units dealing with amputees. The earlier these patients can be treated by a therapist the better, as encouragement at this stage is very important. The therapist may also be able to explain future treatment to the patient, especially with regard to the fitting and use of a prosthesis. Patients will normally be referred when the wound has healed, though in some cases, such as mutilated hands, they may be referred earlier. These patients may often be able to use the affected limb with the provision of a gauntlet.

The principal aims of treatment for patients with traumatic amputation are:

1. to maintain a full range of movement in the remaining joints of the affected limb

2. to maintain strength and function of the affected limb

3. to make and fit gauntlets, where required, to enable the patient to use the affected limb

4. to improve and maintain strength and function of the opposite limb and encourage skills, such as writing, which were previously performed by the other hand.

The best material for gauntlets is a fine, soft leather which should be shaped directly on the stump and cut on the cross to give maximum stretch. For difficult shapes the leather may be dampened slightly. The gauntlet should be comfortable and acceptable to the patient. It may be necessary to make a cast of the stump in which case the leather can be dampened, then stretched on the cast and left to dry.

Arthrodesis- fixing joint in given position. Results in pain free stable joint.

To make a gauntlet for a through-wrist amputation, cut an oval shape to fit the end of the stump and secure this in position. This may have to be padded, depending on the sensitivity of the stump. A piece of leather is then moulded around the stump, overlapping the oval piece a little. Fasten this in position, leaving an opening in the desired place; stitch, trim and adding straps (Fig. 14.16). The gauntlet should fit snugly to allow the use of implements. These can most easily be attached by strapping the article, e.g. a pen, to the gauntlet for correct alignment, and then stitching the appropriate socket on (Fig. 14.17).

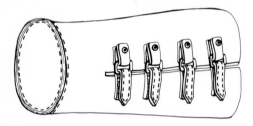

Fig. 14.16 Leather gauntlet

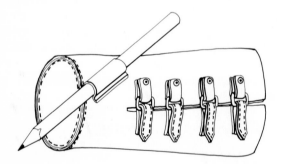

Fig. 14.17 Gauntlet with pencil socket

A gauntlet should always be used if the stump is long enough to take one. This not only helps to toughen the stump, but also to prevent the otherwise inevitable one-handed syndrome. This may be very important during the time before the fitting of a prosthesis. It may make all the difference between acceptance and rejection of the prosthesis by the patient.

Traumatic amputation often leads to psychological trauma. Some patients find it very difficult to re-adjust to the loss of a limb and the use of gauntlets will enable them to use the affected limb at an early stage and therefore to re-adjust more quickly.

The therapist will be able to decide which activities are suitable at this early stage. Activities for strengthening the limb and maintaining full range of movement, such as adapting tools and printing, will no doubt be used. The more successful these are, the more likely it is that a good function will be achieved with a prosthesis.

Patients with brachial plexus lesions can develop behavioural problems and may feel resentment toward the limb. They often suffer extremely distressing, intractable pain. These patients, almost always young men and boys, need a great deal of understanding and support to help them to accept their disability.

If damage to the brachial plexus is extensive, with no prospect of recovery, amputation may be considered. This may happen at a comparatively early stage or at a later date. The therapist should be able to discuss amputation and its implications with the patient. If the advantages and disadvantages are discussed freely and the patient understands the likely result of amputation, he will be in a better position to make a decision. Patients should never be persuaded to agree to amputation and although it is a hard decision, it is one that only he can make. Many patients prefer to keep the limb, even when it is flail, and are often successfully rehabilitated. This of course depends entirely on the intelligence and circumstances of the patient, as well as on his job.

Disease

Malignant disease. Patients who have had, or are about to have, amputations for this reason will need a great deal of sympathy and understanding, as the emotional shock and the physical effects of operation can be severe. The patient is sometimes referred to the therapist before surgery so that he may be reassured and may discuss his future prospects and expected level of recovery with the use of a prosthesis. The therapist should always be optimistic and enthusiastic.

The level of amputation will depend on the site and type of malignancy. Some amputations can be restricted to the hand or forearm. Unfortunately, however, many patients will require a through-shoulder or forequarter amputation. The latter is a radical operation involving removal of the limb, shoulder, scapula and clavicle. After the initial shock most patients adjust very well to this operation. Often these patients are young and many of them are women.

Patients with a forequarter amputation urgently need help with cosmesis, since this operation is mutilating. The most important consideration is restoration of the shoulder contour. A temporary compensating prosthesis can easily be made by the therapist out of foam rubber or moulded plastazote. In an emergency this can be done without the patient, though it is obviously better if the patient can be seen to determine the size. However, this can usually be adjusted during fitting.

To make the appliance, either cut out a piece of foam rubber and trim to shape or mould a piece of ⅜ inch plastozote to the shape of the shoulder. A strap passing from the front of the appliance to the rear via the opposite axilla will hold it in place (Fig. 14.18). Lycra is a good material as it needs no fasteners and is very comfortable. Another and better model can always be made later when the patient has recovered from the operation and is more mobile. The appliance may be covered in flesh-coloured material and other modifications

may be carried out. All this may appear to be a lot of work, but the patient is usually extremely grateful for this help. We have had a patient who would not see her husband after the operation without this appliance. It was fitted before full recovery from the anaesthetic and she never went without it after that. Some patients even prefer this operation to the appearance of a stump.

At a later stage, the patient will be fitted with a permanent prosthesis by the Limb Fitting Centre. This may be a shoulder cap without or with an attached limb (Fig. 14.19). Many patients prefer to wear the shoulder cap only, as they find the limb

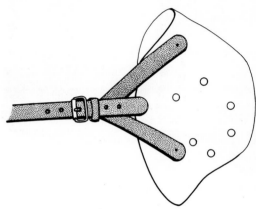

A without arm attachment

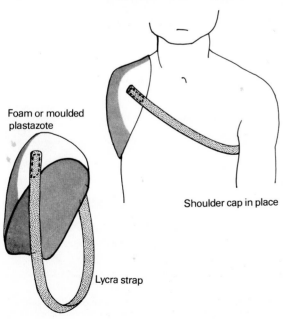

Foam or moulded plastazote

Shoulder cap in place

Lycra strap

Fig. 14.18 A shoulder cap

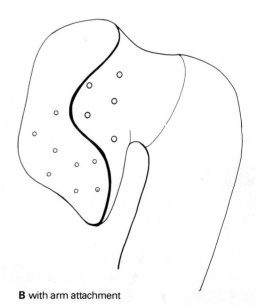

B with arm attachment

Fig. 14.19 Two types of shoulder cap supplied by the Department of Health and Social Security

cumbersome with a tendency to swing around. Although the limb can be used with different attachments, it is mainly used in stabilising and is limited in function.

Scleroderma. This can be a very distressing disease and patients are often treated on a long-term basis. They may need repeated operation, losing a little more of the hand each time. Healing is commonly delayed (Fig. 14.20). Consequently

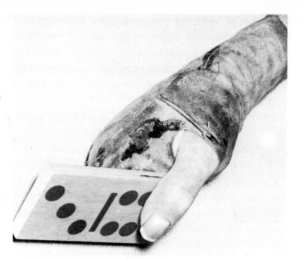

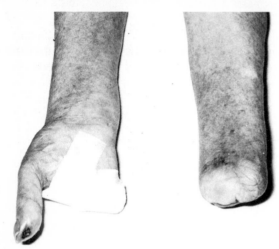

Fig. 14.20 Amputation as a result of scleroderma. Left: through-wrist amputation. Right: amputation at the metacarpal joints

patients tend to become very depressed and the therapist must be able to give them hope for the future by explaining the possibilities of later treatment. It may be decided that temporary appliances should be fitted even before healing has taken place (Figs. 14.21, 22). Their design and production will be left largely to the skill of the therapist. Usually, some form of gauntlet is needed or a simple opposition plate.

Even a small degree of function can improve morale. Some patients who have lost most fingers manage to become almost fully independent with the help of appliances (Fig. 14.23).

If the condition stabilises, a more permanent prosthesis may be fitted by the Limb and Appliance Centre. There is no doubt that the use of temporary appliances can help and influence this part of treatment. Some patients, however, continue to use the temporary type of appliance as they prefer it to more sophisticated ones.

Fig. 14.21 A leather gauntlet padded with plastazote and moulded over the unhealed stumps of the fingers to give opposition to the remaining thumb

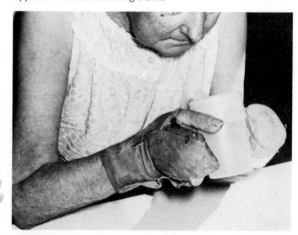

Fig. 14.22 Bilateral leather gauntlets enabling the patient to hold a drinking vessel

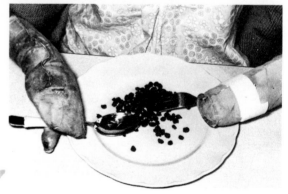

Fig. 14.23 The left gauntlet gives opposition to the thumb, enabling the patient to hold a padded spoon. The right gauntlet has a slot for holding a fork

Raynaud's disease. Fortunately, this condition only rarely warrants amputation of the fingers or hand. Treatment is similar to that for scleroderma, but even more care must be taken in the fitting of appliances so as not to impede the circulation further.

Congenital deformities

Congenital deformities are not uncommon. Children are often seen by the therapist at a very early stage. It is essential that support and encouragement be given to the parents as well as the child. The aims of treatment should be explained to them, so that they can carry on any necessary activities at home. This also applies to the correction of any adverse deformities which may need splinting.

Various abnormalities may be seen, for example absence of one border of the hand or arm, absence of fingers or part of the hand, or absence of the limb with rudimentary fingers at the shoulder (phocomelia). The most common deformity is absence of part of the forearm.

Overall treatment will be decided by the doctor in charge, but the therapist should always have the patient's independence as her primary aim of treatment. Deformities which may impede progress should also be watched for and treated if necessary.

Contact with the local Limb and Appliance Centre should always be made at an early stage. The limb fitting doctor will decide which type of appliance is necessary and when it should be fitted. The therapist should know what may be done so that suitable measures can be taken and deformities corrected before fitting.

In some cases, the fitting of a simple opposition plate may enable a child with finger deficiency to grip objects. This is a plate fitted over the hand to give opposition to the thumb. It can be made by the therapist if necessary, but it is preferable to use the expertise of the Limb and Appliance Centre.

Many children with absence of the forearm are treated in an Arm Training Unit. Often they come at an early age — about three years — when play should be directed towards bilateral activities. The parents should be encouraged to take part in at least some sessions, so that they can carry on with the treatment afterwards. It may be necessary to see the child before he attends school, in order to start some school activities. By far the largest number of children are between 9 and 14 years old when they attend. At this age they are very adept at learning new skills, whether at school or during arm training. It is always advisable to contact the school teachers to inform them of progress, so that they may help the child and report back where necessary.

The role of the occupational therapist

The therapist will see many patients who have had amputations for various reasons. It is important that contact with these patients is made as early as possible, since the therapist may be the link with future treatment, even if this will be carried out elsewhere.

When treating an amputee for the first time one should never assume that he has been seen by an occupational therapist before. Occupational therapy might not have been available at the hospital to which he was admitted initially. It is therefore necessary that all patients are fully assessed before treatment commences and that each patient is given the opportunity to discuss his fears, hopes and needs with the therapist. An optimistic outlook should always be encouraged, but undue optimism curbed.

Where possible and relevant, the plan of treatment to be carried out by the surgeon and the limb fitting doctor should be ascertained, so that treatment can be coordinated. The early stages of treatment for upper limb amputees normally consist of:

● mental and physical assessment of the patient
● support and encouragement for the patient's future
● maintenance of full range of movement in all joints of the remaining limb and strengthening exercises for existing musculature
● increasing dexterity of the unaffected limb and provision of any aids necessary to independence
● supply of temporary appliances for the injured limb
● work assessment. For instance, if a patient with a low amputation and a suitable job is able to return to work at an early stage, treatment should be directed toward this.

Arm training is carried out in many centres throughout the country, which have been established by the Department of Health and Social Security at Area Artificial Limb and Appliance Centres. Most centres have out-patient as well as in-patient facilities. Patients are referred by the limb fitting doctor. Arm training usually lasts one week, 9.30 am to 4 pm daily, though longer periods may be needed for patients with above-elbow or higher amputations.

The number of upper limb amputees attending for arm training is comparatively small and it seems that some of them never come for training at all. It is not possible to say how well these patients do, but experience in this centre suggests that all referred patients certainly need training and feel that they derive great benefit from it. It is quite possible that a therapist may be asked to see patients who have never been referred for training before. The therapist should therefore know where training can be done and, where necessary, do some part of it. In every case it is essential that contact is made with the local Limb and Appliance Centre.

At this centre we have never treated a bilateral upper limb amputee, and it may well be that these patients require the expertise of the Limb and Appliance Centre at Queen Mary's Hospital, Roehampton. This also applies to the use of powered limbs, which need specialised training.

The initial session of arm training is very important, as this is the time when a full assessment is made. It is necessary to explain to the patient that, even if he has used the arm previously, he will feel fatigue and soreness. This is particularly true in the first few days of arm training when exercises are used to manipulate the prosthesis and to build up

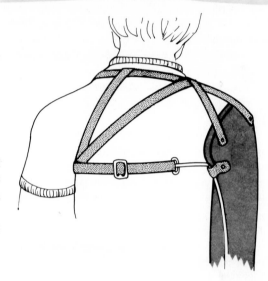

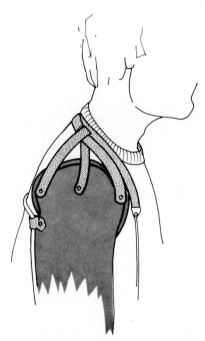

A Bowden cable operating cord for a below-elbow prosthesis

Fig. 14.24 Operating mechanisms for upper limb prostheses

B above-elbow mechanism

shoulder muscles. The shoulder harness of an upper limb prosthesis is never entirely confortable and the patient will have to learn to tolerate it.

At the first session, the patient should be asked to remove his top clothes and his prosthesis so that the stump can be examined. Likely pressure areas should be noted, as well as scars and the condition of the skin. This inspection should be repeated at the end of each session, at least for the first few days. Areas most liable to pressure or friction should be treated by rubbing with soapy water, then surgical spirit. The patient may be taught to do this himself. It is advisable to wear a vest or T-shirt to prevent rubbing from the prosthesis or harness, though not all patients wish to do so. Stump socks are normally worn and are supplied by the Limb and Appliance Centre. It is important to avoid wrinkles in vests or stump socks.

The principle mechanism of the upper limb prosthesis is fixation of the harness under the opposite arm and leverage on the prosthesis by the stump. This is done by abduction of the scapula and forward protusion of the shoulder. This produces tension on the 'op-cord' of the prosthesis, which in turn moves the appliance on the prosthesis (Fig. 14.24).

Careful attention must be paid to the correct tension of strap A (above). This must be tight enough to keep tension on the 'op-cord' which must be free-running. Strap B (above) sometimes requires attention as it is fixed and often causes

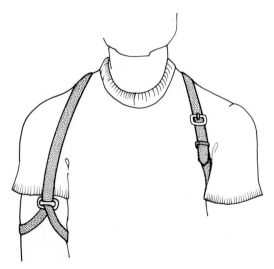

C non-corset mechanism for a below-elbow prosthesis

soreness under the arm. A sheepskin cover replacing the plastic one normally supplied will prevent this.

The most important function of the prosthesis is to operate the split hook, which is the most versatile appliance. Nowadays, the old type of rubber-covered split- C hook is usually replaced by the less cumbersome Dorrance hook (Fig. 14.25).

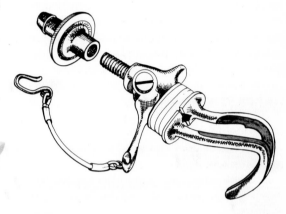

Fig. 14.25 A Dorrance hook

The grip of the split- C hook depends on (a) the relaxation of the 'op-cord', (b) the number of rubber bands on the hook. Opening of the hook is achieved by tension on the 'op-cord'.

Unilateral control is the first aim, using one rubber band on the hook only. A programme of remedial ganes is worked out, consisting of exercises in picking up items and putting them down. This should be done with pieces of varying size and carefully timed. Games like solitaire or draughts are suitable for this purpose. The patient should always sit on a fairly high chair, so that he is well above his work.

As dexterity improves, more difficult exercises may be added. Dowel pieces are often used, as they have to be turned in the hook before they can be put into a hole. This encourages control of the hook. For different sizes and resistance glass-headed pins on a plastazote board and clothes pegs are useful. Variations of these exercises can be designed by the therapist.

At the next stage another rubber band may be added and in some cases a third band may be required. These exercises should form the start of every session. In some cases it may be necessary to start training with a light alloy split- C hook and then progress to the heavier Dorrance hook.

After the first day, bilateral exercises may be started. Any suitable equipment may be used for this, e.g. Lego, Meccano, nuts and bolts, depending on the dexterity of the patient.

Other activities for training are carpentry, metalwork, typing, kitchen work, gardening and electrical wiring. The choice will obviously depend on the needs of the patient, but should include as many as possible. Activities of daily living, such as eating, writing and personal care, must also be dealt with in detail (Figs. 14,26 and 27).

For some of the above activities other appliances may be needed. A selection of these should be kept so that the patient may try them out. Those found to be most useful are:

1. universal tool holders, used for carpentry and other tool work

2. spade grip, used mostly for gardening, but may also be used to hold cricket bats or a cycle handgrip

3. driving appliance consisting of a steering wheel ball and socket which fits on to the prosthesis

4. various types of pliers, for holding nuts and bolts when working with a spanner

Many other appliances can be supplied for different types of work. However, the success of arm training depends largely on success with the split hook and too many extra appliances are not recommended. All patients are provided with a cosmetic hand, usually when the prosthesis is fitted.

Patients with an above-elbow prosthesis are treated in the same way. The elbow on the prosthesis should be locked manually at first, even though the patient has usually been shown by the fitter how to use the automatic lock. This can be used once proficiency with the hook has been achieved.

Patients with a through-shoulder or forequarter prosthesis follow the above treatment programme as far as they are able to.

It will be appreciated that every patient has different needs and abilities. The programme for arm training should therefore always be adjusted to suit the patient, his age, intelligence, circumstances and work requirements. When treating children, the parents should be fully informed about their progress, so that they become aware of the child's ability. If the child is at school, a report, including any necessary recommendations, should always be sent to the teacher who in turn should be encouraged to report back if necessary.

Many adult upper limb amputees return to their former occupation, although sometimes in a dif-

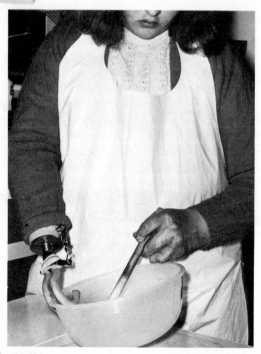

Fig. 14.26 A rubber covered split C hook used for mixing

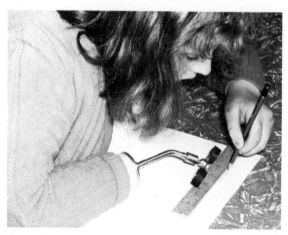

Fig. 14.27 A writing aid in use

ferent capacity. For others the possibility of re-training may have to be considered.

At the end of arm training, a report is sent to the limb fitting doctor with a list of recommended appliances. When approved, these are sent to the patient. Patients should always be told that they may return for help when they need it.

REFERENCES AND FURTHER READING

Humm W 1977 Rehabilitation of the lower limb amputee, 3rd edn. Balliere Tindall, London
Murdoch G (ed) 1976 The advance in Orthotics. Arnold, London
Robertson E 1978 Rehabilitation of arm amputees and limb deficient children. Balliere Tindall, London
Vitali M Robinson, Andrews Harris 1978 Amputations and prostheses. Balliere Tindall, London

15

Burns

Although only a few occupational therapists work with acutely ill burns patients during the early stages, it is important to understand both the regime for the early treatment of burns and the principles of later treatment, i.e. after the initial healing, when most occupational therapists will be asked to treat such a patient.

When considering the treatment of a patient with burns it is essential that the therapist remembers:

● the burnt patient is part of a family and should therefore not be treated separately from them
● every aspect (i.e. medical, social, psychological and physical) of the patient's well-being has to be considered and the whole treatment team must therefore work in close cooperation with each other, the patient, his family and his employers
● because of the nature of the treatment, the patient will often have to bear pain, discomfort and possibly long periods of inactivity and she must therefore be able to gain his cooperation and trust. The relationships built up between all staff members and the patient in the acute stages of his illness will be of mutual benefit later on.

CLASSIFICATION OF BURNS

1. Thermal. Such burns are caused by hot gas (flame), hot liquid (scalds) or hot metal.
2. Electrical. These burns may be caused by low-tension (domestic) or high-tension (overhead cables) currents or by thermo-electrical appliances (e.g. electric fire bar).

3. *Chemical.* Burns caused by acids or alkalis are included here.

4. *Radiation.* Burns caused by sunlight, x-ray or thermo-nuclear radiation.

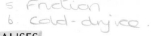

5. Friction
6. Cold - dry ice.

CAUSES

The two main areas in which burns occur are domestic and industrial.

Domestic. Burns caused in the home are frequently the result of carelessness, such as a child pulling boiling liquid from a stove or a woman burnt by hot fat. Contributory factors include:

(a). poverty, often linked with a low standard of housing, heating and education

(b). lack of supervision of young children

(c). faulty heating guards, appliances and electrical wiring, plugs and sockets

(d). diminished responsibility or stress, for example of the psychiatrically ill, the deprived and epileptics.

It is important to remember that some burns to children may not be accidental.

Industrial. Burns at work are also frequently the result of carelessness, disregard or ignorance of safety rules or use of faulty machinery. They are commonly electrical or chemical burns.

Emergency treatment

Correct and quick first aid given at the time of the accident can save further damage. Small burns should be immersed immediately in cold water and left for at least 5 to 10 minutes in order to ease pain and reduce heat. The person should then be taken to hospital if necessary. With large burns, the first priority is to cool the area. Flames should be extinguished by smothering and hot, soaked clothing removed. With electrical burns it is vital to switch off the current before touching the patient. Chemical burns should be placed under running water and an antidote applied if available, for example bicarbonate of soda for an acid burn and vinegar for a caustic burn. The burn should then be covered with a clean piece of cotton, such as a laundered sheet or towel, and the person taken to hospital. Where damage has occurred to the respiratory tract a clear airway must be kept.

TREATMENT

Patients with major burns, i.e. those involving more than 10 per cent of the body surface, have to be treated in hospital. Treatment can be divided into three phases:

I. 'Burn shock'; first 48 hours
II. Healing; can take up to three months
III. Rehabilitation

Phase I. Keep the wound sterile. Loss of protein, salt and water from the circulation results in shock. The replacement of body fluids and electrolyte balance is essential.

Phase II. Avoid infection. The wound is treated by exposure, closed dressing and/or skin grafts. A high protein and calorie diet is necessary to promote healing. Anaemia and dehydration must be corrected and infection, e.g. pneumonia, septicaemia or pyelonephritis, controlled.

Phase III. Correct any flexion contractures, extensor ulcers or disfigurement. Any remaining functional or psychological impairment will be treated by physiotherapy, occupational therapy, psychotherapy and speech therapy. The social worker may need to be called in and convalescence may be necessary.

Control of infection

The dead tissue of a burn wound provides an ideal medium for the growth of bacteria and the entry of infective agents into the body. The risk of infection must therefore be reduced as far as possible during the healing phase.

Environmental control. If the patient is barrier-nursed in a clean, isolated room, the risk of infection is reduced. It is important, therefore, that the therapist also adheres to such a regime should she be treating a patient who is being cared for in this way.

Surface control. The burnt body surface is treated either by exposure or closed-dressing techniques such as bandaging or the 'plastic bag' method (especially useful on the upper limb as a full range of movement can be maintained). Non-touch nursing techniques should be employed and the application of a topical antiseptic such as Hibitane or silver compounds will help to prevent the proliferation of surface bacteria. The early excision of dead tissue and covering of the wound with a skin graft is the ideal solution for burns destroying the full thickness of the skin.

Systemic control. Should systemic infection occur this must be treated with appropriate antibiotics.

Healing of the burn wound

Whereas a superficial partial skin loss burn will heal in 7 to 10 days and a deep partial skin loss burn in approximately three weeks, a wound in which the whole skin thickness has been lost will require grafting in order to promote healing and reduce scarring. There are two basic types of skin grafts.

Free skin grafts. These are cut thinly from an unburnt area of skin known as the donor site, which heals like a graze. They are applied once the wound has been cleared of all dead tissue (i.e. a vascular bed has formed at the base of the wound from which the graft can take its blood supply), when there is minimal infection and no haematoma. Following grafting the area is immobilised in order to promote healing.

Pedicle skin grafting. This type of grafting is used to cover exposed, avascular tissue such as tendons, cartilage and cortical bone, for example over joints or the back of the hand. For this graft a flap of skin, along with its subcutaneous fat, is raised from another part of the body and stitched over the wound (Fig. 15.1A). It retains a blood supply from its base at the site of origin and develops a new blood supply at the recipient site. When this new supply is established the flap can be detached from its donor site (Fig. 15.1B). This process takes about three weeks during which time immobilised joints may become stiff.

Complications

Problems arising during and after healing can seriously affect and delay recovery and the restoration of full function.

Bedsores. These may appear either at pressure sites, i.e. where the body comes into contact with the bed surface, or where skin breakdown is caused by the dragging of delicate skin as the patient is turned. The use of a 'low air-loss bed'

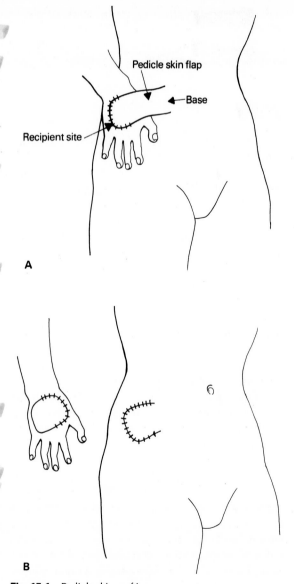

Fig. 15.1 Pedicle skin grafting

which supports the patient on air-filled cushions can reduce such damage by distributing the pressure evenly over the whole surface of the body in contact with the bed. (Fig. 15.2).

Oedema. Immediately after burning oedema begins to form in the surrounding tissue. As well as causing pressure and taking fluid from the circulation it will reduce mobility. It is therefore important that oedema be reduced as soon as possible. Elevation of the limb and rhythmical exercise through the full range of movement of the affected

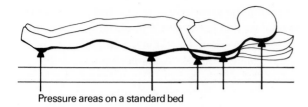

Pressure areas on a standard bed

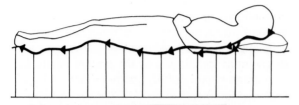

Pressure evenly distributed on a low air-loss bed

Fig. 15.2 Distribution of pressure when lying in bed

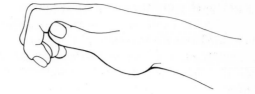

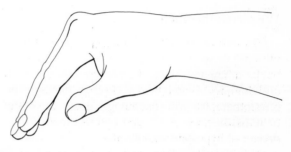

Fig. 15.3 Positioning of the hand to prevent contracture. Above: non-functional position — collateral ligaments are shortened, thumb adducted and wrist held in a neutral position Below: functional position — collateral ligaments are stretched, thumb abducted and rotated and wrist slightly extended

joints are necessary, provided this does not interfere with other treatment such as drips or skin grafts.

Scarring and associated problems. Scar formation may cause problems because of its avascular, white appearance and non-elasticity. Scar tissue has no sweat glands and this may lead to additional problems, particularly if the scarred area is large. Much advance has been made in controlling the final cosmetic appearance and mobility of maturing scar tissue by the use of pressure garments and continuous exercise regimes. As scar tissue contracts, it is essential to prevent joint deformity in the area of the maturing scar by maintaining a full range of movement and by using splints. Finally, the formation of keloid or hypertrophic scarring (i.e. scar tissue which after initial normal formation begins to itch, becomes red and lumpy and overgrows the original confines of the scar) may also occur. Although many treatments have been tried to reduce keloid scarring none has proved entirely successful.

Damage to tissue beneath the skin. Damage to tendons, especially on the dorsum of the hand, can complicate the restoration of full function. It is important, therefore, to place the hand in a functional position if it needs to be immobilised and to keep all other joints as mobile as possible. Similarly, any joint which is immobile should be carefully positioned in order to prevent contracture (Fig. 15.3).

Psychological problems. Considering the shock of the burns accident, the painful and prolonged treatment and the resultant scarring with possible loss of function, it is not surprising that psychological problems arise in some patients. Such problems, which are not necessarily directly related to the degree of damage incurred, may take the form of withdrawal, lack of motivation and associated depression. Fear, especially of pain, and anxiety over the outcome of treatment and of the future, may also occur. Not uncommonly the patient or his family feel guilty about the accident and this can result in rejection of or by the patient and his family, or an exaggerated state of dependence in a previously independent person.

THE ROLE OF THE PARAMEDICAL TEAM

When discussing the treatment of a patient suffering from burns it is impossible to separate the medical, surgical and therapeutic treatments, as all overlap. It is also difficult to distinguish clearly between the roles of the different medical and paramedical workers because, as already mentioned, they all work as members of a team and the areas covered by particular team members will vary from one centre to another. It is intended, therefore, to discuss the possible roles of each team member.

The physiotherapist

Respiration. If the respiratory tract is burnt, blistered or swollen, the physiotherapist may carry out breathing exercises, chest percussion and postural drainage. Even if there is no chest damage, the physiotherapist will encourage good breathing patterns, because prolonged bed rest leads to the danger of hypostatic pneumonia.

Joint mobility. Immediately on admission, or as soon as is medically permitted, the physiotherapist will begin exercises to maintain a full range of movement at all joints, those unaffected as well as those affected by the burn, and this will continue until full scar maturation is reached. As movement often becomes more uncomfortable as the scar develops, it is necessary for the physiotherapist to form a good relationship with the patient and gain his cooperation for prolonged and often painful treatment sessions. In order to encourage full joint mobility and prevent scar contracture causing joint deformity, positioning in bed during the early stages of treatment is especially important, as is the supply of splints jointly with other team members.

Walking. As soon as the patient is allowed out of bed walking is encouraged, even if the legs are burnt. Usually the only period of enforced immobility is immediately after grafting. Full mobility and muscle strength are aimed at after initial healing.

The social worker

As already mentioned the result of having a member of a family burnt can cause extreme psycholo-gical trauma to the whole family and the role of the social worker is extremely important.

On admission, the patient is frightened and in pain; later, frustration, anger, guilt, shame or withdrawal may set in. The patient's family are often equally shocked and frightened and their reactions may also be anger, guilt, shame and rejection or over-protection. The medical social worker aims to help the patient to accept his problem and to cope with it by:

● being aware and tolerant of emotional turmoil
● giving help and/or advice little and often
● giving as much help as the patient needs, but encouraging him and his family to face and solve their own problems
● supporting the family, especially when more than one member is injured, if the house has been gutted in a fire and new accommodation or extensive renovation is necessary
● preventing the family from being over-protective to the patient by explaining the dangers of this and reinforcing the importance of maintaining physical and mental independence
● telling the truth and explaining, in simple terms when necessary, what is going on
● discouraging blame, guilt and rumination by the patient and his family
● encouraging questions to enable both the patient and his family to fully understand the implications of the injury and to participate actively in planning
● giving support and advice during the difficult period of discharge.

The occupational therapist

The occupational therapist will be working with the patient from shortly after admission until he has been resettled at home and work.

Treatment while awaiting healing

In the acute stage and while initial healing is taking place, the occupational therapist will be concerned with splinting, activities of daily living and helping the patient to maintain a full range of movement.

Building a relationship with the patient and his family will aid cooperation later on when treatment becomes more uncomfortable and demanding. It is felt that, at this stage, the therapist should be relatively non-demanding of the patient, as constant demands are already being made on him by doctors, nursing staff, physiotherapists and others. The patient should be given the opportunity to express his anxieties, fears and anger freely.

It is important that the family understand the role of the occupational therapist. They should be asked about activities that interest the patient so that these can be continued in hospital and act as an incentive to recovery. It is especially important that children should be surrounded by familiar objects.

The value of supportive therapy in these early stages cannot be denied. Activities to absorb the patient and take him out of himself may lead him from depression and introversion. Books, radio, television, games and other hobbies will not only provide interest and stimulation, but will encourage movement and conversation and discourage introspection.

The occupational therapist must remember that the patient will probably be barrier-nursed to prevent the spread of infection and everyone in contact with him will be gowned and masked. This not only inhibits normal relationships, but dictates that all equipment used must be washable or cleanable.

Splinting. In the early stages, positioning splints may be necessary to prevent deformity and maintain range of movement.

1. *Neck.* To prevent the chin from being pulled down to the chest the patient may have to wear a collar. Correct positioning of the head when the patient is in bed is important. It may be necessary to extend the neck over a pillow (Fig. 15.4).

2. *Axilla.* In cases with burns in or around the axilla abduction will be lost if tight scarring is allowed to form. Positioning with Orthoplast or similar material will help to prevent this. In less severe cases foam padding held in place by bandaging may suffice.

3. *Elbow.* To prevent flexion deformity at the elbow the three-point extension splint can be used (Fig. 15.5). A similar splint can be used to prevent contraction at the knee.

4. *Wrist and hand.* For adults whose hands are covered with dressings, a paddle or cock-up splint

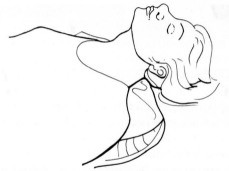

A Correct: the neck is held in extension over a pillow

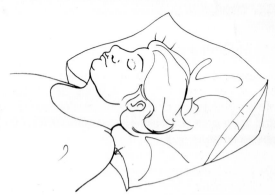

B Incorrect: the chin is allowed to bend towards the chest

Fig. 15.4   Positioning of patient with burns to the neck to prevent contracture.

can be used (see Ch. 11). If the hand is enclosed in a plastic bag to prevent infection, splinting is unnecessary as full range of movement can be maintained through active and passive movements. For children with burnt hands conforming gauntlet splints are sometimes used. These are moulded from a casting of the hand and fit the hand exactly, holding it in extension. It has been found that even when these have been worn for the required time, children are able to regain full range of movement; this is not possible with adults.

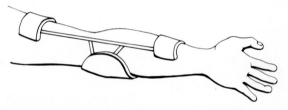

Fig. 15.5   Three-point extension splint to prevent flexion deformity at the elbow

5. *Ankle.* It is vital that foot drop is prevented by use of a padded foot-drop splint or correct use of a foot board while the patient is in bed.

Independence in activities of daily living. The highest possible level of independence in personal activities must be maintained at all times, for physical as well as psychological benefit. It is fairly easy for a patient with burnt hands to continue to feed himself and perform other basic activities, if he is treated by the 'plastic bag' method, although it may be necessary to pad the handles of implements used. If the hand is splinted or bandaged, it may be possible to attach eating utensils to the splints so that the patient can at least continue to feed himself.

Maintaining range of movement. As mentioned previously, the occupational therapist's contribution at this stage will be providing motivation through activities and maintaining independence, both of which will encourage maintenance of movement patterns.

Treatment during the grafting period

Occupational therapy at this stage will depend on the size of the area being grafted and the type of skin graft.

Restoration and maintenance of independence in the activities of daily living. If split-skin grafting is used it must be remembered that, even after the initial period of immobilisation, the grafted area will be relatively unstable and equipment and activities should therefore offer little resistance. Clothing should be lightweight, of natural fibre to allow free circulation of air and loose-fitting. Belts, cuffs and other tight fastenings should be avoided.

Eating and writing utensils may need light, soft padding if the hands are affected.

If full skin grafting is used it is important to ensure maximum independence during the longer periods of immobilisation.

The patient may well be discharged between each grafting period and so a home visit will be necessary. Prior to this, domestic activities should be carried out in the occupational therapy department to maintain and regain skills and confidence. In the case especially of burns which occurred at home, it may take the patient a long time to regain full confidence in the kitchen. Obviously, empha-

sis on safety in the home will be just as important as restoring function.

Splinting. This will be continued, as required, to prevent scar contracture causing joint deformity. Dynamic splinting may be introduced after the initial healing of the grafted area.

Restoration and maintenance of the range of movement. Activities should initially be light and aimed at giving the fullest range of movement at the affected joints (see also Ch.20, 28). Rhythmical, bilateral activities will encourage full range of movement and as healing progresses, more resistance can be added. Do not forget that both donor and wound area may need treatment and that coordination and stereognosis activities may also be necessary.

Restoration of confidence and the ability to cope socially. The occupational therapist is often the first person who takes the patient out of the secure and protected environment of the ward in which he has been treated since admission. Although the patient may have seen a reflection of himself on the ward and therefore coped with the shock of seeing extensive damage, it may well be that this is the first time he makes contact with people other than staff or family and close friends.

If damage is gross and/or visible, the patient should be introduced gently into a small group of understanding (and possibly prewarned) patients and staff. Initially he should not be asked to participate in the group and demands made on him by the group should be gradually increased. His first visit to the department, for instance, may just involve a conducted tour and explanation of the activities he will be doing, or he may sit in the department reading or working with the therapist, but in a position where he can see and be seen. Later he may accept hospitality from another patient in the department, for example one who has been working in the kitchen, or sit in on a group activity, such as a quiz or discussion, before he feels able to take an active part in the group.

Once the patient is confident enough to meet others in the hospital, the therapist must gradually introduce him to society outside the hospital. Walks, shopping trips, bus journeys and other necessary outings should be made by the therapist and the patient before discharge. It may be appropriate for the therapist and patient to visit his place of work together as a preliminary to return to work and outings with people other than hospital staff, for example a trip to the pub at lunchtime with a group of patients, may also help the disfigured person to face society outside.

Hospital self-help groups for patients and relatives are often invaluable in giving support to the patient and his family during and after discharge.

Treatment after healing

The patient will by now be discharged home. Treatment, however, should continue until full scar maturation has occurred. This may not be until 12 to 18 months after healing and, obviously, treatment sessions will become less frequent.

Maintenance of range of movement and prevention of contractures. Activities demanding a full range of movement in the affected areas should be continued and resistance should now be added to regain muscle strength. The therapist should remember that it is vital to maintain full range of movement even though the process may be painful and some surface splitting may occur. It must be explained to the patient that these are relatively minor problems which can be dealt with more easily than loss of movement.

Appearance and skin condition. In recent years the use of pressure garments, such as those made by Jobst, during the period of scar maturation have proved most successful. These garments, worn for 24 hours a day for up to 18 months after healing, help to prevent scar hypertrophy and keep the scar supple and white, thus reducing the danger of loss of movement. These garments should be renewed about every three months as they gradually lose their tension.

The skin should be watched carefully for hardening and shrinking, and a lanolin-based cream or bland, all-purpose cream such as Nivea should be rubbed in regularly. The cream not only helps to keep the scar tissue soft and mobile, but the rubbing action also encourages coordination and sensory input, which is especially important for the hands.

Special make-up products and advice for both men and women are available from cosmetic firms such as Elizabeth Arden and Revlon. Larger branches of Boots often have a cosmetic advisor to give assistance with disguising visible scarring and recently help has been available through the NHS from the London Jewish Hospital. The Red Cross are also training volunteers to give advice in this field.

Resettlement. As mentioned earlier, contact with the patient's employer is necessary from the early stages of treatment so that his progress and likely ability to return to his previous work can be discussed. Many burnt patients return to work with little problem, especially if there is only little visible scarring and full range of movement has been maintained. Difficulties that may be encountered include:

1. unsettled compensation claims, especially if the accident occurred at work. This may delay return to work and the patient may become apathetic.

2. inability to return to the previous job. When this occurs the occupational therapist will need to carry out a work assessment (see Ch. 12) in order to find the exact level of function available for work, and the Disablement Resettlement Officer should be contacted. Further assessment and retraining schemes may be appropriate.

3. lack of motivation to return to work. After a long period of sickness the patient may be reluctant to return to work. In such a case the Job Centre staff, hospital staff and employers must work closely together to persuade the patient that he is fit to work and explain to him the benefits he will derive by returning.

Throughout the often long treatment of the burns patient the therapist must remain conscious of the fact that the patient and his family have undergone severe trauma, followed by extensive and frequently painful treatment. Therefore, the physical as well as the psychological and social aspects of the patient's well-being must be considered and dealt with positively.

REFERENCES AND FURTHER READING

Muir I F K, Barclay T L 1974 Burns and their treatment, 2nd edn. Lloyd-Luke, London

Shopland A et al 1979 Refer to occupational therapy. Churchill Livingstone, Edinburgh

Wynn-Parry C B 1973 Rehabilitation of the hand, 3rd edn. Butterworths, London

16

The elderly

Geriatric medicine is the term used to describe the study and treatment of the diseases of old age. As far as most government bodies are concerned the term tends to mean the treatment and care of those aged over 65 years.

This is a very arbitrary age limit, since ageing people vary widely in their attitudes and abilities — some are 'aged' at 50, while others are still young at heart at the age of 80. The World Health Organisation has classified the ageing population into four groups.

1. Middle age: 45 to 59 years
2. Elderly: 60 to 74 years
3. Old: 75 to 90 years
4. Very old: 90 years and over.

There are obviously dangers in such a classification, as labels tend to create preconceived ideas and therefore a stereotyped approach to the individual. We must accept, however, that when treating elderly patients the general problems associated with that particular age group must be understood. It is therefore intended to discuss these problems and the principles underlying treatment. The chapter primarily discusses the role of the occupational therapist working with the elderly person in hospital, but many elderly people are supported at home and the principles and aims mentioned in this chapter and in Chapter 8 can be applied when treating clients in the community.

THE AGEING PROCESS

As a person ages, certain physiological, functional

and mental changes take place, which are normal processes of ageing. The therapist must understand these changes and plan treatment and approach to the patient accordingly.

Appearance

As a person ages, he begins to look old, i.e. the skin becomes dry and wrinkled and the hair becomes grey or white and dry, with loss or thinning of body and head hair. Clothes will no longer be of the latest fashion, but will be bought for comfort, economy and warmth. Hairstyle may be chosen for ease of care and economy. Clearly, appearance alone should never be used as a guide to the age of a person, as it varies widely from one individual to another, but normal standards and attitude to appearance must be considered when, for example, the therapist is advising on clothing, adaptations and personal care. She must take particular care never to impose her own standards or expectations on the person she is treating.

Skeletal system

Normally during ageing joints remain mobile, although there may be stiffness after a period of inactivity. Bones become brittle and muscle bulk is lost, resulting in weakness. Posture may be poor due to general weakness, aching and a lowered level of activity and there may be a slight reduction in height owing to loss of elasticity of the intervertebral cartilage.

Special senses

Hearing. Acuity is lost and high, low or soft sounds become more difficult to detect. Hardness of hearing is often mistaken for obstinacy, loss of concentration or interest, or mental impairment and the therapist should be aware of this. Although a hearing aid may have been provided, the old person may be reluctant or unable to use it and these aids should therefore be checked regularly. The inability to communicate normally, can lead to isolation and apathy, and the inability to hear a bus, car, telephone, doorbell or kettle can be dangerous as well as isolating.

Sight. Vision becomes less acute and the ability to accommodate to different light levels is decreased. Although wearing spectacles has now become socially acceptable, it is important to remember that a patient may have difficulty with certain activities simply because he cannot see clearly. The elderly person must be reminded and encouraged to have regular check-ups to ensure that his spectacles are of the correct strength. If the patient is admitted to hospital, or receiving treatment in the department, be sure to check that his spectacles are available and used as normal.

Smell and taste. These tend to deteriorate with age. Although this may not cause immediate problems, prolonged and serious deterioration of these senses may result in poor appetite as the three are closely linked. Dangers might arise if loss of smell leads to the inability to detect fire or gas leaks, or if loss of taste and smell leads to the inability to pick out bad or undercooked food.

Temperature control. The ability to control temperature, which depends among other factors on the level of activity and the amount of body fat, is reduced in the elderly. They are therefore less able to cope with changes in temperature. Appropriate heating and clothing are important, both indoors and outdoors, but especially when changing from one to the other.

Metabolism

As the metabolic rate decreases the elderly person becomes less active and tires more easily. Although this is a problem in itself, it may lead to loss of appetite, joint stiffness, apathy and related problems. The elderly person should keep to a well-balanced daily routine with short periods of regular exercise and rest and maintain an adequate diet. The sleep pattern will alter, as older people rarely sleep continuously through the night and therefore need short periods of sleep during the day. This should be borne in mind when arranging a treatment programme and time should be allowed for rest and sleep, especially after the midday meal.

Mental changes

Concentration and memory for recent events will diminish with age, although memory for events long passed will remain and often be quite vivid. The old person finds it more difficult to adapt to change in routine or environment and therefore may often appear confused when in new surroundings. Mental processes will be slower and reactions when answering questions, watching television or crossing the road will take longer. The old often become very self-centred, especially if they are inactive all day long, and can become over-anxious about their food, bowel movements, possessions and other personal concerns.

DISORDERS COMMONLY ENCOUNTERED IN THE AGED

The process of ageing itself is not an illness. However, there are certain disorders, which in the elderly give rise to additional problems and thereby complicate treatment and possibly alter the prognosis. An outline of the common disorders affecting the elderly is given below.

Respiratory diseases

Pneumonia. This is the term used to describe inflammation of the lung. Patients may develop pneumonia after prolonged bedrest as secretions accumulate in the lungs during periods of inactivity and the lungs become infected (broncho- or hypostatic pneumonia). Patients may also develop pneumonia as a result of cross-infection, i.e. through exposure to organisms present in the hospital ward or elsewhere. Rehabilitation following pneumonia will be complicated by joint stiffness, muscle weakness and the loss of independence if the elderly patient is confined to bed.

Bronchitis. Bronchitis is an inflammation of the mucous membranes of the bronchial tubes. In the elderly the disease is usually chronic with coughing, production of sputum and breathlessness as the main symptoms. Air pollution, cold and damp weather and cigarette smoking have been shown to exacerbate the condition.

Emphysema. The alveoli of the lungs become over-distended with air and the walls degenerate, losing their elasticity and thus affecting the efficiency of respiration. The condition is often associated with chronic bronchitis.

Skeletal disorders

Osteoarthrosis. This is a degenerative disease usually affecting the larger weight-bearing joints, i.e. hip, knee and spine (see Ch. 22). Although a high proportion of the elderly show some evidence of osteoarthrosis, the condition may become severe, giving rise to pain, deformity and limited mobility.

Rheumatoid arthritis. This is a systemic disease affecting the joints and resulting in pain, deformity and muscle weakness. Small joints, especially in the hand and wrist, are most commonly affected (see Ch. 26). Although the onset is usually in early to middle adult life, deformity and weakness are often not apparent until old age although pain and exacerbations may be less acute.

Paget's disease of bone. This is a chronic disease occurring in middle and old age, resulting in bone pain and deformity. Headaches and deafness may occur.

Osteoporosis. In osteoporosis the bones become porous and brittle due to lack of calcium deposit.

Circulatory disorders

In the elderly, several interrelated conditions affecting the circulation may occur.

Arteriosclerosis. Hardening of the arteries is due to proliferation of fibrous tissue, infiltration of fat and/or deposit of lime salts and leads to loss of elasticity and contractability of the artery.

Atherosclerosis. The narrowing or occlusion of blood vessels is sometimes associated with high cholesterol levels in the blood.

Thrombosis. Clotting of the blood within the vessel. The resulting clot, called a thrombus, affects circulation distal to its site.

Embolism. A clot, or part of a larger clot, carried by the blood from its place of origin and lodged in a smaller blood vessel, thus obstructing circulation.

All can result in ischaemia, i.e. lack of blood supply, in the tissues beyond the affected area. The resulting damage will depend on the site of the affected vessel; e.g. in prolonged *cerebral* ischaemia the main symptoms are giddiness, loss of memory and mental changes. Gait is affected and there may be muscular rigidity. Sudden occlusion of cerebral arteries by an embolus, or by thrombosis, i.e. a cerebro vascular accident (CVA), may result in hemiplegia.

If *coronary* arteries are affected, the resulting lack of blood supply to the heart muscle leads ultimately to degeneration and congestive (chronic) heart failure, i.e. the inability of the heart to maintain efficient circulation. Angina pectoris (or angina of effort), i.e. the inability of the coronary vessels to cope with the extra demands of effort, emotion etc, and myocardial infarction (coronary thrombosis), i.e. the lodging of a thrombus in a coronary artery which may cause sudden death, may also occur.

In the *lower limb* the tissue beyond the affected area will degenerate leading to intermittent claudication and occasionally gangrene, which may necessitate amputation. The risk of a deep vein thrombosis (DVT) is increased by prolonged bed-rest.

Aneurysm. This is a persistent dilation of the artery due to damage or imperfection of the vessel wall. The aneurysm may rupture, leading to haemorrhage. Damage will depend on the site of the haemorrhage, e.g. a ruptured cerebral aneurysm will lead to a CVA (stroke) and hemiplegia.

Varicose veins. The veins, usually of the lower limb, become dilated due to the inefficiency of valves and muscular tissue in the walls of the veins. It may lead to pigmentation of chronically congested skin and ultimately to ulceration. The veins may rupture.

Hypertension. Blood pressure is raised above normal. In persistent hypertension symptoms of throbbing in the head, headache, giddiness and palpitations may arise. Cerebral haemorrhage in already-damaged vessels may occur.

Hypotension. The blood pressure is lower than normal. This condition may be the result of damaged heart muscle or of the inability of the coronary vessels to maintain adequate circulation. The symptoms are general weakness, fainting and giddiness, especially on rising (postural hypotension), and depression.

Disorders of the nervous system

Few disorders of the nervous system begin in old age, although there are some exceptions.

Cerebro-vascular accident (stroke). Some of the causes have been described above. The extent of damage may differ, but some degree of unilateral paralysis, mental, speech and visual impairment is common (see Ch. 19).

Parkinsonism. This disease occurs in middle and old age and affects the central nervous system. The symptoms are muscular rigidity, tremor and associated incoordination and speech difficulties (see Ch. 24).

Motor neurone disease. This is a progressive muscular atrophy in which muscles of the hands and feet are affected initially. Later, paralysis involves arms, shoulders and legs and the patient becomes wheelchair- and eventually bed-bound.

Senile dementia. This may arise in elderly people and lead to loss or diminishment of normal cerebral functions such as memory and concentration.

Other disorders

These may occur either as primary or as secondary conditions.

Incontinence. The inability to control the passing of urine and, less commonly, faeces.

Constipation. An inability of, or difficulty with, defaecation.

Retention. An inability of, or difficulty with, micturition.

The treatment team

As can be seen from the problems described, treatment of the old person includes medical, social and functional aspects and it requires a wide range of skills and personnel to return the sick geriatric patient to his fullest potential.

The roles of the different members of the treatment team are described briefly below.

The consultant

The geriatrician is the team leader whilst the patient is in hospital. He is responsible for decisions about admission, discharge, diagnosis and medical and surgical treatment. His ability to understand and use the expertise of other staff, and above all his attitude, will determine the efficiency and enthusiasm of both his staff and patients.

The general practitioner

The general practitioner plays a vital role in the care and treatment of the patient. Ideally this should be one of prevention and information, but where this is not possible owing to pressure of work, he should endeavour to see each elderly patient on his list regularly (either at home or in the surgery) so that problems can be dealt with as soon as they arise. He should be well aware of community services for the elderly and of the help for which they may be eligible.

The nurse

The district nurse's role is vital, as she sees the patient regularly in his home surroundings and may therefore recognise problems before they become serious enough to necessitate hospitalisation. Her day-to-day contact with the patient will be for general nursing duties such as dressing sores and ulcers, giving injections and helping with bathing.

The hospital nurse is the only person in the team who sees the patient for 24 hours a day while he is in hospital. For this reason she can support him in any task he finds difficult and, if working relationships are well established, she can also encourage skills taught by the occupational therapist, physiotherapist and speech therapist. She can, for example, reinforce the dressing and feeding techniques shown by the occupational therapist and the walking patterns and communication skills taught by the physiotherapist and speech therapist. Moreover, the importance of specific nursing techniques, e.g. establishing an independent routine, preventing bed-sores and contractures, dispensing medication and teaching the patient to manage his own medication prior to discharge, cannot be underestimated. It is the nurse on whom the newly-admitted, sick patient will rely most heavily for understanding, help, information and comfort.

The social worker (SW)

An active and well-informed SW will make all the difference to the smooth running of a geriatric department. By liaising between hospital and community, by knowing and organising community help and support for patients and by dealing with any problems arising from financial, legal, social or personal difficulties, the SW will make the patient's stay in hospital, and his admission and discharge, much easier.

The physiotherapist

Occupational and physiotherapists in a geriatric department must work closely together, as disagreement over treatment programmes, techniques, aims of treatment or exchange of information will only hinder the patient's progress. The physiotherapist will be concerned with the mobility and activity level of the patient and this will be closely related to the functions the patient will need to perform in order to maintain or regain independence. She will work with individuals as well as groups and concentrate on exercising balance, walking, muscle strength and joint mobility.

The speech therapist

Communication, by whatever means, is an essential part of life. The speech therapist works with patients whose powers of communication have been impaired or lost, mainly as a result of an illness such as a stroke or Parkinsonism. The occupational therapist should work closely with the speech therapist, encouraging the patient to use his communication skills, and at the same time inform the speech therapist of occupational therapy methods, e.g. adaptations of writing instruments, so that these, in turn, may be used during speech therapy sessions.

Relatives (staff of hostel or old people's home)

The hospital team must remember that the elderly person is in their care for only a relatively short period and that, on discharge, the patient will be supported or cared for by relatives. It is of the utmost importance, therefore, that contact is made with the relatives whilst the patient is still in hospital. They must be shown how, when and when not to help the patient and should be informed of the help available to them and the old person. They should be encouraged to visit the patient and, where possible, assist with his hospital routine, and their own worries and suggestions should be discussed in ample time to prevent problems arising on discharge.

The patient

Rarely is the patient himself seen as part of the treatment team, but his help or hinderance during treatment can radically alter his progress, prognosis and discharge placement. The therapist must remember that the patient is her *raison d'etre* and that he has a right to be informed about what treatment is planned, what arrangements are being made and what is expected of him. Too often the patient is left in ignorance of his discharge, pension, drugs, pets and so on. Frequently he is taken for treatment to a department and asked to perform strange activities he neither enjoys nor understands. We must always regard the patient as an individual with rights, fears and opinions, and not just as a cog in a wheel or 'the hemi on ward B'.

THE ROLE OF THE OCCUPATIONAL THERAPIST

The role of the occupational therapist working with the elderly is fourfold:

1. Assessment of functional level
2. Establishment and maintenance of maximum level of independence in activities of daily living
3. Stimulation of social, communication, mental and physical skills through group work
4. Treatment of physical, psychological, personal and social problems through individual work.

Assessment of functional level

It is advisable to obtain basic information about the patient before meeting him. The following information is necessary before initial contact is made or treatment can be planned:

Patient's name. Forename, surname, marital status

Address. If in-patient, note his ward

Date of birth

Diagnosis. Also any relevant related problems, e.g. deafness, diabetes

Prognosis. Where possible, ask the doctor how he feels the patient is likely to progress, as this will help the therapist gauge her treatment programme

Doctor. Both the consultant treating the patient and the patient's general practitioner

Hospital number. So that the patient's notes and X-rays can be obtained for further information if necessary.

Reason for referral. It is both time-saving and practical to state the aim of treatment for the elderly person. If treatment is required for one specific area only, e.g. a Colles fracture or difficulty with putting on a shoe and caliper, the therapist can estimate how much time and what equipment will be necessary for the treatment session. If, however, a patient with a similar diagnosis needs to be assessed for his ability to cope at home or in Part III accommodation, the therapist will organise her treatment quite differently.

The place, time and manner in which the initial interview is conducted are all vital for good rapport.

Place. The therapist should meet the patient initially in surroundings in which he will feel secure, i.e. his own territory. This may be by the patient's bed or in the ward day-room, rather than in the department where the patient may feel insecure and therefore less able to concentrate fully or to trust in the therapist.

Time. Try to see the patient at a time when he is at his best. This may be during morning coffee or after his lunchtime rest. The therapist should try to see the patient before the start of the first treatment session. It is not a good idea to arrive at the patient's bedside for the first time at 8.30 am and expect him to get up immediately and get dressed.

Manner. It is most important to introduce yourself by name and profession and to explain your aims briefly and in terms the patient can understand. Try to keep the initial meeting short and informal. All questioning should relate directly to the patient's problem. For example, if a patient has been told that the occupational therapist will help him to 'look after himself again', it is not relevant to ask him who owns the house he lives in (see also Ch. 1).

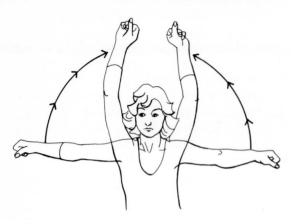

A Elevation through abduction

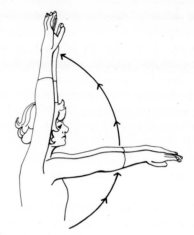

B Elevation through flexion

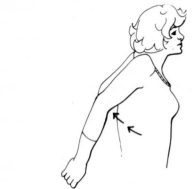

C Extension

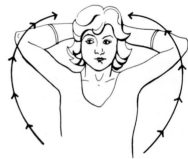

D Lateral rotation

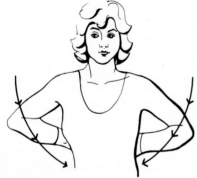

E Medial rotation

Fig. 16.1 Shoulder movement

There are four main areas of assessment: physical, personal, psychological and social. The majority of the assessment can be done by observation during activities and only when a specific problem arises should it be looked at more closely. The older person will find a full, formal assessment tiring and worrying, so observation may take place over several sessions.

Physical assessment

Whereas with the younger patient, or in the case of a specific disability, e.g. a Colles fracture, the therapist will make a formal measurement of the joint involved, with the older person, for whom functional ability takes precedence over full range of movement or muscle strength, a simplified assessment is usually sufficient.

Passive range. Put the joint through a passive range of movement first to estimate any limitation in joint mobility.

Active range *in the upper limb*

Shoulder

1. Take arms out to side and touch hands above

head (elevation through abduction — Fig. 16.1A).

2. Take arms up straight in front until they touch the ears (elevation through flexion — Fig. 16.1B).

3. Lift both arms backwards, elbows loose, as high as possible (extension — Fig. 16.1C).

4. Touch hands behind neck (lateral rotation — Fig. 16.1D).

5. Touch hands behind waist (medial rotation — Fig. 16.1E).

Elbow

1. Stretch arms out in front or reach out to touch therapist's hand placed at arm's length (extension — Fig. 16.2A).

2. Touch thumbs on shoulders (flexion — Fig. 16.2B).

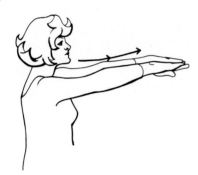

A Extension

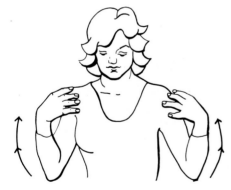

B Flexion

Fig. 16.2 Elbow movement

Forearm

1. Tuck arms into waist, elbows at right angles, turn palms upwards (supination — Fig. 16.3A).

2. Tuck arms into waist, elbows at right angles,

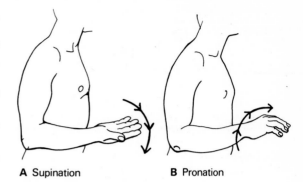

A Supination   **B** Pronation

Fig. 16.3 Forearm movement

turn palms downwards (pronation — Fig. 16.3B).

Wrist

1. Tuck elbows into side, with forearm in pronation, raise hand (extension — Fig. 16.4A).

2. Tuck arms into waist, with forearms in pronation, push hand down (flexion — Fig. 16.4B).

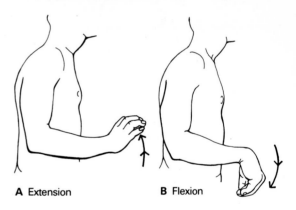

A Extension   **B** Flexion

Fig. 16.4 Wrist movement

Hand

1. Ask the patient to grip your wrist and squeeze (gross grip — Fig. 16.5A).

2. Ask the patient to grip just one of your fingers and squeeze (fine grip — Fig. 16.5B).

3. Pull on a piece of paper held between index finger and thumb (pincer grip — Fig. 16.5C).

4. Ask the patient to touch each finger tip in turn with the thumb of the same hand (opposition and coordination — Fig. 16.6).

5. Place a piece of paper between each finger in turn and ask the patient to hold the paper whilst

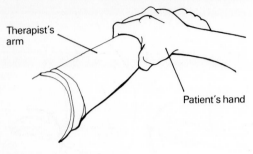

Therapist's arm

Patient's hand

A Gross grip

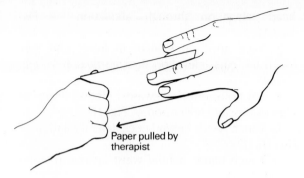

Paper pulled by therapist

A Adduction

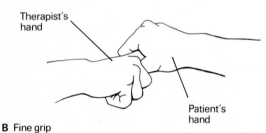

Therapist's hand

Patient's hand

B Fine grip

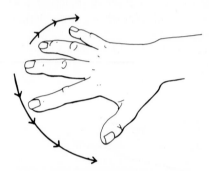

B Abduction of fingers and extension of thumb

Fig. 16.7 Movement of fingers and thumb

Paper pulled by therapist

C Pincer grip

Fig. 16.5 Hand grips

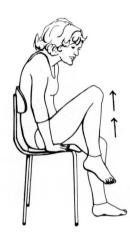

Fig. 16.8 Hip flexion

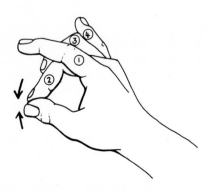

Fig. 16.6 Coordination and opposition

it is pulled by the therapist (adduction — Fig. 16.7A).

6. Span hand out into star shape (abduction — Fig. 16.7B).

The range of movement may be observed even more informally during other activities. Dressing

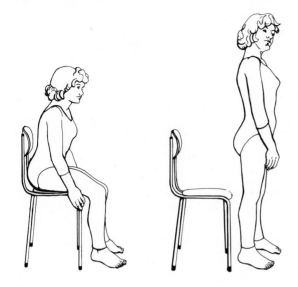

Fig. 16.9 Hip and knee extension. Note balance when standing

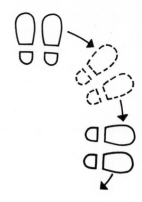

Fig. 16.10 Medial and lateral rotation of the hip

Active range in the lower limb

A slightly less rigid assessment is made of the lower limb as the therapist will be noting stability and balance as well as limb mobility.

Hip. Note first how the patient is sitting. Is he leaning to one side because the hip will not flex or is painful? Is he slumped in the chair with a rounded spine because the hip is fixed?

1. To test the hip flexors ask the patient to sit up straight in the chair, knees together, and then to raise one foot off the ground at a time (Fig. 16.8).

2. To test the hip extensors ask the patient to stand upright from sitting (Fig. 16.9).

3. Ask the patient to turn a circle while standing

practice, for example, will demonstrate most upper limb activites. It is advisable for the therapist to sit opposite the patient when assessing and demonstrate the activity to be copied or explain it in a way he will easily understand. For example, for elevation through abduction ask the patient to take his hands out to the side then raise them until they meet above his head.

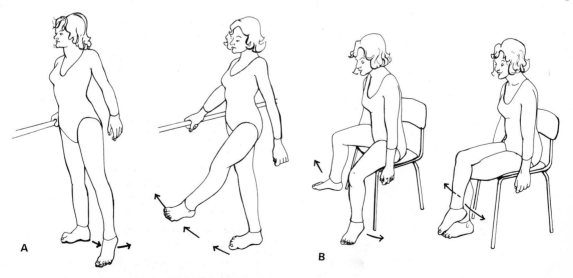

Fig. 16.11 Abduction and adduction of the hip (A) while standing (B) sitting

on the spot, note medial and lateral rotation (Fig. 16.10).

4. While standing — and using support where necessary — the patient raises each leg in turn to the side (abduction) then brings it back and across over the other foot (adduction Fig. 16.11A). Note: if balance is not good enough to allow this, assessment can be made while the patient is seated by asking him to place his feet as wide apart as possible (abduction) then crossing each knee over the other in turn (adduction — Fig. 16.11B).

Knee

1. While seated, the patient straightens his knee (extension — Fig. 16.12A).

2. While seated the patient pulls his feet well back and lifts them off the floor (flexion — Fig. 16.12B).

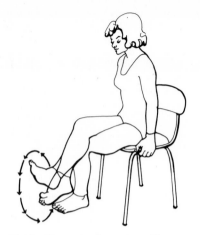

Fig. 16.13 Circumduction at the ankle

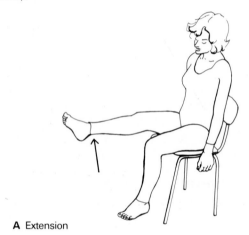

A Extension

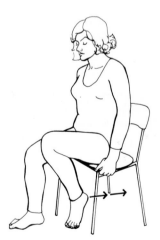

B Flexion

Fig. 16.12 Knee movement

Ankle. With his knees crossed, the patient circles his foot (dorsiflexion, eversion, plantarflexion, inversion — Fig. 16.13).

The patient should also be observed when rising from sitting, walking and climbing stairs. This will show his degree of stability and balance, as well as his ability to bear weight through joints. Functional muscle strength of hip flexors and extensors, knee flexors and extensors and dorsi- and plantar-flexors can also be assessed.

Active range in the spine

Cervical spine. The patient is asked to perform each of the following movements:

1. Touch the chin on the chest (forward flexion — Fig. 16.14A).

2. Look up to the ceiling (extension — Fig. 16.14B).

3. Look over each shoulder in turn (rotation — Fig. 16.14C).

4. Touch each ear to the shoulder in turn (side flexion — Fig. 16.14D).

Thoracic and lumbar spine. Note: these movement are best performed whilst the patient is seated to prevent dizziness or lack of balance.

1. Note ability to touch feet (forward flexion — Fig. 16.15A).

2. Ask the patient to arch his back (extension — Fig. 16.15B).

3. The patient twists to the right and the left in turn (rotation — Fig. 16.15C).

4. Ask the patient to lean over to touch the

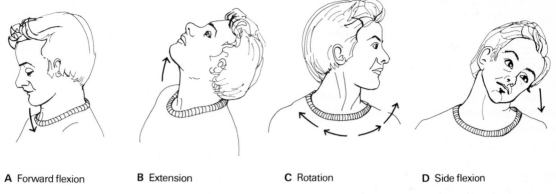

A Forward flexion   **B** Extension   **C** Rotation   **D** Side flexion

Fig. 16.14   Cervical movement

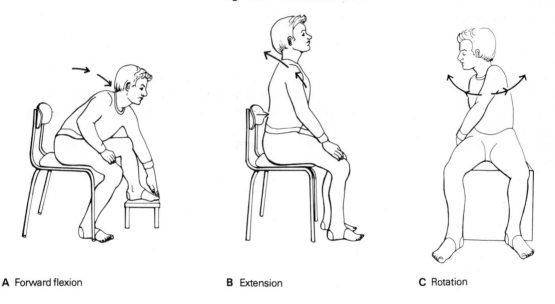

A Forward flexion   **B** Extension   **C** Rotation

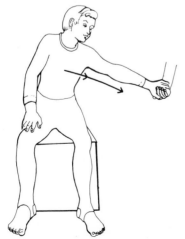

D Side flexion

Fig. 16.15   Spinal movement

therapist's hand to left and right in turn (side flexion — Fig. 16.15D).

The range of movement in the spine may be observed more informally during other activities, e.g. during music-to-movement sessions (see later), while bending to put on shoes or stretching to hang up a coat.

Personal assessment

The ability of the older person to be as independent as possible in all activities of daily living is of prime importance to the occupational therapist. An initial verbal assessment is often useful, as the therapist can discover the patient's attitude to independence and also something of the circumstances in which he lives. The therapist must beware of taking all information given as strictly accurate as, for reasons of privacy, memory or wishful thinking, the patient may not present a true picture. Verbal assessment should always be backed up by practical assessment and where possible the therapist should also check with relatives or friends.

Assessment should be made during the normal daily routine where possible and attention should be given to any particular difficulties.

Dressing. Preferably this should be done on the ward in the morning as part of ward routine. Do not forget that the patient should be assessed during both dressing and undressing.

Washing. A reasonably accurate assessment can be made by observing the patient washing on the ward, usually from a bowl placed on a bed table. Although this is not the way most people wash, the therapist can see how a facecloth, soap and towel are handled and also how the patient manages with razor, comb or make-up. If at home a patient usually washes standing at a basin, this should also be assessed.

Toilet. Again, observation can be made on the ward. During assessment, it may be necessary to accompany the patient to the toilet to ensure not only that he can transfer on/off the toilet, but also that he can reach and use the paper, handle clothing and flush the chain. Remember, that if the ward toilet has rails or a raised seat and the patient's toilet at home does not, he should be seen to manage without these aids.

Bathing. The therapist can observe and/or help the patient in his bath on the ward. Remember that he must be assessed during the whole process of bathing and not just getting in and out of the bath. He should approach the bath from the same side as at home. If he lives alone he should be safe and competent enough to manage on his own.

Cooking. It is advisable to assess the patient's ability in the kitchen during an individual session rather than in a larger group in order to get an accurate picture of how he can manage. However, if the therapist is fairly confident of her patient's ability to manage from previous observation, a group session of washing up, vegetable prep-

aration or similar task will be sufficient to judge his balance, his ability to manoeuvre in the kitchen, handle tools, carry objects, plan work and so on. The therapist can rarely, if ever, simulate the patient's home circumstances beyond providing the same type of fuel for cooking and if it is felt necessary to assess the patient in his own home, this must be done during a home visit.

Eating. This can be observed during mealtimes. The therapist will need to note not only how the patient handles cutlery and cuts food, but also his ability to chew and swallow and the speed at which he eats.

Laundry. This is often difficult to assess beyond seeing how the patient copes with washing his underclothes, nightclothes and other personal items used in hospital. The therapist should find out how the patient plans to cope with his laundry at home and take this as a guideline for assessment. In departments where laundry facilities are available for patients, the problem of assessment is minimised.

Shopping. During discussion and kitchen assessment the occupational therapist should have gathered enough information to tell her how the patient manages with budgeting, shopping, household chores and so on. Any specific difficulties that arise, or are anticipated, should receive special consideration. As these activities require a higher level of ability, the therapist will not be able to assess the patient until later in the treatment programme. By this time a good enough relationship should have developed between patient and therapist for the problems to be discovered and discussed.

Mobility. The therapist can observe the patient's ability to transfer to and from bed, chair or toilet during normal daily routine. Walking and climbing stairs may be noted while the patient is moving around the department. If the patient is very immobile the occupational therapist and the physiotherapist must use the same methods of assisting the patient during walking, standing and transferring and encourage maximum independent mobility at all times.

Psychological assessment

In old age, as indeed in any stage of life, the ability

to perform certain activities is not only determined by physical capability. Old age, and the ability to manage one's daily affairs when old, have been referred to as a 'state of mind' and every therapist has cases to relate of patients who remain independent in spite of severe disabilities and of others who find it difficult to cope with even a relatively minor handicap.

When assessing the patient's psychological state the therapist should note the following:

Orientation. Is the patient orientated in time, place and person? Does he know where he lives, that he is in hospital and why he is there? During the first meeting with the patient the therapist should make an accurate assessment of his level of orientation; she may want to ask a standard set of questions so that an additional assessment can be made at a later date to assess improvement.

Memory and learning ability. Memory and learning ability can be observed informally. Does the patient remember the therapist's name from day to day? Does he keep 'losing' his possessions? Does he remember how he has been taught to put on his clothes, rise from a chair, use his walking aid etc?

For longer term memory the therapist should also note how well the patient responds when participating in quizzes and how he can relate his management of certain activities before his illness. However, she must check that the patient is, in fact, remembering the period he is being asked about, not how he managed 20 years ago, and that he is not confabulating to cover his inability to remember or his embarrassment at not being able to manage. As well as recall, i.e. remembering without any clue to the required answer as in the above examples, the therapist must check the patient's ability to remember through recognition, i.e. with the help of some clue. The therapist may use such methods as asking the patient to collect the equipment he was using the day before from various items in a cupboard; to collect his coat from the hooks in the corridor or show her his bed when he has been away from it for a time.

Attitude. Any assessment of a patient's attitude to his disability, recovery and anticipated dependence is likely to be subjective on the part of the therapist. It is usually gleaned from remarks made by the patient and from observation of the effort and enthusiasm he puts into his treatment. It is often difficult, if not impossible, to change attitudes in the elderly, as they tend to be stereotyped and rigid. The therapist must remember, however, that a patient who is dejected and apathetic may be suffering from depression related to his sickness and inability to cope, and that, as he recovers and finds that he is once more successful in self-care and other activities, this may well change. She must also remember that the patient may be finding it difficult to be treated by a therapist young enough to be his grandchild and be acutely embarrassed at having to be watched or helped while attending to his personal needs. Many elderly people still regard being in hospital as charity, or feel that they are in a workhouse (especially with old hospitals which they remember as such in their childhood) and when asked to perform an activity that they are being 'put to work' in order to earn their keep.

Social assessment

During her early contact with the patient the therapist should discover with whom he lives, what help he is receiving (from relatives, neighbours, home helps etc) and what social contact he enjoys. Often, elderly people who have difficulty with mobility may not leave their home for several months or years and although the therapist should never force or insist that a patient joins the local Darby and Joan Club or attends local functions, she should try to evaluate whether the patient protests about not wanting to join any social events because he really does prefer his own company or because he has no transport, no knowledge of the events, no clean clothes to wear or no money for his tea when he arrives.

Treatment

Having assessed and recorded the patient's abilities and problems, the occupational therapist must organise a programme to deal with specific areas of difficulty. Three important considerations have to be taken into account:

Previous lifestyle. A patient's functional level is much coloured by his previous lifestyle. If, for example, he is the type of person who has always worn a tie or attended church services, he will expect, and should be encouraged, to do so again before he can be considered to have made a complete return to his 'normal'. A person who has a particularly high standard of dress will be distressed if alterations to clothing leave his garment looking less than smart; a person who has always worn corsets will feel most uncomfortable if, because she now finds them difficult to put on (and the therapist cannot find the method or time to make this possible!), she is advised to use garters for her stockings instead. The therapist should not impose, either consciously or otherwise, her own expectations on the patient. If the patient has only been used to a washdown once a week, the therapist should not turn up her nose just because she baths every day !

Wishes. In any institution the wishes of the residents tend to get overlooked and although this cannot be avoided where the choice of bed position, companions and diet are concerned, the occupational therapist must always consider the wishes of the patient when planning for his discharge. She should not, for example, feel that a home help is the automatic answer for the patient who cannot manage to shop for himself, if he would rather rely on neighbours or pay for groceries to be delivered; neither should she arrange for the local task force to decorate the patient's home if he is quite happy to live with peeling wallpaper.

Finance. Often, the therapist can see solutions to problems that, on further investigation, prove to be impractical because the patient's finances will not cope with the demand. It is true that some large items of equipment, or supportive services, can be supplied through social services departments, but the therapist who suggests that an arthritic patient should buy a duvet 'They really cut down on bedmaking' or should eat plenty of high-protein foods like beef and cheese clearly has not understood the problems of living on a pension.

Establishment and maintenance of the maximum level of independence in activities of daily living

The occupational therapist based in a geriatric area can do much to influence the ward/depart-ment routine. To encourage personal independence she can, for example:

● arrange that patients' clothing is not taken away on admission so that dressing practice can be started as soon as possible and establish that getting up and dressed becomes part of normal daily routine (as it is elsewhere).

● see that patients are encouraged to use normal crockery, cutlery and drinking vessels as soon as this is possible. The use of spoons, mashed food and feeding cups should be discouraged unless absolutely necessary, and all those who can should eat at a table rather than from a tray on the bed table.

● ensure that the patient is told that he is expected to take himself to the toilet and to wash himself each morning in the bathroom as soon as he is sufficiently mobile. Even if not sufficiently mobile to manage alone, he should be encouraged to ask for assistance to walk or be pushed, rather than continuing to rely on a bedpan or urinal.

● check that walking and mobility aids are labelled and kept within reach so that patients capable of independent mobility can use the aids and those who still require assistance can be helped with their own aid each time and not just any aid that happens to be around.

● ask that such items as combs, tissues, handbags and pipes are within the patient's reach and that he is encouraged to look after them himself.

● make sure that the ward itself, especially if it cares for long-stay patients, provides a stimulating and helpful background to rehabilitation. There are several aspects of the ward environment which the occupational therapist can influence.

Basic equipment. Make sure that extra razors, combs, handmirrors and clothes are available, clean and functional.

Entertainment. See that newspapers and magazines are available and that they are current copies, that calendars and clocks are large, plentiful and properly adjusted, that table and card games are easily available and complete and that patients are told that they exist. Radio and television certainly have their place, but not everyone appreciates them being on continuously. They should be in a separate area, where possible, and patients encouraged to choose their viewing.

Furniture. Although fewer wards now retain

their military appearance, the therapist can still ensure that the furniture is arranged to aid easy communication, mobility (especially in the day area) and privacy (especially by the patient's bed). Attention should be paid to the things that often hinder communication, such as bedtables, flowers and lockers, as these often block a view.

As with the assessment of the activities of daily living, treatment of specific difficulties should be carried out in relation to daily routine.

Dressing. Do this at the time the patient normally gets up. Ensure his privacy, and sufficient light and time. Tackle problems as they arise, remembering that the patient will tire easily and may get cold if the process takes a long time. It is important to ensure success on the first occasion, regardless of the amount of help that needs to be given. If there are several problems, they should be tackled one at a time, ensuring the patient has mastered one process or aid before attempting the next.

Washing. Most difficulties can be overcome by practice on the ward. Aids such as washing gloves, should be given to the patient to be tried out when he next washes and not as a specific exercise.

Toilet and bathing. When a problem in this area is discovered the occupational therapist should explain to the patient what help is available. Different aids and methods can be tried either on the ward or, where this is not possible, in the ADL section of the occupational therapy department where a selection of aids and adaptations should be available. It is always advisable to arrange that toilet and bathing aids are available on a geriatric ward, as this is an area where patients frequently have difficulty. Once the patient has discovered that he can be independent when using the aids in the occupational therapy department, he can continue using similar aids on the ward.

Cooking. The degree of emphasis on independence in the kitchen will depend on the amount of cooking the patient will have to do after discharge. New skills and methods will take time to learn, but the patient should continue to use the remedial kitchen until he has reached the necessary levels of mobility, concentration, planning, handling of tools, safety and confidence, or his maximum functional ability.

Eating. The first essential is to ensure that the patient can feed himself independently by some method, as being fed is both frustrating and degrading. If aids or new methods are to be introduced, a session outside mealtimes is useful, as the patient will probably be slow and clumsy the first time and his food will get cold and unappetising as he struggles. Once he is more competent the aid or new method should be introduced for part of a mealtime only at first; for example, give a Manoy knife for cutting cheese or dessert and gradually increase its use until the patient feels quite happy with it.

Laundry. Where possible, encourage the patient to look after the laundry of his personal clothing himself. Labour-saving methods or devices can be tried out and other problems discussed either during a home visit or in the department.

Shopping. As the patient becomes more mobile, begin with visits to the hospital shop or purchases from the mobile trolley which visits most hospital wards. Later, progress to shops near the hospital and then to public transport into town, if the patient will have to use this after discharge.

Mobility. As already stated the highest level of independent mobility should be encouraged at all times. Especially ensure that patients who should walk do not become too dependent on a wheelchair and that those who can only walk with assistance have the opportunity to use a self-propelled wheelchair when help is not available.

Note: Treatment of specific problems is described in the appropriate chapters, but remember that there is no 'correct' answer to any problem, especially in the elderly.

Group activities

Whilst treating people as members of a group may not be concentrating fully on the individual requirements, there are several important advantages:

Members of a group with the same or similar problems are often encouraged by seeing the progress of others who are further advanced than they and can measure their own progress by comparison with more disabled members of the group

Similar problems and their possible solutions can be discussed and demonstrated

Communication, social habits, attitude and knowledge can be raised and maintained by influence from the group

Group activities stimulate the reluctant and encourage a wide range of ability and therefore a higher level of achievement

It is time-saving for the therapist, who can observe individual problems and progress of the members and note how they relate within a group

It provides an environment in which the occupational therapist can gain an accurate idea of the realistic effect of her patients' progress.

Group activities can be divided into four main types: orientation, education, social and physical. When planning group activities the therapist, following assessment of each member, should bear in mind the needs of each individual and balance the programme to cover the needs of the majority.

Orientation.
1. *Quizzes* of all varieties and levels can be used to assist long- and short-term memory, orientation in time, place and person, current events and mental abilities. Do not forget that, as the majority of information is taken in through sight rather than the spoken word, all formats of quizzes should be included (see later).

2. *Newspapers and magazines,* which should be current editions, can form the basis for discussions on prices, current affairs, fashion, attitudes, budgeting or sport and can be used for collages, scrap books, quizzes and so on.

3. *Television and radio,* can also act as a basis for discussion, music appreciation, current events and projects. Used discriminately, programmes such as schools and Open University broadcasts, documentary films, panel games and local news can be a great source of stimulation.

4. *Calendars* should be large. Give the responsibility of keeping them up to date to a patient who would benefit from this.

5. *Clocks* can be used in quizzes about timekeeping. Give a patient the responsibility of keeping the clocks wound and to the correct time.

Education. This should not be a case of teaching an old dog new tricks but should serve to stimulate interest and participation, and to update and improve old skills and interests and possibly introduce some new ones.

1. *Talks and demonstrations* should be on a subject relevant to the group. They should be short, with visual aids and audience participation where possible. Topics may include local history, indoor gardening, bird watching in towns and many more. It is often useful to invite speakers from local clubs, day centres and welfare services so that patients can learn of these before discharge.

2. *Outings* are always rewarding, enjoyable and hard work! Ideally patients are taken in groups with similar levels of physical fitness so that the outing is not cut short for some, or too drawn out for others. As well as coach, bus or car outings to local places of interest, concerts and so on, the occupational therapist should remember the less ambitious outings for small groups, such as visits to local parks, churches, shopping centres, exhibitions, fetes or even just round the hospital grounds.

3. *Film and slide shows.* Although it is often easy to ask a member of staff to show her holiday slides and films this can become boring and frustrating for those who rarely leave their own house. In this category the occupational therapist should also include specific educational/interest films and slides on such subjects as home safety, welfare services and keeping fit. Shows should be fairly short and should be followed by a discussion or demonstration. Remember that the occupational therapist who times the activity to take place immediately after the lunch period will soon find any commentary drowned by a chorus of snores!

4. *Quizzes.* It is often a good idea to have a weekly theme, such as budgeting or gardening, for group activities in a geriatric department and quizzes should be related to this theme. In addition to the basic question/answer quizzes the occupational therapist should consider other types, such as pictorial, musical, sound, tactile, smell/taste or object-based quizzes like 'Kims game' or 'What's it for'. It may also be advantageous for some patients to help compile and run the quiz session.

Social activities. Perhaps the most misunderstood and misused aspects of occupational therapy are activities used to improve and maintain the social outlets of the patient's life. They should not, however, be overlooked and activities that can be used in this field are many and varied.

1. *Communication* skills include basic activities such as passing and naming objects as well as more complex ones which need explanation and assistance. Music appreciation, object explanation, charades, singing, play reading and recitals are only a few examples.

2. *Relaxation* will help sleep, reduce pain and aid mobility. Music and movement and relaxation exercises may be included and the importance of diet, time to relax and planning a day should be stressed. Specific relaxation techniques need to be explained and demonstrated.

3. *Constructive use of leisure time.* Any therapist who blindly sticks to bingo and beetle sessions should look to her own old age (and to her grandparents') for the value and popularity of such activities! Although they may well have their place, the therapist should be looking more towards activities that can easily, and fairly cheaply, be carried on after discharge. Examples include:

a. Stamp collecting, related to study and interest in a particular region or period

b. Indoor gardening; many varieties of flowers, fruit and vegetables, can be grown

c. Pen pals, either with a person of similar age or 'find a granny' schemes

d. Table games, e.g. dominoes, whist or chess, which can be enjoyed at home or club

e. Model making, including kits, wood carving and hard toys

f. Sewing, e.g. soft toy making, rag and period dolls, patchwork, nail and thread work, crochet and sewing clothes for bazaars

g. Flower arranging, including flower pressing and making mats and bookmarks.

Physical Activities. Group activities to encourage general and/or specific areas of physical fitness can well be used by the therapist who plans her programme wisely. Sessions of physical activity not only encourage muscle strength, joint mobility, general agility, walking and balance but also circulation, digestion and appetite, respiration,

relaxation and sleep. Exercise sessions can often help to break the viscious circle of inactivity.

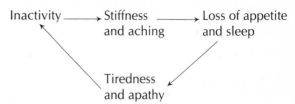

Activities can include music and movement, walks (which can be made purposeful by linking with another activity such as collecting flowers for pressing or pricing of items in various shops for budgeting) outings and shopping, singing, dancing (including wheelchair dancing), skittles, billiards, croquet and bowls.

Individual treatment sessions

Having assessed each patient individually, the therapist must plan her programme to include individual as well as group treatment sessions. Once problems have been identified, treatment can be planned according to the principles described for that particular condition.

Physical. The occupational therapist should arrange treatment of physical difficulties along the principles described for that particular condition, i.e. for the elderly person suffering from osteoarthrosis see Chapter 22, for patients with hemiplegia see Chapter 19.

Personal. Individual treatment should be along the lines described earlier in this chapter for activities of daily living.

Psychological. Where problems of orientation, memory and learning are a particular difficulty, the therapist must treat them on an individual basis as well as with help from group activities. These processes can be treated by repetition of a series of activities in which the patient is asked to use and build up the affected faculty.

1. Orientation. Begin by asking and using basic information about time, place and person, remembering to use visual and other stimuli to aid where necessary. Ask, for example, 'What is your name?', 'Can your write your name down?', 'Can you spell your name?', 'Where do you live?', 'Show me the number of your house', 'Where are

you now?', 'Is it morning now?', 'Which meal will we eat next?'. As the patient improves, the therapist should extend the processes used in the activity. For example, she may ask: 'What are the names of your grandchildren?', 'Place the hands of the clock to show the time you take your next lot of tablets', 'Which bus do you have to catch from town to take you home?'.

2. Memory. Again, begin with simple exercises in recognition and recall.

(a). Recognition. 'What is this item?', 'Which of these two is your comb?', 'Which of these brushes is used for washing up?'

(b). Recall. 'What did you eat for breakfast?', 'What is my name?', 'What is the name of the person in the bed next to you?'.

As with orientation, activities should increase in difficulty as the patient improves.

(i) Recognition. 'Can you collect your work from the cupboard?', 'Please, fetch your green dress and blue cardigan from your wardrobe.'

(ii) Recall. 'Show me how you would make a cottage pie.', 'What is your home help/neighbour called?'. Kims game can also be used here.

3. Learning. This will be superimposed on other activities where needed, e.g. learning to use a new walking aid, understanding a new diet. If learning is a particular problem, the therapist must break down the activities into simple stages and work through repetition to aid the learning process. Only activities that have to be learned should be used and learning not undertaken for its own sake.

Social. Although it may seem an anomaly to treat the patient's social problems on an individual basis, the therapist will find that several aspects can be practised during a one-to-one relationship. If, for example, the patient has communication difficulties, basic activities to aid this, such as practice at explaining the use of an object, reading from a newspaper or matching written words to pictures, can be used. Should appearance, social conduct or personal hygiene be a concern, these are best discussed with the patient privately, during individual treatment. From these few examples it is easy to see that it is indeed possible, and often advantageous, to treat a patient's social problems on an individual basis.

With all the above activities the therapist must keep in mind at all times the level which the patient needs to reach in order to cope with the lifestyle to which he will return and not try to attain higher levels than the patient can manage or will need.

Discharge from hospital

Following a period of sickness, the patient may be discharged home, to relatives or some form of sheltered accommodation. When deciding the most suitable environment for a particular patient, the team must take into consideration his physical and mental fitness, help needed and that which is available, his financial position, his own wishes and those of his relatives, and his prognosis.

Home alone to the same house. The ultimate wish of most old people is to return home to the house they left. When assessing the patient's ability to cope alone at home, the therapist must consider the following points:

Is the patient fully personally independent? If not, can aids, adaptations and/or help be made available to make him independent?

Is he safe to be living alone? If the patient was admitted as the result of a fall, hypothermia, burns, injury following dizziness or blackout or malnutrition, has the cause, as well as the result, been tackled to ensure that the same thing does not happen again?

Is he financially able to cope with the additional demands such as heating, convenience foods, a newly acquired hobby, diet or laundry costs?

Home to family or friends. Points to consider when arranging this:

Is the person as fully independent as the situation demands and if not, are aids, adaptations, outside or family help available?

If friends, relatives or neighbours are going to help, do they know how and when to help? Are they prepared to provide this help over a long period if necessary? Are they aware of services that they can call on for additional help or a break?

Can the household accommodate additional demands on expense, space, time, equipment, diet, laundry and emotions?

Part III accommodation. This accommodation is so called because it was set up under Part III of The National Assistance Act, 1948. In this all local authorities were required to provide accommodation for old people no longer able to live within the community. The criteria for entry are statutory, although local variations may occur from home to home. As a general rule, Part III will not accommodate those who are incontinent, who wander or who are bed-bound. Payment is laid down nationally and the person will be required to pay a percentage of his income towards his keep. The type of care given is similar to that normally expected of a family, i.e. laundry, food, help with bathing and basic nursing care are available.

Warden controlled accommodation. The type of accommodation varies from area to area and may consist of flats, maisonettes or bungalows. However, all have the advantage that a warden is resident in the complex should help be required. Residents are generally self-sufficient and can maintain complete privacy if they wish, although some places have a common meeting area for those who wish to use it.

Old people's bungalows and flatlets. Each local authority housing department is required to provide housing specifically for the elderly in their district. Such accommodation varies, but may be small bungalows, ground-floor flats and maisonettes. Unfortunately, waiting lists are usually long and it is rare that the old person can be discharged directly to such accommodation. Residents are independent, paying rent as any other citizen.

Nursing homes and rest homes. A proprietor who earns the whole or main part of his income from providing accommodation and/or care for the elderly must register with the local authority (under Section 37 of the National Assistance Act, 1948) as a nursing or rest home and must comply with certain regulations and standards of safety and hygiene. Such private accommodation tends to be more expensive than local authority accommodation and will vary in requirements of personal independence, services offered and so on. Therefore, both the team and the patient shoud be satisfied that these points are acceptable and appropriate for the patient. They should also remember that hotels, guest houses and 'homes' that do not earn the main part of their income from elderly residents do not have to register and are therefore not governed by the same regulations as establishments known to the local authority.

Charities and other organisations. Many trusts, organisations, companies and fellowships provide old people's accommodation for their members. The therapist should bear in mind that the patient may be entitled or able to join, for example, ex-servicemen's organisations like the Chelsea Pensioners, Distressed Gentlefolk Association and others. Again, accommodation, criteria for entry and cost will vary and these must be investigated carefully.

Long-stay hospital care. If the patient requires long-term medical and nursing care, a long-stay hospital ward may be considered. The therapist must remember that the ward has now become the patient's home, where personal comfort and possessions should be valued and that such patients should not be 'written off' as being unable to participate in the life of the ward community. A programme of activities to make the life of the individual as enjoyable and purposeful as possible should be arranged. Remember also that, after a period of care, regular food, warmth and exercise, the patient may well become fit enough to transfer to accommodation outside the hospital and all staff must encourage patients along the path of rehabilitation where appropriate.

Community support

As already mentioned, the old person may require some community support after leaving hospital. Indeed, in many instances he may not have been admitted to hospital during the period of sickness but may have been able to remain in the community helped by certain support services.

Day hospitals. These provide medical, nursing and therapeutic care for patients who may otherwise need to be admitted to hospital. They may also provide a stepping stone for the discharged patient and, although the primary aim is one of rehabilitation, valuable social support may be derived by those who live alone or have limited social contact. Day hospitals often allow the patient's family to continue to look after him as:
● he is not left alone during the day if members of the household are out
● the centre can provide social contact for him with people of his own age and interests
● the family is relieved of 24-hour care of the

patient which may put too great a strain on them

● transport and meals are invariably provided.

Day centres. These are usually run by local authorities, church organisations or clubs. Their role is slightly different from that of day hospitals in that they are aiming to:

● provide social contact for their members

● organise activities such as talks, outings, visits, games and crafts

● relieve the family of 24-hour care.

The therapist should check whether transport is provided. Such centres are usually open for a full day and meals are often available.

Clubs, associations and organisations. These are often run by bodies such as residents' associations, church organisations, Darby and Joan and Women's Institutes. They provide social, educational and other activities for their members. They are usually not open all day and transport is not always available; it may be possible to obtain lifts. Members are usually required to be personally independent, refreshment is often available and an enrolment and/or attendance fee payable.

Home help service. Run by the local authority (Social Services) department set up under the Chronically Sick and Disabled Persons Act of 1970. The main duties of the home help are cleaning and shopping, but they are also asked to look out for any change or deterioration in the client's condition. Some home helps will undertake other tasks like cooking and washing, but this is in addition to what is normally expected. The client may be asked to pay towards the cost of the service.

Meals on Wheels. A voluntary organisation providing, for minimal cost, a hot midday meal for the elderly person who cannot provide his own. Meals are delivered to the door.

The value of the home help and Meals on Wheels services cannot be overemphasised. As well as providing an essential service that enables the person to continue living in the community, their members are the regular contact with elderly people who may otherwise be alone, with unreported difficulties, for days on end.

District nurse. As an alternative to hospital admission, routine medical care such as dressings, injections and bathing, can be carried out by a district nurse, thus avoiding the upset caused by

admission to hospital or having to travel to daily clinics.

Health visitor. A routine visit from a health visitor to ensure that a patient discharged from hospital is managing to remain fit and safe can often serve as a follow-up. In this way too, relatives and the patient himself can discuss any unforseen problems that may have arisen since leaving hospital.

Community occupational therapist. The role of the community occupational therapist should not be forgotten, for as well as being a link between hospital and patient after discharge, providing aids and arranging adaptations, she can provide:

1. regular follow-up visits for the chronically sick and disabled to ensure that they are continuing to manage

2. treatment in the patient's home, e.g. mobility training and basic self-care, either as a follow-up to hospital treatment or following an illness, such as a minor stroke, that has not necessitated admission to hospital

3. information on equipment and assistance available (see also Ch. 8).

The therapist should also be aware of other services in her area, such as mobile libraries, talking books, task force and good-neighbour schemes. She should know also how to put the patient in touch with services providing information on rent and rates rebates, travel, theatre, hairdressing, chiropody and dental concessions.

Community physiotherapist. This is a growing service aimed at providing physiotherapy in the patient's own home without the necessity and expense of hospital outpatient treatment.

REFERENCES AND FURTHER READING

Brocklehurst J C 1970 The geriatric day hospital. The Kings Hospital Fund for London, London

Goldberg E M 1970 Helping the aged. Allen & Unwin, London

Hawker M 1974 Geriatrics for physiotherapists and the allied professions. Faber & Faber, London

Hooker S 1976 Caring for elderly people. Routledge & Kegan Paul, London

Irvine R E, Bagnall M K, Smith B J 1978 The older patient — a textbook of geriatrics, 3rd edn. Hoddar & Stoughton — Unibooks, London

17

The hand

A bridge of stone is a thing of architectural expertise and often of great beauty. The hand at rest is an equally finely calculated piece of functional architecture. Looking at its structure it is found that the 'lines' of the hand meet at a point beyond the ulnar border (Fig. 17.1), the distance of which is shortened acutely when the hand makes a tight fist. There is a natural ulnar deviation at the metacarpophalangeal joints on gripping, which is accentuated when the lumbricals pull the fist even tighter. In writing, the ulnar border guides and steadies the pen, while the median side works and manipulates it. When hammering, the ulnar side grips and holds while the median side guides the stroke. The hand works so like an ideal team that

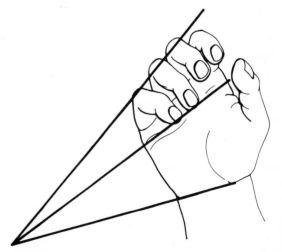

The 'lines' of the hand meet at a point beyond the ulnar border of the hand

Fig. 17.1 The hand at rest

movements are often impossible to isolate. One finger cannot fully flex while the others remain extended. It needs concentration to abduct two fingers while adducting the others. Instructions to isolate thumb abduction and opposition have to be clear indeed to obtain those precise movements. But the hand is more than just a complex structure. It has great strength and amazing dexterity. It can hack coal for 40 years and row across the Atlantic. It can tie flies and play the harp or violin. It can discriminate differences in temperature and pressure and the distance between two points until they are so close they are as one. The hand can express more than can be said by a small gesture or a gentle touch. The hand is at the mercy of its owner and investigates his world. It is the eye of the blind. And the human is at the mercy of his hands, for he receives all the blame when they are clumsy or too hasty and all the praise when they achieve masterpieces or touch to soothe or share. The hand is a small miracle.

The functions of the hand can be described as grip, manipulation, investigation and expression.

Grip

Grip can be divided into power grips and precision grips. Power grips include the cylinder grip as when pulling on a rope, the span grip as when holding a large ball and the hook grip as when carrying a suitcase. The precision grip can include the pinch (or pincer) grip as when picking up a pin, the adductor grip as when turning a key, the tripod grip in use when writing and the plate grip as when holding a plate or when reading a newspaper.

All grip is valueless without release, or extension and abduction of fingers and thumb. All grips need some power and therefore require strength in the muscles involved in flexion, adduction and opposition, and also stability in the whole arm. In any grip the wrist is also stabilised. As more power is needed the elbow and shoulder are involved and often the whole body.

Investigation, manipulation and expression

The hand is 'into' everything throughout life. It manipulates, feels and weighs. It assesses for temperature and texture. It silently gestures its meanings and by a quick movement can reveal hidden anxiety or content. It is a supplement to speech and often a substitute for speech and there are national patterns of both the conscious and unconscious use of the hands.

The hand is so often exposed for such a wide number of reasons that it can become vulnerable to injury. A hand has been known to investigate the red bar of an electric fire, the moving parts of a motor bike engine, a live electric cable, the heat of a candle flame, the sharpness of a circular saw and the length of time a firework takes to light, all with dire results.

The hand as a means of expression is lost when injury occurs. It tends to be 'pocketed' and the hidden trauma pocketed away in the mind. A scarred hand, like an injured face, can change the human who owns them. We need to remember how much of ourselves resides in our two hands.

OCCUPATIONAL THERAPY

Assessment

It is important that each patient is assessed according to his needs and disability. Primarily you assess to discover the condition of each hand and plan treatment. You also assess to record progress. You may assess to plan ahead and recommend surgery or joint replacements, or to return to work. You rarely use all the forms of assessment described here. When you know who you are assessing and why, you can choose your weapon.

1. Examine the injury

Seat the person comfortably at a table with the forearms supported so that both hands can be seen. Compare both hands. Establish which hand is dominant. Note any previous injuries and the possible limitation of movement or strength or sensation they already impose on the hand. Consider the skin condition. Following nerve injury the skin may be thin and papery with some loss of sensation. Run your finger tips over the patient's hands, asking if he can feel normally. This action will also give a quick test of any temperature changes. Look at any scarring. Note the stage of healing, for instance, whether a scar has yet healed, or is over healing into a keloid. Note the position and extent of any bruising and of any odema and check for signs of infection or poor circulation.

2. Examine the movements of the hand

With the person in the same position, get him to make a tight fist with both hands. Then 'spread' the hands into full abduction and extension. Then get him to touch the tips of each finger with the thumb. Also do a quick bilateral check of shoulder, elbow and wrist movements. Examine the strength of the grip by crossing your hands and asking him to squeeze two fingers with both hands. This produces a more natural and comfortable position and aids recording as right hand squeezes right hand and left hand the left. The strength of individual movements can be assessed in the following way: ask the patient to abduct his thumb and hold it there while you press it back into adduction, saying 'Don't let me do it, don't let me'. Ask the patient to flex all the fingers not quite into the palm and hold them there. You lock your fingers under his and attempt to straighten them, saying 'Don't let me straighten them, don't let me'. The same technique can be applied to any movement you need to test.

3. Now measure

Movement

Always measure the uninjured side first and from your previous examination you will know which joints are limited and therefore which to measure for comparison. Any limitation from the shoulder to the distal interphalangeal joints should be recorded in order to show progress.

The principles of measurement are explained in Chapter 2. The same apply for the hand with slight variations. Ensure the forearm is supported and the elbow at right angles.

Measure with a goniometer. For the finer joints, lay a small goniometer over the joint (Fig. 17.2). If a small goniometer is unavailable, use two small Perspex arms only and put them against a normal size goniometer after being placed over each joint. Remember, full flexion means that the nails are hidden in the palm. It is usually easier to get the patient to attempt this with all fingers and then run the goniometer along all four metacarpophalangeal (MCP) joints, then all four proximal interphalangeal (IP) joints. To get to the distal interphalangeal joints the MCP joints will have to be

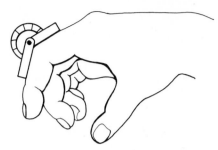

Fig. 17.2 A small goniometer to measure individual joints of the fingers

extended, but flexion at the IP joints maintained. Thumb flexion and extension at the IP and MCP joints are measured in the same way. For abduction, measure the angle between the first and second metacarpals (Fig. 17.3). For full extension measure the same joint, but in a different plane (Fig. 17.4). Measure the wrist (see Ch. 2).

Odstock tracings. Alternative and equally accurate methods of recording are the Odstock wire and tracings. Place soldering wire over the finger at its maximal joint range and record by drawing along the wire (Fig. 17.5). The use of different colours clarifies progress.

Hand tracings. Abduction can be recorded by drawing round the hand on paper (Fig. 17.6). Different colours show progress. A card placed between the fingers can be used to trace flexion and extension of the fingers directly (Fig. 17.7).

Use of a ruler. Abduction can be measured along a ruler, recording the distance between the finger tips. Thumb opposition can be recorded as the ability to touch the finger tips and then the base of the little finger. If this cannot be done at first, measure along a ruler the distance between the

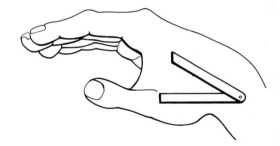

Fig. 17.3 Measuring abduction of the thumb. (Note: the axis of the goniometer is on the first carpometacarpal joint. The thumb is moved at right angles to the palm)

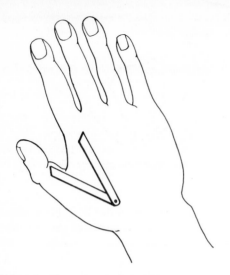

Fig. 17.4 Extension of the thumb is measured as abduction, but with the goniometer on the back of the hand

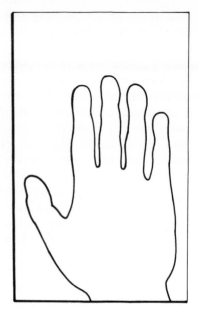

Fig. 17.6 Abduction and adduction at the metacarpophalangeal joints of the fingers are measured by drawing round the hand as full movement is attempted

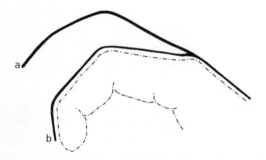

Fig. 17.5 Measuring joint movement by placing wire over the dorsum of the finger at maximal range and tracing

thumb nail and the base of the little finger. A ruler at right angles to the palm from the base of the finger can measure general flexion (Fig. 17.8).

Photographs. Particularly with severe injuries, photographs provide a graphic record of progress.

Sensation

Touch the area with gentle pin pricks and cotton wool. Let the person see and feel what you are going to do then ask him to close his eyes. Work from the de-sensitised area towards the normal as this gives a more accurate representation of the de-sensitised area. Differentiate between no feeling, blunt feeling and full sensation. Record as in Figure 17.9.

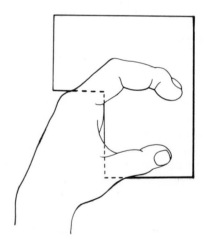

Fig. 17.7 Measuring range of joint movement by tracing directly onto a card held between two fingers

Strength

Use a sphygmomanometer or dynamometer to record the poundage of the grip. The sphygmomanometer can record very weak grip. A torquometer will record twist grip.

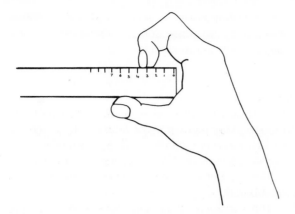

Fig. 17.8 Measuring total finger flexion with a ruler

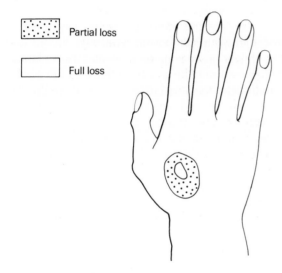

Fig. 17.9 Recording lack of sensation on an outline chart of the hand

Function

A hand that can perform many movements may not be 'functional' due to lack of strength, co-ordination or motivation to use it, but, in contrast, a grossly deformed hand with rheumatoid arthritis causing degeneration and derangement at many joints may be functionally efficient (see Ch. 26).

Have a box with the listed articles ready.

For the power grip use a hammer or saw.

For the cylinder grip ask the person to grip a cylinder or pour from a filled tea pot or pull on a rope.

For the span grip undo and do up screw top jars.

For the pincer grip pick up a pin and a pen.

For the adductor grip turn a Yale key.

For the tripod grip write with a pen or screw in a screw with a small electrical screw driver.

For the plate grip hold a plate.

For a more extensive functional assessment actual tasks should be performed. The following are suggested: write, cut paper, strike a match, put a safety pin through material, thread a needle, pour water, deal cards, hammer in a nail, use a comb, use a knife and fork or get coins out of a purse. These tasks will test co-ordination of all movements in a more realistic way.

For stereognosis testing, ask the patient to identify the same articles with the eyes closed.

Oedema

The circumference of the hand can be measured with a tape measure. Place the tape measure immediately proximal to the metacarpophalangeal joints. Where relevant place it round the wrist and then round all the fingers together, though this is not usually necessary. Lister recommends jewellers' sizing rings to record diminishing oedema of individual fingers. It is important to record where the tape measure or the ring is placed and to ensure that it is in the same place on the uninjured hand and in the same place when next being used as an assessment. These are not accurate measures of oedema as other factors are involved, but they may be effective in showing improvement. The hand can be dipped into an Archimedes bath and water displacement measured. The bath can be a bowl of water as long as the test is well administered.

Finally, check for independence, advise and provide temporary aids if necessary.

Treatment

The aim of all assessment is to enable the treatment programme to be planned. The hand is to be restored to the fullest possible functional use. Other factors must be remembered, e.g. if there is oedema it must be reduced in the early stages.

Prevention and correction of deformity are vital and function must be related to each person, his personality, his home and his work.

Sensation retraining

If there is any numbness or loss of sensation, specific stimulation and retraining will also stimulate motor return. Sherrington expounded the theory that sensory bombardment excited both posterior and anterior horn cells and facilitated motor response. Activities for sensory stimulation are fully described in Chapter 25.

Oedema

If the hand is oedematous it must be treated in elevation, which means at or above shoulder level. Games can be elevated on a table or fixed to the wall on adjustable frames. Use of a fixed electronic drill, overhead adaptations on printing and elevated stool seating can also be included. At rest the arm should be in a sling to keep the hand elevated (see Fig. 25.2).

Prevention and correction of deformity

This is achieved by good positioning of the person during activity so that movements are full, free and bilateral. The advantage of bilateral movements is that the injured hand will be facilitated by the normal movements of the uninjured parts. Work in elevation will prevent oedema occurring. Close work with the physiotherapist and frequent treatment periods are especially important at this time. Should there be a contracture or the possibility of one occurring, work against it exercising to stretch out the contracture. Oil or lanoline massage can be carried out by one of the treatment team. Stretch (serial) splintage may be necessary with both dynamic and resting splints. The sequence of treatment should be (i) massage, (ii) passive movements, (iii) active movements, (iv) splint. With rheumatoid arthritis the strengthening of the first dorsal interroseous muscle will help to prevent ulnar deviation at the metacarpophalangeal joints. This can be achieved by picking up large objects which encourages abduction of all fingers. This helps the index and ring fingers more than the little

and ring but assists in general function. A strong pinch or tripod grip action also strengthens the first dorsal interroseous muscle.

Flexion

Full flexion is achieved when the finger nails are hidden in the palm, and the thumb across them. In reality however patients are discharged when they can do their work, often long before full flexion is achieved, but this ultimate goal needs to be remembered.

The treatment of flexion starts with gross grip and pinch, continues to fine grip and pinch and then can concentrate on interphalangeal and metacarpophalangeal flexion, and power.

Grip and pinch are treated by any activity that involves the thumb opposing to the fingers. It can start by playing draughts using large pieces and end with composing type with thumb and little finger or weaving on a pin and thread board. Activities should be graded so that they are always a millimetre too small to be easy. Reduce the size of all articles and activities as flexion improves. Include sawing, and the use of a mallet and chisel with handles of the appropriate size. Use large draughts, weaving and stool seating with large shuttles and handling large off-cuts of wood, and work down to pin solitaire between thumb and little finger. Between these two extremes use all sizes of remedial games and all types too, to maintain interest. Include draughts, solitaire, halma, chinese chequers, three-dimensional noughts and crosses and peggoty. Chess and Nine Men's Morris are splendid games, but the thinking time belies their value as treatment.

Interphalangeal joint flexion may need to be isolated, especially with fractures affecting these joints. The patient should grasp a disc so large that only with the relevant interphalangeal joint flexion can he reach over it. This could become a home exercise, or could be attached to printing or weaving. The wooden disc can be reduced in size as flexion progress.

Large draughts, built-up saw handles, a disc on the front of a jack-plane, large tongs for picking up pieces of remedial games, hand cutters for cutting the edges of grass and large scissors will also help. Macramé, especially netting and Solomon's knot, can isolate interphalangeal joint flexion if the shuttles are of the required width. Gripping with cylindrical objects of increasingly smaller size produces metacarpophalangeal movement with the interphalangeal joint flexion.

Printing adaptations with a rope, FEPS roller or dowel; sawing, planing and wood carving are also useful as long as the size of the handle is just too small and therefore encourages a little more flexion than was possible yesterday. Puff football is possible now, and great fun. MCP flexion need rarely be isolated as a movement, except in nerve lesions and activities to achieve this are given in Chapter 25. When powerful flexion is needed, strength is built up by increasing resistance on activities such as printing and sawing and by introducing more powerful static activities such as lathe work and digging, cement mixing and cross-cut sawing.

Extension and abduction

These are weaker activities, but are vital for grip release and for full function. Active extension can be achieved by picking up large objects in remedial games, picking them up with extension tongs and using a large FEPS disc attached to weaving or printing. Rolling clay for coil pots or rolling pastry also need active extension. The use of large scissors, typewriters (particularly for the thumb), puppets, ball games using a large netball, flick bagatelle, Karam, jacks or five-stones and cat's cradles also need extension. Cat's cradles can be built up into Indian string games which can be both absorbing and entertaining. Passive extension is sometimes needed. Pressing down on a board with both hands achieves this well. It can be used in printing, sanding or polishing bridge boards or table tops and for lino or fabric printing.

Co-ordination

This vital factor to function is again treated by grading activity. Gross bilateral movements are encouraged to begin with. Activities are gradually made smaller and finer. Large draughts and polishing and sanding of transfer boards can be upgraded to stool seating and large sawing and planing. This in turn can be graded to weaving and

wood carving, to composing print and marquetry, with many gradations between each one.

Skin toughening

A patient with skin grafts to his hands needs graded toughening to ensure that the new skin can cope with work demands. A labourer who is off work with a hand injury will now have soft skin, which will need thickening before he can return to work. The art is to grade and observe so that skin breakdown does not occur, but gradual toughening does. Grade material used from smooth to rough. Stool seating can be graded from nytrim to seagrass. Woodwork can be graded from polishing furniture to rough sanding. Any activity that gives vibration to the hand will aid toughening. This can start with feeding wood through a fretsaw and end with sanding lathe work and cross-cut sawing.

Specific areas of function

These may be needed and their lack may well prevent discharge. They may be dexterity or speed, span or even hyperextension and should be considered throughout treatment. Simulate the action as near as is possible, while maintaining the other movements. A railwayman with fractures of the proximal interphalangeal joints needed full extension to get his hand between two blocks where there was only just room for a hand. Active and passive extension had to be encouraged to achieve this. This was done by the pressing down of both hands, with the injured hand underneath, on a disc whilst polishing transfer boards and active extension by rolling clay and other activities such as those already mentioned.

Although all these separate treatment areas have been listed as separate items, the amount of stress or omission of any one from the treatment plan is entirely dependent on the individual and his injury. It is the therapist's skill to find and maintain the individual priorities.

Complications

Hidden trauma

A young and upright man lost his ulnar three digits. The hand recovered well and soon became functional, but it was always pocketed and he would not be seen out with his wife and child. Once this was discovered a smart glove prosthesis completed his rehabilitation. This is by no means a universal reaction, though it does appear that men are more sensitive to the appearance of their hands than women. The hand is an unacknowledged part of the personality. To shake hands, to express affection or disgust with the hand is part of the person, and a hand that cannot shake hands, a hand that is unusual or deformed needs some mental adjustment, both of the individual and of his family. A good therapeutic relationship will find such trauma early. The use of group discussion and acceptance by others will also help.

Pain

Pain can be intractable, especially after crush injuries, and the fact that it can be tied to both compensatory and cultural factors leads to much misunderstanding. Pain has a reason to be present. It can indicate that the treatment is inappropriate for that stage, or that there is some underlying, undiscovered cause. However, if the treatment team decides to work through the pain to restore essential function, principles to be followed are:

Relax. A good, warm, atmosphere, both physically and psychologically, will promote relaxation. Activities which are bilateral and rhythmical are less tense and therefore less painful. Specific relaxation exercises may be used.

Distract. Although all occupational therapy 'distracts', this is especially relevant where pain is present. The activity needs to be more important to the patient than the pain which causes it.

Compensation

It is difficult to get full recovery when partial disability will lead to massive compensation claims. Fear of returning to the place where the accident occurred may also delay rehabilitation. An understanding of what the 'mind' is doing to the hand may help. So may the brutal realisation of how useless the hand may become if allowed to suffer neglect with consequent oedema and stiffness.

Specific injuries

(for information on nerve injuries affecting the hand see Ch. 25)

Crush injuries

If part of a finger or a whole hand is crushed between two hard objects, gross oedema is the immediate result. The hand may swell to four times its normal thickness. Because there is no room for swelling among the tightly-packed internal structures, the hand stiffens immediately and once fibrinogen is laid down the stiffness becomes irreversible. Instant and constant elevation and movement are vital. However, there is also pain and often damage to other tissues. Fractures are a frequent side issue as is nerve damage. There is then enforced immobilisation and possibly poor skin condition due to arrested innervation, and the early movement regime has to be delayed. Adhesions may occur.

Interphalangeal joint flexion must be treated before full grip is attempted, or a loose fist only is made with the finger tips over the thenar eminence instead of hidden in the palm. Full recovery may take six months or longer.

Burns

Burns frequently occur to the hand especially with children and in the elderly. They can be superficial (dural), partial thickness (epidural and dural) of full thickness which is to the bone. If a whole hand is burnt, both palmar and dorsal surfaces, it is classified as 2 per cent of the whole body area. Burns are now usually treated with closed dressings which are changed frequently; and early splinting especially if the burn is over a joint. The early resting splints using Plastazote or Orthoplast are not a close fit as they are moulded over the dressings and it is often not possible to mould them on to the hand because of the extent of the burn. The splint is being continually remade as the dressings change. As soon as the burn is clean and the dead skin sloughed off skin grafting is carried out. When the graft has taken, usually in 2 or 3 weeks, exercise is begun. When the graft is well established, anithypertrophic pressure gloves are fitted and are worn 24 hours a day for 12 months. This is to make any scarring pliable and elastic. Occupational therapy is given in the early stages to assist feeding and any other ADL problems, and to identify and assist with any psychological problems. As soon as the condition is stable, the person is encouraged to attend the OT department which provides evidence of early public acceptance of the injury. Activities are very gentle and progress is very slow. It is vital to avoid dirt, fluff, anything sharp and any activity involving friction.

Tendon injuries

The palmar tendons are most frequently cut by a minor slip of a tool. The tendon is sutured and the finger immobilised in mid-flexion. Bunnell maintained that a well-repaired tendon could be encouraged to work the day after suture. Three weeks' immobilisation is said to secure the suture while preventing the possibility of adhesions. Six weeks' immobilisation ensures a secure suture that will not rupture. All three policies of immobilisation time are practised. Surgery is rarely performed between the distal palmar crease and the crease over the metacarpophalangeal joints because of the narrow tendon sheaths in this area. However, skilled surgeons have been known to tackle this 'no man's land' with impunity. Tendon transfers are reconstructive surgery done when a tendon has been badly damaged or when its muscle has been paralysed. If flexor pollicis longus is damaged flexor digitorum sublimis from the ring finger may be transferred to restore function. The ring finger maintains its function with profundis and the patient has to be re-educated in the use of the transferred tendon. A tendon graft is the insertion of an entirely new tendon. Palmaris longus and plantaris are most commonly used. Treatment needs to be highly specific to the tendon injured. General function and isolated joint movement need to alternate in the treatment programme. Treat for the movement of the tendon first until it is working well. The tendon must be able to pull through before the other movements are encouraged, even when this is an extensor to the fingers or the thumb. If adhesions occur, they need to be treated as contractures.

Fractures

After fracture, the fingers are usually immobilised in mid-flexion by plaster or strapping. Kirschner wires, for instance, are used in the hand that also has rheumatoid arthritis and would deteriorate quickly during immobilisation. Strapping only may be used for fractures of the metacarpals. Recovery is fast, except when the fracture involves a joint. If full movement does not return, compensatory movements can be taught. For example, hyperextension of the MCP joint will enable the hand to press down on a flat surface when PIP extension is limited. Hyperflexion of the MCP joint will bring a finger down to the palm even with very little PIP flexion.

soft tissue damage → release fibrinogen into surrounding tissues ↓ oedema to prevent permanent fibrosis, elevation & debigub.

Dupuytren's contracture

This is a contracture of the palmar fascia. It starts with a small nodule and can eventually cause one or all digits to be firmly and fully flexed at the MCP and PIP joints. This condition is usually bilateral and familial. Most research confirms that it correlates inversely with work done with the hands. It is of unknown origin, though the theories related to this are both original and prolific. The contracture may take years to develop or three months. Early stretching has given preventive results. Surgery is usually attempted. The contracted fascia is cut (fascectomy) or removed (fasciectomy). The contracture may recur. Open wound healing with the fingers splinted in extension seems to result in less recurrence, as does skin excision and palmar grafting. Treatment is aimed at function, as always, and not solely at restoring extension, unless this is vital to a particular person.

Sudeck's atrophy

This may occur after a minor injury or surgery. The hand swells and does not pit on pressure. Osteoporosis of the joints shows on X-ray examination. There is often some psychological overlay. The treatment should be carefully graded with controlled rest periods, otherwise oedema may recur. Bilateral activities seem to be particularly beneficial.

Amputation

This is usually traumatic amputation, that is, occurring at the time or as a result of the injury. Surgical trimming may also be necessary after finger-tip injuries, tumours or other disease. The stump is sensitive and the hand weak and the patient is often very aware of the appearance of the hand. The stump may need percussion or tapping by one member of the treatment team and general toughening. The surgeon may tidy the hand by removing an awkward stump and its attendant metacarpal, leaving a neat and unnoticeable three-fingered hand. Reconstructive surgery or the restoring of fingers is possible but less often done, as unless sensation is also restored the new digit will not be used.

However, the loss of the thumb is considered a 50 per cent disability. It can be replaced by the swinging over or pollicisation of the ring or index finger with its tendons and nerve supply. A toe may also be used to replace the thumb with surprisingly good cosmetic results. Treatment must include toughening and acceptance of the deformed hand as well as restoring function.

For details of treatment of the rheumatoid arthritic hand see Chapter 26.

Conclusion

When treating hand injuries the therapist needs to summon her ingenuity and empathy. She will use her ingenuity in finding many relevant activities that will absorb and interest the patient while teaching him to perform both highly specific and general functional movements. Her empathy is essential for finding out how much of the total person was damaged with the hand injury. She must show she understands the injured mind as she tackles the injured hand and give to both her total professional expertise.

REFERENCES AND FURTHER READING

Jay P, Jones M 1979 An approach to occupational therapy, 3rd edn. Butterworths, London
Haddon K 1974 String games for beginners. Heffer, Cambridge.
Lister G 1977 The hand: diagnosis and implications. Churchill Livingstone, Edinburgh
Sherrington C 1906 The integrative action of the nervous system. Yale University Press, New Haven
Shopland A et al 1979 Refer to occupational therapy. Churchill Livingstone, Edinburgh
Wynn-Parry C B 1973 Rehabilitation of the hand, 3rd edn. Butterworths, London.

18
Head injury

Damage done to the brain and the consequences of the injury can be so diverse and affect such a variety of physical and mental abilities that no two head injuries are ever alike. Apart from the actual lesion or lesions, personality plays a big part in the ability of the patient to make a good recovery. Age is also important, as the younger person has a more adaptable brain; on the other hand he may have a less responsible personality and, therefore, be less receptive to the hard work involved in recovery.

It is often difficult to locate the exact site of the lesion, as trauma to one part of the head may cause damage in a more remote part of the brain. For instance, a blood vessel damaged at the site of the trauma, may disrupt the blood supply to another area of the brain; a contre-coup lesion may damage the base of the brain.

PATHOLOGY

Head injuries can be classified under two main headings:

1. Closed head injury. The skull may be fractured but the coverings of the brain remain intact.

2. Open head injury. The brain and meninges are exposed.

Closed head injuries may appear to be less traumatic, but the consequences may be quite as serious as in open head injury as a result of damage to underlying structures.

Fractures of the skull

(a). Simple fracture: the skull is fractured but the skin is intact (b). Compound fracture: the skin is also broken

(c). Comminuted fracture: the skull is broken into several pieces

(d). Depressed fracture: the fractured bone is driven inwards.

The seriousness of the fracture will depend on the type of fracture and also on the site; e.g. fracture through the base of the skull may affect the pituitary gland.

Open skull fractures bring the danger of bacterial meningitis, although this risk has been reduced with the advent of antibiotics. Damage to the underlying brain has now become the major complication.

Injuries requiring surgery

The following complications may occur with or without fracture of the skull:

Subdural haematoma

This is a common and serious complication. Only slight trauma may be sufficient to cause rupture of blood vessels between the dura and arachnoid. The bleeding causes a haematoma which will in time produce cerebral compression and cause the patient to become drowsy and to complain of headaches. If the clot irritates the cerebral cortex he may have fits. There is usually a reduction or loss of conjugate or upward movement of the eyes. Eventually the patient's level of responsiveness will deteriorate. Subdural haematoma can develop rapidly (acute subdural haematoma) or slowly and is the chief reason why anyone who has had a head injury should be kept under observation for at least 24 hours. Acute subdural haemorrhage can be suspected if the patient no longer responds to painful stimuli. Exploratory burr holes are made or if available a CAT scan is done to locate the haematoma. Once found, the haematoma is evacuated.

Subdural hygroma

This may follow a subdural haematoma. The blood is removed by phagocytic cells. The resulting walled-off area may produce straw-coloured fluid unrelated to cerebrospinal fluid. Treatment is the same as for haematoma. The fluid may re-

accumulate and have to be aspirated again.

Extradural haematoma

This most commonly occurs in the frontoparietal region when the middle meningeal artery is torn e.g. by fractured bone, causing bleeding between the skull and the dura. The ensuing haematoma usually collects quickly and as it grows the patient becomes increasingly drowsy and restless. There will be dilatation of the pupil on the side of the haematoma with increasing paralysis of the opposite side of the body. X-ray examination will show a shift of the midline structures of the brain by the calcified pineal body being pushed away from midline. Surgery should be immediate. Burr holes are made in the skull or a CAT scan performed, and once the haematoma is located the hole can be enlarged so that haemorrhage can be stopped by coagulating diathermy current, by inserting a silver clip or by a transfixion suture.

Intracerebral haemorrhage

This usually occurs soon after injury when there is continuous bleeding into the brain substance. It is not very common. The patient will show a reduced level of responsiveness. The site of the haemorrhage can be determined by physical signs in relevant parts of the body. A burr hole is made over this site and the dura opened so that the haematoma can be removed.

Compound depressed fractures of the skull

There may be no urgent need to operate in these cases if there is no intracranial haemorrhage or cerebral compression. Antibiotics should be given to prevent infection and X-rays taken to assess the extent of the fracture before operating. A burr hole is made through unfractured bone adjacent to the fracture. This is enlarged if necessary so that bone fragments can be raised. Great care has to be taken not to damage underlying structures.

Other types of brain injury

Shearing injuries

The supportive tissue of the brain, the glia, is not able to withstand violent changes of position and movement so that it may be torn when this occurs, particularly deep in the brain where there is a lack of firm supporting tissue. The glia carries blood vessels and nerves and these will also be torn. The resulting small haemorrhages will heal by glial scarring. This may lead to paralysis and long periods of coma or episodes of grossly disturbed consciousness.

Cerebral contusion

This term implies that part of the cerebral cortex is damaged resulting in laceration of blood vessels or bruising. Contusion may be direct, as under an impact fracture site, or indirect when it is known as a contre-coup lesion (Fig. 18.1). Here the damage may be diametrically opposite the point of impact or both at this point and at the point of impact. There may also be damage to structures at the base of the brain.

Contusion may cause death of cortical cells giving rise to loss of function or feeling in the opposite side of the body.

Acute cerebral oedema

This is a complication of the initial head injury and is due to anoxia which damages blood vessels. The small vessels become permeable to plasma proteins and a large excess of fluid passes into the brain. Because the covering of the brain, i.e. the skull, is rigid, intracranial pressure will quickly rise, causing herniation and arterial compression. There is only one point of exit, the foramen magnum. Herniation in this area may quickly lead to death. Cerebral oedema cannot be treated until intracranial haematoma has been excluded. The oedema can then be resolved by treating the initial cause and by giving doses of dehydrating agents.

EARLY SEQUELAE

To a considerable degree, the outcome of recovery after head injury depends on the treatment given at the site of the accident. Immediate treatment consists of keeping the airway clear and preventing further blood loss from other injuries. Speed is essential so that the patient can be given surgery as soon as possible, if this is necessary. If a patient

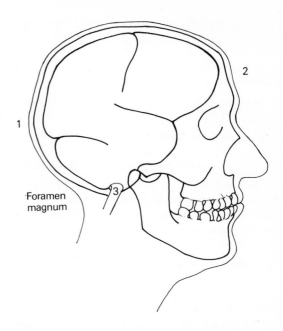

Fig. 18.1 Contre-coup lesion, As the head is thrust forward, damage may occur (1) in the occipital area (2) in the frontal area (3) at the base of the brain

has had a head injury severe enough to cause concussion he should either be admitted for observation, or relatives should be instructed to monitor him for the first 24 to 48 hours and report back if any untoward signs develop.

Concussion

Any trauma to the brain, mild or severe, may cause temporary arrest of function of brain cells resulting in unconsciousness. The nerve cells may not be permanently damaged in which case recovery will occur comparatively quickly. In severe cases, there may be extensive damage to nerve cells and their branches. This will become apparent both by the clinical state and by the dilation of the ventricles which can be seen through air studies. The central reticular formation, a network of cells and fibres in the brain stem, is responsible for keeping the brain in a state of activity. When this is damaged unconsciousness will occur. It is damage to the brain stem which causes some patients to lie in coma for weeks or sometimes years; but consciousness may return after a few days.

Assessing the severity of head injuries

The period of unconsciousness and post-traumatic amnesia (PTA) is a recognised yardstick for assessing the severity of head injuries. It is often difficult to assess exactly when the patient has fully come out of PTA, but he should no longer be confused and have a continuous memory of events. Degrees of head injury can be described as follows:

Slight head injury: unconscious less than 1 hour

Moderate head injury: unconscious from 1 to 24 hours

Severe head injury: unconscious from 1 to 7 days

Very severe head injury: unconscious for weeks.

The severity of the effects of head injury will also depend on other injuries incurred at the time of the accident, for example burns, fractures or internal injuries. These need to be treated in conjunction with the problems produced by the head injury itself and this combination of problems may well produce far more serious consequences. The patient may already have some disability which now becomes aggravated or more difficult to manage. His age will also affect his recovery and reflect on the actual severity of the injury.

Management at this stage involves good nursing care of the unconscious patient. Observation is essential so that complications such as subdural haematoma are recognised as early as possible. Treatment is designed to prevent complications as far as possible as these may prevent or limit recovery.

Damage to respiratory organs

This may involve obstruction of the airway either through the accumulation of secretions, blood or vomit, or through fractures of adjacent bones compressing the airway. This obviously calls for immediate treatment and an airway may have to be passed. The patient may need frequent suction to clear the airway. If he does not regain cough and swallowing reflexes after twenty-four hours a tracheostomy will be performed so that suction and ventilation can be carried out through the tracheostomy tube. A ventilator may need to be used in cases of severe respiratory insufficiency.

When treating patients with respiratory problems, the occupational therapist should understand the use of resuscitators. She should be aware of environmental factors which may aggravate the patient's condition (e.g. dry atmosphere).

Skin

The immobile patient may quickly develop sores, particularly if he is incontinent, or if he is restless, as he may rub skin off prominent areas such as over the ankle bones. Sores will delay recovery and may lead to infection. Incontinence can be dealt with by catheterisation or condom drainage and all vulnerable skin pressure areas must be treated.

Atrophy and contracture

Disuse atrophy of muscles and contracture must be avoided. The patient's limbs should be put through the full range of passive movements regularly by the physiotherapist. Night splints may be required to prevent deformity. Treatment can be difficult in those with disturbed muscle tone or decerebrate rigidity and in those who are grossly disturbed. Myositis ossificans is common in head injury patients; calcification and bone formation appears in muscles and around joints.

Other fractures

There may have been other fractures at the time of the accident. These cannot always be treated in the normal way, particularly if the patient is very disturbed.

Peripheral nerve injuries

Because of their position some nerves are easily damaged, particularly the ulnar, median, sciatic and lateral popliteal nerves. Injury to these nerves may cause weakness in the muscles they supply and loss of sensation over the relevant area of skin. These nerve injuries must be sought after consciousness has returned as they may be missed during the acute life-saving stage.

Incontinence

In the early stages, the patient may have had to be catheterised to control incontinence and reduce the danger of sores. There is always a risk that catheterisation will cause infection of the urinary tract and it should therefore be discontinued as soon as possible. Bladder training should be instigated and the patient asked to pass urine at regular intervals day and night. This requires a great deal of work and coordination on the part of all staff concerned with the patient in order for it to be successful. A system of rewards, if behavioural problems are the cause, can be useful once minimum cooperation has been achieved.

Visual impairment

Any part of the visual pathwas may be affected by head injury (Fig. 18.2).

In addition to hemianopia the patient may have impairment of either the upper or lower fields of vision or of any of the visual quadrants. He may have diplopia (double vision) or nystagmus (inability to coordinate the movements of the eyes). Both mystagmus and diplopia may be helped by covering one eye with a patch so that visual input or ability to coordinate is reduced. The patch must cover each eye alternately. It is extremely important for the occupational therapist to understand the visual problems her patient may have so that these are not mistaken for other causes of inability to function (see later).

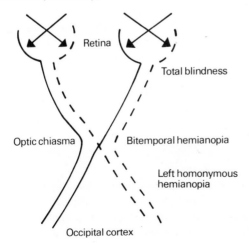

Fig. 18.2 Common lesions of the visual pathway

Epilepsy

Epilepsy occurs in a large number of patients particularly where the frontal lobes have been involved. The healing lacerated tissue leaves a scar which can act as an irritant and result in fits. Fits are particularly likely after damage to the frontoparietal or temporal lobes. They may occur at any time after injury and should be treated with anticonvulsant drugs. These should be continued for at least three years after the last attack.

The occupational therapist should be aware of procedures to keep the airway free and prevent the patient from damaging himself during a fit. She should observe the patient during the fit and report her observations to the ward sister or doctor concerned. Treatment may need to be modified so that the patient is not unsupervised in potentially dangerous situations.

Fits can be very distressing for both the patient and his relatives, who should be given the opportunity to talk about their worries. Difficulties can also arise in returning to employment. Some occupations will obviously be ruled out, such as working at heights or with moving machinery. Employers and workmates may also need help in understanding and coming to terms with the problem.

Post-concussional syndrome

This is more commonly noted after minor injuries. The patient complains of headaches, intolerance of noise and irritability. He may have some impairment of memory, be unable to concentrate and complain of inability to work. He may suffer from insomnia. This usually clears up fairly quickly but in some cases it persists and is known as chronic brain syndrome. In these cases it is relevant to note if there is any compensation case pending.

CLINICAL FEATURES AND TREATMENT

Because of the nature of head injuries clinical features are rarely demonstrated in isolation, neither can the treatment of each feature be carried out in isolation. The principles of treatment should be aimed for, but the methods by which they are achieved must be adapted to the individual patient, that is, to the combination of features demonstrated by him.

The team is of utmost importance in cases of head injury, as these present physical and mental problems which the patient may not be able to understand. The team must comprise all those who are concerned with his management, including the patient himself and his family. It is very important for the occupational therapist to decide on her methods of treatment with the other therapists and nursing staff so that all methods are coordinated, as inconsistent treatment may disrupt progress and thoroughly confuse and frustrate the patient.

In spite of the increasing number of head injuries, there are only few specialised units dealing with the many and varied problems requiring attention in order to rehabilitate these people. Therefore, these patients spend much of their time in the wards of acute hospitals from where they should be referred to the remedial professions. It is the job of the therapist to do the best she can for her patients with the facilities available. There is very little equipment on the market suitable for use with the mentally damaged adult, as it is important that simple basic activities should not appear childish. So the therapist may have to make much of the equipment necessary to fulfil the specific needs of patients at each stage of recovery.

Neuromuscular dysfunction

Paralysis

This may involve all limbs but is usually hemiplegic. Muscle tone may be lost, reduced or increased as a result of damage to higher centres of the brain which are responsible for muscle tone and integration of muscular reflexes. This initial loss of tone (hypotonus or flaccidity) is usually replaced by an increase of tone (hypertonus or spasticity). Where higher centres are damaged reflex activity will predominate. Additionally, loss of sensation and proprioception can also affect control of movement.

Treatment

Methods of treatment depend on a number of factors unrelated to the patient's physical condition. Some methods of treatment cannot work without the full cooperation of all members of the treatment team. The need for speed in emptying hospital beds has to be considered in some areas. The age and ability of the patient to cooperate must also be considered.

The emphasis of treatment is increasingly moving away from encouraging the patient to use his unaffected side leaving him as a one-sided person, to helping him to feel and be, as far as possible, a symmetrical whole person again. In the hemiplegic patient, emphasis should be on the affected side from the earliest stages and techniques can be used to inhibit reflexes and facilitate movement wherever possible. Bobath, Rood, Brunnstrom and others have written of their approaches to the problem. It is for the therapist to choose the method or combination of methods which produce the best results for the individual patient.

Initially, she may help with correct positioning of the patient in bed. Once he is able to sit up out of bed, it is very important that he is given the opportunity to relearn the feeling of normal position. In sitting, the head and trunk should be in the mid-line and weight taken through both buttocks. The affected scapula should be protracted so that the arm is brought forward out of the spastic pattern. Activities may be carried out bilaterally or with the non-affected hand. In the latter case the affected arm should either be resting on a table, resisting associated reactions, or the hand may be placed on a chair or table beside the patient so that he can lean towards that side in performing an activity, thus providing proprioceptive feedback and aiming towards stability at the shoulder and elbow joints. Feet should be squarely placed on the floor. Treatment will vary, depending on whether the patient is at the flaccid or spastic stage.

Flaccid stage. At this stage, treatment is aimed at normalising tone and establishing the ability to bear weight. Icing and vibrating techniques may help facilitate the increase of tone. Joint approximation can also assist in achieving this. It may also be possible to use synergic movement (stereotyped flexor or extensor patterns of the whole limb) as a precursor to normal movement, for example, through sanding (Fig. 18.3) or

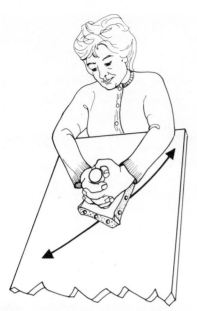

Fig. 18.3 Sanding into the synergy in the early stages of recovery

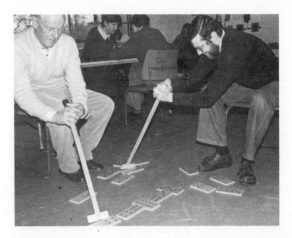

Fig. 18.4 Floor dominoes used to increase balance through leaning forward and to encourage bilateral arm activity

polishing diagonally into the extensor synergy. Any movements into flexion should be discouraged as this is the strong movement. As soon as possible movements should move out of the synergy into the anterior/posterior plane. Once trunk stability has been achieved, treatment should concentrate on stability of other joints so that weight can be taken through them. Great care must be taken not to increase tone to the extent of causing hypertonus.

Spastic stage. At this stage there are three main aims of treatment: (i) to inhibit increased tone, (ii) to facilitate normal movement patterns and (iii) to give the patient the sensation of normal position and movement.

Increased tone should be inhibited by putting the patient into reflex inhibitory postures, i.e. into positions out of the spastic pattern (see Fig. 18.6). If patients can move the affected limb, they can only use gross movements, as they lack the variety of motor patterns necessary for normal movement and the ability to combine them. To improve these movements, the patient should be taken right back through the developmental sequences to try to gain control at each level. Facilitatory techniques of icing over spastic muscles may help to bring limbs into the weight-bearing position. Activities

which require weight transfer will help to increase stability and balance. The ability to lean forward is very important (Fig. 18.4) in order to stand from sitting and for activities such as putting on shoes and socks. The patient must be able to return to the upright position. Trunk rotation (Fig. 18.5) should then be encouraged either sitting or standing.

All positions and movements achieved should be used to perform some activity which must be chosen with all the patient's disabilities in mind. For example, a patient capable of only gross arm

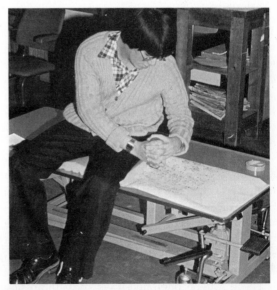

Fig. 18.5 Bilateral stamping to practise trunk rotation. The patient sits on a low plinth with his feet flat on the floor and turns from the ink pad on one side to the paper on the other side

movements with additional visual perceptual problems may be given symmetry domino pieces to slide into the appropriate places on the table. This can be done bilaterally, with the patient sitting or standing, or taking weight through the affected arm and leaning towards that side to place the pieces.

Ataxia

This term implies disturbance of muscular contraction and tone. Apart from an inability to coordinate movement of the limbs, it may cause disturbance of speech (dysarthria) due to an inability to coordinate the muscles of the mouth, and disturbance of eye movement (nystagmus) for the same reason. Ataxia is caused by damage to the cerebellum which regulates muscle contraction and joint position thus affecting and controlling balance. Muscle power, however, is not usually affected. Damage to the cerebellum results in incorrect spindle interpretation and will lead to uncoordinated corrective movements with inaccuracies in speed and timing and direction. Loss of sensation and proprioception will considerably exacerbate the situation and the patient will try to compensate through vision.

Treatment

Treatment of patients with ataxia has still not been resolved. Weights attached to wrist, waist, thigh or ankle have been found to produce some control of coordination in some patients. Weights should be added gradually so that the patient learns to adjust. In patients with some loss of position sense, added weight has been found to improve this, probably due to increasing proprioception through joints.

Patients can often be taught to compensate for their lack of coordination to some extent. For instance, if activities can be done sitting down, the patient has to coordinate his limbs only from the hips; if hand activities can be done with the elbows resting on the table, the patient only has to control movement from the elbow instead of from the shoulder.

These patients often find it very difficult to slow down their speed of activity. They try to work at

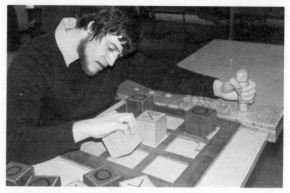

Fig. 18.6 Noughts and crosses used to treat ataxia. The spastic left arm is brought forward into a spastic inhibitory position while the right arm is used for gross coordinating movements

their normal speed which is now impossible. They should be taught to work within their present ability and to control movements of their limbs and eyes. 'Putting' activities, using wood blocks which must be lifted from one place to another, provide good initial training, allowing the patient to work at the required slow pace and control the tremor between each move (Fig. 18.6). This simple activity can be made into a number of games such as noughts and crosses, draughts or dominoes. With improvement, the size of pieces can be reduced and the precision and speed increased.

Extrapyramidal tremor

Damage to the extrapyramidal system, in particular to the basal ganglia, manifests itself by a continual tremor caused by fluctuating tone in opposing muscle groups.

Treatment depends on other clinical signs so that it may be necessary to incorporate treatment principles of hypertonus and ataxia.

Disturbance of equilibrium and righting reactions

Treatment will again depend on associated clinical features.

The centres of the brain concerned with these mechanisms may be damaged resulting in an inability to place and maintain the body in the required position against gravity. Postural adjustments to maintain balance, such as stepping reactions, are upset.

Sensory disturbance

Damage to the sensory area of the cerebral cortex and the posterior column tracts in the brain may cause lack of appreciation or distortion of sensation. Loss of sensation and proprioception can considerably increase all the patient's disabilities described. For instance, if a patient has sensory loss in his left side, inattention of that side will be considerably increased due to poor input. Loss of sensation in the foot or loss of proprioception in the knee will make walking very difficult without using sight as an aid.

It is therefore important for the occupational therapist to assess for loss of sensation and proprioception. Training may help the patient to discriminate hot, cold, different textures and shapes, and also to become aware of his limbs in space and to appreciate different weights. Activities which involve taking weight through the affected limbs will increase proprioceptive feedback; joint approximation can also help to increase this. The use of the vibrator and ice will provide additional sensation, as well as facilitate movement.

A patient with spatial disturbance has problems of body image and awareness of himself in space. Successful management depends on a good understanding of his specific problems. How much of his problem is due to sensory and proprioceptive loss and how much to perceptual disability? In either case the patient can be given guidance through all his senses, for instance by verbal instruction, by tapping an object to be picked up (auditory) and by feeling the movement (sensation, proprioception and vision).

Activities of daily living such as dressing, washing, shaving or putting on make-up will help the patient with body image problems and give sensory feedback. All these activities are 'overlearned', thus now helping the patient to achieve them through habit. Spatial problems may be overcome by everyday activities and by activities in the department which help the patient to see himself in relation to objects and objects in relation to each other. Jigsaws, peg and board games and joining dots or mazes are some examples.

Perceptual problems and memory

Perceptual dysfunction occurs when the sensory end organ is intact but the area concerned with interpretation in the cerebral cortex is damaged.

Perceptual problems are often present in the severe head injury, but they can be missed in assessment because of the many other personality problems and physical difficulties. In a diffuse head injury the perceptual problem may be less clearly defined than in a cerebrovascular accident. In order to assess for perceptual problems it is essential to eliminate all other possible causes of functional disability. Sensation, proprioception eyesight and hearing, must be carefully tested and speech must be assessed for receptive and expressive loss.

The categories of perceptual disability are described more fully in Chapter 19. In cases of head injury it is particularly important to understand perceptual problems. If a team member does not understand why the patient responds in a particular way, she will not be able to adapt her treatment appropriately and treat the patient to the best advantage.

Apraxia and agnosia are also important and may be misunderstood because they do not show con-

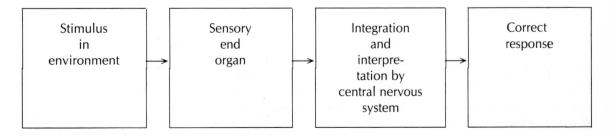

sistently. Apraxia is the term used to describe an inability to carry out required movements, even though the patient has little or no loss of power or control over his limbs. If this inability is not consistent, the patient may be accused of being lazy and uncooperative, which may or may not be the case. Agnosia is the sensory counterpart and is most recognisable in visual agnosia when the patient is unable to recognise familiar people or objects. The sensory end organ is intact and the mental image is unimpaired but the correct response is lost. (For further detail see Ch. 19)

Principles of treatment are described later in this chapter and in Chapter 19. Only when perceptual and speech problems have been resolved to whatever degree this has been possible, can residual intellectual ability be finally assessed. Reduced intellect may be due to poor concentration, poor memory or some degree of general confusion and inability to reason. In severe cases with gross intellectual impairment, there has obviously been widespread cortical damage.

Memory

This has already been mentioned and may be a persisting problem. Loss of memory can be aggravated by life in hospital as the patient tends to be told what to do and where to go so that he need not bother to remember for himself. There are many ways in which the patient can be helped and the therapist must communicate with other staff so that they all encourage the patient to be independent and think for himself. The patient can be given certain jobs in the department, e.g. changing the calendar each day when he first comes. He should be encouraged to find his own work and put it away at the end of the session. He should follow his own timetable and find his own way from one department to the next, with some support at first, but then on his own, perhaps using a map which he has made himself.

Personality change, changes of mood and behaviour problems

After severe head injury, patients frequently undergo some personality change. This may simply be due to the frustration caused by present disability or to specific brain damage. Patients may show changes of mood and inability to control emotions.

They may be emotionally labile which means that they show their emotions very easily and that their emotional response is often exaggerated and inappropriate. This is most often shown through crying, which may be provoked just by their efforts to do what is required of them. These tears do not usually require any comment from the therapist, but may be taken as a sign that the patient is reaching his maximum tolerance level.

Behavioural problems may be an exaggeration of pre-morbid behaviour. In young patients the head injury may have been the result of irresponsible behaviour so that the therapists cannot expect great changes in this respect after the injury. However, it may be possible to control behaviour to an acceptable level.

Behaviour modification

This is used in all walks of life to produce the required behaviour from a person. It is a technique used to discourage or encourage certain behavioural patterns by altering the consequences of existing behaviour. For example, favourable consequences will reinforce specific behavioural responses.

1. A common approach must be adopted by all hospital staff and must also include his family.

2. The reasons for therapy must be clearly understood by all concerned, including the patient. There must be close communication between all members of the team so that ideas can be pooled and aims discussed, making treatment as effective as possible.

3. Targets should be set low and increased very gradually. If the patient does not achieve success initially he will become discouraged and perhaps cease to cooperate. Success in the early stages will help the patient to understand what is required of him.

4. Reward for favourable behaviour must be given as quickly as possible after the required behaviour.

Rewards. These should be appropriate for the

particular patient. Material rewards are often more acceptable in the earlier stages, but should later be replaced by social rewards. A points system may be suitable, i.e. points can be awarded for achieving the target on a set task and perhaps deducted for inaccuracies and shoddy work. These points can then be exchanged, for example, for extra time on a favourite activity or exemption from a set task when the maximum target has been achieved. Some patients appreciate charts showing their achievements so that they have some visual method of measuring their progress. Whatever form of reward is chosen, it must be easily controllable within the hospital environment. Every care must be taken by all members of the team that the programme is strictly adhered to and the patient is not manipulating events.

The therapist's aim is the patient's return to full independence. She must encourage and praise all attempts towards greater independence, initiative and more responsible behaviour. This is extremely important, as attention given to the patient only when he has given up, will encourage him to seek attention by giving up. In a busy department, it is very easy for the therapist to find this is just what she is doing. It requires thought and planning to ensure therapy is effective in all respects.

Whatever system is chosen to modify a patient's behaviour, it must be simple and easily adhered to, otherwise it will fail in a busy department.

Finally, the patient must fully understand what is happening. He must be able to accept the programme and want to achieve the targets with the ensuing reward. The programme should not appear childish and the patient's inclusion in planning the programme may be helpful to both the patient and the team. Appraisal of progress should be carried out by the instigator of the scheme at regular intervals and the programme modified if necessary.

Insight and motivation

Many head-injured patients do not have insight into their disability, either as a result of brain damage or because of their inability to come to terms with their present problems. In either case this may lead to poor motivation and an inability to cooperate. Here again, an understanding of the patient's problems and the ability to provide activities which are within the patient's capability and which he will find interesting to do is of utmost importance.

Depression, euphoria, irritability, inertia or anxiety may be displayed by the patient. These moods may pass quickly or remain for various reasons. They may require medical treatment such as antidepressants, but as far as possible they should be treated as a normal result of head injury. It would be abnormal not to feel depressed periodically after an accident.

The therapist should show understanding and patience, but should nevertheless insist on an acceptable level of performance so that the patient can get some satisfaction from his achievement. It is perhaps easy in a hospital environment to be too sympathetic of the patient's poor performance but this should be resisted.

Speech and communication

Communication problems are common in the early stages after extensive injury of the dominant hemisphere, but only persist when the lesion affects the more highly localised areas of the brain. Recovery may take a long time, in some cases several years.

Patients may have a wide variety of communication problems. These may be expressive or receptive.

Speech problems may include:

Aphasia. Loss of expressive and/or receptive language

Dysphasia. Difficulty with language
(a). Inability to produce nouns, e.g. 'the thing you write with'
(b). Inability to use prepositions, e.g. 'I go home Friday 6 o'clock.'
(c). Inability to use verbs, e.g. 'I home Friday.'

Jargon. The patient carries on long conversations which are incomprehensible. He is often unaware of this

Perseveration. The patient repeats a word or phrase and has difficulty completing the sentences or in stopping

Dysarthria and anarthria. Inability to control and coordinate the muscles used in speech so that the patient can speak, but is often difficult to understand (cerebellar damage)

Dyspraxia. Inability to perform purposeful movements in the absence of any paresis or muscular weakness

Dysphonia and aphonia. Loss of voice power. An inability to produce power and modulation of the voice is comparatively common after head injury.

These problems should be treated by a speech therapist who will communicate with all departments as to the best method of dealing with the problem.

For the occupational therapist it is important to give the patient the opportunity and encouragement to speak. The patient may need time to find the words or to coordinate the muscles of speech and it takes courage to attempt to speak under these conditions. To put words into the patient's mouth and brush aside his own attempts will discourage progress and confidence. Opportunities to use normal everyday language should be seized so that, for example, a regular greeting can be used with increasing confidence.

The principles of 'see it, say it, read it, write it' can usually be adopted. It is easier to produce a noun in speech if the object to be named can be seen. For the literate, this noun can then be reinforced by writing it down and then reading it back. Useful nouns, for example the names of ingredients used in the cookery session, can be practised before, during and after the cookery session.

Some words have been over-learned, such as the days of the week and numbers. These can therefore be used with confidence and so encourage the patient to try other words. Words can often be produced by 'triggering', for example 'here is a cup of . . '; the patient can then say the word 'tea'. This is by no means useful speech, but it does serve the purpose of giving the patient confidence in himself.

It is always daunting to be expected to perform on a one-to-one basis and the patient may find it much easier to produce words in the more relaxed atmosphere of a game. Games also have the merit of bringing a person who is normally isolated through lack of speech, into a group. While it is the patient's turn to play he is temporarily 'in control' of the group. Games such as sevens provide an opportunity to practise number and counting.

Writing may be important for the individual. In some cases, but by no means all, it may be a means of communication where speech has failed. It may therefore be helpful if the occupational therapist can provide writing practice. This may involve learning to write with the non-dominant hand.

Some patients learn to copy well, but cannot 'compose' a required word, although they recognise it when seeing it written down. This ability to read can be put to good use. For instance, in writing a shopping list the patient can copy the required items from the list of household goods supplied by the therapist.

It is important that some method of communication is found for patients who cannot verbalise. Simple aids such as an alphabet board, a pad and pencil or pictures showing the patient's major needs (to which he can point) may be helpful. Some patients can use the electronic communication aids on the market, but this depends on the individual's comprehension and physical ability to use the machine. Most firms will allow the patient to try their machines before purchase.

Patients who speak in jargon sometimes have no insight into this. They should be encouraged to name objects and use short sentences and phrases, perhaps describing pictures, as this will make the patient conscious of what he is saying.

Perseveration does not only occur in speech, movements and actions, for example, can also be repeated. Patients may only be able to utter one word or to name one object and then not be able to move on to the next. Repetitions should be discouraged, perhaps by increasing the time lapse between naming two items.

Dysphonia means that the patient must make more effort to make himself heard and this effort must be encouraged.

It must be stressed that with regard to speech or communication problems the team should work under the speech therapist's guidance.

SEVERE AND VERY SEVERE HEAD INJURIES

Early treatment

The occupational therapist has a part to play even while the patient is in the very early stages of recovery. Initially this may involve no action on the part of the patient apart from maintaining correct position in bed, but the therapist can start to build up a useful relationship and begin to stimulate interest through her own conversation or activity. These patients, who may still only be semi-conscious or in PTA, find themselves in a confusing world in which people are always 'doing' things to them, when all they want is to be left alone. The occupational therapist can be the one person who does not 'do' anything to them except talk of familiar and interesting things. A little later the therapist gradually draws the patient into some familiar activity in a very small way.

At this stage treatment sessions should take place in the ward. Patients with injuries nearly always show a lack of security and regression in years so that the patient's bed becomes the womb and the ward his home. Like a child, he will have to learn to stand on his feet in the outside world, but this must be done gradually and with the support of the therapist. Short visits to the department should be made with the therapist who should keep him informed of what is happening and where he is. This is particularly important if the patient is still in PTA and disorientated.

As the patient's tolerance increases, longer periods can be spent in the department. Particularly for the more insecure and restless patient, it is important that the therapist tells him how long he is staying in the department and that she always does exactly what she has said. In this way a relationship of trust can be built up.

Suitable activities

As a result of brain damage the patient may have a variety of disabilities such as perceptual impairment, lack of ability to concentrate and lack of ability to reason in addition to any physical problems he may have. In the early stages after the injury it is vital to catch the patient's interest and to start to build up his confidence in his ability to achieve something, however small. Early activities must be within the patient's ability without appearing childish. They must be completed within the patient's concentration span. It is very important that activities should be completed within the allotted time and that the patient should succeed; he can only accept failure when he is feeling more secure.

Even though the patient may only be able to achieve very simple tasks, he may be very aware that he should be performing at a higher level. Great care must therefore be taken not to present childish activities or to present simple activities in a childish manner. It may be helpful to present a mental activity as a physical one, for example sorting differently shaped blocks with a physically affected arm. Too much exposure of perceptual or any other intellectual disability may lead to behaviour problems.

Environment

The patient's ability to complete activities may be influenced by his environment. On first coming to the department he may fail simply because of the unfamiliar surroundings. He may be influenced by his position in the room. If he faces other occupants in the room his concentration may be disturbed by watching them, but if he sits with his back to the room he may be disturbed by the noise and continually need to turn round to see what is happening. Which is best for your patient? The therapist must be aware of the patient's problems and experiment. The patient may be disturbed by others at his table. Another restless person or somebody creating noise can be very distracting, but a person who is quietly getting on with his work can encourage others to work too.

Some patients in this early stage show disturbed and aggressive behaviour. These patients may still be in PTA, in which case their behaviour is often a result of insecurity and fear. They do not understand what is happening to them or where they are; and any unexpected movement or noise may be sufficient to produce an apparently aggressive outburst. These patients should, as far as possible, be treated by one therapist so that they can learn to feel 'safe' with one person. They should also be treated in the same area of the department and familiar material should be used and reused in treatment sessions.

Head-injured patients may show impulsive behaviour and display an inability to foresee the results of their actions. This may necessitate some quick thought and action from the therapist in averting drastic results. Any patient who has these problems must be in a suitable environment and be given adequate supervision. These problems must be resolved before the patient is put in a workshop environment where the results of impulsive behaviour could have serious consequences.

Supervision

As the small child needs his mother, so the severely head-injured patient needs his own therapist. The same therapist should treat the patient. However, she must be aware of becoming too indispensable. Once the patient has become more secure and confident, the therapist should begin to wean herself away. She should always tell the patient where she is going and return within the specified time.

Initial assessment

It is often not realistic to attempt formal assessment with severely head-injured patients in the early stages, as their concentration span is very short. Information about their abilities can only be gleaned through a series of treatment sessions. However, it is important to establish some sort of base line from which to measure improvement. The results of all activities should be recorded noting date, activity, how long it took to achieve, whether the patient needed continual supervision and what problems he had in completing the task. In order to do this the therapist must understand exactly what task she has given the patient to do. For example, to complete a simple mosaic pattern the patient had to employ three skills, recognition of shape, colour and spatial relationships. In which area did his problem lie?

PRINCIPLES OF ASSESSMENT AND PLANNING TREATMENT

The following points should be borne in mind when assessing and planning treatment at any time after brain injury:

Date of injury. The results of assessment should be evaluated with this in mind when planning future treatment programmes. Improvement after head injury may continue for several years particularly in the younger person. The therapist must take this into consideration when deciding whether her therapy should aim at further physical and/or mental improvement or whether she should be concentrating on resettlement at home and thinking of future occupation.

Previous intellectual ability. The therapist must not expect more from her patient than he could have achieved before the injury.

Other illness. The therapist must be fully informed of any medical problems, perhaps unconnected with the head injury, which may hinder his progress.

Age of patient. Older patients may tire more quickly and therefore achieve less.

Length of session. Achievement may decline as the session goes on. Should you have done the assessment in two sessions instead of one? Is treatment becoming less effective towards the end of the session? Head-injured patients tire quickly and need frequent rests.

Environment. Noise and activity may distract the patient so that he cannot concentrate and his performance level is reduced.

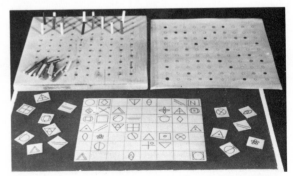

Fig. 18.7 Assessment of colour, spatial awareness, attention and concentration. The patient is asked to place the coloured pegs into the holes corresponding to the chart on the right (top) and to match the shapes on the bottom chart

Instruction. The therapist must provide clear instructions which can be understood even with receptive speech loss. She must understand how much speech and how much demonstration she is using in presenting the activity.

Number of skills involved. We must all be able to cope with more than one skill at a time, e.g. to recognise colour and shape. If the patient cannot cope with colour and shape together, he may be able to sort them separately (Fig. 18.7). We must find out what the patient can do and then gradually try to increase his ability.

Quantity of materials. As with skills, the patient should eventually be able to cope with a wide variety of materials. But what is his limit now?

Unfamiliar materials. We all feel more at ease with familiar objects and activities. Assessment and early treatment materials should be chosen with this in mind.

Emotional disturbance. Nobody performs at his maximum if upset for any reason. So the therapist must have some knowledge of the patient's background.

Interpretation of results. The therapist must be quite sure she has considered all points already mentioned and others which may affect the patient's ability to perform, e.g. cultural factors or the need to wear glasses.

The results of each assessment must be recorded accurately and dated. It is ideal if occupational therapy assessment or reassessment can be done within the same period as physiotherapy and speech therapy so that the team can meet to discuss the outcome and plan future treatment. A carefully planned and coordinated treatment programme is of vital importance, particularly for patients with head injuries, as timing and approach can affect outcome.

Aims of treatment

The long- and short-term aims of treatment should be basically the same in all departments. Long-term aims will probably change as progress continues. Initially, they may be quite unforeseeable, as the early short-term aims are very basic, such as getting the patient to swallow or to participate minimally in an activity. Later, the long-term aim may be to make the patient as independent as possible with a view to returning home, so that the short-term aims at this stage should be, for example, balance and coordination and relevant activities of daily living. Later still, the long-term aims may be to return the patient to some sort of open or sheltered employment and the short term-aims to develop speed, manual dexterity, accuracy, or whatever is relevant to the employment being considered.

It is important not only to communicate within the treatment team, but also with the patient and his family. Treatment and aims must be explained so that both the patient and his family understand as much as possible of what is happening.

Recovery from a head injury can be prolonged. It is not ideal for the patient to remain in a hospital ward after the acute stage, but there is often no alternative. A rehabilitation centre may be the next step, if there is one not too far from the patient's home. It can provide a period of concentrated, coordinated therapy where the patient learns to look forward into the future. But rehabilitation after head injury can take years — years which cannot be spent in a rehabilitation centre and should not be spent in idleness at home. Much depends on the individual combination of problems. In some cases, the patient may be able to return to some form of work which can be used as a step towards more ambitious employment in the future. Otherwise, he may be able to attend a day hospital or day centre where activity, and maybe improvement, can continue.

Intermediate stage of treatment

This stage may go on for a very long time with the patient's condition remaining fairly static at some stage of recovery from which he may or may not finally progress. It will be beneficial for the patient to continue with active therapy for some time, but if this stage continues, decisions may have to be taken for longer term treatment, involving perhaps attendance at a day hospital. These patients should be regularly reviewed so that if they show any sign of improvement, further, more concentrated therapy can be prescribed.

The occupational therapist will need ingenuity during this period in order to maintain and encourage progress. She must be able to offer a suitable variety of activities to maintain interest. She must continue to encourage the patient to use his initiative and to develop responsibility and independence within what must be an institutional environment. Relatives will need a great deal of support and explanation at this stage so that they understand how they can help. It is particularly difficult for relations to watch a member of the family regain his independence, to see him struggling slowly to perform a task or taking what seems to be a risk, e.g. as by going out to the shops alone. It may be helpful for the family to attend various treatment departments with the patient so that both patient and family know that the other knows exactly how and what can be done independently.

PSYCHOLOGICAL AFTER-EFFECTS

People react to accidents in many different ways, but their response to accidents involving the head is often particularly complicated. The head is a very important part of man, it is man's conscious self, so that damage to the head can produce great anxiety as to the damage which may have been done to his self-image.

Superficial damage to the head, particularly if it affects the face, can cause great problems for the patient. Damage to the face may lead to withdrawal from society and a wide variety of neurotic or even psychotic states.

The psychological response to head injuries will be conditioned by upbringing and past experience. The patient may have known other people who have had head injuries, so that now he compares himself to them. His expectation for recovery will partly depend on his intelligence and morale. In some cases more primitive ideas come to the fore and the patient may have feelings of fate and guilt. He may have the feeling that he is being punished for something he has done. He may have fears of permanent incapacity, or of going insane.

It is most important for members of the team to understand these feelings which the patient may be afraid of or unable to express. He may need to be given information; over-protection of the patient can cause more anxiety and do more harm than good. We must help the patient to face reality

and not hide from it. Many patients cannot face the truth until they have adjusted mentally to the effects of their injury. After brain damage there is even more need for care in presenting patients to situations gently so that they can understand gradually and come to terms with their disability.

Some physical effects of brain damage may persist and become a chronic problem. Chronic brain syndrome is a collection of symptoms which are often present in the recovery period and normally disappear quite quickly, e.g. headache, irritability, apathy and inability to sleep. These symptoms may persist and should be a warning that the patient needs more support.

In cases where a claim for compensation for the injury is pending, patients may show poor recovery until a settlement has been reached. They may then improve or deteriorate, depending on the result of the settlement. This may be known as accident neurosis and is far more likely with industrial accidents when the patient feels he has a target to sue, than with sports injuries.

Epilepsy has already been discussed. An understanding of the problems this may produce and the way in which these are tackled, may be enough to ensure they do not give rise to more serious problems. But much will also depend on the patient's home and employment.

Patients may have personality changes as a result of head injury and this may cause more problems for the family than for the patient. Unfortunately, it is often the less desirable traits which become exaggerated and the patient often shows less inhibited behaviour.

It would not be natural if the head-injured patient did not periodically become depressed. However, this can become chronic and is then known as post-traumatic depression. This may be directly due to the head injury or it may be a result of the patient grieving for something which he has lost. Schizophrenia after head injury and is then known as post-traumatic or symptomatic schizophrenia.

WORK RESETTLEMENT

Planning for the future of the head-injured patient requires as much thought and care as any other part of his rehabilitation. By now, the patient has in many ways become the leader of the team and the members of the treatment team can only guide and advise. The patient should be achieving independence in all respects, although he may retain some effect of his head injury. The patient has reached the stage where, whatever disabilities he still has, only minimal further improvement is expected. The end of active rehabilitation is in sight and a future away from the rehabilitation regime must be sought.

Future prospects

What possibilities are open to the patient?

Return to previous employment. This is obviously ideal, but will depend on whether the job is still open and whether the patient still has the ability to do it.

Return to his previous employer but in a different capacity. It is much easier to return to a familiar work scene; pension schemes can be continued.

New work with a new employer. The Disablement Resettlement Officer should be asked to help in these cases as he knows all the local employers. Depending on the patient's ability and age it may be worth considering retraining. This may be undertaken at local centres, but the patient may also attend a suitable centre away from home if he is willing to travel and spend some time away from home. These centres, Employment Rehabilitation Centres (ERC), are only for assessment for open employment. The assessment covers a period of from 6 to 12 weeks of which the first part will be probationary. At the end of the assessment period the centre will make recommendations for future work which may involve a further specific training course at a Government Skills Centre.

Sheltered employment. This may be a good introduction to returning to open employment or, in some cases, it may have to continue on a long-term basis.

Because head injuries will continue to improve gradually over a long period, it is important to help patients to understand that their first job after the accident need not be permanent. Once they are back in employment with a good record they may progress to other jobs.

Points to consider in planning the future

1. *Previous employment.* It is often helpful to contact the employer (with the patient's permission) so that the patient's job description can be fully understood.
2. *Patient's work records.* A good past work record will now pay dividends. The employer may keep his job open or make efforts to find another suitable job in his firm. A poor past record may help the therapist to plan future job prospects realistically.
3. *Educational standard.* In planning a change of employment, what was the patient's educational standard? Has he any qualifications and is he still functioning at that standard?
4. *Expectations.* What does the patient hope to achieve and is he realistic?
Can he accept guidance from you or anybody else?

Assessment

Previous assessments of the patient during his rehabilitation have shown up all his problems as well as monitoring his improvement and increasing abilities. As only little further improvement is expected at this stage his capabilities now have to be assessed and matched to a job and possible future problems should be faced.

Physical assessment. Mobility. Is he mobile or chairbound? How practical is his mobility in relation to his previous work; to what extent will his mobility restrict future work prospects? Is his balance normal?

Upper limbs. Can he use his arms/hands efficiently? Has he normal power, stamina, speed and accuracy of movement? Is sensation normal?

Vision. Will his eyesight impede him in any way?

Does he have fits?

Mental problems. Adaptability. Does he have insight into his problems and is he able to adjust to residual disabilities and their consequences?

Loss of self-confidence. After a period away from work it may not be easy to return. The work habit may be lost and this point should be borne in mind when planning a realistic programme for the patient.

Lack of motivation. Some patients have little or no insight into their problems and this can produce lack of motivation. It can also be produced by an underlying lack of self-confidence and a fear of returning to normal life and employment.

Poor memory.

Loss of noise tolerance.

Loss of concentration. This can be caused by loss of noise tolerance and can affect speed and accuracy.

Behaviour problems. Aggressive, irresponsible or impulsive behaviour must be controlled.

Inability to communicate easily. In order to return to work some form of communication must have been found, but the patient may still find this an embarrassment.

Types of work which can be considered

Academic work. Return to any type of work requiring concentrated thought and fine work should be gradual. It may be necessary to assess the patient's ability to return to academic work and cooperation of the employer may be useful in providing suitable work exercises. Patients wishing to go on to re-training usually have to attain a prescribed level of English and arithmetic so that tuition may need to be provided by the occupational therapist.

Clerical work. Clerical work varies from very responsible, personal secretarial posts to less responsible, routine and more manual jobs. Having seen the job description the occupational therapist should be able to provide suitable practice, gradually building up the patient's ability.

Skilled/unskilled work. It can be most helpful for the patient to have some experience in a workshop before returning to open employment. The tempo of his daily programme should be gradually stepped up so that he does not find fatigue added to his list of difficulties in returning to work.

Contract work may provide a useful alternative. Many jobs are very repetitive, and require varying degrees of manual dexterity, speed and concentration. In the hospital, it is usually quite easy to find suitable work such as assembling hospital folders, packing CSSD packs or printing stationery.

Activities in heavy workshops can also provide an opportunity to practise previous skills and so regain confidence, or to try new ones so that future work prospects can be assessed. Again, contract work may be useful, or work on individual projects which may provide more skills.

Whatever the future work prospects, the patient and his immediate family must be closely involved in discussions and plans at this stage, as they should be at every other stage. If the patient has to learn to accept disability and change of life-style, he must have the support of his family and they must all have the opportunity to discuss and understand.

In conclusion, perhaps three points should be made. First, there are no exact rules for treating a head-injured patient. The therapist must assess all aspects and then try various methods to see which works best. Second, think of each patient as an individual. What was his past ability? What are his needs and our aims? Are we being realistic? It is all too easy for the therapist to decide on aims of treatment without really considering the patient's needs. This leads to the third point, which is to consider how far the patient's problems are going to affect his life and, therefore, how much importance needs to be attached to them. Look at each problem in relation to all the patient's disabilities and to his particular needs.

REFERENCES AND FURTHER READING

Bannister R 1972 Brain revised. In: Clinical neurology, 4th edn. Oxford University Press, London

Bickerstaff E R 1971 Neurology for nurses, 2nd edn. English Universities Press, London

Bobath B 1978 Adult hemiplegia: evaluation and treatment, 2nd edn. Heinemann Medical, London

Briggs M 1975 Management of patients with head injury. Physiotherapy 61(9):266

Cash J 1974 Neurology for physiotherapists. Faber & Faber, London

Holmes G 1971 Clinical neurology, 3rd edn. Churchill Livingstone, Edinburgh

Miller E 1972 Clinical neuropsychology. Penguin, Harmondsworth

Potter J 1974 The practical management of head injuries, 3rd edn. Lloyd Luke, London.

19

Hemiplegia

(resulting from a cerebro-vascular accident)

Hemiplegia or hemiparesis (*hemi* — half, *plegia* — paralysis, *paresis* — weakness) is paralysis or weakness of the limbs, and often of the face and trunk, on one side of the body. It is the consequence of damage to the upper motor neurones innervating the affected muscles. It is commonly caused by a stroke. This has been defined by the World Health Organisation as 'the rapid onset of the clinical signs of a focal disturbance of cerebral function of presumed vascular origin and of more than 24 hours duration'. Disease or trauma to the brain may damage the upper motor neurones at the cortical level, i.e. the motor cortex where the motor nerve cell bodies are sited, or interrupt the long motor nerve fibres in their pathway through the cerebral hemisphere or brain stem. Interruption of the upper motor nerve pathway causes complete or partial loss of active movement in the affected muscles. In the lower part of their course, upper motor neurones decussate at the junction of the medulla and the spinal cord. The majority of them continue their pathway down the spinal cord in the lateral corticospinal tract. They terminte in synaptic connections with the cell bodies of the lower motor neurones whose fibres pass to the innervated muscles through peripheral nerve trunks.

Unilateral weakness or paralysis is not the only impairment or loss of function occurring in strokes. The clinical picture depends on the site and extent of brain injury. Other structures, such as the sensory cortex, sensory nerve fibres, optic tract or visual cortex, may also be damaged. Damage to either or both cerebral hemispheres may result in loss or impairment of higher cerebral function, as will be described.

Hemiplegia may be unilateral or bilateral. Unilateral strokes are commonly the result of damage to one hemisphere of the brain. Brain-stem strokes may be associated with bilateral hemiparesis or quadriparesis. Cranial nerve lesions leading to bulbar palsy, in which there is difficulty in swallowing (dysphagia), slurred speech (dysarthria) and difficulty in coughing, are also common in brain-stem strokes. Inco-ordination of one or more limbs is often present and is due to the interruption of cerebellar pathways in the brain stem.

CAUSES OF CEREBRO-VASCULAR ACCIDENTS (STROKES)

Cerebral haemorrhage

Cerebral haemorrhage may occur at any age due to abnormal intracranial arteries, particularly if there is coincident hypertension. Angiomatous arterial malformation and aneurysmal dilatation of an intracranial artery may be the cause, particularly in younger patients. Hypertension and arteriosclerosis increase the likelihood of strokes. As these conditions become more common with increasing age, many of the patients suffering from strokes are elderly. Haemorrhage may occur from small aneurysms in arterio-sclerotic cerebral arteries in patients with hypertension.

Cerebral embolism

Patients with diseases of the heart or major arteries may have embolic strokes. An embolus is a piece of a thrombus which has broken away from a vessel wall into the circulation and finally lodges in a smaller vessel, through which it is unable to pass. Several fragments may break off from a thrombus or blood clot formed on the wall of a major artery in the neck or in the left atrium or ventricle of the heart and cause more than one embolic incident. The patient may have a history of multiple strokes.

Cerebral thrombosis

Intracranial arteries impaired by degenerative atherosclerotic changes may be blocked by the formation of a thrombus on the damaged endothelial lining. The affected artery becomes occluded and, as in the case of embolism, the brain tissue beyond is deprived of its blood supply and therefore becomes infarcted.

Damage to the brain tissue adjacent to the cerebral infarct may resolve gradually during the first three to six months following the stroke and this probably accounts for the more rapid recovery of function in the early months after the onset of the stroke. Reduction in cerebral blood flow may result from a reduction in cardiac output which is believed to be a contributory factor in the onset of strokes in some people, particularly if there is already generalised atherosclerosis of the cerebral arteries.

Onset

A sudden onset is more likely with cerebral embolism or haemorrhage. There may or may not be loss of consciousness.

Onset which is gradual is sometimes described as a 'stroke-in-evolution', or a stroke of 'stuttering' onset. The symptoms and signs develop in a series of episodes over a period of time varying from several hours to several days. A slow, insidious development of symptoms and signs may be due to cerebral tumour. The nature of the symptoms and signs is determined by the site of the brain damage.

Common clinical features (Fig. 19.1)

Disorders of higher cerebral function (perception)

Anosognosia. Anosognosia, or denial of disease, is associated with neglect of the hemiplegic side, lack of recognition and sometimes delusions concerning the affected limb. The patient may deny or be unaware of his disabilities. In its less severe form, there is some awareness, but also some forgetfulness or inattention to the affected side.

Agnosia. The patient is unable to recognise what he perceives and to organise sensory impressions

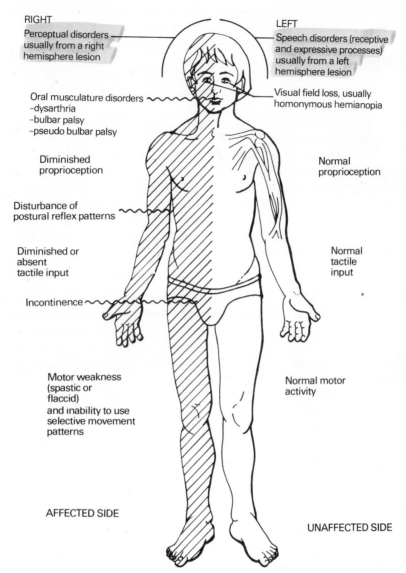

RIGHT

Perceptual disorders usually from a right hemisphere lesion

Oral musculature disorders
-dysarthria
-bulbar palsy
-pseudo bulbar palsy

Diminished proprioception

Disturbance of postural reflex patterns

Diminished or absent tactile input

Incontinence

Motor weakness (spastic or flaccid) and inability to use selective movement patterns

AFFECTED SIDE

LEFT

Speech disorders (receptive and expressive processes) usually from a left hemisphere lesion

Visual field loss, usually homonymous hemianopia

Normal proprioception

Normal tactile input

Normal motor activity

UNAFFECTED SIDE

Fig. 19.1 Common problems associated with hemiplegia (a left CVA leading to a right sided weakness is illustrated)

into a recognisable form, although the appropriate sensory organs and nerve pathways are intact. This disability may involve visual, auditory or tactile impressions.

Disorders of visuo-spatial perception. These are demonstrated as difficulty with drawing, figure-ground discrimination, assembly, non-verbal, constructional tasks shape and size recognition.

Neglect and disturbance of body image of the hemiplegic side and impairment of visuo-spatial perception are often associated with injury to the parietal lobe of the non-dominant (usually right) brain hemisphere.

Apraxia. Apraxia is the loss of ability to perform a previously learned pattern of movement, although there is no evidence of loss of muscle power, comprehension, coordination or sensation essential to the action.

1. Idoemotor apraxia — is the loss of connection between the idea of the action and its execution.

2. Gait apraxia occurs with bilateral frontal

lobe injury. The patient is unable to walk and to correct postural errors.

Difficulties in sequential thinking may also be present.

Speech disorders

Aphasia. This is the partial or complete loss of language ability. It may involve both expressive and receptive speech, impairment of reading and writing, gesture language as well as spoken speech. Aphasia and apraxia frequently occur together.

Apraxia

1. *Buccofacial apraxia.* Voluntary movement of oral musculature is impossible, but reflexes e.g. swallowing, are preserved.

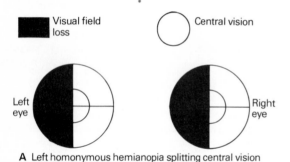

A Left homonymous hemianopia splitting central vision

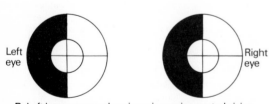

B Left homonymous hemianopia sparing central vision

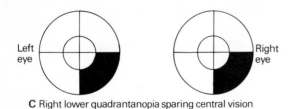

C Right lower quadrantanopia sparing central vision

Fig. 19.2 Homonymous hemianopia

2. *Articulatory apraxia.* Voluntary movements of the oral musculature are possible, but the patient is unable to utilise these movements to produce articulate speech.

Dysarthria. Difficulty in speaking clearly due to muscle weakness, although there is no language loss.

Other associated disorders sometimes manifested are impairment of memory, loss of orientation in place and time and of emotional control. This causes easily provoked crying or laughing and is one of the more distressing symptoms of a stroke. Problems associated with concentration, personality and intelligence may also occur.

Disorders of vision

Homonymous hemianopia. Loss of half of the visual field results from trauma to the optic tract or to the visual cortex of the occipital lobe on the side opposite to that of the visual field loss. The same side of the visual field is lost for each eye. It is commonly the same side as the hemiplegia. It may be peripheral, sparing central vision, or it may 'split' or divide the central field of vision. In some patients vision is lost in only one quadrant, giving rise to quadrantanopia (Fig. 19.2).

Visual inattention. There may be some inattention to visual stimuli on the affected side, with no evidence of visual field loss.

Extraocular muscle weakness or paralysis. This may cause blurred or double vision.

Motor disorders

There is commonly impairment or loss of voluntary movement of the hemiplegic limbs. Initially, the affected limbs may be hypotonic (flaccid), but after the first two or three weeks, muscle tone may increase causing a characteristic resistance to passive movement, i.e. spasticity. Other disorders of muscle tone may be present and may involve the opposite, unaffected side. This will be determined by the site and extent of brain damage.

Voluntary movement tends to be better preserved and to recover more readily in the proximal muscles of the limbs. The hand and foot are often slow to recover and may remain permanently weak. Weakness or eversion of the foot on the affected side often persists and causes instability in walking. A below-knee caliper may be required to stabilise the ankle and foot and to correct foot drop and the tendency to inversion of the foot on standing and walking.

Ataxia or incoordination may result from muscle weakness or injury to the cerebellum or cerebellar pathways.

Other disorders

Sensory loss or impairment. Loss of postural or position sense (proprioception) is a significant handicap when learning to walk again and to perform practical tasks. A combination of, for instance, incoordination and loss of position sense may deprive a hand of much useful function, even if power is well preserved. Loss of superficial pain sensation is a handicap in the kitchen where the patient is likely to handle hot objects.

Unilateral facial weakness. Unilateral facial weakness is common and results in a disfiguring drooping of the mouth on one side. If combined with extraocular muscle weakness and a squint, the altered appearance can be distressing and of some consequence in social rehabilitation. Loss of muscle power to tongue, cheek and face on one side can cause problems with chewing, swallowing and dribbling. The lower eyelid may droop.

Bulbar and pseudo-bulbar palsy. Difficulty in swallowing (dysphagia) and coughing, and slurred speech (dysarthria) occur in bulbar and pseudo-bulbar palsy. The symptoms are due to muscle weakness and sometimes incoordination. Bulbar palsy results from lesions of the cranial nerve nuclei and pathways in the lower part of the brain stem.

Pseudo-bulbar palsy results from bilateral upper motor neurone disease and is often accompanied by loss of emotional control. It is commonly associated with bilateral, widespread cerebral arteriosclerosis, for instance in patients with hypertension.

INCIDENCE AND PROGNOSIS

The incidence of strokes of various types is approximately 1.8 to 2.0 per thousand population per annum. Most are over the age of 65 years, about 20 per cent are below retiring age and about 70 per cent of patients have hypertension. Mortality varies according to age and the presence of associated disease such as heart disease and diabetes mellitus. Mortality increases with advancing age and over 70 years of age is about 50 per cent. About 50 to 70 per cent of the survivors will learn to walk independently, 20 to 30 per cent will be more handicapped.

Factors influencing prognosis

Research has made it possible to identify some of the factors which may allow a more accurate prognosis in individual cases. Strokes are more common in late middle-aged/elderly patients, who also have a higher incidence of cardiovascular disease than younger people. With advancing age there is a greater likelihood of coincident disabilities and disease, for instance degenerative joint disease or heart disease, making rehabilitation more difficult, complex and prolonged.

Features associated with a less good or poor prognosis are unconsciousness and any combination of impaired consciousness, severe weakness of the affected side, failure of conjugate vision towards the weak side, severe hemiplegia and advancing age.

During the period after the onset of a stroke several factors may adversely affect prognosis:

1. Receptive dysphasia and dementia.

2. Accompanying homonymous hemianopia and sensory neglect.

3. Denial of the hemiplegic side and disturbance of body image and spatial perception. These symptoms often occur in lesions of the non-dominant hemisphere and make rehabilitation more difficult. Improvement in independence may follow in the succeeding months, but it is important that the patient is encouraged early on to overcome these difficulties by correct management by therapists, staff and relatives.

4. A hand which is still useless three weeks after the stroke is unlikely to regain useful function.

There is more hope of recovery of useful function in the affected leg if the patient can lift the extended leg off the bed two or three weeks after the stroke and dorsiflex the affected foot after four to six weeks.

Finally, it is most important that great caution is exercised in assessing the prognosis, because patients vary in their response and may not conform to the described pattern. Discussion with the patient concerning his prognosis is primarily the responsibility of the physician caring for him. It should not be undertaken by therapists and other people caring for the patient, except in consultation and cooperation with the physician in charge.

Emotional and psychological factors are of the utmost importance in the successful rehabilitation of patients. A depressed patient who is unable to succeed in most of his undertakings in the rehabilitation department, who has poor motivation, or is being rejected by his family, is at a serious disadvantage.

THE ROLE OF THE OCCUPATIONAL THERAPIST

The hospital occupational therapist may frequently have contact with the stroke patient from the early days following his admission. If working in the community, she may find the patient referred whilst at home being cared for by his relatives (having not been admitted to hospital), or when he is about to be discharged or has just been discharged from hospital following initial rehabilitation. It is important that she maintains an overall picture of the patient's recovery and social circumstances in order that treatment priorities can be linked to those activities most essential for the patient and his family.

The assistance given to the stroke patient and his family must therefore follow a detailed assessment of his difficulties and be based upon the demands of the environment in which he lives or will live when discharged from hospital. The overall aims of occupational therapy may be summarised as follows:
- to help the patient to adjust to his disability
- to assess his difficulties
- to facilitate maximum independence in the activities of daily living
- to prevent deformity
- to encourage maximum return of function

- to work with and reinforce the work of other members of the treatment team
- to resettle the patient within the community and at work, where appropriate.

Adjustment to disability

As the therapist may be involved with the patient soon after his stroke, it is important that she helps him to begin to adjust to his difficulties as early as possible. To suddenly be changed from an active individual to one unable to speak, sit unaided or even eat food without difficulty can obviously be extremely distressing for both the patient and his family and it is essential that the therapist conveys her understanding of the situation by handling and moving the patient efficiently and without causing discomfort and by giving practical advice on immediate problems and long-term worries. The therapist should always treat her patient as an adult by ensuring that she does not 'baby talk' to him or raise her voice when addressing him simply because he cannot respond. She should give the patient ample time to reply to questions if he has speech difficulties or is confused, and, where appropriate should phrase questions in such a way that they can be answered by 'yes' or 'no' or with only a nod or shake of the head.

Activities or equipment used for assessment and treatment should not appear childish, although they may be simple to use. The therapist should approach the patient with confidence and be sure of her knowledge so that he will trust her judgement and treatment. Where possible, it is helpful to treat stroke patients in a group, not only so that they can see the progress of other members, but also in order that common problems can be discovered and discussed and encouragement given by other group members.

The therapist should emphasise essential activities such as eating, drinking, communication and toilet transfers early on in treatment so that the patient does not have to rely on others for help with these personal activities. Similarly, the therapist, along with other members of the treatment team, should note whether the patient recognises his limitations and can begin to check his own safety by ensuring that his affected limbs are well positioned and will not be damaged by sharp or hot objects.

Assessment of disability

It is essential that the occupational therapist has a thorough knowledge of the difficulties resulting from her patient's stroke in order that a realistic and comprehensive treatment programme can be planned. Clearly, it would be undesirable and impractical to try to assess all the patient's difficulties in one session and frequently assessment is carried out over a period of time, closely linked with treatment of essential and obvious difficulties. It is equally impractical for each therapist to carry out assessment of all areas of difficulty and where a detailed assessment of a particular aspect has already been performed and reported, the therapist need only carry out a brief assessment herself. The therapist will often find that assessment and treatment activities overlap and that the amount of formal testing can therefore be reduced. For example, the patient's memory and physical ability can be well observed during dressing practice, his level of sensory appreciation noted when practising washing techniques or cooking and his speech and visual skills during group activities and normal conversation.

Bearing these points in mind a description of some basic assessment techniques is given below.

Anosognosia/neglect. Observe any difficulties the patient has in perceiving his own body. Does he, perhaps, 'lose' his foot or arm, get his arm caught in the spokes of his wheelchair, fantasise about or disassociate himself from his weak limbs? When dressing, does he attempt to put both feet down the same trouser leg, put his pants on over his hands, or neglect to clothe his affected side altogether?

When asked to draw or copy a picture of himself or an article such as a clock, does he fail to complete one half by pushing all the numbers of the clock over to one side, by adding detail only to one side of the body, or by drawing two right arms or only one leg (Fig. 19.3)? The therapist may also note an accompanying or alternative disturbance of body image.

Agnosia. If a patient is unable to handle and use an object correctly, even though he has the physical capacity to do so, it is possible that he is suffering from a visual agnosia. The therapist may notice, for example, that a patient accepts a cup of

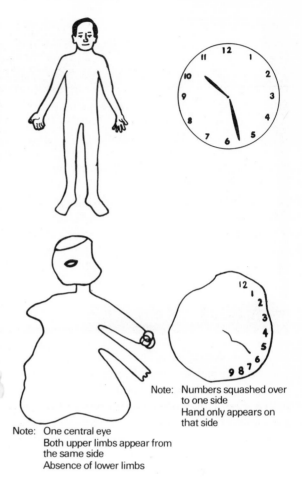

Note: One central eye
Both upper limbs appear from the same side
Absence of lower limbs

Note: Numbers squashed over to one side
Hand only appears on that side

Fig. 19.3 Testing for neglect and/or body image disturbance

tea but then turns it upside down to inspect the bottom or that, when given a razor, he attempts to use it to comb his hair, or puts it in his mouth. Where auditory or tactile stimuli are affected, speech and stereognostic skills can also be disturbed.

Apraxia. If the patient is unable to perform a previously known task in spite of intact motor and sensory pathways, he may be suffering from apraxia. If he is unable to respond to a request within his physical capacity, an assessment may need to differentiate between his inability to understand the command and his inability to perform the task. Facial expression can afford a clue here. Does the patient look as though he understands the command or not? The therapist may notice that the patient's automatic responses remain. For exam-

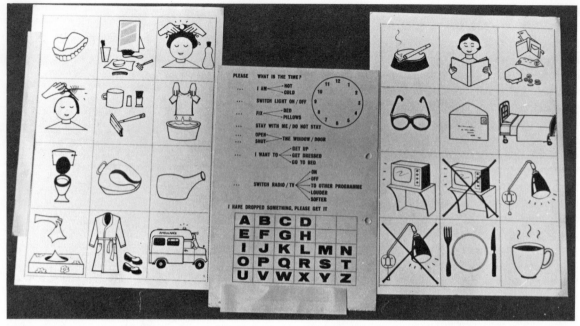

Fig. 19.4 Communication cards

ple, he may not be able to respond to a request such as 'drink your tea', but will perform the action if the cup is placed in his hand. However, the therapist must be aware of the patient's inability to respond positively to a command. She must also explore all channels of expression for response to a request, such as verbal, motor, gesture and writing.

Speech disorders. A full assessment of speech difficulties will be carried out by the speech therapist. The occupational therapist should, however:

be aware of any severe speech difficulties before meeting the patient. Where such problems exist she should bear in mind the points mentioned earlier in this chapter.

observe any receptive disorders by simple tests in which the response to a command can be made without speech, for example 'Pick up your brush and brush your hair.' or 'Show me where you keep your toothbrush.'

find out, where possible, a method through which the patient can communicate his needs. This may involve writing, drawing, gesticulation or the use of communication charts (Fig. 19.4). With the patient whose speech is still present the therapist should encourage conversation in order

to observe any particular areas of difficulty.

Disorders of vision. The therapist may test for hemianopia in several ways. An initial assessment can involve asking the patient to describe a wide picture or frieze, to describe objects or people in the room around him or to pick out objects from a selection placed on a wide table in front of him. For a slightly more accurate assessment the therapist stands behind the patient and brings two objects (such as pens) round on either side of him at eye level, asking him to say when each object comes into his field of vision. This will give some indication of visual field loss. It must be remembered, however, that unilateral neglect may give a similar result.

Motor disorders. It is vital for the therapist to obtain an accurate picture of the level of motor function in her patient. This may be affected by an alteration (often an increase) in the muscle tone of the affected side, the patient's ability to correct his posture and the presence of abnormal associated reaction patterns. The therapist should be aware of the functional use to which the patient puts his affected limbs, for perceptual disturbance, as well as sensory loss, can hinder the functional use of the limb. She should also note any incoordination which will hinder motor activity.

CEREBRAL FUNCTION TEST

Section 1

A. Name   B. Age

C. Address   D. Day or date

E. Where are you now?   F. What time of day is it?

G. Remember 4 items – Horse   skirt   apple   hand

    (To test orientation and memory)

Section 2

A. Write your name   B. Close your eyes
   (Graphic ability)   (Ability to follow verbal instructions)

C. Perform this action   D. Read this aloud
   (Card 'show me your tongue')   (Card with short sentence)
   (Ability to follow written instruction)

E. Check memory test

    (To test language skills)

Section 3

A. Trace the triangle with a red pencil   B. Place these cards in the appropriate order
   (Figure-ground and colour recognition)   (Sequential thought)

C. Draw a man   D. Show me how you would use these (cup and saucer)
   (Body image)   (Object recognition)

E. Pick out all the triangular bricks and post them
   (Post box with bricks placed in an arc)
   (Hemianopia, shape recognition)

    (To test perception)

Fig. 19.5 A

Sensory disorders. Proprioceptive disturbance can be assessed either by asking the patient to position his limbs while his eyes are closed (for example the therapist holds and positions his affected limb and then he imitates this position with his strong hand) or by observing how the patient uses his affected limb when it is out of sight. Can he, for example, turn down the back of his collar or tuck in his shirt accurately, or does his hand get 'lost' when he cannot see it?

Sensation impairment is of particular importance to the stroke patient, as many activities, such as cooking, bathing and smoking, can prove hazardous if sensation is disturbed. Sensory problems may be noted during sessions in the kitchen or in washing or bathing when the patient finds it difficult to appreciate different temperature or textures. A more accurate assessment can be made by formally testing the patient's reaction to different textures, pinprick, light touch (such as cotton wool) and temperature.

Emotional disorders. It is not uncommon for a patient who has suffered a stroke to become emotionally labile. Where this occurs the therapist will note an exaggerated mood response to a slight change in the patient's emotional level. He may, for example, cry when asked about his home life or giggle when asked to perform a slightly difficult task. The patient may also become depressed, i.e. apathetic and unresponsive and his face will become expressionless and lifeless. Where speech is present, this may also lack expression. The patient will show no hope for, or interest in, the future. Such a patient will find the demands imposed by rehabilitation particularly taxing and may withdraw altogether from his surroundings.

Finally, the therapist may find that her patient, not unexpectedly, becomes extremely frustrated, especially if his speech has been greatly affected. It is not uncommon to hear a patient swear or shout out in anger, or to react by banging furniture, crying or hitting out at those near him.

Other thought and perceptual disorders. The inability to distinguish an object from its surroundings (figure-ground disturbance), may show itself in the patient's inability to pick out a single item from several in a drawer, or to distinguish one item of clothing from a pile placed on his bed. Sequential thought disturbance (i.e. the inability to think in a logical order) may show up when the patient

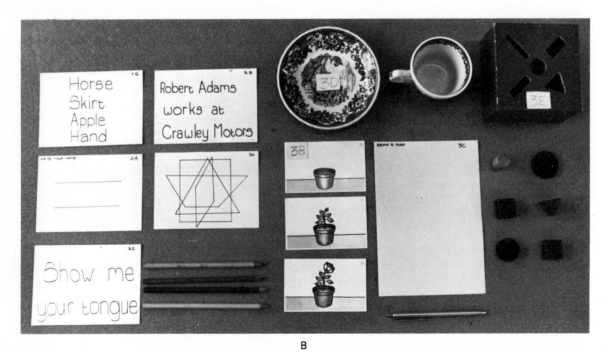

B

Fig 19.5 A & B Introductory test for assessing perceptual and thought disorders

tries to put on his top clothing before his under-wear or attempts to drink from an empty cup before pouring liquid into it.

The therapist may find that in some centres initial assessment (especially of thought processes) is performed using a introductory test (Fig. 19.5) and only where some pronounced difficulty is encountered will a more detailed test be carried out.

The therapist must remember that the difficulties arising as a result of a stroke cannot always easily be distinguished one from another as functions often overlap. For example, if a man only shaves one side of his face or ignores items placed in his affected hand, the cause may be a combination of hemianopia, the inability to move or feel the affected side, the loss of proprioception or stereognosis in the weak limb, a disturbance of body image or neglect of the weak side. Similarly, a patient who does not respond to a request may be hindered by a lack of understanding of the command, an inability to perform the task physically, by apraxia which inhibits his initiation of the activity, or he may simply be so depressed that he lacks the motivation to comply. What must be clearly assessed and recorded are both the results of specific tests to distinguish particular problem areas as well as the patient's functional ability.

Independence in activities of daily living

Maximum independence in ADL is vitally important for the stroke patient, as many become completely dependent on others for all daily living activities in the acute stages of their illness and, as recovery occurs, all activities must be relearned within the physical and psychological limits of the patient. The therapist must also remember that, as the majority of patients are over 50 years old, they may be living with an elderly spouse who is unable to accept heavy demands from his partner. As the ability to learn new tasks and agility also decrease with age (see Chapter 16), the patient will need competent and reptitive teaching in order to relearn his old skills.

As learning faculties and perception may be disturbed, it is important to introduce aids only when absolutely essential.

Eating. It is important to start the patient feeding independently as soon as possible. Being fed is not only degrading to the patient, it also emphasises his complete dependence and is time-consuming for the staff. Assessment and treatment of eating and drinking problems can be done on the ward, even when the patient is still confined to bed; it is one of the first problems that should be tackled. It is often appropriate to have the first session outside mealtimes so that the patient can become used to new methods and aids slowly and does not have to cope with the added frustration of trying to eat fast enough to prevent a tepid hospital lunch from becoming stone cold before he finishes! The following points should be remembered:

He should be able to drink from a normal cup or mug, but do not fill it too full or have liquid too hot. Try to educate other staff not to provide spouted containers.

Avoid letting the patient eat with a spoon; if he can only cope with one utensil a fork is far better.

Resume the use of a knife and fork as soon as possible. It may be necessary to support the weak limb in a beneficial position, to pad the utensil in the weak hand or to sue commercially available lightweight, enlarged cutlery.

If aids are necessary consider the use of a plate guard or Manoy plate, a Manoy or Nelson knife, Spork and/or a non-slip mat such as Dycem (Fig. 19.6).

If the patient eats very slowly a double shelled 'warming' plate may be useful. The therapist should note the patient's chewing and swallowing abilities, the fit of his dentures and his ability to 'find' his mouth if proprioceptive mechanisms are disturbed.

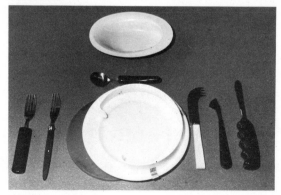

Fig. 19.6 Eating aids

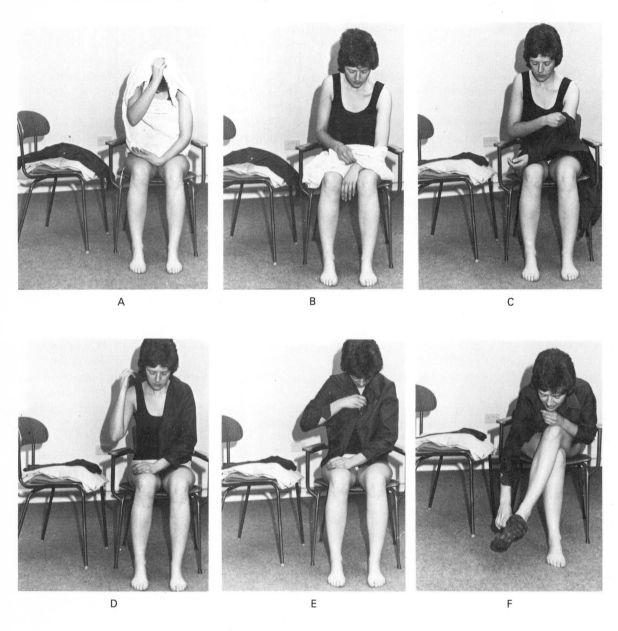

Fig. 19.7 Dressing sequence for the hemiplegic patient

Fig. 19.7A The patient sits with both feet firmly on the floor. A nightdress or pyjama jacket is pulled over the head as shown

Fig. 19.7B The garment is removed first from the strong arm, then from the weak

Fig. 19.7C Sleeves are put over the weak arm first

Fig. 19.7D The garment is pulled up high onto the shoulder and across the back by reaching round the neck for the collar

Fig. 19.7E The strong arm is then put into the sleeve, the garment adjusted for comfort and the buttons fastened. Note: A bra can be adapted to open at the front and fasten with velcro

Fig. 19.7F Socks, stockings or tights are put on by crossing one leg over the other

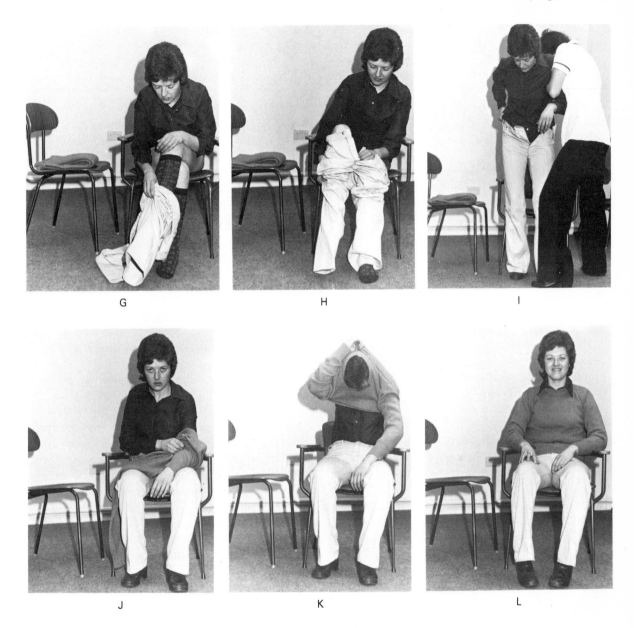

G

H

I

J

K

L

Fig. 19.7G When putting on trousers and pants cross the weak leg over the strong leg first and pull the garment up to the knees so that it comes right over the foot

Fig. 19.7H Put the strong leg in and pull the garment up to the knees as before

Fig. 19.7I When all lower garments have been put on, the therapist helps the patient to stand and to adjust clothing over the hips

Fig. 19.7J Garments put on over the head are placed on the patients lap with the welt towards him. The weak arm is put into the sleeves and this is pulled well up until the hand is free

Fig. 19.7K The strong arm is put into the other sleeve and the garment pulled over the head as shown

Fig. 19.7L Garments are then adjusted for comfort. Don't forget spectacles and hearing aid if these are needed

Dressing. The patient should begin getting dressed completely as soon as he is sitting out of bed for a reasonable length of time, for example a morning. However, it is useful to begin dressing practice earlier with, for instance, a pyjama jacket, so that the patient begins to learn the method and is able to control his own temperature, at least to a limited degree. Several other points should be remembered:

Use familiar, everyday clothes, not hospital garments or the patient's Sunday-best.

Use as few clothes as possible in the beginning.

Dressing practice should take place at the appropriate time of day, i.e. in the morning when the patient is getting up, not in the middle of the afternoon.

Ensure privacy and good light.

The patient should either sit on the edge of the bed with his clothes placed on his weak side or on a chair with his clothes laid out nearby.

The clothes should be laid out in the order required with bra/vest on top. If the patient has problems with figure-ground discrimination garments should be presented to him one at a time.

Practice is essential, and the patient should not be rushed.

The principles of dressing are basically that the weak limb is put in the garment first when dressing and comes out last when undressing (Fig. 19.7A–L).

Beware of problems associated with poor trunk balance when sitting and leaning forward.

Toilet. As well as making the patient physically independent in using the toilet it is important to establish a routine which suits the patient and his family, especially if he is being retrained to control his bladder and/or bowel after a period of incontinence.

Where support is needed, e.g. grab rails, this should be provided on both sides of the toilet as the patient usually has to turn round having entered the bathroom/WC. It may be possible to use a washbasin or *strong* towel rail as support on one side, but this is not advisable if the patient is very unstable.

Make sure that the patient can manage his clothing, and can clean himself and flush the toilet as well as get off and on the WC.

A commode may be necessary at home for night use or if the toilet is upstairs and the patient is unable to reach it. A urinal for men may be useful for use at night.

A raised toilet seat may be necessary, but it must be very secure.

Washing and bathing. Remember that *safety* is of utmost importance in the bathroom. When assessing the patient's ability to use the bath remember that it is essential to see him actually have a bath, as his stability when wet and slippery may be very much reduced.

Consider the use of a bathboard, bath seat, grab rails, non-slip mat and shower unit fixed to bath taps.

Will a strip wash be safer?

Is it appropriate to ask the district nurse to help?

Consider aids such as a washing glove, suction pads for soap and nailbrush, looped towels for drying, or long-handled aids for reaching toes and back.

Do not forget associated activities such as shaving combing hair and cleaning teeth.

If the patient regains reasonable use of his affected lower limb, can he manage to get in/out of the bath without aids as shown in Figure 19.8?

If help is necessary for part of the bathing procedure, can the (elderly) spouse manage what is required and is he willing to give the help?

Transfers. When moving a person with a unilateral weakness it is important to remember not to put strain on the weak limb in such a way that it causes pain or possible damage. This is especially important at the shoulder joint where upward pressure in the axilla can cause great discomfort and may injure an unstable shoulder by pulling on weak muscles.

If support is necessary during transfers it is important that the therapist finds, and uses, the method most acceptable to the patient and his family. There are several ways of moving a stroke patient; the pelvic or scapular holds may be preferred in units where the bilateral approach to treatment is used and the 'through-arm' hold when support is needed for the weak side without pressure being put on the axilla. The various holds are described in Chapter 4.

Kitchen and household activities. The severely disabled hemiplegic patient has a lot of hard work ahead of him when he begins his rehabilitation

Weak side

Strong side

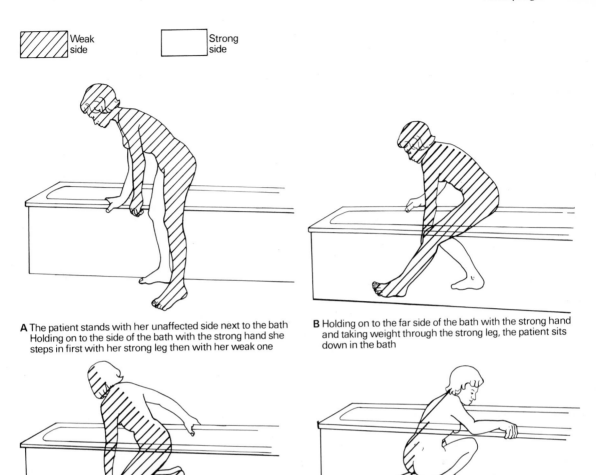

A The patient stands with her unaffected side next to the bath Holding on to the side of the bath with the strong hand she steps in first with her strong leg then with her weak one

B Holding on to the far side of the bath with the strong hand and taking weight through the strong leg, the patient sits down in the bath

C After bathing, the water should be drained. The patient holds the side of the bath behind her with her strong arm

D The patient swings round towards the sound side ending in a kneeling position

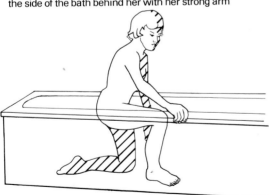

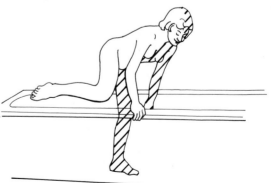

E The patient pushes up into a standing position using the strong leg and holding on to the side of the bath

F Holding the side of the bath with the strong hand she then steps out

Fig. 19.8 A–F Bathing without aids. (Note: the patient must be able to rise from sitting through kneeling. A non-slip bath mat is essential)

and, although household activities are an essential part of many patients' daily activities, the therapist must remember that not all patients will have to learn to cope with these. She must guard against the family's reluctance to allow the patient to continue his domestic activities and explain to them that the patient can relearn to be safe and competent to a degree and that this is important for his self esteem.

Points to consider during treatment:

Begin with activities that will be successful and can be done seated e.g. weighing ingredients, filling tarts, chopping vegetables and putting out biscuits.

Introduce the patient into a small group with similar difficulties so that he can see that progress is made and can begin to become familiar with the methods and aids used.

As the patient improves, increase the length and complexity of the activities and introduce basic equipment such as oven and hotplate, and simple tools for weighing, chopping, mixing, spreading, carrying, washing up and drying.

Remember that safety is vital in the kitchen and should be emphasised from the beginning, especially if there are perceptual, sensory or gross balance problems.

The patient's main difficulties are likely to be balance, stabilisation of work or problems connected with perceptual loss. Many aids are now designed specifically for this purpose and these are available commercially. Commonly used aids in the kitchen are spike boards, non-slip mats, bowl stabilisers, chopping and cutting aids, cards giving large and concise instruction and mobility aids such as trolleys, but there are many other aids, either designed especially for the disabled or ordinarily available in department stores, which the therapist should consider (Fig. 19.9).

Do not forget that the patient will tire more easily after a stroke and labour saving equipment and advice are therefore important.

Progress only as necessary for the patient to cope at home and remember that kitchen and household activities can also be used for other aspects of treatment, such as coordination, general mobility in a confined space, and ability to follow instruction and use initiative.

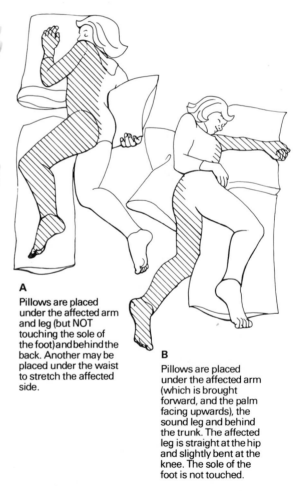

A Pillows are placed under the affected arm and leg (but NOT touching the sole of the foot) and behind the back. Another may be placed under the waist to stretch the affected side.

B Pillows are placed under the affected arm (which is brought forward, and the palm facing upwards), the sound leg and behind the trunk. The affected leg is straight at the hip and slightly bent at the knee. The sole of the foot is not touched.

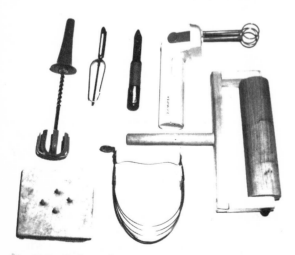

Fig. 19.9 Kitchen aids

Fig. 19.10 Positioning at rest to reduce spasm. (Note: the sole of the foot is not touched)

Prevention of deformity

As the majority of patients suffering a stroke ultimately have an increased muscle tone in their affected limbs it is important that the limbs should not be allowed to remain in a position of spasticity. A deformed limb is not only non-functional, but also unsightly, and difficult to dress and use as a weight or stop for steadying work. If movement begins to return, it will be much more difficult, if not impossible, to remobilise as spasticity must first be overcome. This may at best be slow and painful, and at worst impossible.

Points to consider during treatment:

Encourage normal positions both during activity and at rest.

Inhibit spasticity, working proximally first, into inhibiting positions (basically the opposite of the spastic pattern) before treatment and during activity as necessary.

Weight bearing through the affected side reduces spasticity.

Reduction of stress (physical and/or emotional) will reduce associated reaction patterns.

The patient and his family should be encouraged to accept responsibility for his own rehabilitation.

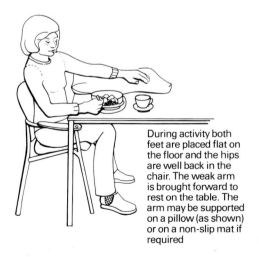

During activity both feet are placed flat on the floor and the hips are well back in the chair. The weak arm is brought forward to rest on the table. The arm may be supported on a pillow (as shown) or on a non-slip mat if required

Fig. 19.11 Positioning during activity to reduce spasm

Encouraging maximum return of function

Motor difficulties

Before and during recovery, the affected limb must be encouraged and used to its maximum efficiency during all treatment sessions. The therapist must remember that the patient will need a relatively less mobile, but more stable lower limb in order to regain reasonable function, whereas for the upper limb a greater level of movement, coordination and sensation is necessary. The main function of the upper limb is to place the hand (its working unit) in a position of function, and a mobile shoulder, elbow and wrist are of little use unless they are supported by a functional hand. By contrast, providing the level of recovery in the lower limbs gives *stability*, especially at the hip and knee, the patient's chances of learning to weighbear and walk are better.

The therapist will note that, as recovery begins at the proximal joints, i.e. the hip and shoulder, and progresses distally to the foot and hand, the controlling unit of the lower limb (the hip) has a greater chance of regaining functional use than the working unit of the upper limb (the hand).

Therapists working in hospitals with specialist approach to treatment may find that methods and principles vary. Many centres, for example, have swung right away from the traditional treatment of calipers, unilateral walking aids and sling supports for the affected upper limb and now use a bilateral approach to encourage awareness and movement of the affected side; rigid external support is discouraged. The methods most commonly used are briefly described below. Should the therapist work in a centre where they are practised, she will have to gain additional practical and theoretical knowledge in order to become familiar and competent with them.

1. *The bilateral approach.* This technique was described by Dr Berta Bobath and aims at inhibiting primitive reflex activity and facilitating the righting and equilibrium reactions. Emphasis is placed on bilateral activity and particular attention is paid to careful positioning during lying, sitting, working and walking in order that spastic reflex patterns do not inhibit activity.

2. *Proprioceptive neuromuscular facilitation (PNF).* This technique is based on use of the

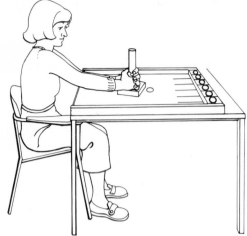

A Shove ha'penny using a pusher

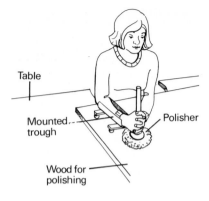

B Polishing with the aid of sliding trough on mini-castors

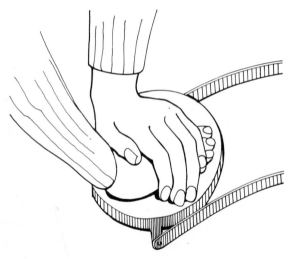

C Printing—the strong hand is placed on the weak one for support

Fig. 19.12 Bilateral upper arm activities

natural diagonal and rotational movements which are facilitated by touch, pressure and stretch.

3. *Brunnström.* This is a traditional method aimed at controlling flexion and extension through mass movement patterns and reflex movements.

Upper limb. Even before functional use has returned it is important that the affected limb is considered during all activity. It should be placed so that the patient can see it and therefore remain aware of it when seated at a table, for example during writing or eating (see Fig. 19.11). Alternatively, weight can be taken through it so that

it supports the patient whilst the other limb is used, for example, for dressing or working with the other limb. In this way rotation and righting reactions can be encouraged.

Bilateral activities with the hands clasped can help to retain range of movement at the affected shoulder, elbow and wrist, to promote awareness of the affected side and to prepare the upper limbs for individual function. Useful activities are: rolling (e.g. making coil pots or rolling pastry), pushing (e.g. sanding, polishing, cleaning a blackboard or playing simple table games with large 'men'), lifting large, light objects (e.g. solitaire pegs) or rotating (e.g. painting, varnishing or stirring) (Fig. 19.12A–C and Fig. 19.13).

As movement improves, activities involving an individual action from the affected limb can be encouraged. Such activities should initially involve a large range of movement, offer little resistance and, where possible, be rhythmical. Additional activities which encourage supination and extension (especially of the fingers, wrist and elbow) are particularly valuable. Numerous activities come to mind, and bagatelle, printing unadapted, making coil or slab pots, correlating, guillotining, planing, finger painting and pastry making are just a few which could be considered.

Where good recovery occurs, late-stage activities should aim to increase coordination, dexterity and strength in the affected limb. Finer activities should be used, and macramé, composing type, wood carving, rubbing in pastry or cake mix, playing small table games and clay modelling may be useful.

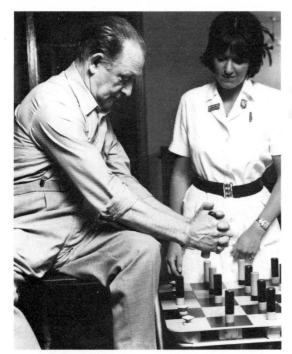

Fig. 19.13 The patient sits sideways to encourage spinal rotation and balance

If recovery is slow or incomplete, dexterity and independence with the remaining strong hand must be improved. The therapist should still remember to ensure that the affected limb is safely and positively positioned and that it is used as a 'prop' or support where appropriate. Remember also that if the patient now has to cope with his once non-dominant hand, fine-control activities, such as writing or sewing, need only be pursued to the level required by that patient. For example, it would seem unnecessary to spend a long time practising writing or stitiching if the patient will in all probability only ever have to sign his name or possibly sew on a button.

Aids as an assistance to returning function should be kept to a minimum. Stablising aids seem the most necessary, and non-slip matting, bowl stabilisers or suction pads can prove invaluable.

Lower limb. Again, in the early stages of recovery good positioning is important, especially when the patient is working. When seated, both feet should be flat on the floor and weight taken evenly through both limbs. When standing, support from a Sutherland harness across the pelvis will help maintain a good posture; support to the front of the

knee to prevent flexion may be necessary. If the patient is unable to stand unaided he can sit on a Camden stool set high to encourage the feeling of weight being taken through his limbs. A mirror may help some patients correct their posture but self education through response to sensory feedback is preferable.

When standing, activities should encourage even weight distribution and the transference of weight from side to side and later from front to back, when one leg is placed in front of the other. Correlating, planing, sanding, playing large table games, weaving and printing with the paper piled on each side of the press may be done standing or sitting, as can activities to encourage speech, sensory or perceptual problems.

As movement increases, activities that encourage walking, coordination and greater balance can be introduced. Many activities come to mind, including lathe work, a tyre for balancing, skittles, remedial floor games and the pottery wheel. The therapist will find that some centres actively discourage activities which require great effort from the strong limb (e.g. the bicycle or treadle fretsaw) as it is felt that such effort increases spasticity in the affected limb.

Throughout treatment the therapist should ensure that the patient maintains a good posture and walking pattern. Where walking aids or supports such as calipers are used she should check that these are correctly adjusted and, in the case of calipers, not causing discomfort or chafing.

Sensory and speech difficulties

It is important that a positive and organised approach is made to the treatment of sensory difficulties. The therapist must guard against a concentration of the treatment on the immediately obvious motor problems to the exclusion or detriment of her patient's other dysfunctions. Some methods of treating sensory problems are described below.

Anosognosia. This neglect is treated in several ways. The therapist can, for example, sit opposite the patient and ask him to identify and touch different parts of the body by saying 'Lift your right arm', 'Touch your nose' or 'Touch my shoulders'. The patient should be asked to distinguish between left and right as well as to demonstrate

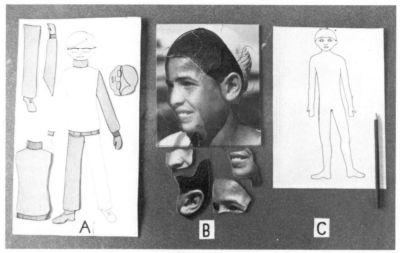

Fig. 19.14 Activities to treat anosognosia and/or body image disturbances. A. Body block matching B. Face puzzle C. Body outline tracing

different areas of the body. The therapist may also use body block or face puzzle completion activities or ask the patient to trace and then copy a body drawing (Fig. 19.14). During activities which require the specific use of parts of the body, such as dressing, washing or bathing, the therapist should emphasise both verbally and physically the parts involved by rubbing or patting the limb at the same time as saying 'Put your weak arm into your sleeve' or 'Wash your strong leg'. Bilateral work and good posture will also help to encourage use and awareness of the weak side. For some patients a mirror may help. If the patient ignores the weak side, for example when combing his hair or putting on clothing the therapist should draw attention to his neglect and physically assist him to correct it.

Agnosia. Where visual agnosia is present the therapist should physically encourage the correct use of objects by placing them in the patient's hand and initiating the movement pattern for him. Familiar objects such as the patient's own clothing, toothbrush or flannel should be used as they may be more easily recognised. Commands should be simple and clear and recognition assisted by the use of many stimuli such as the sound of the word, the feel of the object, a clear view of it and, where appropriate, the smell and the taste.

Apraxia. Here again, the patient needs to be physically and verbally assisted to initiate his

activity. When dressing, for example, the therapist may say 'Put on your shirt' and then take the patient's arm and help him pick up the garment. Similar help can be given during most other activities. Activities and instructions should be kept simple so that a single command requires only one positive response. Encourage automatic responses.

Speech disorders. If the patient has difficulty in understanding instructions (receptive dysphasia) the therapist should ensure that visual or tactile stimuli are given to help the patient's comprehension. For example, when working in the kitchen, cards with clear drawings and simple written instructions can help to reinforce verbal commands. If the therapist wants the patient to weigh out some sugar, for instance, she can ask him to weigh the sugar, at the same time showing him an instruction card. If the sugar, and scales are also easily visible these will act as visual clues.

Where expressive difficulties exist (expressive or nominal dysphasia) communication through writing, gesture or word cards should be encouraged in order to avoid frustration. Continual encouragement to speak should be given, and word matching activities, singing, reading aloud, object recognition and pair matching (for example 'brush and . . .') can also assist.

If the patient has difficulty with the mechanics of speech (dysarthria), activities that involve blowing and sucking (such as the use of straws and blow football using a straw and ping pong ball) will help

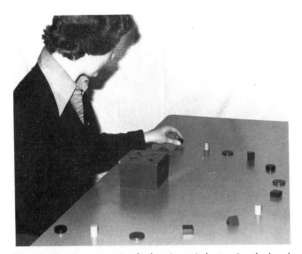

Fig. 19.15 Compensation for hemianopia by turning the head

to stimulate muscle action. Where appropriate, activities to encourage the use of speech control such as singing or miming may be used. The therapist should encourage the patient to always speak as clearly as possible.

Disorders of vision. For the patient with hemianopia the therapist should first ensure that he is aware of his problems and learns to compensate by turning his head to scan the area around him. To reinforce this she can ask him to describe large pictures, to describe the room he is in or to pick out objects from those placed in a large arc in front of him (Fig. 19.15). Assistance can be given

by the use of activities such as Pelmanism, large table games, stoolseating, weaving or painting wide surfaces. When treating the patient, the therapist should stand or sit on the blind side and pass or place objects on that side. Once the patient is aware of his problem, positioning during group activities should be considered so that he must actively make himself aware of other group members (Fig. 19.16). In reading or writing, a ruler can help the patient to work along the whole line, and a heavy margin drawn on both sides of the paper will help him to see its edges as he scans.

Care must be taken in the early stages, that the patient's lack of ability to appreciate objects on his blind side does not lead to ignorance of food, drink, 'Get Well' cards, flowers or people on that side (Figs. 19.17 and 18).

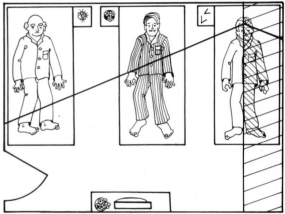

Fig. 19.17 Positioning in the early stages. The patient has a good view of the room, other patients and television

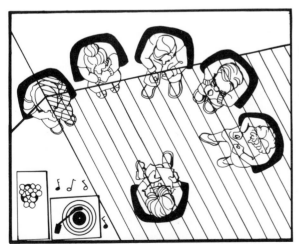

Fig. 19.16 Positioning of the hemianopic patient during group activities. (Note: he must turn his head to see other members of the group)

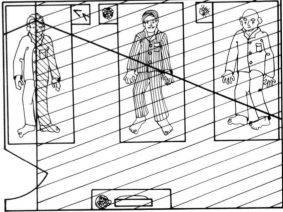

Fig. 19.18 Later positioning. The patient is encouraged to look to his affected side

Other disorders. A patient with proprioceptive problems should be encouraged to compensate visually for his lack of positioning sense. Bilateral activities are important and he should ensure that his limbs are safely and comfortably placed after he has changed his position. Activities such as exercises to music and those requiring a specific placing skill (e.g. the span game or playing cards) can help.

Lack of sensation can be specifically treated by the use of texture dominoes or texture boards. As many different materials as possible should be used, e.g. wool, flour, paper, marbles, soil or water. Activities which give a particularly high sensory input, such as rubbing in pastry, potting plant cuttings, kneading dough, using clay, finger painting or weighing flour and sugar in handfuls, can also help. The appreciation of temperature can be encouraged during washing, cooking, art or pottery.

Figure-ground discrimination can be encouraged by asking the patient to identify single and, later, collections of items placed on a plain background. Identification of object outlines may be used. As his discrimination improves objects can be jumbled together or placed so that they overlap, and a patterned background can be introduced (Fig. 19.19).

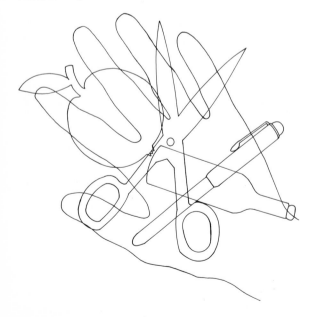

Fig. 19.19 Card used for figure-ground discrimination

Emotional lability usually settles as the patient recovers; while he is still labile the therapist should accept his emotional outbursts, which are usually expressed through crying. She may cope with them by:
● allowing the patient to cry and then recompose himself
● pausing and giving comfort, either verbally or by physical contact such as putting a hand on the patient's shoulder or holding his hand
● pausing slightly and then continuing to talk to allow the patient recompose himself.

The therapist should neither make a fuss about the incident nor ignore it altogether. If should be explained to the patient and his family that such inability to control emotion is quite normal. Some patients are afraid that they have upset and/or embarrassed staff or relatives and should be assured that this is not so.

Depression. The therapist must emphasise activities which the patient can do, and be in a position to show the patient exactly what progress he is making. Group treatment makes it easier for the stroke patient who is depressed to realise that progress can be made. Give activities within the patient's capability or, if hoping to progress and to introduce a new activity, ensure that the new activity is successful, even if some help is given. Instructions should be clear and simple.

Frustration. It is inevitable that the stroke patient will sometimes get frustrated by his performance. The therapist can help him by:

explaining that this is normal and allowing him to express his anger

helping him overcome the problems causing the frustration

not allowing him to continue to reject or ignore unsuccessful situations, but to return to them and help him with them.

Cooperation with other members of the treatment team

As the patient will be treated by members of several different disciplines it is important that all should work with one another. The following are particularly important to the occupational therapist:

All staff treating the same patient should work

out a daily programme to ensure that there is no overlap of treatment sessions. It is not only important, for example, to work out treatment times for occupational therapy, speech therapy and physiotherapy, but also to check whether the patient is required for bathing, X-rays, enemas or other investigations or treatment. Staff meetings help.

Remember when organising the programme that the patient should not be over-tired and that he will need time to rest and see his visitors.

Be aware of which stage the patient has reached in mobility and walking, and always ensure that you use the correct methods for each stage and make the right level of demand.

Ensure that all staff use the same principles of treatment.

If the patient has speech problems allow him time to express himself and if he has difficulty in comprehension give clear and simple instructions. During other activity encourage the patient into conversation, naming objects and describing what he is doing. If resting or relaxing, and at meal times, it is helpful to place the patient with speech problems in a group who will help him and speak to him. Explain to them, if necessary, that he has difficulty in expressing his needs or understanding what is said to him, and that this makes it all the more important to try and include him in conversation.

Report any signs of skin breakdown and difficulty or change in bladder or bowel control as soon as they are noticed.

Avoid asking the patient unnecessary questions. For example, it is unfair if the doctor, social worker and occupational therapist all ask questions about patients' home and social circumstances. Use the patient's notes for information and ask the patient only for information which is needed to fill in gaps.

Resettlement within the community and at work

Throughout treatment it is important to keep in mind the situation to which the patient will be discharged. Remember to teach relatives how to cope and when and when not to help. The hospital occupational therapist should make a home visit as soon as it is possible to assess what degree of mobility and comprehension the patient will have on discharge and where he will be discharged. Avoid a last-minute home visit as, if any alterations will be needed, discharge may be delayed while these are carried out. It is advisable that the hospital occupational therapist, community occupational therapist and patient visit the house together (preferably when the patient's relatives are at home) so that the situation can be accurately assessed and the patient and community occupational therapist can meet each other prior to discharge when the community occupational therapist will probably take over responsibility for the patient's ability to cope at home.

If the patient lives alone or with an elderly relative, gradual introduction back home for a day or weekend may be appropriate. If assessment shows that the patient is unable to return to his former home the alternatives may be considered: Part III accommodation, long-stay hospital care, private or charity nursing homes, warden-controlled accommodation or rehousing. (For further details see Chapter 16). Remember to use community support services where necessary, as these frequently mean the difference between the patient being able to return home or not, and before discharge ensure that all aids/adapatations are ready for use.

Some kind of support is often advisable after discharge. This may come from stroke clubs, day centres, day hospitals, or other associations such as luncheons clubs or Darby and Joan clubs. If the patient was a member of a society or organisation before his stroke, encourage him to return and maintain social contact. It is often reassuring to the patient and/or his relatives to have the name and telephone number of a member of the treatment team who is familiar to them so that they feel they can contact them should difficulties arise.

Treatment can be continued on an out-patient basis after discharge so that recovery can be monitored and helped. It is important to remember, however, that this should only continue until recovery has slowed down or reached a plateau. Support should then be continued away from the hospital. Do not allow a busy department to take the place of a day centre where the patient comes for social support. Recovery can be expected to continue for some time and this should have been explained to the patient and his relatives as soon as possible after the stroke. It is also necessary to explain that hospital support (apart from regular doctor's appointments) will not continue for that length of time. Do not forget to make firm transport arrangements with the patient before discharge so that he has a definite time and date on which to return for further treatment. Remember, however, that the patient should be encouraged to make his own travel arrangements as soon as possible.

If the patient is still of working age it is important that contact be kept with the patient's employer and a work assessment made as soon as the condition has stablised (see Ch. 12). Even if it appears from the assessment that the patient will be unable to return to his old job, the patient's previous employer will be more likely to be sympathetic towards finding him a lighter job within the same firm than a new employer confronted with a 'disabled worker'.

The community therapist may find that very often a person with a mild stroke has not been admitted to hospital and will therefore receive all his medical and other care from the community care team. In such cases she must not only make a clear assessment of the person's abilities and dificulties and solve them through treatment within the home, but also:

involve the client's family by asking for their help in supervising and teaching ADL techniques and other treatments such as exercises, walking and communication skills

make the house as safe as possible so that the client is able to develop his maximum mobility potential

bring in community support services as soon as possible to relieve the family from some of the additional burden

refer, or ask the general practitioner to refer the client for out-patient treatment at his local hospital if it is felt that this would be complementary to treatment carried out at home.

It is clear that the occupational therapist can do much to help the person who has suffered a stroke. It is not only important that she gains experience in the specific skills required to help such a patient, but also that all aspects of the previous lifestyle are considered and helped before the person is considered to be as independent as possible.

The following words from J. G. Somerville, Medical Director, Camden Road Rehabilitation Centre, London should be borne in mind:

There is no point in adding years to life unless you add life to those years.

REFERENCES AND FURTHER READING

Bobath B 1978 Adult hemiplegia — evaluation and treatment, 2nd edn. Heinmann Medical, London

Dalton P 1975 Learning to speak again. The Chest and Heart Association, London

Jay P, Walker E, Ellison A 1966 Help yourselves — a handbook for hemiplegics and their families. Butterworths, London

Johnstone M 1976 The Stroke patient — principles of rehabilitation. Churchill Livingstone, Edinburgh

Light S 1975 Stroke and its rehabilitation. Waverly Press, Maryland

Parry A, Eales C 1976 Hemiplegia. Nursing Times (Series of 5 articles October–November)

Ritchie D 1960 Stroke — a diary of recovery. Faber & Faber, London

Somerville J G 1974 The rehabilitation of the hemiplegic patient. In: The handicapped person in the community — source book. Tavistock ch 41, 350, London

Todd M J 1974 Physiotherapy in the early stages of hemiplegia. Physiotherapy 60 (11): 336–342

Trombly C, Scott A 1977 Occupational therapy for physical dysfunction. Williams & Wilkins, Baltimore

20
Lower limb injuries

An even gait and upright posture require strength, coordination and mobility in the lower limbs, and when one of these is impaired the performance of basic functions such as walking, sitting, standing, running, squatting and climbing can be seriously disturbed. When treating the lower limb, therefore, the therapist must ensure that she aims not only to restore the physical properties of range of movement and strength, but also balance, coordination and control, which are necessary for the activities described above. It is important that, during rehabilitation of a patient with lower limb dysfunction, the therapist encourages correct methods of walking, use of aids, transfers and weight bearing at each stage of recovery, as the development of poor posture and gait can delay or prevent the return of maximum function.

Whatever the disability within the lower limb, the following points should always be considered during treatment:

Although the lower limb can perform adequately without the return of a full range of movement, stability is vital for effective function and may therefore take priority during treatment.

The degree of recovery reached will determine whether full, partial or no weight can be taken through the limb, and this rule must always be observed, whether the patient is receiving treatment or resting.

It is important that the patient wears appropriate, comfortable footwear during treatment sessions. Should the foot itself be affected, plimsolls or other light shoes are advisable and where hip and knee are being treated, low-heeled shoes with a firm support across the instep should be encouraged. Slippers, flip-flops, clogs, boots or shoes with built-up soles and/or heels should be avoided. For some forms of treatment trousers or bare feet are most appropriate and the patient should be informed about this so that he arrives for treatment suitably dressed.

It is useful to have a full length mirror in a department where lower limb injuries are treated so that the patient can observe his own posture and gait.

As with the upper limb, the lower limb should be treated as a functional unit with emphasis on the affected joint.

During immobilisation, joints which are not immobilised should be kept active in order to prevent joint stiffness and disuse atrophy. In some cases, for example at the knee, static exercise of the muscles around the immobilised joint should be encouraged. Although this is usually carried out under the supervision of the physiotherapist, it is important that the occupational therapist reinforces (and on occasions supplements) this treatment.

The therapist should work within the regime preferred by the doctor in charge of each patient.

Following injury, some pain on movement and weight bearing must be expected. The therapist can help to reduce this by using bilateral, rhythmical activities in a warm and relaxed atmosphere. She should emphasise that, although the avoidance of weight bearing through limping or uneven posture will temporarily ease pain, it will have an adverse long-term effect.

Although all joints which have been immobilised will be stiff and the muscles controlling them weak, the joint distal to the site of injury will be particularly affected because of the presence of oedema and possible injury to soft tissues overlying the damaged area.

When strength is being increased, activities offering maximum resistance in the mid-range of movement should be used.

THE HIP JOINT

Stability of the hip joint is vital for an upright posture, as each hip joint bears two-thirds of the body weight when standing and up to four times the body weight during walking. If the hip joint is unstable, walking and movement become uneven and balance is affected. Should the hip extensors be affected, movements such as climbing stairs and standing from sitting become a problem.

By contrast, a stiff hip can be reasonably functional, provided that it flexes sufficiently to allow comfortable sitting (about 90° flexion) and climbing of stairs (between 65° and 70° flexion). Should one hip be fixed, walking, sitting, transfers and stair climbing are still possible, although awkward, provided that the other hip is reasonably functional. This stiffness will, however, add extra strain on the spine and opposite hip joint.

Conditions treated

The following conditions may be referred to the occupational therapist for treatment:

1. *Results of trauma*, such as fractures and dislocations involving the pelvis and the proximal end of the femur; nerve lesions affecting the muscles which control the hip joint. Pathological fractures may occur in elderly patients.

2. *Other conditions*, such as arthrodesis or pseudoarthrosis of the hip joint, some congenital disorders, and non-progressive types of muscular weakness such as anterior poliomyelitis.

Other conditions affecting the hip should be treated according to the principles described in the relevant chapters.

Complications of trauma around the hip include delayed or non-union of a fracture, or malunion; injury to urethra, bladder and bowel with possible subsequent infection, thrombosis, nerve damage (especially to the sciatic nerve following hip dislocation) and avascular necrosis of the femoral head. Elderly patients may become confused and disorientated while in hospital.

Treatment principles

Treatment of conditions affecting the hip will vary according to the age of the patient and the type of disability. The therapist may be asked to treat an elderly person who has suffered a fracture, often as the result of a fall. Internal fixation allows these patients to be up and mobile almost immediately, thus preventing the complications of prolonged bed rest. The therapist's main aim will be the restoration of personal independence and confidence in mobility. Treatment should commence once a comprehensive assessment of the patient's functional ability and level of mobility has been made, and instruction and help with dressing and transfer techniques can prove a sound starting point.

Dressing should be attempted with the patient either sitting on his bed or on a firm chair with both feet firmly on the floor for support. Aids may be needed to help the person reach and put items over his feet and he may need support to boost his confidence during initial attempts at transferring and walking. Principles for assisting such a patient in the activities of daily living are described in detail in Chapter 22. A home visit should be made if appropriate, as many patients often find it difficult to remember in detail the layout of their home and also to transfer the confidence gained in walking on a flat, spacious hospital ward to a more confined and uneven floor at home. During the home visit, the therapist should pay particular attention to the patient's ability to transfer on and off the toilet, bed and favourite chair, his ability to climb stairs and steps, the type and security of floor coverings, and whether he can cope with getting in and out of the bath, reaching high and low shelves and performing basic kitchen and household chores. Should the patient live alone or feel particularly unstable, alternative methods or supportive services should be considered (see Ch. 7). It is especially important to investigate the cause of the accident, particularly if it occurred at home, in order to prevent a recurrence. Falls in the elderly occur not only because of tripping, e.g. over a loose mat or down the stairs, but also because of dizziness following sudden movement of the head and neck. This is particularly common in patients with arthritis of the cervical vertebrae, or those with poor nutrition or similar associated medical conditions. Should the patient complain to the therapist of feeling faint or dizzy on occasions, this should be reported to the doctor.

Although in the elderly the hip itself is rarely treated through specific activity, the therapist may feel it appropriate to help to increase the patient's confidence and balance by simple activities in-

volving standing, walking with a walking aid and sitting on a Camden stool with weight taken evenly through both legs. Familiar activities related to the patient's needs and everyday life, such as cookery, remedial games, craft activities or gardening, can be used. An even gait and good posture should be encouraged throughout treatment. This regime can also be adopted for those suffering from pathological fractures.

The treatment of a younger person with trauma around the hip will involve specific activities aimed at restoring stability and movement of the hip joint and lower limb. The younger person will possibly spend several weeks on traction while his injury is healing and may be referred when walking, partially weight bearing, on crutches. However, the therapist may also be asked to provide supportive therapy during the long period of bed rest and, although many may 'prickle' at the idea of providing something to 'occupy his mind', there can be no doubt that an enforced period of bed rest can be boring and extremely frustrating and may, as a result, delay healing. The therapist, along with other members of the treatment team, will often need to decide on a general policy for her particular hospital. Frequently I have found that the patient is seen by an occupational therapy helper or technician and that realistic activities, regularly supervised, can provide a challenge and talking point for the patient in his restricted environment. It is important that everyone concerned with the patient takes part, and the therapist, helper, nurses, relatives, friends and other patients can all contribute. Activities suggested should be realistic (offering soft toy making to a 19-year-old motorbike rider can hardly be considered appropriate), and if messy, wet or dangerous activities involving sawdust, matches or fumes are considered, these should be carefully organised and supervised. Activities that offer a challenge and/or help the patient to maintain social contacts can be rewarding, and correspondence courses, typing, writing to pen-friends or stamp collecting may make a welcome change from endlessly playing Scrabble or listening to Radio 1!

Once the patient is mobile the therapist should undertake a full physical and functional assessment in order to form a base line for treatment. If there is any extension lag (an inability to maintain

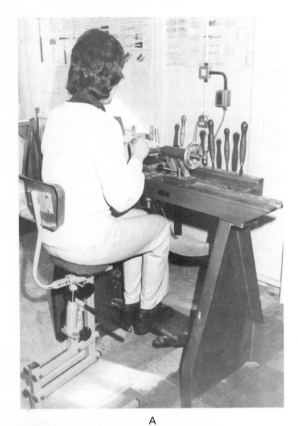

A

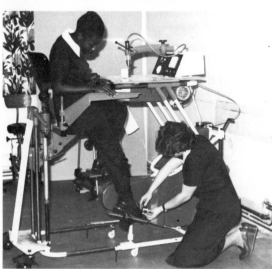

B

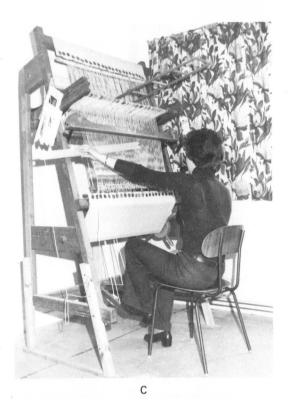

C

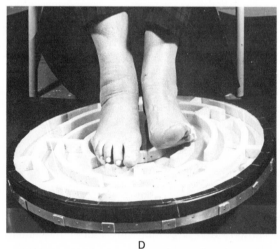

D

Fig. 20.1 Activities suitable for treating the lower limb during the partial weight bearing stage. (A) Wood-turning lathe (B) Electronic cycle (C) Upright rug loom (D) Footmaze

the knee in full extension against gravity), this should be eliminated first in order to ensure stability at the knee; flexion of the knee should be kept to a minimum during this period to avoid overstretching the weak quadriceps muscles (see later

for further detail). Once extension lag has been eliminated, activities to treat the hip and knee joints simultaneously are advisable, as both are likely to be stiff and weak. While the patient is partially weight bearing, work at the wood-turning or pottery lathe while seated on a Camden stool (Fig. 20.1A), the use of the electronic cycle (Fig. 20.1B) in a mid-range of movement with some resistance, bench work with the patient supported on a Camden stool, work on the upright rug loom using the foot pedal change (Fig. 20.1C), and remedial games such as foot noughts and crosses and the footmaze (Fig. 20.1D) (either standing on the strong leg or seated on a tall stool) can all be used.

When full weight bearing is permitted, activities can be upgraded to offer more resistance and an increased range of movement. The electronic cycle can continue to be used with increased range and resistance, as can the woodwork lathe and remedial games. Activities to improve standing tolerance and balance may be introduced, e.g. bench work, printing, cookery or similar work involving standing, leaning and walking. Balancing on the walls of a large tyre for activities such as darts, hoopla or ball games can also help once balance has begun to improve (Fig. 20.2).

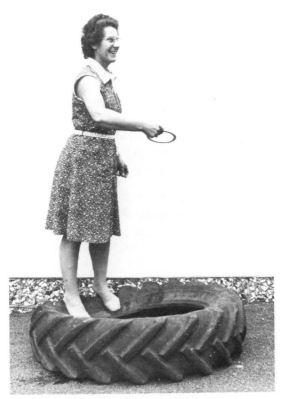

Fig. 20.2 Using a tyre to improve balance

During the final stages of treatment greater resistance can be added and as full a range of movement as possible encouraged. Balance, crouching and work tolerance should also be increased. Use of the bicycle fretsaw can be continued with added resistance and range of movement and the wood turning lathe can also continue as part of the treatment programme. It can now be used by treadling with the weak leg, using a full range of movement, and also by standing on that leg and treadling with the other to increase balance and standing tolerance. Printing may be adapted to offer resistance to hip flexion, extension and abduction (Fig. 20.3), and the footmaze or wobble board can also be introduced (see Ch. 10).

Where appropriate, work assessment should be carried out, and the patient should be encouraged to participate in leisure activities such as active sports, gardening, climbing, swimming and cycling, all of which will continue to strengthen his hip. As already mentioned, a good walking pattern with or without aids should be encouraged throughout treatment.

Where joint arthrodesis has taken place, independence in the activities of daily living will be the primary aim of treatment.

THE KNEE JOINT

Stability of the knee joint is essential for an upright posture, to allow an even gait, to raise, lower and control the body weight for climbing or descending stairs and for kneeling, bending, twisting, crouching, running and jumping.

Should the knee joint be weak or unstable, the above activities become difficult and some may prove impossible. Some problems, such as climbing stairs, may be overcome by locking the knee into extension manually or ascending with the strong leg first and descending with the weak one first, but this procedure is tiresome and slow, and if rehabilitation techniques cannot restore stability, mechanical means such as splints or calipers may need to be considered. By contrast, a person whose knee flexes only to 90° can function adequately in most activities, provided the knee is stable. Should the joint have been arthrodesed

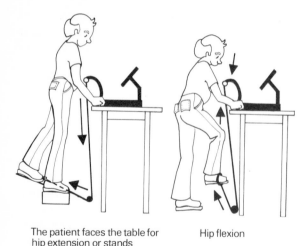

The patient faces the table for
hip extension or stands
sideways on for hip abduction

Hip flexion

Fig. 20.3 Printing adapted to treat the hip joint

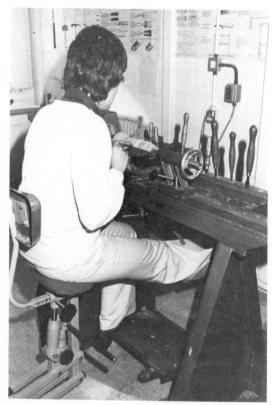

Fig. 20.4 The wood-turning lathe used to encourage
reciprocal action of the quadriceps in the slung limb

because of gross instability, it will remain reasonably functional (as it is now stable), although
rather awkward socially, for instance when sitting
in a car, bus, cinema or crowded room.

Conditions treated

A wide variety of conditions affecting the knee
joint is treated by the occupational therapist.

1. *The results of trauma,* such as fractures of the
mid- or distal section of the femur, of the proximal
or mid-section of the tibia and fibula, and of the
patella; tearing of the menisci (often resulting in
removal) and of the cruciate or other ligaments
around the knee; nerve injuries.

2. *Other conditions.* These include problems
associated with bursae, burns and other skin damage resulting in scarring and/or loss of movement,
and non-progressive muscular weakness.

Other conditions involving the knee should be
treated according to the principles described in the
appropriate chapters.

Complications of injury around the knee include
delayed, non-union or malunion of the fracture,
gross and/or prolonged oedema and nerve damage
(especially to the common peroneal nerve). Weakness and instability may persist, and flexion contractures can occur if the joint is not kept fully
mobile.

Treatment principles

The therapist should make a thorough physical
and functional assessment of the lower limb, noting particularly whether there is any extension lag
at the knee. If this is present, activities should aim
first at strengthening the quadriceps group of muscles in order to eliminate the lag before flexion is
increased. For this purpose the quadriceps switch
(see Ch. 9) can be used, as can bench work or the
lathe set up with the patient's weak leg slung
underneath the work surface to encourage reciprocal action of the quadriceps group whilst treadling. The patient should be seated on a bicycle-
type seat (Fig. 20.4). Weaving can also be adapted
to encourage the outer ranges of contraction of the
quadriceps muscles.

Once extension lag has been eliminated, flexion
— within the limits permitted by the surgeon —
may be encouraged. Initially, flexion should be
gentle and rhythmical; the potter's kick wheel, the
bicycle fretsaw set to gradually increase flexion,
treadling with the weak foot whilst standing, or
bilaterally when seated at the wood-turning lathe,

remedial foot games such as noughts and crosses (see Ch. 10), weaving adapted to encourage knee flexion and the upright rug loom using the foot pedal charge can be introduced. To continue to encourage full strength in the extensors, the quadriceps switch set up with increased resistance and printing using the knee extension adaptation (Fig. 20.5A) can be alternated with these activities. If balance has been greatly affected by the injury, activities to encourage walking, leaning, standing (either unaided, supported by a hip band whilst working at a high bench, or seated high astride a Camden stool) and twisting may need to be included during treatment whilst good posture and a correct even gait should be encouraged throughout.

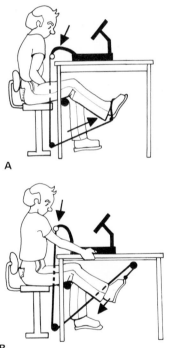

A

B

Fig. 20.5 Printing adapted to (A) strengthen the knee extensors. (B) strengthen the knee flexors. Note: a popliteal bar is used

The activities described above can be used while the patient is still partially weight bearing. Once full weight bearing is permitted the treatment programme can be extended to activities demanding a full range of flexion with greater resistance. The wood-turning lathe can now be set to give full flexion (see Ch. 9), as can the bicycle

fretsaw and printing (Fig. 20.5B). Weaving can also be adapted to encourage full flexion, and weights may be added to the circuit to add resistance to an otherwise lightweight activity (Fig. 20.6). Activities to encourage balance, twisting, crouching and leaning can also be continued, and the wobble board, tyre and skittles can be used. In order to continue to strengthen and increase movement of the injured knee, the patient may be encouraged to play football, swim, cycle, climb and work in the garden.

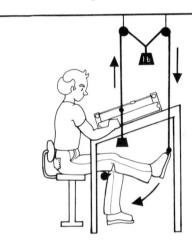

Fig. 20.6 Weaving adapted to encourage knee flexion

In some cases, the therapist will find that her patient does not make a textbook recovery and that his knee continues to be stiff and swollen. If this occurs, treatment should not be too vigorous as this may aggravate the condition; the therapist should aim to improve the gait, balance and work tolerance of her patient and, where possible, encourage the knee to flex to at least 90°, as this will allow adequate function for most activities. Here again, extension lag should be eliminated and the knee made as stable as possible. Attention should be paid especially that flexion contractures do not occur.

THE ANKLE AND FOOT

The architecture and ligamentous support around the ankle and foot combine to give a very stable, yet mobile, functional unit. Considering the shoes we wear — ranging from plimsolls to platform soles, clogs to carpet slippers and winklepickers to wellingtons — and the strain we put on our feet by weekly bursts of vigorous exercise and sudden sprints for the bus — it is a wonder that our feet do not protest more often! Many people are notoriously negligent of their feet and rarely think about them until some injury or disability befalls them.

Any disability of the ankle and foot, whether leaving it stiff or weak, will affect the gait, and sometimes also balance. A weak ankle may 'give way' unexpectedly, especially while negotiating rough ground, turning, twisting or running. Weakness of the foot itself can affect the arches within the foot, and the resulting flat foot can lead to a painful and waddling gait in which the normal heel-toe pattern is lost.

By contrast, a stiff ankle or foot may present little problem if it is stable, provided that the metatarsophalangeal joints are mobile enough to allow a 'push off' during walking. The absence of inversion or eversion in a stiff foot may not be noticed until the patient attempts to negotiate rough ground or drive a car.

Conditions treated

Conditions affecting the ankle and foot are often referred for treatment by the occupational therapist.

1. *The results of trauma.* These include fractures (with or without dislocation) of the distal end of the tibia and fibula (Pott's fracture), of the shafts of the tibia and fibula, and those of the and os calcis (calcaneum). Other fractures within the foot may not be referred for treatment, but rehabilitation may be required following rupture of the Achilles tendon, after crush and nerve injuries and after burns.

2. *Other conditions.* These include some congenital deformities and severe sprains. Although vigorous treatment may be inappropriate for those with rheumatoid arthritis, osteoarthritis, diabetes, hemiplegia and other conditions of the foot, advice on foot care may be necessary.

Complications of ankle injuries include delayed or non-union and malunion. Volkmann's ischaemia may result because of interrupted blood supply, especially in fractures of the tibia, and avascular necrosis can occur, particularly with a

fractured talus. Skin may break down or be slow to heal and pain, swelling and stiffness may persist.

Treatment principles

Where active treatment is appropriate, for example following a fracture or nerve lesion, activities should aim to stabilise and mobilise the ankle and foot as, although stability is vital and must therefore be increased as soon as possible, mobility is often difficult to regain and therefore should be encouraged from the beginning. As oedema often persists around the ankle, rhythmic pumping activities and treatment of the limb in elevation are also important. Problems associated with activities of daily living are rare unless the knee has been affected. A physical assessment of the ankle, foot and knee is necessary, as this latter joint may also have become stiff or weak if it has been immobilised during the early stages of healing. Should extension lag or weakness of the quadriceps be present, this should be treated along with the ankle and foot.

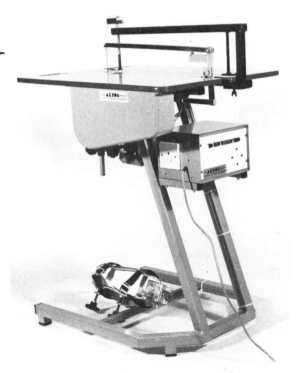

Fig. 20.7 The PIED saw is used to encourage dorsi- and plantarflexion, and inversion/eversion at the ankle

Initial activities should encourage mobility, stability and the reduction of any oedema. Sitting to use the lathe or pottery wheel, remedial foot games, the footmaze, the treadle sewing machine and the PIED saw can all be employed (Fig. 20.7). If the knee is also affected, the bicycle fretsaw (with the seat set high and back to encourage knee extension and plantarflexion at the ankle), bench or lathe work (with the affected leg slung to encourage reciprocal action of the quadriceps muscles and reduction of oedema), weaving adapted to encourage contraction of the outer range of the quadriceps muscles and the quadriceps switch can all be employed to treat ankle and knee simultaneously.

As the ankle and foot improve, activities offering greater resistance and range of movement can be used. The treadle fretsaw can be introduced and activities such as lathe work, use of the bicycle fretsaw and PIED switch can be continued. To encourage active inversion and eversion, and movement of the toes, activities such as games using large cylinders or other objects (to be picked up between the soles of the feet or with the toes) and foot drawing can be performed barefoot by adults. Where appropriate, wedges can be attached to the foot rests of equipment such as the lathe and treadle fretsaws to increase these movements passively (Fig. 20.8). For children modelling, painting, sand play and writing using the feet can add some light relief to treatment. In the final stages of treatment the treadle fretsaw and PIED switch can be continued and the ankle rotator introduced. For balance and coordination the wobble board, use of the tyre and activities en-

couraging squatting or crouching (e.g. skittles or indoor bowls) may be considered. Leisure activities such as cycling, gardening, climbing and dancing, and sports performed barefoot, such as judo, karate and gymnastics, will all continue to increase function of the ankle and foot.

Throughout treatment an even, heel-toe gait should be encouraged and foot care emphasised. Where machinery is used, the foot can be supported and protected during the early stages of treatment by a plimsoll or similar lightweight shoe. Towards the latter stages of treatment, however, muscle work within the foot may be encouraged by leaving the shoe off. Where protection is needed, for example when working on machinery, a thick sock can be worn.

Where active treatment is not appropriate, for example in those suffering from rheumatoid arthritis, osteoarthritis or in the elderly, foot care should be emphasised as part of an overall treatment programme. The wearing of shoes which give support across the instep and do not rub the skin or cramp the toes is important, and the size of socks, stockings or tights should be checked to ensure that they do not cramp the feet. Shoes and socks of natural materials, which allow the feet to 'breathe' and absorb perspiration, are preferable to nylon or plastic footwear but, obviously, finances may cause restriction here. Foot hygiene, however, costs little and it is important that feet should be regularly washed and thoroughly dried. Talcum powder can help, and skin breakdown, especially in the elderly or diabetic patient and those with diminished sensation, should be attended to immediately. It is especially important for those with foot problems to keep toenails short and this may prove quite a problem to the elderly, arthritic or paralysed patient who cannot reach his feet. Aids are rarely successful for this task and frequent attention by a relative, nurse or friend is probably the best answer. Regular exercise and a good walking pattern will help to maintain the tone in the muscles around the feet and ankles; this is especially important in order to preserve the arches of the foot. Exercise will also help to stimulate circulation and thus keep the feet warm. Finally, where overweight puts extra strain on the feet, a weight-reducing diet should be recommended.

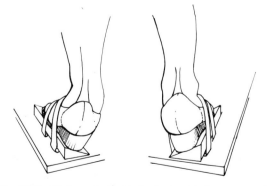

Fig. 20.8 Wedges attached to the foot rests to increase passive movement

REFERENCES AND FURTHER READING

Adams J C 1978 Outline of fractures, 7th edn. Churchill
  Livingstone, Edinburgh
Adams J C 1981 Outline of orthopaedics, 9th edn. Churchill
  Livingstone, Edinburgh
Jones M, Jay P, 1977 An approach to occupational therapy, 3rd
  edn. Butterworths, London
MacDonald E M 1976 Occupational therapy in rehabilitation,
  4th edn. Balliere Tindall, London
Shopland A 1980 Refer to occupational therapy, 2nd edn.
  Churchill Livingstone, Edinburgh
Trombly C A, Scott A D 1977 Occupational therapy for
  physical dysfunction. Williams & Wilkins, Baltimore

21
Multiple sclerosis

Multiple sclerosis (MS) or disseminated sclerosis, is a chronic disease in which degeneration of the white matter of the brain and spinal cord leads to progressive weakness and disability. During the course of the disease the myelin covering of the nerve fibres is destroyed in small patches and the axons become thin and may disappear. These patches eventually become sclerotic and shrunken in appearance, and result in the destruction of the nerve fibre or in its conductivity being seriously affected.

The disease usually attacks young adults between 20 and 40 years of age and appears to be slightly more common in women than in men. It is characterised by remissions and relapses and is the most common disease of the central nervous system in Great Britain.

Causes

The cause of the condition is unknown although several theories have been put forward. It has been thought that the disease may be the result of an infection, an autoimmune reaction or a circulatory disturbance causing transitory or permanent ischaemia in the affected areas. Several factors, however, such as trauma, influenza, sepsis and surgery are known to precipitate a relapse.

As the disease has its highest incidence in temperate climates and is rarely been seen in the tropics, theories relating its cause to climate, lifestyle or diet have also been formulated. In addition, there appears to be an increased familial incidence.

Course

The first manifestations are usually local symptoms such as sudden weakness in one or both lower limbs, visual disturbances or numbness and paraesthesia. These symptoms may disappear after a few days or weeks, and a long period of remission often follows. However, as more plaques appear more attacks occur and permanent symptoms develop depending upon the areas involved. As further symptoms develop, the person becomes more seriously disabled.

Although the course of the disease is usually spread over a period of years, the onset may be acute; widespread involvement can lead to death within a few months.

Diagnosis

Diagnosis is often difficult and many patients may have to wait a considerable length of time before the diagnosis can be confirmed by study of test results together with a history of the condition.

Symptoms and signs

In the early stages of the disease the symptoms and signs may be widespread.

1. *Visual disturbances.* Involvement of the optic nerve and chiasma may give rise to blurring of vision, tenderness of the eyeballs on pressure and pain on movement. Diplopia (double vision), ptosis (drooping of the upper eyelid) or strabismus (squinting) may also be present. These visual disturbances may disappear after a short while and not reappear for several months or years.

2. *Motor and sensory disturbances.* Weakness in one or both lower limbs, accompanied by a feeling of 'dragging' and heaviness, may appear. Paraesthesia giving rise to numbness and tingling in the hands and feet is also common and may be so severe as to become painful. Proprioceptive impairment may accompany these disorders.

3. *Disturbances of bladder and bowel control.* Frequency and urgency of micturition or incontinence of urine can cause particular problems and embarrassment. Retention of urine (or constipation) may also occur.

4. *Mental changes.* Euphoria, though not com-

mon, is perhaps the most striking alteration of the mental state.

As the condition advances and symptoms and signs become more permanent, the problems which arise will depend on the area of the nervous system which is affected. Where, for example, the cerebellar system is disturbed, hypotonus and ataxia will be the main problems.

With pyramidal involvement problems of spasticity (leading to flexor spasm and contracture) and exaggerated reflexes will occur, and with posterior column involvement there will be sensory ataxia and postural control disturbance.

However, in the majority of cases these symptoms and signs are present to a varying degree with only one or two predominant manifestations. Commonly, the condition presents a mixed picture with a jerky ataxic gait, intention tremor, weakness and incoordination in the upper limbs and lack of postural stability in the trunk and proximal joints. Walking and daily living activities become difficult. Frequently, the person suffers extreme weakness and fatigue; if the muscles of speech are affected speech becomes slurred. It is not uncommon for the sufferer to become irritable or depressed.

In the latter stages of the disease extreme weakness, ataxia and loss of movement confine the patient to a dependent existence in bed or wheelchair, and even basic activities such as eating and drinking have to be assisted. Death usually occurs as the result of intercurrent infection.

Treatment

As there is no known cure, the condition is one which must be managed rather than treated. Specific symptoms can be relieved, however. For example, flexor spasms causing problems can be treated by anti-spasmodic drugs or tenotomy. As dietary insufficiency has been thought to be connected with the condition, special diets have been recommended. Those containing sunflower seed oil (either neat or in the form of Naudicelle capsules), or gluten-free diets, are said to be effective in some cases. Some success has been reported with spinal stimulation techniques which seem to particularly improve bladder control, dexterity and mobility. The administration of drugs such as ACTH and cortisone can also help.

The role played by the remedial professions is of great importance. Physiotherapy is invaluable in maintaining and improving balance, coordination and mobility skills, and occupational therapy aims to keep the patient mobile and personally independent for as long as possible. The speech therapist, community nurse and social worker also play an important part in the patient's treatment.

THE ROLE OF THE OCCUPATIONAL THERAPIST

As multiple sclerosis is an incurable, progressive disease occurring primarily in the young and middle-aged, it is clear that the role of the occupational therapist is one of providing long-term assistance and support. As with all progressive conditions, it is unnecessary for the patient to receive continuous active treatment from the therapist. Once a good relationship has been established, an initial assessment performed and immediate problems solved, contact will be maintained at regular intervals so that the therapist can help to maintain the patient at his highest level of physical, personal and social function. The interval between each period of treatment will depend to a large extent on the rate of progression of the disease. For example, if the patient's condition is deteriorating rapidly, it may be necessary to maintain more or less continuous contact with him in order to ensure his continued comfort and maximum ability; if, however, his problems increase more slowly, the stages of treatment described in this chapter may take place over a period of many years. The occupational therapist must at all times work closely with the other members of the treatment team so that a comprehensive and integrated programme of treatment can be offered.

As with all progressive conditions, the therapist will find that the patient will not be admitted to hospital or long-term care unless the problems involved in looking after him become too great for his family. It is essential that a sound working relationship is established with the patient's family so that help and advice can be given to them at all times, as well as relevant information on, for instance, the availability of holiday relief admission to hospital, or attendance allowance.

Aims of treatment

It is extemely difficult in such a short space to discuss in full all the problems associated with multiple sclerosis. Indeed, many of the suggestions made in this chapter can apply, in principle, to the treatment of any progressive paralysis. A case history showing the problems posed by one particular MS sufferer, is given in Chapter 8.

When treating a person with multiple sclerosis, the occupational therapist should aim to:
● assess and maintain the patient's maximum level of personal independence
● advise and support the patient and his family
● maintain and, where possible, restore the patient's fullest physical, mental and social capacity, especially during remissions
● give help and advice with employment.

The initial interview

The first meeting between the therapist and patient is of great importance as it is likely that the relationship established will continue over a period of several years. The therapist should endeavour to gain as full and clear a picture as possible of the patient's family, home and work situation so that priorities for assistance can be established. In addition to this, it is essential that the therapist discovers the patient's attitude towards and knowledge of his condition. Because the onset of multiple sclerosis can be variable in its symptomatology and flitting in nature, it is possible that the patient is referred with only a tentative diagnosis and that he himself has not yet been told of the doctor's suspicions. It is unwise, therefore, to automatically expect the patient to be aware of the nature of his condition; he should be given the opportunity during this first meeting to express the depth of his knowledge and his attitude towards the complaint.

The early stages of treatment

When giving advice and assistance in the early stages of the condition, it is important for the therapist to help the patient and his family to adopt a realistic outlook towards the future. The knowledge that he is suffering from multiple sclerosis may come as a great shock to the patient. He may feel that the future for himself and his family is hopeless and intolerable. However, much can be done to overcome this despondency, and the therapist can help the patient to make the most of his remaining abilities by giving appropriate advice, treatment and support. She must realise that there is no single solution to all the problems which may arise, that changes which may be necessary in the patient's life should take place slowly and that equipment needed to make life easier can be bought over several months or even years; there is no need for the patient or his family to rush out and buy all useful items at once. Problems must be tackled as they arise, and with careful planning many can be minimised or prevented for a considerable period of time.

By contrast, the therapist may find that confirmation of the diagnosis comes as a relief to some patients who have previously been accused of malingering or of imagining their problems. This new certainty can lead to a more positive attitude towards their condition.

Lastly, the therapist, the patient and his family must bear in mind that the confirmation of a diagnosis of multiple sclerosis does not necessarily imply a steady, downhill decline. Often, symptoms remit for long periods and the condition can remain stable for many years. It may be that after an initial period of treatment the patient and therapist will not need to meet again for several years; it is therefore not right to paint a gloomy and pessimistic picture of the future.

Personal independence

As weakness and incoordination of the limbs accompanied by a lack of sensation can seriously affect the level of personal independence, early assistance and advice can not only relieve immediate problems, but also help the patient to choose the most suitable clothing and equipment for future use. As with all patients, aids should be introduced only when absolutely necessary. New methods and suitable equipment will frequently eliminate the necessity for specific aids.

Dressing. Clothing should be lightweight and easy to launder, and styles which are roomy and easy to put on are advisable. Garments should have as few fastenings as possible positioned so that they are easily managed. Where existing fastenings are too small or awkward to handle, adaptions using velcro, large buttons, zips and other methods requiring little effort or coordination are advisable. The material and construction of clothes should be strong, as they will have to stand up to pulling and stretching, particularly where weakness and tremor make dressing difficult. Clothes with a certain amount of 'give', such as those made from knitted, biased or elasticated material, will be easier to put on and take off. As few garments as possible should be worn in order to make dressing easier.

No therapist can expect a patient to completely change his wardrobe; when new clothes are bought, however, she should point out that dressing and undressing will be less tiresome if clothes are easy to put on and take off. Because of lack of coordination and sensation, dressing aids are often ineffective.

Eating. Tremor and loss of sensation in the hands can make eating and drinking a messy and prolonged activity. Insulated mugs will not only protect the hands from burning, but will also keep drinks warm for a longer period. If strength and control in the hands are weak, mugs or cups with two large handles or specially designed mugs such as the Manoy (which requires little precision gripping and can be easily supported in both hands) are advisable. Cups with a lid or the use of a straw may also help.

Plates and dishes can be stabilised on non-slip mats, and if the patient finds it difficult to put food on a fork or spoon, a plate guard or built-up plate can be used. If grip is seriously affected, cutlery with large handles or a loop attached to the handle can help (Fig. 21.1). Lightweight, picnic or padded cutlery may also be tried and weighted bracelets may help to control tremor.

Personal hygiene and use of the toilet. If holding the soap or flannel is hindered by incoordination or weakness, a suction soap holder and washing mitt can often prevent a frantic scramble for the soap bar. For some women, cream cleanser may be easier to use, if a little more costly, than soap; a 'soap-on-a-rope' or a push-button liquid soap dispenser may solve the problem for others.

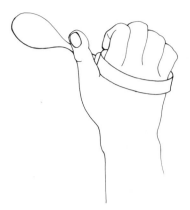

Fig. 21.1 A spoon with a hand strap to help those with poor grip

Shaving can be difficult especially if the person is used to a wet shave and an enlarged looped handle may help in gripping the razor. Electric or battery razors may not be the answer for all patients, as they are heavier to hold, and do not give as close a shave. However, should they be considered, a holder can help the patient to grasp the razor.

Hair care and make-up are other areas where problems may be encountered, as tremor and weakness can make combs, lipsticks, eye pencils and other small objects difficult to handle. Here again enlarged handles may help, but often a change from, for example, a foundation and powder make-up to an all-in-one liquid based variety, or from a liquid to a cake eye-shadow can overcome a difficulty more effectively. A change of habit or style, for example from long to a short haircut or from a style requiring regular setting to one which will fall easily into shape, may also be considered. These points may seem minor and obvious ones to the therapist, but for any person who wishes to remain well-groomed, advice on how to stay smart and fashionable with only minimum effort can be extremely valuable. The therapist may seek help for her patient from a beautician in order that problems such as the growth of facial hair or weight increase due to steroids can be discussed.

When considering problems related to bathing, the main criterion should be the patient's safety in the bathroom. The installation of appropriately placed grab rails by the bath or toilet will help to steady the person during rising, sitting and trans-fer. A non-slip bath mat will help considerably to steady a wet, slippery body in the bath. Baths should not be too hot, as heat weakens the multiple sclerosis patient and if they lack sensation there is a danger of scalding. A hoist may also be considered at this stage, and a self-operated hoist, such as a Mechanaid auto-lift, may allow independence in some cases. As the patient's condition deteriorates, bathing aids may be introduced. An inside bath seat, bath board and/or shower attachment to the taps may solve the problem for some, whereas for others the installation of a shower unit may be appropriate as a long-term solution. This can make washing easier not only in the early stages but also later when the person becomes more disabled and may need a plastic chair, stool or wheeled shower chair for safety and easier bathing.

Home management

Cooking The ability to remain safely independent in the kitchen for as long as possible is important for the patient suffering from multiple sclerosis, as this will allow him to retain a useful role in the household and not feel a total burden on his family. It is difficult to enumerate all the problems which may arise and impossible to give definite solutions. However, the therapist should consider the following principles when assessing a person's level of function in the kitchen:

If mobility is affected, an easily managed and cleaned kitchen with an open lay-out will be a great advantage. Aids to mobility such as a firm trolley or stable work surfaces can eliminate the need for a walking aid which may clutter the kitchen. If fatigue, weakness and incoordination affect mobility, the therapist should help the person to plan his daily activities so that energy is reserved. Where possible, tasks such as ironing, vegetable preparation and washing up which are usually done standing, should be practised sitting as this gives better stability and is less tiring. If the person uses a wheelchair, special features such as domestic arm rests and trays may increase his mobility in the kitchen.

The floor surface should also be considered. A wall-to-wall floor covering is ideal; but where this is impossible, non-slip polishes can be used to help prevent slipping; loose edges should be secured. To minimise stretching and bending, long-handled tools, such as brushes and dusters can be suggested, and items in everyday use should be stored at the most convenient height. Electric switches and points can also be made more accessible by raising them from the skirting board or by replacing knobbed wall switches with modern rocker or pusher designs. The use of a perching stool may help to save the energy of those who are still mobile.

For safety, all members of the family should be encouraged to wipe up any spills as quickly as possible.

If sight is affected large, clear labels on storage canisters may help with identification. Colour coding can be used to save confusion, and handles and knobs on cupboards and drawers may be easier to see if they are painted in a contrasting colour. Much supervised practice may be necessary to help the patient gain confidence in the kitchen.

If tremor affects coordination and if sensation is impaired, equipment should be carefully checked to ensure that it is securely made, easy to handle and not likely to cause burns. Large wooden handles placed over existing metal or enamelled handles of saucepans, colanders or similar items will not only make them easier to hold but will help prevent burns. Guards on the stove to prevent saucepans being knocked over can prove invaluable, and a continuous level work surface, especially between sink and stove, will eliminate much lifting. Special care must be taken when putting food into the oven or taking it out. A well-designed oven-glove and a small wooden stool, placed in front of the oven, on which to put items for basting, stirring or steadying before carrying them to the work surface can be very useful. Basic tools such as vegetable knives and wooden spoons may need adapting with enlarged or lengthened handles and, again, hints about labour-saving equipment such as electric mixers and toasters can be dropped before Christmas and birthdays!

Owing to the long-term management problems presented by multiple sclerosis it may well be wise for the family to plan ahead to the time when the patient may not be able to play his full role in household management. It may be advisable to start saving for large items of equipment such as washing machines, cookers and cleaners early on, not only so that the patient can learn to use them at this stage but also because the family may find that they are financially better able to cope with major expenditure at this stage.

Cleaning and laundry. Here again, no one solution is 'correct' for any particular problem or circumstance and the therapist must learn to treat each case individually. Splitting the weekly washing, ironing and cleaning into smaller parts so that a little can be done each day may be the answer for some patients, while for others using a laundrette once a week and the services of a home help to tackle major cleaning jobs may work well. Again, the therapist and family must discuss long-term solutions. It would be unsuitable, for example, to suggest that the family use a private laundry service for sheets and towels 'for the moment', when it is clear that their budget cannot cope with such expense over a long period. Planning is an important consideration in many areas; for example, as bedding wears out it may be replaced by non-iron sheets or a duvet. The purchase of easy-care clothes and the use of fabric softeners can also reduce the washing and ironing load. The use of a duvet may also help those who find that the weight of blankets makes moving and turning in bed difficult.

Transport and shopping. Much will depend on the area in which the patient and other family members live, when problems associated with shopping arise. It is true that frequently other members of the household take over the main weekly shopping, but where this cannot be arranged or if the patient wishes to continue to shop at least for more personal items such as clothing, furniture or presents, the therapist should be aware of the services available to help.

1. *Mobility aids.* Combined carrying and walking aids are now available and, where appropriate, should be discussed with the patient, It may be advisable to supply a wheelchair for outdoor use so that, even if a person is able to walk around inside a shop, he can be wheeled around the town or to the shops in order to save effort.

2. *Transport.* Help is available for both the disabled driver and a disabled passenger (see Ch. 6), and the therapist must be aware of facilities

such as parking concessions and the mobility allowance which may be available to her patient.

3. *Purchasing goods..* Although few shops will deliver groceries these days, some stores will supply goods such as clothes or shoes on approval to a disabled customer. Mail order catalogues are obviously a useful method of purchasing some items and not only overcome shopping problems, but can also serve as a source of pocket money and a means of social contact if the patient becomes an agent for the mail order firm. Similarly, home purchase schemes such as those run by 'Avon', 'Tupperware' and 'Pippa Dee' can serve a useful purpose.

General mobility and housing

Very often, quite minor alterations to the home lay-out or daily programme can help the sufferer from multiple sclerosis to stay mobile. For example, furniture can be arranged to allow as free a passage of movement as possible, especially when walking aids or a wheelchair need to be used indoors. If stable furniture is thoughtfully arranged the need to use such an aid around the house can often be eliminated, as the furniture can provide the necessary support. Where this is not possible grab rails can be fitted. These are especially useful where transfers or steps are negotiated, for example by the toilet or near an internal step from hall to kitchen. An additional bannister may be necessary and the therapist should ensure that this is long enough to provide sufficient support both at the top and at the bottom of the stairs.

If the person tires easily or finds walking up and down stairs especially trying, his day should be planned so that as few trips upstairs as possible are needed. Should the patient only feel safe to use the stairs when someone else is around, the therapist must decide whether a commode or urinal should be supplied for use downstairs during the day.

When the supply of a wheelchair seems advisable to aid mobility, the therapist will need to choose an appropriate time to tactfully suggest this. Many people see the reliance on a wheelchair as 'the beginning of the end', and if the subject is not broached well it may be rejected out of hand.

Access to the home must be considered, along with associated items such as door handles and locks. Looking at long-term solutions to mobility problems, the family may consider major changes such as an extension to their home in order that the patient (and spouse) can sleep downstairs and also have a suitable bathroom/toilet on ground level. The therapist must be aware of grants and assistance available for moving to a flat, bungalow or other suitable accommodation. Where council property is concerned, application for suitable housing, backed up by a letter from the patient's doctor, may mean that the family can settle into an easily run home as soon as possible. Considerations such as applying for a specially designed home for the disabled, or moving to a house nearer relatives, friends, work, school or shops are equally important.

Social interaction

If problems such as loss of mobility and coordination, impairment of speech or difficulty in controlling the bladder make social intercourse difficult, the therapist should discuss with the patient and his family the help available to them and explain the importance of maintaining an active social life for as long as possible.

Communication. As the patient finds it increasingly difficult to go out and maintain contact with friends and relatives, the ability to keep in touch with them from home is important. If the house has no telephone the patient may be entitled to some assistance with its installation not only for social reasons, but also for emergencies, especially if he is left alone during the day. If the patient already has a telephone, but finds it increasingly difficult to use, the GPO can help to find the most suitable model for him. The patient should be advised to speak more slowly if troubled by dysarthria, and liaison with the speech therapist is important.

If writing has become a problem, a change of pen, for instance from a ball-point to a felt-tip pen, may help for a while. If the patient finds it difficult to hold the paper steady, a writing board, non-slip pad or magnetic support can be suggested. An electric typewriter may prove the answer, and the patient may find that learning to type will keep him both socially active and at work. A guard may help the patient in the use of his typewriter.

Interests and pastimes. The patient may find that

active hobbies such as some sports, or those requiring fine coordination, e.g. dressmaking or car maintenance, quickly become impossible for him. The therapist must realise that in all progressive conditions the ability to occupy leisure hours productively and enjoyably will become increasingly important, especially if the patient finds that he can no longer continue in his role of wage earner and homemaker. Interests that involve the patient and his family are particularly rewarding, for it is so easy for the family unit to become isolated, especially if they have no common interests outside the home. Interests that can be continued even when the patient becomes more handicapped are particularly helpful and ornithology, stamp collecting, the study of local history, fishing, photography, home brewing, radio hamming and the joining of a local debating society or language circle may be considered.

Clearly, the choice of a new hobby will depend greatly on the interest and financial ability of the patient, and no therapist should be heard to remark 'Well, I think you should take up ...'. However, it is important that she does not ignore the social aspects of the patient's life. She should be aware of clubs, associations or societies in her area, and ready to give advice, assistance and information about taking up a different hobby. Some areas run clubs especially for handicapped people and these may be appropriate for the patient, but it is very likely that he will prefer the company of able-bodied people at this stage.

All efforts should be made to help the person to continue with his existing hobbies for as long as he can. Sport and other outdoor pursuits should be encouraged as they not only help the patient maintain a normal life, but also keep him physically fit and mentally alert and challenged. A family with young children may join a baby-sitting circle in order to have some free evenings. If the mother is the MS sufferer, relief from looking after the children for part of the day, either by baby-sitters or play-groups is particularly important in order to give her a rest or allow her to shop or visit friends without the additional constraints imposed by youngsters.

Figures show that the divorce rate amongst MS sufferers is high, and the therapist may find that her patient is lonely and isolated. In this case the purposeful fulfilment of leisure time is especially important. She may find it necessary to help a man who now has to cope alone with basic homemaking techniques.

Physical function

The therapist should encourage the patient to remain as active as he can for as long as possible. He may need periods of intensive specific treatment in the occupational therapy and physiotherapy departments in order to maintain maximum level of function, especially after an exacerbation.

Coordination. Activities to regain and improve coordination can greatly assist the patient's confidence. Large, bilateral lightweight activities such as weaving, pottery, work on the bicycle fretsaw, woodwork and stool-seating can be used. Large table games are also valuable and at the same time encourage social contact, especially for those embarrassed by speech problems.

Mobility. If the patient is to remain active walking aids may be necessary, and the community therapist may be required to assess for and supply a suitable aid. She should check heights of bed, chair and toilet for ease of transfer. Good posture should be encouraged and a normal heel-toe gait maintained for as long as possible. Correct standing and sitting (i.e. without crossing the legs) should be encouraged; sideways lying in bed will help reduce spastic patterns. The use of standing tables may also be helpful.

Stamina. A rest-exercise programme (REP) has been shown to increase the level of physical function in some MS patients. This programme consists of two or three periods of strenuous exercise a day, each followed by a rest period of 10 to 20 minutes. The occupational therapist may find that the activity programme could be planned in this way.

The Multiple Sclerosis Society (which has a junior branch called 'Crack') aims to help sufferers from multiple sclerosis, and their families, by raising money for research, organising local branches to provide social contact and practical advice, and running holiday homes for patients and their families. The therapist should inform the patient of the existence of the society and be able to outline the benefits of joining the local branch.

The society produces a magazine which each member receives. This gives information on new developments in research and also on the society's own activities. The society may also help with the provision of specific larger aids such as standing frames and exercise bicycles.

Work

If the patient can continue to go to work for as long as possible he will not only benefit physically and financially, but also by maintaining his wage-earning role in the family and retaining contacts with friends and colleagues. Once the patient's existing job becomes difficult for him, or he becomes unsafe or hinders others (because of lack of sensation, coordination or reduced mobility), alternative employment needs to be considered. If at all possible he should remain with his current employer, as the goodwill, pension rights, familiarity and social contact already established will be a great advantage. As the patient with known MS may find it difficult to be accepted for retraining, he should discuss the possibility of a transfer to a lighter or supervisory job, or to part-time work with his employer and the Disablement Resettlement Officer. It is more likely that a firm in which the patient is well known will make allowance for his problems, and his workmates will no doubt be more tolerant towards his awkwardness. The therapist should ensure that transport to and from work is as easy as possible and that if help is required at work, e.g. with adapted tools or equipment, the patient's case is presented to the appropriate authorities.

The later stages of treatment

As the condition progresses and the patient becomes more disabled the therapist will find that he and his family are having to come to terms with his changing role both at home and at work. He will find that because of increased immobility, weakness and tremor he will probably have to give up work, unless he can continue in an advisory or supervisory capacity. His family will have to help him more and more at home and socially, and if the patient has been the major bread winner and has had to cease work, the other partner may need to find work in order to support the family. This arrangement, added to the financial strain imposed by the disabled person, can put tremendous pressure on the household, especially if there are young children and no relatives close at hand to relieve the stress. Mental changes such as euphoria, depression and intellectual deterioration can also strain relationships and make the patient unrealistic about his capabilities.

Personal independence

As the ability to remain personally independent decreases the therapist will need to deal with each presenting problem in the way which is most suitable to the patient and his family. Once dressing becomes a prolonged or impossible task the patient's relatives should be shown the easiest way to support, dress and move the patient to make him comfortable. If the patient is incontinent suitable protective clothing should be discussed and the availability of laundry services investigated. Incontinence affects a great many MS patients and can be a source of acute embarrassment and worry. Easy access to the toilet (or other facilities) is vital and personal hygiene must be stressed. Catheterisation may be considered in the later stages (see Ch. 3). Where dressing, washing or settling the patient becomes too difficult for the relative or spouse, it may be appropriate to arrange nursing or similar services. It is important that the patient does not spend too much energy on these activities, as there are other, more enjoyable or important things to do, e.g. a trip to the shops or visiting friends. Regular attendance at a day centre can help the patient to retain a degree of independence for as long as possible.

Eating. The indignity of being fed is often very distressing to the patient. It is obviously important that independent feeding is prolonged as long as possible, and easily held spoon and feeder cups may be considered.

Washing, bathing and use of the toilet. When the patient becomes too heavy to be helped in and out of the bath or too incapacitated to use bath aids, an attendant-operated hoist should be considered and the family taught how to use it. A shower or commode chair can be extremely helpful, as it can be wheeled into the shower so that the person can be washed from a sitting position. A bed bath, either from a relative or the community nurse, is another alternative.

When immobility makes use of the toilet difficult, a commode, urinal or commode facility in the patient's wheelchair may be considered. While the toilet remains accessible the relatives should be taught to help the patient with transfers. Supports to assist his posture whilst sitting on the toilet (such as the toilet aid made by Mecanaid Ltd) could be supplied.

Home management

Although the patient will take a decreasingly active role in the running of the home it is important that he maintains a role there for as long as possible. Tasks such as writing letters, planning menus or washing dishes can be done without pressure and may make him feel that he is at least contributing in a small way to home life.

If running a home, providing an income and caring for the patient puts too great a stress on the family, the therapist must be able to call upon the services of other agencies, e.g. the home help and Meals on Wheels services, or other local groups who may visit or take the patient out. The therapist should also consider whether the patient is eligible for such financial help as attendance allowance or housewives' non-contributory invalidity pension. It may be appropriate that the patient attends for an assessment period at a specialist centre such as Mary Malborough Lodge in Oxford, where all problems of independence and mobility can be fully assessed and discussed and specialist equipment recommended as appropriate.

General mobility and housing

When walking even short distances becomes impossible a suitable wheelchair is essential to ease the burden of immobility.

The principles for choosing a wheelchair are dealt with in Chapter 6. The therapist may find that an electric wheelchair is necessary and that restraining straps, heel or toe straps, a head support, sheepskin mat to help prevent pressure sores, commode facilities or U-shaped cushions to take a urinal are features which should be considered. A

gel or ripple cushion may help to relieve pressure areas.

House alterations and mobility aids will now become extremely important. A stairlift or a suitable hoist, for example, may be considered. Ramps to take the wheelchair may need to be fitted and additional heating may be required to keep the immobile person warm. A ripple or electric mattress may help the patient who spends the major part of his day in bed. If it proves impractical to alter the house so that the patient can get upstairs, alternatives such as bringing the bed downstairs, building an extension or moving house may have to be contemplated. Sadly, such major adjustments can be difficult if finance is limited and homes are small with just one living room, or if suitable housing is scarce, and it is often this final stress on family life which dictates long-term care, e.g. in a young chronic sick unit or Cheshire home. Obviously, such a move may have to be made earlier by a single person or one whose marriage has broken down due to the strains imposed by multiple sclerosis. For the family to remain together as long as possible in the easiest of circumstances should be the joint aim of the medical team. All should be aware of the stresses that can occur and of additional services such as marriage guidance counsellors, the 'Sexual Problems for the Disabled' group (SPOD), the Church, Samaritans or other supportive groups. Holiday relief is also important to allow both patient and relatives to have a break from routine, and such facilities as exist both locally and through the Multiple Sclerosis Society, should be made known to them.

Social interests

Social contact is extremely important as the patient's ability to leave the home diminishes. Company at home, whether from pets, visitors or assistants, can prove a great boon to him. Pets that he can look after himself, such as fish, cage birds or hamsters, can give special companionship. Cats, who are fairly self sufficient, or birds feeding at a bird table can also bring company and supply a valuable source of conversation. If friends or relatives find regular visiting difficult voluntary groups such as the Red Cross, Scouts or other youth groups will often visit, not only for company, but also to read or write letters where this may help. To help pass long hours, large-print books, mobile libraries, talking books or educational courses on television and radio should be considered. Again, a telephone can be a valuable source of communication and a POSSUM unit may also be appropriate.

To help the person remain in contact with life outside the home the attendance at a day centre, lunch club or similar can give him an interest and at the same time help to relieve the family. Pen-friends or other correspondence outlets may be considered.

Physical function

Exercises to help maintain as high a level of physical function as possible are usually the province of the physiotherapist at this stage. The occupational therapist, however, may find it necessary to provide positioning splints to reduce deformity; she must ensure that activities are performed in the best position to ensure the patient can fulfil his highest physical potential. Activities which encourage as much movement as possible, such as painting, light cookery, indoor gardening and board games, should be continued for as long as possible.

Work

Even though the person with multiple sclerosis may have to come to terms with the loss of income, status and social contact caused by an early retirement, it may be appropriate to consider employment at home or in a sheltered workshop. Keeping the status and financial benefit provided by work for as long as possible may make it easier for the patient and his family to accept his increasing disability.

The occupational therapist, especially when working in the community, will no doubt be asked to treat a patient with multiple sclerosis at some time, and she will find working with such a patient and his family rewarding and exacting. She will see great relief brought by a sensitive and practical answer to a seemingly insurmountable problem. Similarly, the therapist working in a hospital will be able to give much help and support through a programme of exercise, advice and assistance in personal activities.

REFERENCES AND FURTHER READING

Atkinson J 1974 Multiple sclerosis — a summary for nurses and patients. Wright & Sons, Dorchester
Cash J 1974 Neurology for physiotherapists. Faber & Faber, London
Macdonald E M 1976 Occupational therapy in rehabilitation, 4th edn. Balliere Tindall & Cassell, London, ch 10, p 200
Matthews B 1978 Multiple sclerosis — the facts. Oxford University Press, Oxford
Ribeiro J 1978 Spinal cord stimulation in the treatment of patients. British Journal of Occupational Therapy 41 (10) October: 342-3
Shopland A et al 1979 Refer to occupational therapy. Churchill Livingstone, Edinburgh

22

Osteoarthrosis

Osteoarthrosis (*osteon* — the bone, *arthron* — the joint, *-osis* — relating to a condition or disease process) is a degenerative disease of joint surfaces associated with ageing. Any joint may be affected, but the patient usually presents with problems in the larger, weight-bearing joints.

Osteoarthrosis occurs most commonly in patients past middle age and, indeed, the radiological changes associated with it are almost universally present after the age of 55. The incidence is the same in both sexes, except in primary generalised osteoarthrosis, which is ten times more common in women. The hips, knees and spine are most frequently affected, but any other joint can be involved. Perhaps the commonest incidence in primary generalised osteoathrosis is in the first carpometacarpal and metatarsophalangeal joints.

As surgical treatment of osteoarthrosis becomes more successful, more occupational therapists are asked to treat patients during the period of rehabilitation following joint replacement surgery. However, the occupational therapist is also needed to treat and advise patients who are receiving conservative treatment and those being prepared for surgery. This chapter aims to discuss the role of the occupational therapist during preparation and rehabilitation. Much emphasis is put on the treatment of those having undergone treatment for lower limb disease, although the upper limb is also frequently involved and surgical procedures not uncommon. The role of the occupational therapist in the treatment of the upper limb is discussed in detail in Chapters 17 and 28.

Causes

Osteoarthrosis may be primary or secondary.

Primary Osteoarthrosis arises from no known cause, although there does appear to be some familial tendency.

Secondary Osteoarthrosis arises in response to a number of conditions:

(a) *Congenital causes*. Congential dislocation of the hip, especially if undetected, or other bony or joint deformity can lead to the development of osteoarthrosis in later life due to the continuous abnormal stress put on the joint and the incongruity of the opposed surfaces.

(b) *Acquired causes*. Osteoarthrosis can occur as a result of:

1. conditions causing irregularity of a joint surface, e.g. avascular necrosis, Perthes' disease of the hip or osteochondritis dissecans of the knee

2. trauma, such as fractures which cause malalignment of the joint, fractures in which the joint surface has been involved making it irregular, or those where loose fragments of cartilage or bone have been left within the joint

3. repeated trauma. This is especially related to certain occupational diseases and is particularly important with regard to the upper limb

4. septic or other arthritis. This causes destruction of the articular cartilage

5. obesity. This causes undue wear and tear, especially of the weight-bearing joints such as the foot, knee and hip.

Pathology

Initially, the articular surface becomes rough, and the cartilage degenerates and becomes flaky and worn away. The radiological examination shows a narrowing of the joint space. Eventually the cartilage disappears in some areas, exposing the underlying subchondral bone. This in turn becomes thickened, dense and eburnated (polished), and at the margins of the joint buttressing osteophytes are formed. Where the bone is denuded, synovial fluid may enter and form cysts within the bone. Lubrication of the joint is affected causing it to become dry and creaky. As a protective mechanism muscles close to the joint may go into spasm, or they may waste due to pain and the protective postures adopted by the patient.

Diagnostic investigations

The synovial fluid appears clear, yellow and non-inflammatory, although some debris may be present; laboratory tests are normal. X-rays, however, show the loss of joint space, sclerosis of the underlying bone, subchondral cysts, osteophytes and irregularity of the joint surfaces. Blood tests are normal unless the osteoarthrosis is secondary to a biochemical disorder such as gout or a rheumatic disease such as rheumatoid arthritis.

Clinical features

The condition usually presents in one joint initially and the *symptoms* include:

● pain with or after movement, which is worse at the end of the day and often in bed at night

● stiffness in the affected joints, especially after a period of immobility and in the morning

● deformity, particularly valgus deformity of the knees or apparent shortening at the hip

● referred pain, particularly with spinal involvement. If the cervical spine is affected pain is often referred to the shoulder or down the arm. Similarly, if the lumbar spine is affected sciatic pain can result.

Physical Signs of the condition can include:

● bony deformation and tenderness around the affected joint

● increased warmth, redness and fluid swelling in the joint during acute episodes; crepitus and later deformities

● instability of the joint.

The joint may be unstable due to the loss of the articular surface and cartilage and to associated soft tissue changes. This is especially so in cases where osteoarthrosis has occurred secondary to rheumatoid arthritis.

Swelling may be marked and is initially bony, although acute episodes will be associated with an effusion into the joint. The disease makes slow, relentless progress.

Treatment

Osteoarthrosis cannot be cured. However, symptoms can be relieved both by the patient's efforts and by treatment.

The patient, for example, may naturally avoid aggravating factors. He may hold the joint in a relaxed position and avoid use under load. The hip, if involved, will characteristically be held in a position of slight flexion, external rotation and adduction. The patient will also limp because the hip joint takes a load in excess of three times the body weight during normal walking. This is due to muscle action, especially of the abductors. By tilting the affected joint and thus reducing the effect of the abductor pull, he can reduce this load to almost one times the body weight. The majority of patients also find that a walking stick held in the opposite hand to the affected hip will have a similar effect. Local heat (such as a bath) and proprietary medicines may also relieve symptoms. Obese patients should be encouraged to slim.

Conservative treatment

This should always be undertaken in the early stages of osteoarthrosis.

Diet. The obese patient should be encouraged to lose weight. It should be explained to him that this is most important and that it will reduce pain in the weight bearing joints. Every kilogram of weight lost represents a reduction of three kilograms of load on the joint.

Remedial therapy. Occupational therapy is especially valuable in advising the patient how best to carry out the activities of daily living and to avoid further strain on the involved joints. Together with other remedial staff the therapist may supply walking or other aids which may be considered necessary. Physiotherapy and remedial gymnastics may be prescribed and the patient will be instructed in techniques to build up strength in the muscles around the joint, to increase the range of movement around the joint and to prevent fixed deformities. Hydrotherapy, heat and other mechanical treatments may also give symptomatic relief.

Drug therapy. Simple analgesics such as aspirin are used to relieve pain. Anti-arthritic drugs such as the modern propionic acid derivatives, e.g. buprofen and ketoprofen, have a specific action on the pain causing process. Other specific drugs may be used. During acute episodes, for example, aspiration of the joint and local injections of a steroid may be necessary.

Splints and supports. These may occasionally be used on acutely inflamed joints or to prevent fixed deformity.

The encouragement of general health. A good diet, exercise and the avoidance of fatigue are recommended. This is especially important if the patient is to be fit for later surgery.

Manipulation under anaesthetic. This is performed especially where there is decreased range of movement and muscular contracture.

Surgical treatment

Surgical treatment may be required for severely affected joints when conservative treatment has failed or when the disease has progressed too far. Various surgical techniques are employed. Joint replacement techniques, especially of the hip, have improved dramatically and are being increasingly used. In other joints the same high success rate has not yet been achieved, although joint replacement is possible at the interphalangeal, carpometacarpal and carpal joints of the hand, at the wrist, elbow and shoulder joints and at the toes, ankle and knee. Partial replacement can be employed for the first metatarsal head, the head of the radius, the distal ulna, the femoral head, tibial condyles, carpal bones and the patella.

Joint replacement techniques involve the removal of the patient's own diseased tissue and the insertion of a prothesis. Before this stage is reached, however, other techniques are available, particularly for younger patients:

1. Osteotomy. This can be used particularly to correct deformity and also to relieve pain. At the hip, a subtrochanteric division of the femur is performed and an appropriate displacement carried out to correct any flexion, rotation or adduction deformity. At the knee, a division of the upper tibia or lower femur may be performed to correct valgus or varus deformity. If this would result in an oblique line of the knee joint a double osteotomy of the tibia and femur may be performed (Benjamin's osteotomy). The main advantages of osteotomy are relief of pain and correction of deformity. Osteotomy of the neck of the scapula may reduce the effects of osteoarthrosis at the shoulder.

2. Arthrodesis. Permanent fixation of the severe-

ly affected joint by bony union of the two joint surfaces may be undertaken, provided that other joints in the region are mobile enough to compensate for the lost range of movement. This is particularly valuable in the upper limb, as it will give permanent relief of pain. Of the weight-bearing joints it is most commonly performed at the knee if the opposite knee and the hips are not affected. The procedure may also be performed where osteoarthrosis secondary to an infected process prevents the use of a joint prosthesis, or in younger patients who are going to make greater demands on a joint.

Arthroplasty. Modern techniques of arthroplasty involve the replacement of part or all of the affected joints by artificial components. Not all joints can be replaced successfully, but very good results can be obtained at the hip and often at the

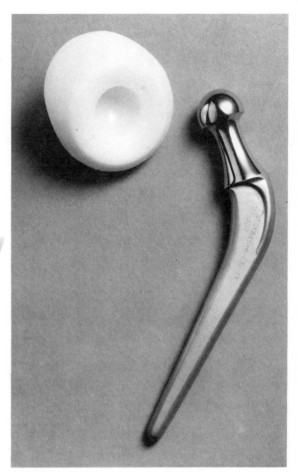

Fig. 22.2 The Charnley low-friction arthroplasty (photograph by kind permission of Chas Thackray Ltd)

knee. The artificial hip joints are made of a metal femoral component and a polyethylene acetabular cup. Many types are now in use (there are over 100 different designs of total hip replacements) and a few examples are illustrated in Figures 22.1, 2 and 3.

Complications include infection or loosening of the new joint which, in most cases, is retained by cement. If this occurs the joint must be replaced again or removed leaving a fibrous pseudoarthrosis. In this latter instance, splints would be used to support the joint in the initial stages following operation. A deep vein thrombosis may occur.

Following surgery an active and progressive programme of rehabilitation is commenced. After a hip replacement, for example, the patient is up two to three days following operation and is

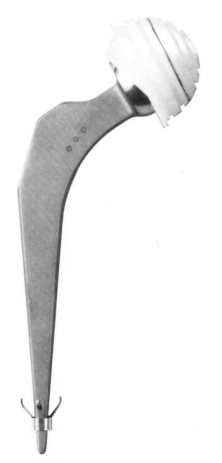

Fig. 22.1 The Exeter (Ling- Lee) total hip joint (photograph by kind permission of Howmedica (U.K.) Ltd)

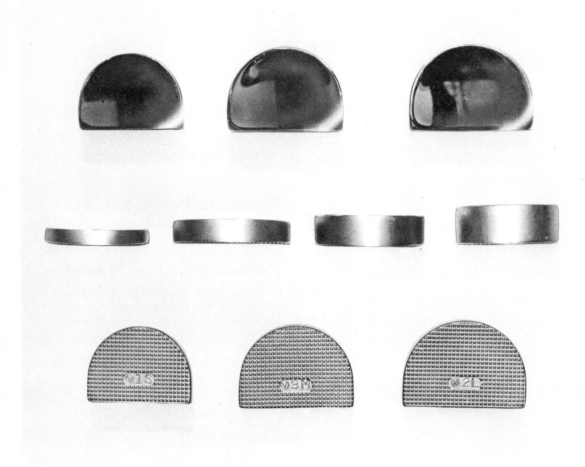

Fig. 22.3 MacIntosh tibial plateaux

allowed to be fully weight-bearing. Mobility is encouraged initially by the use of two walking aids (normally sticks or elbow crutches). On discharge some 10 days later he will return home, using only one walking aid, to resume a normal life as soon as possible. Some precautions, like avoiding flexion with adduction, are necessary, especially during the first six weeks while the soft tissues heal. Figure 22.4 shows an example of instructions given to a patient who has undergone total hip replacement. The leaflet was compiled at the Princess Elizabeth Orthopaedic Hospital, Exeter, Devon.

THE ROLE OF THE OCCUPATIONAL THERAPIST

The occupational therapist may be asked to treat the patient either as part of the conservative treatment by giving advice and helping to preserve and maintain the strength and range of movement of the affected joint, or after surgical treatment in order to help restore the patient to his highest level of function. The role of the occupational therapist varies during these two stages.

During conservative treatment

Activities of daily living. Methods and aids to reduce the strain on affected joints should be introduced. If the lower limbs are affected, aids such as a raised toilet seat, bath board and bath seat, long-handled brushes and mops, a high stool for the kitchen, sock sticks and a stocking gutter (Fig. 22.5), elastic laces and long-handled shoe

A. During the first six weeks following your return home from hospital:

1. Do **NOT** sit in low chairs.

2. Do **NOT** try to force your leg to bend at the hip in an effort, for example, to put on your shoe and sock.

3. Do **NOT** do any exercises to restore movement to your artificial hip joint (a few patients do need exercises, and, if you are one of these, your physiotherapist will instruct you before you leave hospital). Movement will gradually return to the hip with activity and the passage of time.

4. Continue to sleep on your back and do not try to sleep on your side.

5. Do **NOT** discard your elastic stockings until at least three weeks after your operation, and then only discard them gradually provided that swelling of the legs is not tiresome.

6. Do **NOT** try to discard your walking stick.

7. Do **NOT** drive.

8. Avoid gardening.

9. Kneel or stand in the bath or shower and do not sit with your legs out in front of you.

10. Lie prone (i.e. face down) for twenty minutes each morning and evening.

B. After the first six weeks:

1. You may drive, bath normally, sleep on your side.

2. Do **NOT** try to force movement of the hip by passive movements or exercises.

3. You may discard your stick progressively as your ability to walk improves, but it is safer to go on using the stick when walking out of doors. You should hold the stick in the hand opposite your artificial hip joint.

4. Continue daily prone lying.

5. Remember that, even if the new joint feels normal to you, it is an artificial hip joint and over-vigorous use—running, for example—is unwise. With sensible use, the joint should last some years.

6. If you develop any infection, for example, in your chest, kidneys or bladder, it is important that this should be treated promptly and intensively to prevent any spread of the infection by the bloodstream to the hip joint. You should, therefore, contact your doctor immediately under these circumstances.

Fig. 22.4 Instruction sheet for patients who have undergone replacement of the hip at the Princess Elizabeth Orthopaedic Hospital, Exeter

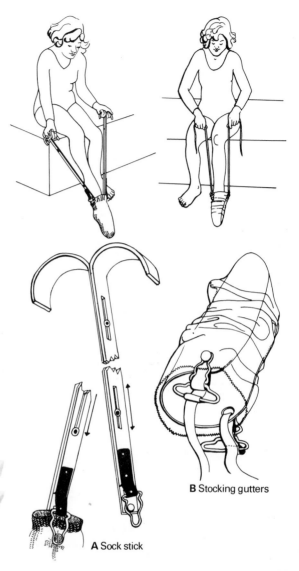

B Stocking gutters

A Sock stick

Fig. 22.5 Aids to reduce strain on the hip and knee

horns can be used. Advice on labour-saving methods and equipment should be given, and the height and support from beds and chairs checked for comfort and ease of transfer. Grab rails or a support by the bed, bath and toilet may be of help. As general stiffness and immobility increase, a hoist, wheelchair and/or a ground-floor flat or bungalow should be considered.

Safety at home. This should be discussed with the patient, and its importance explained. The edges of mats and carpets should be firmly fixed or a non-slip backing applied. A non-slip mat in the bath is advisable and firm shoes with support over the instep and a low heel will encourage good posture and gait. Grab rails by internal and external steps will help security and balance.

Diet. For the overweight patient advice on how to lose weight and maintain this loss is always appropriate, as a reduction in weight will decrease strain on the affected joints.

Splinting. Resting splints for knees, wrists and hands may be requested, as may work splints for hands. A spinal support may be made in the occupational therapy department, and a back support for working chairs or car seats may help posture during prolonged periods of sitting.

Exercise. Regular, rhythmical exercise will help to increase and maintain the range of movement of the affected joints and increase strength in the muscles around the joint thus giving support and relieving pain.

If the hips and knees are affected, the following activities may be used:

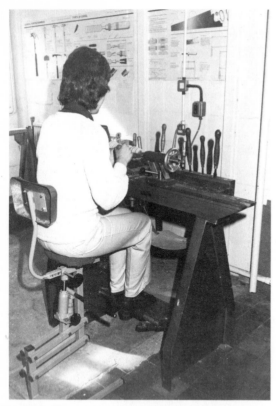

Fig. 22.6 The wood-turning lathe (Note: in the early stages the patient sits on a cycle seat and treadles with both feet)

Bicycle fretsaw. The bicycle should be set to give as large a range of movement as is comfortable and this should be increased as range returns. Strength should be built up by increasing resistance and length of exercise.

Treadle wood-turning lathe. The patient can begin by sitting at the lathe on a Camden stool and treadling with both feet (Fig. 22.6). Later he can progress to standing on the sound limb and treadling with the affected one. Any activity of interest can be done on the lathe.

Pottery lathe. This needs a lighter treadling action than the wood-turning lathe and is normally performed seated.

If the spine is affected the spinal extensors and rotators should be strengthened and a good posture encouraged.

Elevated wall games can be used (see Ch. 10) with the patient either seated or standing.

The upright rug loom can be used with the overhead shed bar to encourage the spinal extensors.

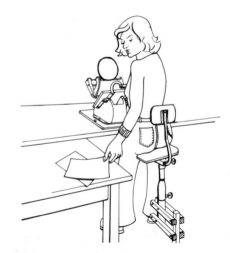

Fig. 22.7 Printing used to encourage good posture and spinal rotation

A standing table or activities sitting upright on a Camden stool are also useful (Fig. 22.7). Weight should be evenly distributed on both feet and a good posture maintained. All activities should be worked between waist and chest height and should encourage rhythmical movement of the spine in extension and/or rotation.

Correct lifting techniques should be taught to avoid back strain.

General activities. The patient should be encouraged to take regular exercise through such activities as walking, gardening and swimming.

Help at work. If the patient is still at work the therapist should check that, where possible, excess strain caused by machinery, working postures or structural barriers is reduced to a minimum. She may, for example, advise on a more suitable chair or stool for the patient to use at work, and it may be appropriate to contact the Disablement Resettlement Officer in order to initiate adaptations for machinery or buildings. Where generalised stiffness and immobility are a problem and are likely to increase, a change or adaptation of occupation may be indicated. As previously mentioned, attention should be paid to labour-saving and lifting techniques and driving posture.

After surgical treatment

The patient will remain in bed for a varying length of time depending on the type of operation performed and the regime favoured by the surgeon.

For example, following pseudoarthrosis of the hip the patient may be put into traction and remain in bed for approximately three to six weeks, whereas after hip arthroplasty many patients are now encouraged out of bed after two or three days. A full weight-bearing gait is taught initially, the patient walking with the aid of elbow crutches, walking sticks or a frame. During this period of rehabilitation the role of the occupational therapist is to increase independence in the activities of daily living and to increase mobility.

Independence in activities of daily living

Dressing. This should be started as soon as the patient is allowed to sit out of bed for a reasonable period. It should be practised with the patient seated on the edge of the bed or on a steady chair with both feet flat on the floor to prevent strain on the hip or knee and to aid balance. Dressing the upper half is generally no problem, although front-fastening garments are advisable if the spine is affected. Everything possible should be put on over the head to avoid excess movement of the lower limbs. Pants, underpants and trousers can be put on with the help of sock sticks, a Helping Hand or other aid, the affected limb being put into the garment first. Some patients can manage by hooking garments over the end of a crutch or walking stick. All lower garments should be pulled up as high as possible and then the patient need only stand once to adjust the clothing. A long-handled shoe horn and/or elastic laces will help

the patient to put his shoes on as lateral rotation, adduction and gross flexion should be avoided in the early stages after hip replacement because of the danger of dislocation. Those with good balance can put their shoes on from behind (Fig. 22.8). Corsets are not advisable in the early days following operation as they will rub the wound. A light suspender belt or tights should be recommended. Garters should be avoided as circulation may be sluggish, and pressure will increase the danger of a deep vein thrombosis.

Toilet. A raised toilet seat and a grab rail or other firm support will help transfers on and off the toilet in the early stages.

Bathing. A bath board and bath seat will help the patient to take a bath when initially discharged home. Transfer in and out of the bath is easier if the weak leg is lifted over the edge of the bath as shown in Figure 22.9. Some patients prefer to use a shower fixed to the taps to save sitting down in the bath. Whichever method is preferred, a non-slip mat should always be used in the bath. It may be considered wise for the patient to wait until his balance has improved before taking a bath or shower, especially if he is elderly or lives alone.

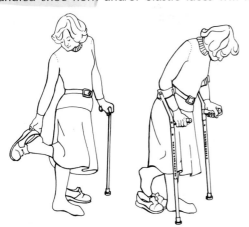

Fig. 22.8 Two methods of putting on shoes to avoid strain at the hip

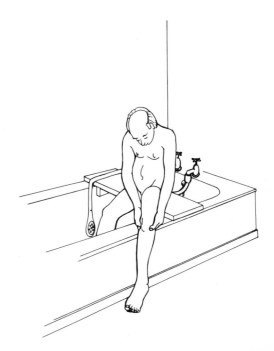

Fig. 22.9 Transfer using a bath board

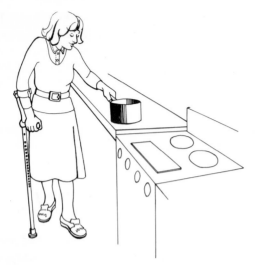

Fig. 22.10 Mobility in the kitchen is easier if only one walking aid is used

Housework. During early treatment sessions the occupational therapist should help build up the patient's confidence in the kitchen if he needs to be able to cope there on discharge. The patient should be shown how to manoeuvre using just one crutch or walking stick and sliding items from one surface to another (Fig. 22.10). The programme should begin with activities to improve mobility and sitting tolerance. A high Camden stool should be used for activities such as ironing, washing up and making light snacks. As confidence and mobility improve, the longer sessions can include bending, stretching and carrying. A trolley may be helpful in a larger kitchen or for taking food from kitchen to dining area. The patient should be able to cope without crutches or sticks once balance, strength and confidence are restored, as support can be gained from working surfaces.

If the patient has not already received advice on labour saving and lifting this should be offered. The patient should be encouraged to use a tall stool for long periods of sitting and standing to avoid stiffness at hip and knee, and if the limb is still swollen, a footstool should be available for use in the kitchen. As before, aids that avoid bending and stretching can be introduced.

The occupational therapist should be satisfied that elderly patients and those who live alone are safe and independent before discharge. It may be necessary to arrange support services such as Meals on Wheels, home help or district nurse for

the early days at home. If this is not possible the occupational therapist may advise a longer period in hospital or convalescence with relatives or elsewhere until the patient is fully independent.

Transfers. The occupational therapist should ensure that the patient can rise and sit safely when using his crutches or sticks (see Ch. 16). The bed should be checked to see that the patient can get on and off with ease and that the mattress gives

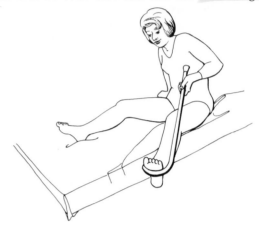

Fig. 22.11 Lifting the weak leg with the aid of a walking stick

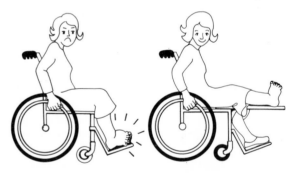

Fig. 22.12 The weak leg is elevated on a fracture board

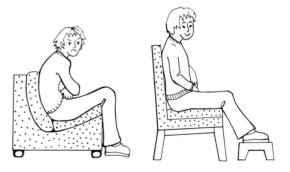

Fig. 22.13 The patient's chair should give firm support and be high enough to allow easy transfer

firm support. While the leg is still weak the patient should be shown how to lift it onto the bed by hooking the crutch or walking stick round the instep (Fig. 22.11). If the leg is swollen he should be encouraged to support it on a footstool, or fracture board in a wheelchair, while resting (Fig. 22.12). The knee should always be supported when the leg is elevated. During a home visit before discharge the patient's usual easy chair should be checked to ensure it is high enough to allow easy transfer and that the seat and the back give firm support and encourage good posture (Fig. 22.13).

Mobility

The occupational therapist should aim to increase the strength and range of movement in the affected joint. The principles are the same as for the conservative stage of treatment, that is, rhythmical, regular exercise should be given. However, the therapist will find that immediatley postoperatively, when the range of movement is limited by pain and the leg may be weak and swollen, lighter-weight activities should be used. These can include activities with the affected leg resting in elevation to reduce oedema, and remedial foot games seated on a Camden stool. She must remember at all times that flexion should not be forced. The range of movement and time spent on activities should be increased as the limb improves.

Standing and sitting tolerance and balance must be improved. The patient's activity tolerance will be low initially, and movements should be restricted to those which do not cause excess discomfort. The therapist should explain that a certain amount of discomfort is inevitable as more and more is demanded from the joint. Activities can include the use of the standing table and Camden stool, darts, elevated remedial games and light domestic and benchwork. These should be started as soon as possible and may need to be continued after discharge. Correct walking patterns and good posture should be encouraged throughout treatment.

The therapist may well find that not all units use specific activities to increase mobility, as it is thought that this will return in time with normal daily and work activities.

As surgical treatment of osteoarthrosis becomes more common, the period spent in hospital is being reduced continually and, for younger patients at least, this may be no more than 10 days after operation. Provided that rehabilitation is started early and continued regularly, the patient should regain sufficient strength and mobility in his joint to enable him to regain full independence and take a more active part in work and social life than before.

REFERENCES AND FURTHER READING

Dick W C 1972 An introduction to clinical rheumatology. Churchill Livingstone, Edinburgh
Jayson M I V Dixon A St J 1977 Rheumatism and arthritis. Pan, London
MacDonald E M 1976 Occupational therapy in rehabilitation, 4th edn. Balliere Tindall, London
Panayi G S (ed) 1980 Essential rheumatology for nurses and therapists. Bailliere Tindall, London
Shopland A 1980 Refer to occupational therapy 2nd edn. Churchill Livingstone, Edinburgh
Trombly C A, Scott A D 1977 Occupational therapy for physical dysfunction. Williams & Wilkins, Baltimore

23

Paediatrics

(Children suffering from Cerebral palsy, Muscular dystrophy and Spina bifida)

HANDICAPPED CHILDREN

Children will always be injured in road traffic accidents and fires, and always suffer permanent damage from certain medical diseases, but will there always be children handicapped by congenital disorders? The answer is probably yes, but the numbers are decreasing rapidly and the nature of the handicaps is constantly changing.

Forty years ago, pulmonary tuberculosis, poliomyelitis and osteomyelitis were common conditions affecting children, but with improved prophylactic measures and antibiotic treatment these conditions have become relatively rare. Improved delivery techniques and more readily available ante-natal care have led to the survival of many more children with cerebral palsy. Twenty years ago the number of congenitally deformed children tragically increased with the use of the drug thalidomide during pregnancy. The advent of new paediatric surgical techniques resulted in the survival of large numbers of spina bifida children who had previously died at birth or awaiting closure of the cyst. More medical and paramedical personnel were required to treat the wide variety of problems which these children presented. Many new units were built to accommodate and treat the children and their families, and paediatric medicine expanded. New treatment procedures and equipment were developed, more special schools were built and others extended. In the next ten years medical, surgical and paramedical treatment improved further to ensure the survival and fullest possible life for handicapped children.

Table 23.1 Normal child development (Note: this table is intended to give a basic outline and it must be remembered that all children develop at different rates.)

Age	Development
2 weeks	Child able to suck well
4 weeks	Beginning to lift head momentarily
6 weeks	Beginning to smile at the spoken word
8 weeks	Following movements with eyes
3–5 months	Turns head in direction of noise
	When prone can hold head and shoulders up
	Can loosen clenched fist and keep hands open
	Able to grasp toys if given to him
	Often drools, precursor to teeth coming
	Can lay on back with head in mid-position
5 months	Starting to chew
7 months	Starting to pass a toy from one hand to another
10 months	Picks up very small objects
	May start to walk
	Sits up well unsupported
12 months	Walking commences. Simple words being spoken
15 months	Able to build brick towers
	Bladder able to retain urine for longer periods
18 months	Memorises simple tasks
2 years	Beginning to dress himself with simple clothing
2–3 years	Bowel control beginning

Following this period, the number of children handicapped by congenital abnormalities began to decrease due to further improvements in antenatal care and diagnostic techniques, and an increase in genetic counselling and selective pregnancy terminations. The position which the medical profession now holds as a result of modern knowledge and legalised abortion has raised the moral question of whether or not it is right to strive to keep a severely handicapped child alive at birth. Thanks to improved prophylactic measures, this decision need not be made frequently.

CEREBRAL PALSY

Occupational therapy with children suffering from cerebral palsy may be divided into two broad categories. These are play therapy and personal care training for children and prevocational therapy and personal care training for older children. Perceptual training is always part of the treatment.

The young child

It is essential to have a basic knowledge of normal child development so that we remain logical in our treatment and realistic in our ultimate aims for the handicapped child, remembering that he will eventually have to cope with living in the community. Table 23.1 shows the normal stages of child development and Table 23.2 the characteristics of the different types of cerebral palsy.

Planning treatment. Following a case conference, the therapist having had a referral from a doctor will plan her treatment. Initial assessment

Table 23.2 Cerebral palsy (No child will conform to the table exactly. He may exhibit some or many of the characteristics to a greater or lesser degree.)

Disability	Area of brain involved	Presentation	Causes
Spasticity	Cerebral cortex Pyramidal tracts	Tongue thrust Scissor gait Stiffness Flexed elbows Swallowing difficulties Speech disorders Perceptual problems Facial contractures Teeth grinding Increased muscle tone Possible mental impairment	Rhesus-incompatability Foetal anoxia Toxaemia Rubella (first 3 months of pregnancy) Prematurity
Athetosis	Basal ganglia Extra-pyramidal tracts	Uncontrolled movements Writhing movements Speech disorder Hearing loss Unable to control saliva Mental impairment less common	Unknown Diabetes in mother Birth trauma Meningitis Cerebro-vascular accident Road traffic accident
Ataxia	Cerebellum	Loss of balance Incoordination Wide gait Poor hand/eye coordination Frequent falls Poor speech Unable to control saliva Loss of tactile sensation	

should include: head control, grasp and release, hand/eye coordination and knowledge of basic concepts (colour, shape and size).

Throughout the assessment period, observe very carefully and try to determine the child's major difficulty and the treatment priority. Aims of treatment may be: (a) to improve head control, (b) to teach basic concepts and (c) to teach simple self care.

Keeping records. Each child requires a personal file where details of his progress should be kept. This will include drawing tests, self-care profiles and work standards. As children progress slowly, it will not be necessary to enter a daily report, but it is useful to have a system of 'work cards' on which the therapist can record daily happenings such as achievements or reactions to new activities.

Although for purposes of discussion it is necessary to categorise children, it must be remembered that first and foremost the child is a person and not an 'athetoid' or a 'spastic', and the occupational therapist's approach should show this.

Testing. It is wise to apply tests very sensitively to avoid increasing nervousness and feelings of failure. Administer tests such as drawing a man (to test body image) more as a game or drawing session, but not without firmness and discipline. It is useful to have standardised tests at your disposal, provided you have the expertise to administer and evaluate them correctly. Intelligence tests can give misleading pictures of a child and it is wise to use the knowledge more as a guide to treatment than as a rigid fact.

Visuo-spatial problems. Many children suffering from cerebral palsy will have visuo-spatial difficulties. An apparently bright child who copes with academic subjects may nonetheless have perceptual problems. These may become apparent when the child is attempting to do ordinary everyday tasks such as dressing or washing up. The difficulty lies not in the 'seeing', but in the perceiving of what is in front of them.

To help to overcome these difficulties the therapist must provide tactile games, memory games, auditory games and any activity which will stimulate perception through as many different channels as possible. For the young child, floor games are extremely useful, for example crawling in and out of furniture, feeling for toys in deep boxes of polystyrene packing material and dressing each other up. Coloured bricks, stacking toys, dolls or soldiers, tea sets, different sized bottles or jars that will unscrew are all very useful; during play, talk about the activity, stressing the colour of things, and their size and feel, so that the child gains a total picture of the world around him. Never assume that a child knows something, always make sure for yourself.

Play therapy

The normal child will instinctively play with toys because he has no physical handicap, nor does he have perceptual problems, and therefore he does not need to be taught how to play. The child with brain damage, however, must be given extra clues to his surroundings and will require time and patience. The first task of the therapist is to establish rapport with the child. Treatment will often take place on a one-to-one basis, according to the severity of the problem. It is wise to alternate individual treatment with group treatment so that the child is able to identify with his peers.

A great deal of play therapy takes place on the floor, as this is where the child feels most secure. With the therapist at his level the child feels no barrier or feeling of being dominated.

Play positions. Discuss the most beneficial body position with the physiotherapist. It may prove beneficial for the child to play in the prone position over a foam wedge (Fig. 23.1A). The therapist may need to support the child from behind, kneeling with the child firmly anchored between her knees (Fig. 23.1B), or it may be possible to sit him in a wooden floor chair or a foam floor chair depending on the degree of sitting balance. A corner seat with pummel is illustrated in Figure 23.2. For standing activities an Amesbury Quadra Table may be used (Fig. 23.3).

Manual dexterity

Hand dominance does not become firmly established until the child is nearing three years of age.

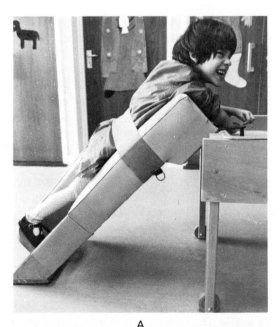

A

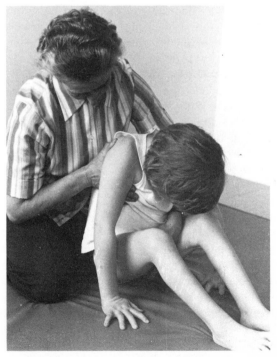

B

Fig. 23.1 Play positions. (A) Prone board enabling a severely handicapped child to use her arms (B) The therapist supports the child firmly from behind

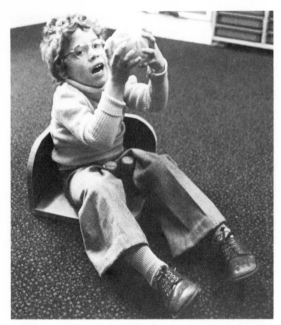

Fig. 23.2 A corner seat with pummel. (Note: this can be used by a child with sufficient balance to increase stability and allow free use of both arms)

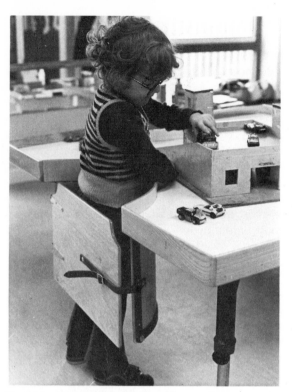

Fig. 23.3 The Amesbury Quadra table

This of course may be later in a child suffering from cerebral palsy. There is also a possibility that it is the dominant side of the body which has suffered more damage and this will pose further problems. It is only by sustained observation of both organised and free play sessions that one will be able to decide definitely which is the dominant hand. The following toys and materials encourage manual dexterity: bricks, Lego, wooden assembly toys, plastic cups and saucers, cotton reels and beads to thread, embroidery cards with large holes, colouring games, plasticine, clay, flour and water dough etc.

Grasp and release. Many children suffering from cerebral palsy will find it very difficult to release the clenched fist and will be unusually sensitive on the palmar surface of the hand. It will be necessary to stimulate the palm of the hand using different textures such as furry fabric, soft brushes and wet sponges in order to lessen the persistent grasp reflex. Another common difficulty is opposition of thumb to fingers, because the thumb adducts strongly into the palm of the hand. A corrective splint to be worn for short periods when the child is working and requiring a functional grip will help. All games needing fine finger

manipulation will aid dexterity. A few examples are threading cotton reels and beads, basketry, weaving, papier maché, solitaire or indeed any game or activity which provides the level of activity required. A spastic child will need to increase his range of movement and requires activities which will stretch him, whereas an athetoid child has too much movement and may need to have his elbow stabilised in order to control hand movement. Try to invite parents into therapy sessions frequently so that they are involved in the treatment and can be given ideas to use at home. Give as much practical support and help as possible to the parents, as they are experiencing the handicap with their child and often feel helpless and depressed. It is wise to refer to the less useful hand as the 'helping' or 'enabling' hand as this is positive, rather than calling it the 'bad' hand, especially when trying to encourage bilateral use of hands. Use games which encourage the child to reach out for objects, holding the object first in one direction and then in another so that the child uses hand/eye coordination as well as grasp.

Sense-training apparatus

When teaching the basic concepts of colour, shape and size, the equipment to be used is too numerous to list. There are always things in the immediate surroundings which can be pointed to and talked about, the most obvious ones being the child's own clothing. Try to use everyday objects as much as possible, as this helps to build up experience which the child may not be able to get on his own because he cannot move sufficiently well to discover in the normal way.

Aids to self-care training. Bows, buckles and buttons present endless difficulties, often because they are in such awkward positions as well as being fiddly tasks. To overcome this difficulty the bow, buckle and button board illustrated in Figure 23.4 is extremely useful.

Contraindications

1. Short sharp strokes, as in sanding down small articles will increase spasticity in spastic children

2. Too much noise and excitement will increase spasm, add to confusion and lead to bad behaviour

3. Too many instructions given at once

4. Different instructions given regarding the same activity

5. Too many toys within reach will cause distraction.

Specific abnormal reflexes

ATNR (asymmetrical tonic neck reflex). The head turns towards the extended arm.

MORO. The startle reflex. The arms are thrown up above the head and the head is thrown backwards.

NRR (neck righting reflex). If the body is turned to the left or right then the head automatically follows.

ET (extensor thrust). When a child is held above the ground under his axillae his body goes into extension, the legs cross and the toes go into plantarflexion.

PR (parachute reflex). When the child is held above the ground by his ankles he makes no attempt to put his hands down to save himself. Normally the arms would extend towards the ground.

Any treatment which increases these abnormal reflexes is contraindicated and should be modified or avoided. For example, an athetoid child walking along a corridor will go into an extensor thrust if someone suddenly walks up behind him and speaks without previously making his presence known.

Self-care training

Dressing

Involve the parents in this from the beginning, and it is more likely that you will achieve lasting results.

Undressing is always easier than dressing as less precision is needed. If it is possible to have the child before his physiotherapy session then there will be a good reason to undress, and the child will also have to be ready at a set time. It has been

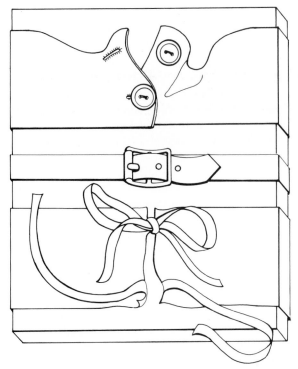

Fig. 23.4 Bow, buckle and button board

found beneficial to make small record books in the form of small home-made books containing pictures of different items of clothing on each page. Beside the drawing or picture the therapist can make brief notes on the method employed, and for the child's benefit there will be a large red tick when he has achieved success. These books should be taken home, and the parents can then keep up with the progress at school or clinic and jot down the performance at home. So often it is found that what happens in the occupational therapy session does not happen at home. Group dressing sessions for the younger age group are very successful and can be presented as dressing-up sessions on occasions to prevent monotony. Depending on the children in the group a competitive spirit may evolve, but the game should not be presented in such a way as to 'show a child up' unless his problem is laziness!

General rules

1. Dress the hemiplegic arm first
2. Ensure that the child is seated safely and comfortably
3. Try to use the same instructions daily, and with mentally retarded children even use the same words and sentences
4. Do not bribe a child, but give praise and encouragement always
5. Generally the child will find it easier to put his head into a jumper first, thus eliminating one of the holes, but this will vary from child to child
6. When tying a bow on shoes or boots, a helpful tip is to do a double twist with the laces prior to tying the bow.

Suitable clothing

1. Raglan sleeves have larger arm holes and are therefore easier to put on
2. Garments one size larger than is actually needed facilitates dressing, and the clothes last longer
3. Front-opening dresses with zippers. (A tab or large ring on the end of the zip enables the child to pull it more easily)
4. V-neck pullovers are easier to pull over the head than the crew neck variety
5. Heel-less socks. These are made in the form of a tube so that it does not matter which way round they are put on
6. Nylon clothing presents two main disadvantages:

(a). it causes the child to perspire which is particularly uncomfortable when confined to a wheelchair
(b) it does not 'give' very much and so causes the child to become stuck in the process of dressing or undressing.

The advantage is that is is easy to wash and dry, which is an asset if the child drools copiously and needs many changes of clothing. Generally speaking, cotton and cotton mixtures are the most comfortable.

Orthoses

Children suffering from cerebral palsy will often need to wear orthoses (calipers) to prevent deformity and give stability for walking or weight-bearing. Orthoses cause many problems to the child who is learning to become independent with dressing. In order to achieve their purpose orthoses must be put on correctly and firmly, and it may be several years before the child has sufficient strength or manual dexterity to do this.

When putting orthoses on a child it may be helpful to use the following guidelines.

Remove the shoes or boots from the calipers and put the boot or shoe on the foot.

Always ensure that the toes are lying flat in the shoe as they have a tendency to curl under.

Once the shoe is on, the irons may be inserted into the slots in the shoe, having first positioned the caliper correctly on the leg.

With full length orthoses ensure that the knee piece is placed accurately. The knee piece generally serves to pull the knee out, but as there are occasions contrary to this, it should always be checked with the physiotherapist.

When placing a child into full-length orthoses it is often easier to unlock all the locking points, i.e. at knees and hips, before attempting to do the calipers up.

When the child is getting out of the orthoses he should undo all the buckles or velcro fastenings, unlace the shoes or boots and manually pull his legs up and out of the shoe, thus leaving the shoes attached to the orthoses.

Check that there are no chafing points on the calipers or orthoses.

A little oil in the shoe slots will help them to remain trouble-free.

Bathing

Discuss bathing with the parents before starting, if possible, and explain the necessity for starting when the child is young and not heavy.

The child who comes daily and is not resident may feel happier if he brings his own towel, sponge, duck or boat and all these things help to increase his confidence.

Bath seats. A child whose limbs are very stiff, but who has reasonable sitting balance, is often able to use the orthodox top seat and inset seat. Check that (a) the seats fit well and will not move, (b) the wheelchair brakes are good, (c) a suction bath mat is firmly fixed in the bath and that (d) you have all the equipment necessary and will not have to leave a child alone in the bath.

Give simple instructions in a calm manner, supplying mental and physical help when it is needed. Withdraw your physical help gradually and give praise whenever possible. Try to make the activity fun, but teach the child how to wash properly before playing. Establish a routine and adhere to it as this will build confidence. When washing himself, try to encourage the child to use diagonal movements, i.e. to wash the right leg with the left hand and vice versa, as this rotates the trunk and helps to break up spasm in the abdominal muscles.

A flannel mitten may be used especially with an athetoid child who may have difficulty sustaining a grip. Long-handled bath brushes and loofahs are also useful.

If the child is unable to use bath seats, the following methods may be tried:

1. A hand rail on the wall. Position the wheelchair so that it faces the bath edge. Before the chair is too close lift the child's legs over into the bath, with the feet placed on the suction bath mat. The child then pulls himself forward and moves onto his knees or bottom depending on what he finds easier. It is always best to allow a child to do what is most natural for him if it means that he achieves the aim safely.

2. For the heavily handicapped child who is unable to assist himself a hoist may need to be used.

If sitting balance is not good enough for the child to support himself in the bath a supportive inflatable bath chair may be necessary.

Toilet use

The major difficulties are access, lack of mobility and poor bilateral use of hands or of one hand.

Access. Lavatories world-wide are notorious for being the smallest and most badly-designed 'rooms' imaginable. This is surprising as they are often the most frequently used room in the building.

If a child can be taught to stand and pivot-turn to sit upon the toilet, the access problem is not so great. A grab rail at a convenient height is usually required. In larger toilets, such as are to be found in some public places, sideways transfer may be possible. In very narrow toilets where there is no room to manoeuvre or for a helper to stand, the problem may be solved by having a zip opening in the back of the wheelchair. The child can then twist around and unzip the chair and slide backwards from chair seat to toilet. If he is unable to undo the zip himself, a helper must do this whilst the child holds tight to the chair arms and is pushed towards the toilet.

Structural alterations. These are a last resort as local authorities are often reluctant to supply grants. It is very important to look ahead and plan for the future as far as possible. Remember that the child is going to grow, he may fit into a shower unit whilst small, but require a bath and hoist when he is older and possibly even more handicapped.

Mobility. One hopes that mobility is going to improve as the child grows and works in therapy, but there will be times when the reverse is the case and stiffness increases. In such cases the occupational therapist must adapt aids and appliances skilfully.

Poor use of hands. Most small children require help to clean themselves having used the toilet. The child with stiff or athetoid hands will need this help for longer if not always. The commercial 'Toilet Hand' is not really of use for the kind of difficulty experienced by cerebral palsied children. It may be more successful to have a special sponge to be used only for this purpose and kept discreetly in the toilet bag. If this does answer the problem, the accent must be on hygiene and cleanliness in washing out the sponge and regularly buying new ones. A bidet may be used, but they are not common yet and are very expensive.

Many children suffering from cerebral palsy tend to be thin and bony, and find the toilet seat uncomfortable because they are almost falling through it. It may be necessary to use an insert which makes the aperture smaller and not so terrifying.

When dealing with any self-care problem, have an up-to-date knowledge of aids and appliances available. Many aids can be supplied free of charge by the local authority, but only if the child is on the local register of the disabled. This is merely red tape and is often avoided by parents who do not wish to register the child as disabled for personal reasons.

Care of teeth and hair

Teeth cleaning. As this requires fine finger movements, it often presents problems. A child with a fierce grip may squeeze too much toothpaste out and may not be able to place the paste on the brush accurately. Hand-to-mouth coordination may be too poor to get the toothbrush into the mouth. The following suggestions may help:

Fix the toothbrush into a stand which can be fixed to the basin either by rubber suction pads or with a clamp.

Make a vitrathene or darvic toothpaste case which will protect the tube. This will have a hole cut into it for the child's finger to control the amount of paste squeezed out (Fig. 23.5).

An enlarged grip on the toothbrush may help.

With some children any stimulation of the tongue will cause tongue thrust and activation of the bite reflex, and these children will probably never be able to clean their teeth thoroughly. In such cases the parents may be well advised to invest in an electric brush to be used on the child's teeth before bed. If inserted into the side of the

mouth (avoiding the tongue) and then switched on, it can be successful. This will help to prevent tooth decay and distressing visits to the dentist.

Occasionally, a child has a continual bite reflex, which can be so severe as to cause damage to the lower lip. A lip guard may have to be used, but is not comfortable. The orthodontist may provide a form of 'gag' to prevent the jaws completing a bite. This would only be used in extreme cases and will depend on the advice of the orthodontist and the dental surgeon.

Hair washing. The major difficulties are access to available basins, poor sitting balance when arms are raised above the head, lack of confidence and fear of water.

1. *Access.* Teach transferring to ordinary chairs as early and as frequently as possible so that the child uses transferring naturally in order to overcome obstacles. The reason for using an ordinary wooden chair is that a wheelchair often cannot get close enough to the basin even with the footplates turned back. The wheelchair may be reversed up to the basin and the head tilted back over the basin. The hair can also be washed in the bath. It is useful to have a soap rack or the inset bath seat on which to place flannel and shampoo so that everything necessary is within reach.

2. *Poor sitting balance.* A grab rail on one side of the bath will help. This will leave only one hand free to wash the hair, which will require practice. Shampoos which will not sting the eyes may be used.

3. *Lack of confidence.* This is normal and needs to be dealt with sympathetically but firmly. The occupational therapist needs to be inventive and patient in this situation.

Water guards which prevent water from dribbling over the face are available commercially, but usually a flannel held over the eyes by the young child will suffice.

Feeding

Although this is specifically the speech therapist's subject the occupational therapist is often involved.

One of the major difficulties for cerebral palsied children is drinking. The therapist may have to give a great deal of assistance at first, even holding

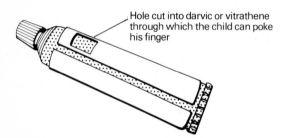

Hole cut into darvic or vitrathene through which the child can poke his finger

Fig. 23.5 Toothpaste tube holder

the lips around a plastic drinking straw with finger and thumb. This initiates the action and, given time and practice, the child will usually grasp the idea and take over himself. Developmentally, sucking comes before drinking from a cup, but with a cerebral palsied child, age is not the determining factor on whether to train with a straw or a cup. It is the level of speech and ability to articulate which decides this. The child with no speech will generally use a straw as this helps to train the muscles required for speech, whilst the child with quite a lot of speech will be more likely to use a cup. It is up to the speech therapist and the occupational therapist together to plan their approach.

When feeding a child with severe tongue thrust, attempt to place the food into the side of the mouth as you do not want to stimulate the tongue. Feed from in front of the child if possible, as he will have more control of head and arms if he holds his head in the mid-position. Try to discourage the tilting back of the head often occurring with

athetoid children, as this may lead to choking. The child will often find that laying his head back aids swallowing but this is very temporary and only helps when eating very liquid foods. There are several plates and adapted knives, forks and spoons available which are of help to some children. Plate stabilisers are essential for many cerebral palsied children (Fig. 23.6). If a plastic straw is used it is wise to train the child to wash his own straw and keep it with him in a bag as there may not always be straws available if he is out.

Splints

There are a few occasions when a splint will help a child suffering from cerebral palsy. Splints must be used carefully and in full consultation with the physiotherapists. Used indiscriminately, a splint may cause the spasm to move from one area to another. For instance, a splinted wrist may cause the elbow and shoulder to go into spasm.

Suitable cases for splinting:

1. The very young child. If he has severe wrist flexion he will be unable to form a functional grip. An extension splint will place the hand in a functional position, but care must be taken not to give too much wrist extension (Fig. 23.7). It may be possible to prevent contractures while the limb is still reasonably flexible. Splints should be worn for very short periods of time only and very gradually upgraded.

2. The hemiplegic child. The child suffering from hemiplegia is not usually too handicapped and can often run around, and because of this he is more likely to fall. He will often fall onto his hemiplegic side, and if the hand is in flexion there is more likelihood of damage and the dorsum of the hand may be continually lacerated. Splinting the hemiplegic hand provides the child with a much more useful second hand.

3. An 'enabling' splint. This may not be an orthodox splint, but it will be what its name implies. The 'cup' of a cup-shaped splint for the fist, for example,, may be attached to the controls of an electric wheelchair. An athetoid child having had some hand movement eliminated will thus have more control.

This brings us to aids made from splinting materials. Because splinting materials are so

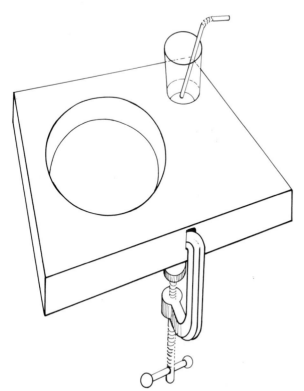

Fig. 23.6   Drinking straw, cup and plate stabiliser

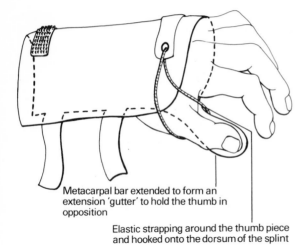

Metacarpal bar extended to form an extension 'gutter' to hold the thumb in opposition

Elastic strapping around the thumb piece and hooked onto the dorsum of the splint

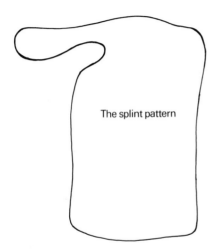

The splint pattern

Fig. 23.7 Wrist extension splint. (Note: the splint leaves the child with more freedom to move and with sensation in the palm and fingers. The ventral surface of the wrist is left free to avoid stimulation of the flexors)

adaptable, they can be used to make gadgets which are not available from any manufacturer. Aids of this type are tailored to the individual and are unique, which is another good reason for the occupational therapist to make them.

Foot splints may be made as night resting splints to prevent deformity or as day shoes which are corrective. One instance when shoes have been of benefit was to prevent the great toe from curling in and under the other toes. The shoes made were in the form of sandals with a toe strap between the great toe and the next toe. Always line the splints with a soft plastazote or velvotex for skin which is especially tender.

Practical experience has shown that it is more successful to put wrist extension splints on the dorsum of the hand. The reason for this is that a splint on the flexor surface stimulates increased flexion.

Writing

It is always better for the child to try to write by hand if possible, as he will be able to perceive the shape of letters with more realism if he has formed them with his own hands before. However, this is not always possible and alternative methods must be found.

Before using typewriters the occupational therapist must observe and assess the exact problem. Why can the child not hold a pencil? What hand movement is he incapable of performing? It is often necessary to sort out the major problem first and then move on to the associated problems. For example, gain wrist extension either by splinting or weighting the forearm and then attempt to establish opposition of the fingers to the thumb. The action of writing is initiated at the shoulder, as may be seen by the person who writes beautifully using only a shoulder stump with a pencil attachment. With an athetoid child we need to eliminate excess arm movement. The elbow may be strapped to the body with a wide webbing band which does not cause any discomfort to the child. If he is also able to rest his forearm on a desk or extension desk fitted to the typewriter he will be even more stable. For the child with intention tremor of the hand a weighted bag may be secured on the dorsum of the wrist to steady the hand and bring it down towards the paper.

Writing aids

1. A 'corkscrew aid' can be made for the child who is unable to oppose his thumb but can sustain a gross cylindrical grip. (Fig. 23.8).

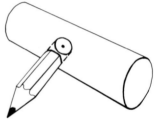

Fig. 23.8 The 'corkscrew' writing aid

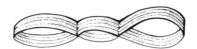

Fig. 23.9 Elastic strapping to fit around thumb, pencil and forefinger

2. Elastic strapping. Ordinary elastic can be stitched to fit around the thumb, the pencil and the forefinger (Fig. 23.9).

3. Padded pencils. Grips must vary according to the individual's need. The grip may be as large as a ball of two and a half inches diameter or may just be a roughened surface. In-between sizes may be made of rubazote of different gauges. Rubazote is very useful because it is quickly removed if the grip is found to be wrong.

4. Head-band with a long dibber attached. These are commercially available, but can be made in the department using splinting materials. They are often useful for athetoid children.

Note: check aids frequently as children can often discard an aid or require a modified one as they develop.

Typewriters

At this point I am referring to ordinary electric typewriters. Several adaptations are available with certain typewriters:

1. Metal finger guard. This screws onto the typewriter over the keys so that the hand may rest on it without depressing the keys, and one finger may then be inserted through the appropriate hole. A child with quite severe athetosis often finds this useful, if he steadies the typing hand with the 'slave' hand and rests the lateral border of the hand on the guard.

2. Wooden arm rest. This is a board which extends from the front of the typewriter. It extends to the full width of the typewriter and is approxi-

mately six inches deep. It is invaluable to children who need to limit their movement in order to achieve accuracy.

3. Typewriter rest. A wooden wedge upon which the typewriter rests will tilt the machine so that the child can see what he has typed (Fig. 23.10).

Typing aids: These are aids which make the action of typing possible, if only with one finger. The most common aid used is a 'dibber'. It may be made as an integral part of a splint or in the form of a 'corkscrew'. They are most successful when used in conjunction with a metal typing guard. Figure 23.11 shows a dibber which consists of a gross cylindrical grip, with the dibber protruding between the two fingers most natural to the individual. Figure 23.12 shows a dibber as an integral part of a splint.

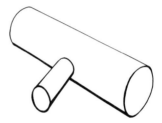

Fig. 23.11 Typing dibber with a gross cylinder grip

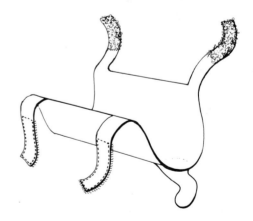

Fig. 23.12 A dibber as an integral part of a splint

Possum typewriters

There are many Possum systems available. They may be operated by the most minute movement, but in the case of a child suffering from cerebral palsy it is more usual to have too much movement.

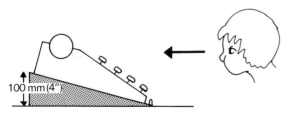

100 mm (4")

Fig. 23.10 A typewriter wedge

An athetoid child may well have more control over his feet, and it is wise to assess controlled foot movement if there is not sufficient control in the hands. The following possum adaptations are commonly used:

1. The wobblestick. The wobblestick will operate the typewriter by being knocked in any direction and is thus very useful for an athetoid child with wide movements.

2. The joystick. This requires a little more control as it has to be pushed into specific slots in order to type correctly.

3. The foot 'skate'. This can be used when the hands have no control, but the feet have a certain degree of control.

4. Knee or head microswitches. These are not so commonly used, but should not be discounted.

The first thing to remember when considering a child for a possum typewriter is whether he or she has sufficient intelligence to use the machine, for it requires a certain amount of concentration, and basic knowledge of the alphabet, sounds, sentence structure and so on. It is for the educationalist to decide which children are eligible and for the occupational therapist to help to find the correct control and work positioning.

When a child first has his new typewriter it may be beneficial to withdraw the child and machine from the classroom where there are many distractions. He will be more likely to succeed if he is taught in a quiet, uncluttered setting on a one-to-one basis, and once he has acquired the skill he can return to the classroom to use the possum typewriter.

Prevocational training

It is essential to start preparing for life after school well before the child approaches school-leaving age. The type of training that the child needs obviously depends upon his mental and physical capabilities. Another almost equally important factor is the motivational disposition of the child, as a child who is hard-working and enthusiastic, but not so academic, will often achieve more than the child with a 'laissez-faire' attitude. It is usual for the Disablement Resettlement Officer to be involved with the child at the age of fourteen approximately, and he will know what is available in the child's own home town or in the area he will be resident in after school. The child may not be capable of open enployment, but need sheltered work, or even work at home. There are many factors to be considered.

1. Home background
2. Mental and physical ability
3. Child's own wishes (provided they are realistic)
4. Residential care available
5. Sheltered workshop available
6. Ability to cope with public transport
7. Ability to cope with personal toileting etc.
8. Ability to communicate with others and be generally sociable
9. Manual dexterity.

If there is no communication with the Disablement Rehabilitation Officer, the Careers Office in the child's locality can often help. If the occupational therapist can visit local factories and establish a working relationship with the personnel concerned with employment this is ideal, but also very time consuming.

Manual dexterity. However poor this is, it will improve with plenty of practice and encouragement. The two main aims are speed and accuracy. In open employment the two must be combined equally so that the handicapped person can compete on equal terms with able-bodied workers. If this is not possible, emphasise accuracy rather than speed. Suitable activities for pre-school leavers are typing and shorthand, telephone work, addressing envelopes, filing, collating magazines and assembly-line work. Use as many varieties of jobs as possible.

Jobs which involve several skills will make it possible for the occupational therapist to assess manual dexterity, speed, the ability to work with others and reaction to pressure.

When operating a work group with young people, try to involve them in the work as much as possible. This may be done by asking one team member to type out the order for more materials or discussing the cost and the selling price of goods produced. Group discussions to sort out 'industrial disputes' or the work group's own party help to bring the group together.

Suitable assembly-line work: Making Christmas

crackers, sorting and packing screws (printing the packet labels), making parcel tags, collating school magazines and folding circulars for envelopes.

Individual or pair work: Making coathangers, chamois mops or pot scourers; craft activities, e.g. enamelling, decorating plain china, macrame, lino cutting, needle work and simple woodwork.

Group social activities. Reading and discussing the daily newspaper, make-up sessions, hair care, clothes sense and grooming, personal hygiene, budgeting, child and baby care, and planning small buffet parties and preparing the food.

Always reinforce talks with practical sessions.

The severely handicapped pre-school leaver. When the handicap is so severe that the young person is unable to control hand movements or to move himself around, the occupational therapist will have to use all her ingenuity. Quite often, if work is clamped securely to the table and a gross activity is given to the person, certain amount of integration into a work team is possible but this will take practice.

For example when making coathangers, position the child at the end of the work line. Clamp a stand with an upright dowel rod to the table. The previous member of the work team having completed the hanger will place it on the table within reach of the child whose job it is to pick it up and place it over the dowel rod until he has the required number in a bundle. The 'runner' or person who collects finished work will remove the coathangers and tie them into a bundle ready for sale. This is a small job but it does include the person in the work team.

Stoolseating may be managed by a severely athetoid child if the stool is firmly clamped to the table and very large needles are used. An upright rug loom may be used with a child who has wide arm movements.

It is always difficult stating what a person will or will not manage, as there will always be individuals who succeed against all odds and thankfully prove the therapist wrong.

Wheelchairs

Physiotherapists and occupational therapists often deal jointly with wheelchairs and it is vital for the occupational therapist to have a knowledge of the type of chairs or at least means of mobility available to children.

The very young child. The Avon Tilting push chair is suitable for the child with little head control. It is available with a padded inset for the very thin child.

The Avon self-propelling wheelchair can be used by the more able small child.

Cindico buggies are similar to the folding buggy made by McLaren but have rigid arm rests and footplates and can have a firm backrest.

McLaren buggies are lightweight folding pushchairs. They are made in different sizes.

Older or larger children. The Everest & Jenning wheelchair is supplied with pummels to keep the knees apart.

Mobility aids

The 'Big T' trike Mark 4 is made by R. C. Hayes (Leicester) Ltd.

The Yorkhill Chariot consists of a wooden box with one opening side and large wheelchair wheels. It is a mobile standing aid.

Rollators are supplied by the National Health Service.

If the child is physically and mentally able he should be shown how to clean and care for his wheelchair, e.g. how to pump up tyres or give it a drop of oil when necessary.

Leisure activities

It is often very difficult to interest somebody else in a hobby, especially if he has little motivation. However, if the occupational therapist can achieve success in this sphere, many empty and frustrating hours may be filled. Handicapped children are bound to have more spare time than able-bodied children, as many outside sports will be impossible to pursue without help, planning and support from the able-bodied community. Physical activities are not ruled out, but it must be remembered that help is required. Sedentary activities are essential if the handicapped young person is to occupy himself independently, Here are some suggested activities: PHAB Club, stamp and coin collecting, painting and drawing, wire craft, pressing flowers, model making, woodwork, weaving, knitting machine work, theatre, music and further education, for instance at the Open University.

Addresses of suppliers

The Spastics Society 12 Park Crescent, London W1
Socks without heels: Burt Bros, Hosiery Ltd, The Poplars, Wollaton Rd, Beeston, Nottingham
Button hooks: Taylor & Law, 10 Yew Tree Road, London W12 0TJ
Soesi Shoe laces: Radiol Chemicals Ltd, Witham, Essex
Crossland Toilet Aid: Crossland Plastics Ltd, Moorhouse Works, Horbury, W. Yorkshire (Toilet seat)
Suzy Air Chair: Newton Aids Ltd, 2A Conway Street, London W1P 5HE
Blissymbolics Communication Resource Centre, South Glamorgan Institute of Higher Education, Western Avenue, Llandaff
Possum Control Ltd, 11 Fairacres Industrial Estate, Windsor, Berkshire

Mobility Aids

Buggies (major, minor, walking aids etc.):
Andrews McLaren Ltd, Station Works, Long Buckby, Northants, NN6 7PF. Also available on prescription
Model 8LC has many features and accessories which may be suitable for children with cerebral palsy. Available on prescription
Tilting Push chair & self-propelling chair (Avon):
Amesbury Surgical Appliances, Southmill Road, Amesbury, Wilts
'Big T' trike: R.C. Hayes (Leicester) Ltd, 65a Main Street, Kirby Muxloe, Leicester

Associations

PHAB Clubs & Camps: N.A.Y.C. Central Council for the Disabled, 30 Devonshire Street, London, W1
Possum Users Association – see Appendix 1

MUSCULAR DYSTROPHY

Muscular dystrophy is one of a group of neuromuscular diseases characterised by progressive deterioration of muscle activity caused by necrosis of muscle fibre. There are a number of different types of muscular dystrophy, all of which are genetically determined.

The most frequent and usually most severe form of muscular dystrophy affecting children is the Duchenne type, first described by Duchenne in 1868. This is transmitted by an X-linked recessive gene and affects only boys. It is carried through the female so that the mother, sisters, aunts and female cousins of one family may be carriers and their male offspring may be affected. There is no known cure for the disease, but genetic counselling has significantly reduced the number of affected children. Each carrier has a one-in-four risk at each pregnancy of having an affected son, a one-in-four risk of having a carrier daughter and a one-in-two chance of having a normal child of either sex. In recent years, tests of muscle enzymes in blood samples have been able to detect female carriers and advice on the risks of producing affected sons or carrier daughters has led to more potential parents adopting children. Unfortunately, as yet no antenatal method of detecting affected or carrier foetuses has been developed, so selective termination of pregnancy is not possible.

Children with Duchenne muscular dystrophy appear normal at birth, but signs of muscle weakness begin to show between two and four years of age. Differences in the rates of development of individual children may cause the first signs of the condition to remain unnoticed, but eventually parents recognise that their child is slightly clumsy on his feet; he may fall over easily and have difficulty in running. Later, running becomes impossible, and getting up after a fall or climbing steps and stairs present considerable problems. Clinical examination reveals selective muscle weakness, particularly in the hip extensors and the muscles of the shoulder girdle and upper arms, although in many cases there is no evidence of muscle wasting. In fact the muscles often appear to be hypertrophic, but this is a false impression and usually due to deposits of fibrous tissue and fat.

The condition is slowly progressive, the weakness spreading down the limbs from the shoulder and pelvic girdles to produce difficulties with mobility and personal independence. Muscle weakness leading to contractures affects particularly the lower limbs, and the child walks on his toes with his lumbar spine lordosed to compensate for loss of hip and knee extension. The child also has problems raising his arms above his head for dressing and personal care. Many boys are unable to walk and become wheelchair-bound by the age of ten to twelve years. Deterioration continues over the next few years; flexion contractures at the hips and knees and plantarflexion at the ankles become fixed, and the upper limbs slowly become weaker causing difficulties in manoeuvring the wheelchair, transferring to and from it, and in daily living activities. Weakness of the spinal muscles results in the child adopting abnormal postures to obtain support thus causing kyphosis and scoliosis. This in turn may distort the chest and cause respiratory difficulties. Eventually the muscles of the face, hands and chest become affected, the heart weakens, respiratory infections linger and death frequently results before the age of twenty five from respiratory failure.

Many intellectual and psychological problems complicate the brief life of the muscular dystrophy child and may upset the family stability permanently.

Experts differ in their findings as to the factors influencing intellectual ability. A high proportion of muscular dystrophy children subjected to formal intelligence test procedures will score below average figures. Some believe this is due to a diminished basic intellectual ability, while others argue that it is mostly due to restricted environmental experience and emotional problems.

Undoubtedly, the stresses of the condition can cause widespread behavioural and emotional problems in the child and the family. The parents frequently experience great feelings of guilt, particularly the mother, if she is aware of the sex-linked inheritance of the disease. They may attempt to compensate the child for their feelings by over protection and over-indulgence in his needs. Consequently, the child is restricted in his emotional development and may become timid and hesitant. In some children this over protection only adds to the frustrations caused by their physical difficulties

and their behaviour may appear aggressive or uncooperative. Other siblings may feel jealous towards the handicapped child if they are overlooked, and may try to compete for their parents attention, or they may support the over sympathetic approach, further restricting the child's progress. The guilt feelings of the mother and father may upset their relationships with each other. The husband occasionally blames the wife for bearing the handicapped child which only adds to her difficulties. In some cases, the husband resents the amount of attention his wife shows to their handicapped child. She may appear to further deny his needs by inhibiting sexual activity for fear of further pregnancy. Parents should be encouraged to express their problems openly and discuss their feelings. All members of the family will benefit if the parents support each other in their approach to their children, and this situation can only be acquired by mutual cooperation of both partners.

The growing awareness of the prognosis of the disease may result in severe depression in the whole family. The child's increasing physical needs place greater demands on the parents' strength and time, and the resulting fatigue makes the parents less able to cope with their emotional difficulties. Many refuse to acknowledge the child's approaching death in the daily hope of a discovery by medical research to cure or arrest the disease. Those who do not bear this hope and accept the present situation with no available cure and eventual deterioration, inevitably need help to approach their problem positively, and all members of the treatment team should work together to support the child and the family to ensure their best integration in the community. Death from respiratory failure frequently occurs quickly, leaving the family in a state of shock. Many families having had to adapt their lifestyle for two decades or more never recover from their emotional upsets. Any frictions or separations cannot be remedied overnight. The child's sister may be contemplating motherhood and suffering the anxiety of being a possible carrier. Parents are frequently left with only their own company after the death of their handicapped child, because their other children will probably be adult by this time. If their own relationships are strained this may continue for the rest of their lives.

Treatment

At the present time there is no known cure for muscular dystrophy, so treatment is essentially palliative. The main aims are to maintain the child's optimum physical ability, to support the child and his family in their everyday physical and psychological needs and to reduce the risk of complications, wherever possible. Despite intensive treatment, physical deterioration will inevitably take place, but early recognition of the problems of the condition by the treatment team, and help for the family and the child, should ensure maximum achievement.

The most important aims of physical treatment of the child are to prevent contractures and deformities, and to maintain muscle strength for as long as possible. Physiotherapy, occupational therapy and parental instruction will all play an important part. The most beneficial way of delaying deterioration in muscle strength is active exercise. The child should be encouraged to walk as much as possible, however difficult and slow this may be, in order to maintain muscle tone. Motivation can be improved by using remedial games in place of formal exercise regimes. Football or similar kicking games, climbing steps or frames, and games involving catching, throwing, pulling and pushing will benefit the muscles of the pelvic and shoulder girdles respectively. Swimming and hydrotherapy are excellent activities. The greatest single factor limiting the child's walking ability is weakness of the hip and spinal extensors, which cause the child to flex, thus altering his posture and centre of gravity. Particular attention should be paid to maintaining tone in the glutei, latissimus dorsi and erector spinae. Prone lying will discourage the development of flexion contractures and passive stretching of the hip flexors also plays an important part.

Deterioration will, however, occur as the hip and spinal extensors weaken and the child spends more time in the sitting position causing the hip flexors to contract. The risk of serious injury from frequent falls, the gross postural abnormalities adopted to retain balance and the negligible benefit of time spent on passive exercises of the hips at the expense of time spent on education and other activities eventually results in the acceptance of wheelchair existence. A tricycle or pedal car may be used as an interim mobility aid if the child is not too large and still has trunk balance. Prone lying will delay the development of fixed flexion deformities for some time. Treatment of the wheelchair-bound child should concentrate on the maintenance of ankle dorsiflexion, upper limb strength for wheelchair propulsion and transfer, and good spinal posture. Fixed plantarflexion deformities of the ankles cause problems with footwear and increase the probability of damage to the feet when manoeuvring the wheelchair. Various methods of encouraging dorsiflexion may be used. These include the use of toe-spring or foot-drop calipers, moulded splint supports, surgical elongation of the Achilles tendon and specific exercise. Modern opinion favours surgical elongation of the Achilles tendon before the child is even walking on his toes, as this helps to retard postural abnormalities to retain balance as the hip and spinal extensors weaken. Undoubtedly, if surgery is left until the child already has great difficulty with walking, the deformities at the hips and lumbar spine will not be reversible, and the postoperative immobilisation required while healing occurs will further weaken the child's muscles and may result in a wheelchair existence earlier, rather than later, in life. Passive stretching of the Achilles tendon, remedial games involving dorsiflexion and treadling exercises are commonly used to support surgery. Activities for the upper limbs should aim to maintain grip strength, elbow and shoulder mobility for wheelchair propulsion and daily living activities. The biceps, triceps, deltoids and pectoralis major muscles are usually the first to weaken. Elevation of the arms becomes more difficult, affecting feeding and dressing. Grip and finger dexterity remain good in the majority of boys until quite late in the disease, and support for the arms to alleviate gravity, by overhead slings or, more popularly, ball bearing arm supports, will ensure maximum independent upper limb activity for as long as possible.

One aspect of physiotherapy which has proved very beneficial is the policy of teaching the child control of breathing very early and maintaining regular breathing exercises throughout the course of the disease. In the late stages when complications frequently result from weakness of the intercostal muscles and chest infection, these exercises can assist the child in overcoming respiratory failure for a longer period.

In the later stages of the disease, treatment should concentrate on the maintenance of alignment of the spine as far as this is possible, passive mobilisation within the limited range of all joints to retard contracture development and active mobilisation where power remains. Breathing exercises should be repeated regularly, and postural drainage may help to keep the chest clear. A lightweight brace to support the spine, used as soon as any postural weakness is detected, helps to allay scoliosis or kyphosis. This brace should not interfere with breathing. When the child is wheelchair-bound a moulded body support with padded lining can help to delay further postural deterioration. Padding inside the support is essential for comfort, and the prevention of pressure sores; freedom of the chest for breathing is imperative.

Independence in daily living

One of the most important aspects of care, which should be the responsibility of all members of the treatment team, is to support the child and the family in their physical and psychological needs in everyday life. Maintenance of the child's optimum physical ability plays an important role not only physically, but also psychologically. Depression in the child is deepened by increased handicap, and the stress and fatigue caused by the child's requirements and emotional behaviour affect all members of the family. Assistance in daily living to maintain the child's independence for as long as possible and advice, aids and adaptations to make home care easier when the child is no longer able to perform tasks alone provide widespread relief. Whenever possible, the provision of assistance should consider the child's future needs without too much morbidity; for example, a shower unit will be of use for a longer period than bathing aids, provided it is conveniently located for the child's access. It will not have the stigma of special aids for the disabled, and all members of the family may benefit from its use.

Physiotherapists, occupational therapists and social workers, both in the hospital and in the community should work together closely to ensure the most suitable help and advice is provided.

Mobility

There are differences of opinion between departments regarding the use of walking aids, because the child may find it difficult to control and steer them due to flaccid weakness at the hips and lumbar spine and because the more stable aids of the frame or rollator type tend to encourage the child to stoop forwards. Walking with the support of another person is much more suitable when this is possible. Rails in the home will assist the child, particularly on steps and stairs. When a wheelchair is required, great care should be taken in the choice of the most suitable chair. Again, opinions regarding the type of chair differ from place to place, some departments preferring an electrically propelled chair for the child from an early stage, with a folding chair for the family to push the child outdoors, while other departments prefer the child to propel himself indoors in a non-electric chair whilst his upper limb strength still enables him to do so. Whichever policy is adopted, there are a number of important points to be considered. The seat of the chair should be of the correct width to enable the child to sit upright without leaning to one side to support the upper half of his body on an armrest. The footrests should be at a suitable height to hold the ankles in dorsiflexion; toe-restraining straps may be necessary to prevent the feet from sliding off the front of the footrests. A cushion allows the child to have a more comfortable ride, and the backrest may be very slightly reclined to help delay flexion and scoliosis deformities. A tray is imperative to ensure maximum upper limb activity whilst the child is sitting in the chair, and later, as spinal extension weakens, the tray may help to support the upper trunk by providing an elbow rest. The chair used by the parents for outdoor journeys must be easily folded for transportation and sufficiently robust to withstand long-distance travel and rough terrain so that the child can participate in normal family outings. The BEC electric chair is particularly suitable for the muscular dystrophy child. It can be folded for transportation, it may be adapted to light fingertip microswitch control and it has provision for two heavy duty batteries to be carried to allow the child to travel greater distances. Help with alterations to the home to accommodate the wheel-chair-bound child can be obtained through the social services department in many cases. Ramped access will allow greater mobility, doors may need to be widened, and the provision of bed, toilet and bathing facilities at ground level overcomes a lot of lifting and carrying for the family.

Personal care

Feeding. The mechanics of feeding present few problems until the late stages of the disease when the upper arms become too weak to lift the hands to the mouth. Obesity should be avoided by a well-balanced calorie-controlled diet. This should be commenced early in life in order to establish good eating habits. This may seem hard on the child, but over-indulging him with sweet foods to compensate for limitations is positively detrimental. The obese child tends to lose ambulation earlier in life as the weakened muscles will not support his weight, and the extra burden placed on the family in lifting and carrying the heavy child is obvious. When the upper arm muscles weaken, pivoting the wrist of the feeding arm on the clenched fist of the other will allow the hand to reach the mouth. Ball-bearing arm supports will also help arm elevation in feeding.

Dressing. Dressing presents many probles as the child deteriorates. The type of clothing will be an important factor. Garments should be loose-fitting and front-opening with the minimum of fastenings. Shoes must be supportive.

When upright balance becomes difficult the child should sit in a chair to dress, standing only to pull up trousers and pants. Braces may make this task easier as they may be slipped over the arms before standing, thus ensuring the garments do not fall to the floor on rising. Shoes and socks can be put on with the feet on a low footstool, the child using the technique of 'walking up his thighs on his hands' to recover sitting posture when the hip and spinal extensors are weak. Substantial help will be required as the child's arms weaken and deformities develop. Calipers and trunk supports are difficult and eventually impossible for the child to put on satisfactorily unassisted. Severe, fixed

plantarflexion deformities at the ankles may cause difficulties with footwear. High-laced shoes or boots will obviously be more successful than slip-on or low-cut shoes. Once wearing boots or shoes becomes totally impossible, thick woollen socks or slipper socks may be used because these will keep the feet warm and comfortable, and provide them with a small degree of protection when manoeuvring the wheelchair.

In the late stages of the disease, the child may be dressed on the bed by being rolled from side to side to pull clothes over the trunk. The spinal support is easier to fit while the child is supine than when he is in a sitting position. The backstrain placed on the parent or assistant in dressing the child on the bed must be considered, and advice on lifting techniques and raising the bed on blocks or similar supports will reduce the necessary bending. Lifting the child from the bed to the wheelchair or toilet facilities becomes increasingly difficult as the child grows heavier and less able to help himself. A small mobile hoist with fully supportive slings is particularly useful for this purpose, and a raised bed will allow easier access. The sling may be placed under the child while he is being rolled on the bed in dressing. The hoist will also be of assistance in transferring the child from his chair to the bath or to the car for outdoor journeys.

Washing and bathing. The greatest difficulties presented when washing and bathing the child are access to the bath, lifting the child in and out of the bath and balance problems caused by postural weakness when in the water. There are various ways of tackling these problems. As already mentioned, the most suitable long-term answer is the installation of a shower unit accessible from a bed-sitting-room downstairs. A mobile shower chair may be used. If this solution is not possible, alternative methods must be considered. A traditional over-bath board and lower seat, preferably combined, and a non-slip mat in the bottom of the bath will help the child who has difficulty with standing balance and some weakness in the shoulder girdle and hip and spinal extensors when getting in and out of the bath. The child should be advised not to lower himself to the bottom of the bath, but to remain seated on the lower seat with his legs extended and feet braced against the end of the bath when washing. As deterioration occurs a moulded bath insert installed over the bath will reduce the lifting required to help the child in and out of the bath and, depending on the shape of the mould, it may also provide some support for the child. It will, however, deprive the child of the comfort and relaxation provided by deep warm water around him as the water level is very much reduced. Another possible solution is the use of a fixed or mobile hoist to lift the child in and out of the normal bath. The slings may remain attached to provide support, or a moulded seat wedged between the sides of the bath or attached to the base of the bath by suction can be employed. A washing mitten, soap on a rope or a suction soap holder, and a long-handled bath brush or sponge will make washing easier for the child. It is usually safer to remove the water before lifting the child out of the bath, but if the sling support technique is used this is immaterial.

If the child is able to sit in a chair he may do so in the bathroom to dry and dress. The severely handicapped child may be taken to the bedroom and laid on a towel on the bed if this is close to the bathroom. The optimum time for bathing the child is in the evening just before he goes to bed. Dressing after bathing is then reduced to pyjamas, and the warmth of the bath helps to relax the child and induce sleep. A morning bath similarly reduces the dressing needs because there are only pyjamas to remove and the bath may ease joints stiffened during sleep. Parents may be assisted with or relieved from bathing responsibilities by the services of a bath attendant from the local district nursing team. When the child reaches puberty, shaving may present a problem. A lightweight electric razor is most suitable. This may be stabilised in a swivel stand if upper limb weakness prevents the child from controlling the shaver manually.

Toilet use. It is fortunate for the muscular dystrophy child that control of bladder and bowel action usually remains good until the very late stages of the disease. Some children never suffer incontinence. The greatest obstacle to be overcome is access to the toilet. Ideally, toilet facilities with rail supports should be provided adjacent to the bed-sitting-room and be accessible to the wheelchair. If this is not possible, a chair commode or a chemical toilet with a frame may be used. A paraplegic cushion in the wheelchair simplifies the use of a urine-collecting bottle. Faecal management may be obtained by the use of suppositories, but these are not often needed because training in regular bowel habits and easily accessible toilet facilities are usually adequate to prevent frequent accidents.

A simple communication system to enable the child to summon assistance when required will help to reduce the need for constant attention and will allow the child some privacy. This system can be particularly useful if the child needs attention during the night for the toilet or for discomfort from cramp or stiffness of immobility. The control should be easily accessible from bed or, during the day, from the wheelchair. The most suitable type is the small portable radio-controlled activator which requires minimum pressure to operate.

Education

Despite the present inevitable prognosis of the disease, every effort should be made to provide the child with the broadest education possible, even though he may never, or at best only very briefly, use his knowledge in employment. The acquisition of formal academic knowledge presents less of a problem than gaining of practical experience.

The possiblity of impaired intellect, the frequent absence from school for hospital visits and the child's emotional state may all affect academic attainment. The child should continue attendance at a normal school as long as this is possible. Once this is no longer practical a choice has to be made between home tuition, which limits the child's social stimulation, but maintains family unity, or attendance at a special school for the handicapped. The latter gives the child contact with other children with difficulties and this may help with his emotional adjustment. Unfortunately, however, not all children are able to attend such a school on a daily basis, and the many problems caused by family separation frequently outweigh the benefits gained. All factors should be carefully explored before a decision is made. Daily attendance at a special school where transport is provided is the ideal for most boys.

Practical problems in academic learning occur

most markedly when the child's upper limbs weaken. Writing may be affected, and the introduction of ball-bearing arm supports, and a typewriter if necessary, prolongs written communication. Maximum use of library facilities and audiovisual aids should be made to widen the child's knowledge.

Education through experience becomes increasingly restricted by the child's growing handicap. For this reason it is important to give priority in the early years to the child's participation in as much experience of life as possible. Family outings, visits, school and neighbourhood friendships, hobbies and practical activities will provide the child with a variety of interests and opportunities which he can maintain and continue as his mobility diminishes.

The majority of children with muscular dystrophy unavoidably lack opportunity or are unable to obtain full benefit from the situations provided. This may be because they cannot participate physically, because of their social isolation or fear of embarrassment or because their knowledge is patchy through previous absences. Parents and all those concerned with the child in the hospital, school and community should help him by providing information and opportunity to further his learning whenever possible. Friends of his own age are particularly valuable for social stimulation.

A few children with muscular dystrophy continue to further education at sixteen or eighteen years of age, but the majority are homebound. This may add to family frictions and to the child's frustrations or apathy. Radio, television and library facilities should be utilised to the fullest to maintain stimulation. Day-centre attendance may also provide an educational outlet, although they usually concentrate on practical and social skills.

Hobbies and leisure activities

Hobbies and leisure activities fulfil a very important need in the muscular dystrophy child's life and that of his family. It is through these activities that the child should be able to achieve happiness and enjoyment, as he chooses when his interests are aroused. He may also gain friendship with other persons who share the same interest, but are not disabled, thus allowing him to widen his horizons beyond his family, the treatment team and his school companions. Some hobbies will also help to unite the family, as all members may be able to participate equally.

It is especially important that the child should be introduced to as wide a variety of activities as possible while he is still young and able to participate physically. This will give him a broad experience on which he can build his future interests.

Many boys are very keen on sporting activities, and although disability may prevent the muscular dystrophy child from continuing some sports, there are a great number which are still available to him for many years as they can be successfully continued, even when he is wheelchair-bound. The British Sports Association for the Disabled and the Central Council for Physical Recreation may be able to help the child by giving advice on sports assistance and contact with local sports organisations. Swimming is a particularly beneficial activity which the child can enjoy for some years. Other less active sports suitable for the disabled child include table games, particularly snooker and billiards, as well as smaller games like chess and dominoes. Target shooting has proved to be popular with quite a number of muscular dystrophy children; the arm can be stabilised on the wheelchair table if the muscles of the shoulder girdle are weak. Fishing is another popular outdoor sport. The introduction of the more active sports such as tennis, squash, badminton and football in the form of television games may help to compensate the child for his inability to participate physically.

Many other interests and hobbies which are not in any way connected with sport can be pursued. Music provides a wide variety of opportunities both as a participant and as a listener. Children with muscular dystrophy are often able to play wind instruments well if they have been taught breathing control as part of their physical treatment programme. Many string instruments, provided they are not too large and do not require a wide range of arm movement, may also be played. In recent years the guitar has become very popular and this is an ideal instrument for the muscular dystrophy child. Listening to music may also provide the child with great pleasure. Cassette and record players enable him to listen to the music of his choice, and outings to concerts can be very rewarding to the child and to the entire family if they share his interests.

In addition to music and sport, there are a large number of normal boyhood interests which may be pursued by the muscular dystrophy child. Model trains, planes, boats and other items can all be made from kits and these, together with background reading, enable the child to enter the world of technical achievement which may otherwise be denied him. Many hobbies associated with nature interest all children. Collecting samples of leaves, flowers or grasses for microscopic or biological study or preservation, bird watching and raised or plant-pot gardening can be pursued. Some children even use this type of hobby to raise money for other activities by selling their plants.

With ingenuity and encouragement many different hobbies can be fully pursued; philately, art, pottery and photography to name but a few. Local authorities have improved access to libraries, cinemas and theatres, and museums, art galleries and many organisations are only too willing to help once they have been approached.

Encouragement of the parents and child to continue in these activities when physical ability diminishes is necessary to alleviate possible despair. Therapists can enable parents to see the importance of leisure activities in themselves and not as secondary needs to education and physical treatment. It is through pursuit of hobbies that the child will gain pleasure, enjoyment and maturity, and will therefore be helped to overcome feelings of depression and apathy which inhibit maximum benefit from formal education and physical treatment. A busy child is a happy child and idleness breeds boredom. If parents and family are involved in the child's interests they will obviously be more able to encourage him, despite their own fatigue, commitments and personal worries. Youth clubs and scout troups bring the child into contact with local children of his own age and thereby assist in his social development. Club members who are willing to transport the child and further his involvement will help the parents considerably in their management of the child. This permits him to 'do his own thing', an essential part of development in boyhood and adolescence.

The highlight of the year for many families is a holiday away from home, and every effort should be made to encourage the parents of the muscular dystrophy child to have an annual family holiday. In the early stages of the disease, this should present few problems, but as the child deteriorates and his mobility decreases, his need for assistance with some everyday activities and the search for suitable accommodation frequently result in his parents abandoning the holiday because of all the preparation and worries involved. It is even more important at this stage, when the family may already be feeling very restricted, that a holiday should be arranged.

There are a number of organisations who provide holidays for groups of handicapped children where help and supervision are available, and recreation and outings cater for the interests and abilities of the child. The homebound child may appreciate a vacation with other children outside his own family to widen his group of friends, and this enables the family to have a break from the burden of continual care.

Children who are away from home for education need the support of other members of the family at holiday times to reinforce the family bond. Many of these children prefer to stay at home and go out for day trips with other members of the family. Families who choose to go away together for a vacation can obtain information and assistance from a large number of different sources. Many hotels and holiday centres are now increasingly aware of the needs of the handicapped and will provide accommodation in adjoining rooms to help with problems of daily care. Motoring organisations, rail, sea and air travel operators provide information on facilities available for disabled travellers, and camping and caravanning clubs publish information on sites suitable for handicapped users. Information on holidays abroad can be obtained from the European Alliance of Muscular Dystrophy Associations, which at the present time consists of nine member countries, who particularly encourage exchange holidays between members.

Financial assistance for families who have difficulty meeting the cost of a holiday can be obtained in some cases through local authority social service departments or from various charitable organisations.

Complications

Complications can occur for a variety of reasons, many of which have already been mentioned. Physical treatment to maintain optimum mobility and muscle tone will help to delay the onset of fixed contractures and spinal deformities. A wheelchair cushion and sensible supports will reduce the risk of skin damage as a result of friction or pressure over particular anatomical areas. Training and practice in breathing control helps the boy to overcome lung congestion as a result of respiratory infection. Chemotherapy plays an important role in avoiding and surmounting other illnesses which may complicate the boy's condition. The normal routine immunisations of childhood should be provided for the muscular dystrophy child and some doctors recommend annual influenza vaccination. If the child develops a cough, cold or influenza most doctors advise early antibiotic therapy to combat the possibility of a more serious respiratory illness.

Obesity should be avoided at all costs. This not only makes lifting the child more difficult, but also seriously reduces the child's independent mobility as weight outweighs muscle strength. Further mobility problems may result from bed rest and this should therefore be avoided except when absolutely essential.

Complications as a result of psychological disturbance require much support and guidance. Full, active participation in as many normal boyhood activities as possible will help the boy and his family to adjust to the situation, but it is impossible for anyone to provide a fully satisfactory solution, and the family of the muscular dystrophy child will bear a permanent scar during the boy's life, which will continue for many years after his death.

SPINA BIFIDA

Spina bifida is usually defined as a congenital abnormality of the spine due to failure of closure of the spinal canal in its posterior mid-line. The contents of the spinal canal may protrude through this gap and the coverings of the spinal cord are frequently maldeveloped. The commonest site for this abnormality is the lumbar region, but it may be present at any level in the spine.

Causes. There is no conclusive evidence at present as to the cause of this condition. Various theories have been put forward, and although it may now be detected *in utero* the initial cause of the defect is still unknown. If both parents suffer from the condition the risk of affected offspring is undoubtedly increased. Many mothers present a history of miscarriages or anencephalic births but, as previously mentioned, the root cause of these is undetermined in the majority of cases. A genetic factor is obviously involved in some cases where the abnormality recurs in blood-related families. Incidences of racially connected abnormality also point to a possible genetic cause, as demonstrated by the fact that one of the highest incidences of spina bifida is recorded in the Irish Republic and reflected in second and third generation Irish-Americans. In other families no such obstetrical or family history exists and the occurrance of the spina bifida abnormality is completely unheralded.

Diagnosis. Modern medicine has, however, enabled obstetricians to diagnose the abnormality *in utero* by analysis of blood samples for alpha-fetoprotein and by ultrasound testing between the fourteenth and sixteenth week of pregnancy. This sophisticated procedure will detect anencephaly or hydrocephalus; enlargement of the ventricles; developmental abnormalities of the kidneys and gross skeletal deformities. The diagnosis should be confirmed by amniocentesis before pregnancy termination is considered. This is the withdrawal by aspiration of a small amount of amniotic fluid from the sac surrounding the foetus for analysis. A raised level of alphafetoprotein is indicative of a spina bifida abnormality. However, the alphafetoprotein level is also raised if there is more than one foetus, and sometimes for no apparent cause. The use of these diagnostic measures in early pregnancy, together with the more widespread acceptance of abortion, has significantly reduced the number of spina bifida babies born in Britain today. In some areas paediatricians have altered their previous policy which was to strive at all costs to ensure the survival of the severely handicapped child, and some babies are now allowed to die. This has further reduced the number of young children with severe spina bifida deformities.

There are two basic types of spina bifida: the occulta, which as its name suggests is not often obvious, and the more common severe type, spina bifida cystica. In spina bifida occulta, the vertebral laminae are defective, but the contents of the spinal column do not protrude. The spinal membranes are frequently connected to the skin by fibrous bands. In early life, there is little or no loss of function in the patient's bladder, bowels or limbs. The condition may remain undiagnosed unless the patient requires a spinal X-ray for some other reason. In other patients, the abnormality may be recognised visually by a covering of horny, pigmented skin or a tuft of hair. Occasionally in later life frequency of micturition or slight paraesthesia in the lower limbs result from traction on the cord by the fibrous bands. Little or no treatment is required in childhood, but awareness of the existence of the condition may help in later life when parenthood is considered, because if two such persons marry, their offspring may be at risk.

Spina bifida cystica

The more severe types of spina bifida are those of the cystica variety. The main abnormalities are meningoceles and meningomyeloceles.

The meningocele is a sac which protrudes through the bony gap in the vertebral column. This sac contains cerebrospinal fluid, but no nerve tissue. It has a narrow neck connecting it to the spine and is usually successfully removed by surgery in the first few hours of life with little or no resulting paralysis below the operation site. Meningoceles occur most commonly in the lumbar region and, depending upon the exact site, the nerves to the bladder and bowel may be involved and slightly damaged causing weakness or frequency in micturition and defeacation.

The meningomyelocele is a much more serious deformity. The sac protrudes through the vertebral column in a similar way to the meningocele but the neck attaching it to the body is wider. The sac is usually larger and contains nerve tissue and cerebrospinal fluid, and the spinal cord may protrude into the sac. Surgery to remove and close the sac is successful in providing a better skin covering

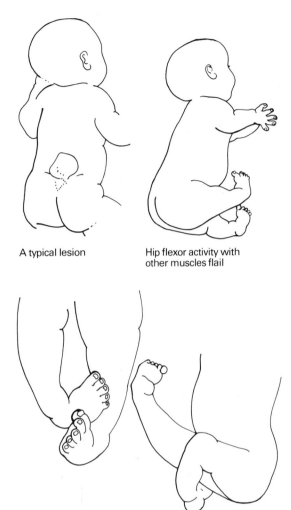

A typical lesion   Hip flexor activity with other muscles flail

Typical lower limb deformities

Fig. 23.13 Typical lesion and deformities in spina bifida

over the abnormality, thereby reducing the risk of rupture and resulting infection, but some paralysis is virtually inevitable. The severity and distribution of the paralysis depends on the site and extent of the lesion (Fig. 23.13).

Complications

Many complications are associated with spina bifida, the most common being *hydrocephalus*, which affects about 80 per cent of all spina bifida children. This is the medical term for increased fluid in the brain, usually caused by a congenital malformation or blockage of the foramen of

Magendie or interventricular foramena, thus restricting the circulation of cerebrospinal fluid and causing distortion of all or part of the brain and surrounding skull (which is soft and ununited) as the pressure of fluid increases. In some babies hydrocephalus is present before birth, causing difficulties at delivery, while in others it develops after birth either spontaneously or as a result of infection. The enlarged head of the hydrocephalic child at birth is easily recognised, but for children who develop it after birth early diagnosis is vital to prescribe treatment or growth monitoring before permanent damage has occurred. Widening of the skull suture lines, bulging of the soft tissue in the anterior fontanelle, unusual enlargement in the head circumference, and crying and general malaise are early symptoms. Treatment to relieve the increase in fluid and pressure build-up in the brain by the insertion of a tube (usually into the right lateral ventricle of the brain) with a one-way valve to control pressure, is very successful. Below the valve is another length of tubing connecting the valve to the blood circulatory system via the jugular vein. The valve will only open when the pressure in the ventricles is above the normal level, and there is no danger of backflow of blood because of the valve's one-way action (Fig. 23.14). The head gradually returns to normal size and grows at the usual rate as the valve controls the pressure. Complications do occasionally occur in the use or installation of the valve. It may become blocked or disconnected, or the subcutaneous tissue surrounding the valve may become infected. Infection or a blocked valve require immediate treatment, and disconnection should also be treated quickly to avoid further complications. Failure to arrest hydrocephalus results in a grossly enlarged head which is difficult to support, in mental retardation because of pressure of fluid in the brain and in blindness due to compression of the optic nerve. As the child grows, it will probably be necessary to replace the lower tube with a longer one to ensure the valve remains connected to the systemic circulation.

Bladder and kidney disorders can also complicate the spina bifida problems. These may be due to malformation of the organs themselves, but are more usually the result of damaged or absent nerve supply from the spinal abnormality (Fig. 23.15).

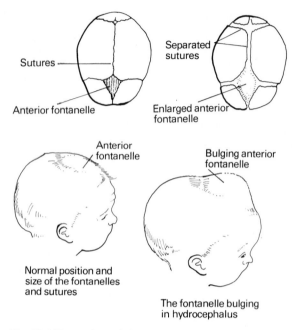

Fig. 23.14A Hydrocephalus

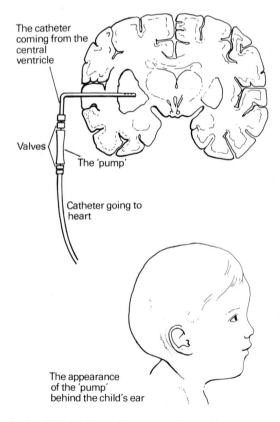

Fig. 23.14B Working of the shunt in the treatment of hydrocephalus

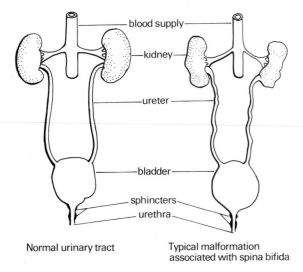

Fig. 23.15 Kidney function in spina bifida.

Dysfunction is caused by lack of sphincter control or by damage to the nerve impulses to empty the bladder and bowels, eventually resulting in overflow. In the former case the child is constantly wet and frequently dirty, and pressure applied to the abdomen to further express the contents of the bladder produces no urine. The child is at risk of ascending infection because the sphincters are constantly relaxed. In overflow incontinence the child may remain clean and dry for some time. Manual bladder expression after dribbling will produce a stream of urine. These children may suffer from damage to the ureters and kidneys due to backflow or urine or pressure build-up by retention. Stagnation of urine in the bladder which may not fully empty without assistance causes an infection hazard. Severe constipation may also be present.

There are various ways of approaching these problems. It is always important to regularly check the child's urine for infection, and if this is present treatment by chemotherapy should follow.

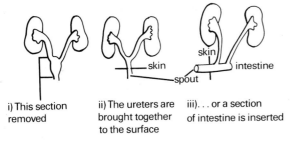

i) This section removed

ii) The ureters are brought together to the surface

iii)... or a section of intestine is inserted

Fig. 23.16 Ileostomy

Teaching manual bladder expression may solve the overflow problem, but this should not be recommended if an intravenous pyelogram shows kidney or ureter damage from backflow. Suppositories will assist in the control of faeces. When incontinence is due to lack of sphincter control good hygiene on the part of the parents in regularly changing and bathing the child will help prevent infection. As a long-term measure nappies are not ideal, and ileal-loop diversion for social reasons may be recommended, particularly in girls (Fig. 23.16). This is the diversions of the ureters to the surface of the abdomen to bypass the bladder and form a stoma to which can be attached a rubber flange and a urinary collecting bag (Fig. 23.17). In boys a penile collecting bag may solve the urinary problem. Ileal-loop diversion is indicated where ureter and kidney damage is present from urine backflow. Suppositories may again be used to help faecal control.

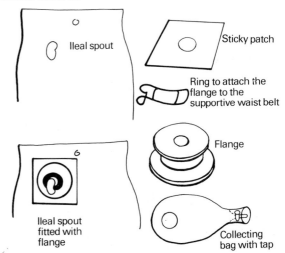

Fig. 23.17 Management of the ileostomy

In addition to the problems of hydrocephalus and bladder and bowel dysfunction there are many other complications which are not critical for survival, but markedly affect the quality of life. The greatest of these problems is the extent of the *paralysis and weakness*, and the associated sensory loss. In the words of the parents the first question is usually 'Will he live?' and this is closely followed by 'Will he walk?' The answer to these questions will depend on a combination of factors, including the extent and site of the lesion, the successful control of hydrocephalus, the provision of operative measures to assist weight-bearing together with the success of intensive physical treatment and bracing, and the motivation of the child. All persons concerned with the management of the child should work together to ensure a well integrated programme for mobility.

Sensory diminution or loss may cause the child to injure himself without being aware of it. This may happen through dragging his legs on a rough floor, entangling them in toys or equipment, or by heat from a hot water bottle, radiator or fire. Injuries in the anaesthetic area take longer to heal than elsewhere and the possibility of secondary infection through the open wound is ever present.

A high proportion of children with hydrocephalus also have visual problems, the most common of these being a squint. Surgery may be needed to correct this. The squint will affect the child's visual perception which may result in further activity problems. Mental retardation associated with hydrocephalus will also have some effect on the child's manual dexterity. In children who do not have hydrocephalus, problems of dexterity, hand control and fine finger movements are not uncommon. This may be largely due to the child using the upper limbs for weight-bearing and support for much of the time, thereby limiting opportunities for the development of fine arm and hand control.

Psychological problems are common in families where spina bifida occurs. Initially, the decision to abort the foetus causes much distress in the hopeful parents. Unless they already have a handicapped child, many of them are unaware of the pressures placed upon their future by the needs of the child, and many people feel that the advice of the 'experts', i.e. the obstetricians and paediatricians, should be followed because of their insight into the problems of other such families. However, it would not be natural if the prospective parents did not suffer feelings of insecurity and bewilderment when making the decision to abort the foetus. In some families this pregnancy may be the culmination of a number of attempts to conceive and deliver a normal child and an abortion may result in them remaining childless or applying for adoption, while in other families it may only be an isolated case and future pregnancies may be uneventful.

The anguish of abortion is far outweighed by the multitude of psychological problems which arise once the handicapped child is born. The initial despair after nine months of waiting is immeasureable. The mother is fatigued by the birth process, and the shock of having a handicapped child, added to this fatigue and the hormonal change after delivery, can result in serious permanent psychological disturbance, however understandingly and compassionately the situation is handled by the medical staff. The decision to isolate the mother from the other mothers and their babies to grieve alone or to allow her to remain in a ward surrounded by the joy of other families and their embarrassment towards her is a difficult one to make, and the mother's wishes should be respected. The father has to face the world of expectant friends and family to break the news of the birth of the handicapped child alone. A decision by the parents at this time as to whether medication should be provided to save the child or whether the child should be allowed to die is very difficult and many parents are unable to give a rational answer because of their own shock and grief and their lack of understanding of the medical facts. The maternal and paternal instinct in most parents to protect the baby from pain and suffering is torn apart. On the one hand, they want to relieve the baby of any distress, but on the other, by helping him to overcome the initial struggle to live, they are usually condemning him to a life of frequent operations, medication and emotional distress. The number of operations required by some spina bifida children is well into double figures, and at each operation there is the inevitable apprehension on the part of the parents and child regarding the operation itself and also the separation of the family, however short this may be.

Many parents feel despair and fear once they are home with their handicapped child who is their responsibility. Frequently, they have had all the medical facts explained to them, but since they were in a state of shock they were unable to comprehend them. It is important, at this early stage, that they are given ample opportunity to ask questions and discuss the management of their child if depression, fear and overanxiety are to be controlled. Neighbours and friends can be a great comfort to them at this time, but often they tell stories of other children they have heard of with a similar condition, or shy away because of their own inhibitions towards the child and mother.

Over the years, as they see other children of the same age walking, out of nappies and playing freely together, the parents realise how the burden of caring for the handicapped child has restricted them. They frequently suffer feelings of helplessness and of being at the mercy of the medical services with frequent hospital visits, long waits for appointments and disagreements over treatment and appliances. This helplessness may change to bitterness and anger in parents, who, besides their natural love for their child, develop an over protectiveness which may stifle the child's freedom for individual expression later in life. Crisis after crisis faces the family throughout the child's first few years of life. There are all the medical and surgical problems, complications which may arise in daily home management, the search for the most suitable type of education, the frustrations of adolescence and the worry of the possibility that the child may not be able to find employment.

The child is not spared from emotional upset. Frequently, many spina bifida children exhibit behavioural difficulties because of their anger and frustrations about the limitations the disability places upon them. They may be timid or apathetic if their parents have protected them from the harsh realities of their struggle in life, or they may rebel against their parents for not allowing them their freedom. Mental retardation, frequently the result of hydrocephalus, may also cause behavioural disturbances.

The emotional problems which may occur in the siblings of the spina bifida child are similar to those experienced in any family where there is a handicapped child. The diversion of the parents' attention towards the handicapped child at the expense of the rest of the family frequently results in the other children suffering feelings of rejection or neglect and therefore behaving in an apathetic or attention-seeking manner. Some parents also attempt to compensate for their own feelings of guilt, inadequacy or disappointment by overburdening the other children with their own hopes and aspirations for attainment.

It is important to reflect the present trend to encourage abortion of an affected foetus in the light of evidence from parents who already have a spina bifida child. While they show great love and affection for their child, many wish the present antenatal diagnostic knowledge had been available at the time of their pregnancy. Those who do become pregnant are only too eager for full investigations and the majority readily accept abortion should the tests prove positive.

Surgery

There are many different forms of surgical treatment for the spina bifida child. In the first few weeks of life, surgery to close the cyst and to insert a control valve should hydrocephalus develop is recommended. Later operative measures concentrate on bladder management and the improvement of lower limb function to aid mobility and ambulation. Tendon transfers at the hips to improve extension and external rotation, release of contractures at the knees or operations to stabilise the knee joint and surgery to correct deformities of the ankles and feet may be necessary. Occasionally, secondary skull surgery to release premature closure of the skull suture lines is required, and the necessity for revision of the valve is not uncommon. It is important to remember that any child with spina bifida may require a number of such operations, bringing them in contact with three of four different surgical teams, each concerned with a particular problem, and close liaison is necessary to integrate the treatment and avoid parental confusion.

Mobility

The main aims of physical treatment of the spina bifida child are to prevent and correct deformities and to build up muscle strength and control to encourage mobility and ambulation. Many children are born with deformities of the legs and feet, and as they grow these will become worse if they are not treated early in life. The commonest deformities are flexion at the hips, hyperextension or flexion at the knees, plantarflexion at the ankles and equinovarus deformities in the feet. In a very young baby whose bones and joints are still very supple, serial splintage and regular exercise can correct some of these deformities. In other children, surgery to correct and stabilise the joint may be required if weight-bearing is to be successful. Exercise concentrates on the maintenance of optimum mobility at all joints. If active movement is not possible because of lack of innervation to the muscles, passive exercise should be regularly repeated to maintain joint mobility. Upper limb and trunk strength is also very important, for the upper limbs will be used to assist in weight-bearing and the spinal extensors to maintain upright posture. Most spina bifida children require calipers for ambulation. These may be supports which extend from the thorax to the feet, pelvic supports or long-leg and below-knee calipers, depending on the site and extent of the lesion. It requires a lot of practice and patience on the part of the child and the therapist to learn balance and control of the limbs with such large calipers. Walking frames, particularly the rollator type, are most popular in the early stages and many children progress to elbow crutches or even sticks. Knee extension and ankle dorsiflexion may be maintained when the calipers are not worn by the use of lightweight splints. Plastazote knee supports are widely used, and thermoplastic foot-drop splints worn between two socks hold the ankles in dorsiflexion. Plastazote may also be used to provide a cushion insole in the surgical boots used when walking with calipers. Mobility training is primarily the role of the physiotherapist, but all members of the treatment team and the family should work together to encourage the child. The occupational therapist may be involved with splintage and she should be concerned with the child's mobility. The invention of the 'trolley' has provided a simple form of independent mobility for the child from a very early age. However the most commonly used trolleys, the ASBAH and the Chailey, have a slightly different merit. The former is particularly suitable for the very young child as it is lighter to manoeuvre. The padded backrest also provides some protection for spinal protrusions. Repositioning of the single front castor approximately halfway along the total length of the seat allows the front corner of the leg rest to tilt to the floor when weight is applied and therefore makes climbing on and off easier for the small child. The absence of a harness as a standard fitting may restrict its use, as may its instability on uneven terrain, notably soft

grass. The Chailey trolley is much heavier, and is sometimes impossible to manoeuvre for young children. The backrest is not padded. It does, however, have a harness, and the two rear castors and bumper bar give added stability. The bumper also saves damage to furniture. Both trolleys, by keeping the knees in an extended position, help to discourage the development of flexion contractures.

As the child grows, the Yorkhill chair may take over from the trolley to fulfil the child's need for wheeled mobility. Most people concerned with handicapped children will be familiar with the merits of this small, neat child's wheelchair. The spina bifida child may benefit greatly from its use, although transfer to and from it can be difficult because of the fixed arm- and footrests. An interesting feature is the ability to use the chair to support the knees in extension by raising the footrest to the highest point and placing the seat cushion on the footrest. Psychologically the child benefits from the higher position which makes communication with other children easier.

A number of small hand-controlled cars and similar toys for wheeled mobility in and around the home are now available. These are suitable for spina bifida children between two and seven years of age. As the child grows, a small Model 8 chair is the most suitable replacement for the Yorkhill, and in later years, although it is hoped by this time wheeled mobility will be supplementary to ambulation, a lightweight standard Model 8 chair may be supplied.

When considering wheeled mobility the needs of the parents must not be overlooked. Anyone who has tried to lift a four-year-old child onto a one-man-operated bus, together with a pushchair and a bag of shopping, and then attempted to pay the fare before finding a seat will appreciate the value of the Baby Buggy or similar lightweight, easily folded pushchair. These types of chair are now universally used for both normal and handicapped children so that little needs to be said of their merits. Their most helpful feature for use with the spina bifida child is that they can be opened and folded with one hand whilst holding the child in the other arm. The position in which the child sits is not particularly good and a lightweight, easily detachable backrest may be needed. Plastazote is useful for this purpose and may be strengthened by the application of vitrathene. If more support is required, a child car-safety seat may be fitted into some folding pushchairs easily, and the child can be lifted out harnessed in the car seat while the chair is folded.

In later years, spina bifida teenagers should be encouraged to make use of the mobility allowance, if at all possible, to enable them to have greater freedom for work and leisure activities.

Architectural barriers to mobility in and around the home should be considered. Steps and stairs may be overcome by ramps, lifts or changing the function of particular rooms, and rails will provide support where ambulant mobility is possible. A strong, lightweight moveable box in wood or plastic can act as a 'half-step' and will assist the child in climbing on and off the bed, chair or toilet when not wearing calipers. This may remain in position as a foot support when the child is seated.

Independence in daily living

Feeding. Feeding should present little mechanical difficulty unless there has been brain damage due to hydrocephalus, but consideration should be given to the child's diet. As with all handicapped children, obesity should be avoided at all costs. Ample fluids should be taken, particularly when urinary infection is present, to ensure the kidneys are kept fully functional. Constipation may also occur and a high-roughage diet may ease its management. Foods liable to cause faecal laxity should be avoided.

Washing and hygiene. Balance in the bath is a major problem for the spina bifida child; this is later joined by the difficulties encountered when climbing in and out of the bath independently. When the child has outgrown the baby bath or sink, a small bath support made from an oval washing up bowl or for a larger child a high-sided baby bath has proved very successful. One short edge is cut away from the bowl or baby bath with shears and the edge smoothed with sandpaper. Four holes are punched into the base, one at each corner, and a single-sided, one-inch suction pad is inserted into each hole. A hole can be punched into each side of the bath to take a long dowelling rod which will act as a front support, and a piece

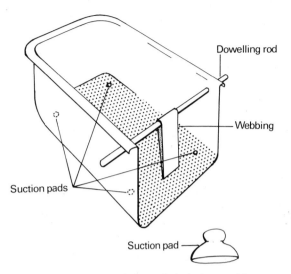

Fig. 23.18 Bath seat made from a baby bath or washing-up bowl

of webbing or similar material looped around the dowelling and through two slots in the base of the seat will provide a groin strap (Fig. 23.18). This is a very simple, easily made seat which is cheap to produce. A number of bath aids suitable for children are available commercially, usually at a greater cost.

The problem of access to the bath, and climbing in and out independently, should be approached in a similar way to that described for the muscular dystrophy child, the ideal solution being a shower unit with a detachable hand-held spray attachment.

Cleanliness and personal hygiene are of prime importance with the spina bifida child to reduce the risk of ascending infection and friction sores. The addition of a small amount of antiseptic fluid such as Savlon or Dettol to the bath water is advisable. Dental hygiene is also very important because of the possible damage to the tooth enamel by long term chemotherapy.

Dressing. The choice of clothing and the level of disability are important factors in determining the extent to which the spina bifida child will achieve dressing independence. Many parents choose to clothe their children, whether male of female, in trousers. These not only cover the caliper splints which may be necessary for mobility, but also provide some protection for the skin. Trousers with elasticated waist bands, although relieving the child of the need to manage fastenings, may prove to be impossible to put on over calipers. A wide waist opening and loose-fitting flared legs should be chosen. The suitability of clothing for the upper half of the body will depend on the site of the lesion and the child's sitting balance. A loose-fitting, V-necked sweater is easy for most children, whilst removing a front-opening shirt may provide difficulties with fastenings as well as with balance for a child with a high lesion affecting trunk control. Underclothes should be loose-fitting. If surgical boots are not worn, footwear should be supportive, with a front opening down to the heads of the metatarsals to facilitate easy placing of the foot in the shoe whilst ensuring that the toes are not turned in under the foot. Protective toe caps made from plastic or steel prolong the life of the shoes.

The most suitable place for independent dressing is on a warm floor near a corner. A low footstool may be of assistance when pulling clothes over the bottom. The child may place his chest on the stool and in a half-kneeling position pull the clothes up or down. If balance is poor, rolling from side to side may be safer for dressing the lower half of the body. Garments may be removed from the upper half of the body most easily by the child sitting in a corner, resting the chest on the outstretched legs and pulling the clothes over the head from the back of the neck, as this is a symmetrical movement and does not affect balance unduly. When dressing the upper half the reverse procedure should be followed, placing the arms in the garment first and then pulling it over the head.

Toilet use. This produces a wide variety of problems depending upon the severity and extent of the physical abnormality and/or the child's intellectual ability. The medical and surgical management of incontinence has already been discussed. The task of explaining the day-to-day care of such problems and discussing possible appliances frequently falls to the nursing staff or the occupational therapist. Manual bladder expression should only be taught on the recommendation of the consultant, because of the dangers of backflow of urine. Patients who are considered suitable for this method of training should be given ample opportunity to practise with supervision to ensure that pressure is applied correctly from the top of the abdomen downwards. Later, the child may be able to do this himself and thereby gain independence.

Children with ileal-loop diversion should be taught to empty their collecting bag from four or five years of age. Again, it is frequently the occupational therapist or nurse who teaches the parents the technique of changing the flange and the importance of good hygiene. It cannot be stressed enough that the parents must be completely familiar with the management of the stoma because the physical consequences of incorrect hygiene and the psychological effect of fear of the stoma can be disastrous for the child and the parents.

Sitting balance on the toilet is a common difficulty. Various designs of armchair potties have been produced and these are extremely useful for the young child. A simple child's wooden armchair can be adapted with a removeable cushion and a cut-out, commode-type base to accommodate the potty. Some armchair potty frames can be transferred to fit over the standard toilet. The spina bifida child who is ambulant will require a rail on at least one, and frequently on both sides of the toilet, and a Mothercare or similar over-toilet seat will help the small child to overcome the fear of falling into the toilet pan.

The value of suppositories to maintain regular faecal evacuation should be clearly understood by the parents and the child, as embarrassment regarding their use is frequently present. Ample opportunity should be given to discuss this problem with the nurse, therapist or doctor.

Recent publications by various bodies, particularly the Disabled Living Foundation, on the variety of incontinence garments available and on methods of odour control have greatly assisted in the management of total incontinence in patients with spina bifida. One extremely useful development has been the one-way incontinence pad which has markedly reduced the dangers of friction sores and infection from permanent dampness.

Education and development

There are many problems regarding education and development of ability in the spina bifida child.

Mental retardation, usually the result of hydro-cephalus, adds to the physical difficulties. Further complications concerning hand function and per-ceptual disturbances can restrict learning ability. It is important, therefore, that every opportunity is given to the child to develop basic skills from a very early age.

Mary Sheridan's booklet *The Developmental Progress of Infants and Young Children* is a useful guide for activity and assessment.

Visuo-perceptual problems occur usually as a result of a squint or similar abnormality in the eyes distorting visual feedback. Surgical correction should be attempted where possible at an early age and if successful, may totally overcome any problems regarding recognition of images. However, many children with spina bifida and hydrocephalus do still have perceptual problems, even when visual correction has succeeded. These particularly affect the organisation of sensory infor-mation into activity, which suggests a more com-plicated perceptual difficulty. Marion Frostig Tests of Visual Perception may be used for assessment purposes. Some children also appear to have difficulty with body-image presentation, but this may be due to gross sensory loss or rejection of the affected limbs. It is important that the therapist is aware of the possible occurrence of such problems and that she liaises with the psychologist to help the parents in assisting the child through play and practice to overcome them.

The development of hand function is closely related to intellectual and perceptual awareness and each is to some extent dependent upon the other. Because of the need to use the arms and hands for support, there is a lack of opportunity to develop fine finger control and dexterity. The therapist should encourage the child and parents to spend some part of every day in dextrous play to help overcome this deficit. Normal childhood construction games, needle and thread activities, and the use of scissors or jigsaws are all suitable for the development of hand function. Writing and typing practice and playing a musical instrument are particularly beneficial for the older child.

In addition to these difficulties there is another problem, which affects all handicapped children — the limitation of experience. The complexity of the problems of spina bifida from birth onwards greatly restricts the child's opportunity for de-velopment through play. The parents fear that the child may injure himself, their hesitancy to allow messy activities because of hygiene and the restric-tions placed upon the child because of poor mobility or balance may grossly curtail his play. The opportunity to help mother or father in their daily activities and thereby learn is denied to many children, and communication with other children of the same age is very restricted. Too many parents err on the side of fear and overprotection which further inhibits the child. The therapist should therefore encourage safe participation for the child in as many activities as possible, and attendance at a pre-school play group can be very rewarding. In the home, the mother should allow the child to join in household activities where possible. Baking, sweeping the floor or dusting low shelves can be easily arranged and weeding or hoeing the garden can be done very successfully from a trolley. There are an infinite number of opportunities for the child to join in the day-to-day family activities and learn through experience.

The choice of the most suitable school is a very difficult problem. In many cases the design of school buildings has played too important a role in this decision. Every opportunity to integrate the spina bifida child into local infant and junior schools has been made, but limited mobility and urinary problems have denied places to many children. The alternatives of special schools, fre-quently requiring the child to live away from home, have far-reaching consequences on the family bond and restrict the child's circle of friends, particularly amongst local children.

Reference has been made to the importance of hobbies and leisure activities for the muscular dystrophy child and the same applies to the child with spina bifida. These add greatly to the quality of life and provide a wider scope for future life experience.

The emphasis in the education of the teenager should be on future employment where possible. The development of practical as well as academic skills is necessary and the occupational therapist can play an important role in this. Training in homecraft is also very important for the child's independent future. Liaison between all persons involved with the child's future development is essential for the best possible integration of the child into the adult world.

Acknowledgement Figures 23.13, 14A and 14B are reprinted by kind permission of ASBAH and Dr John Lorber. They were drawn by Mr A. F. Foster, Medical Artist, United Sheffield Hospitals.

REFERENCES AND FURTHER READING

Allum N 1975 Spina bifida: The treatment and care of spina bifida children. Allen & Unwin, London

Bobath B, Bobath K 1975 Motor development in the different types of cerebral palsy. Heinemann Medical Books, London

Bowley A H, Gardner L 1972 The handicapped child. Churchill Livingstone, Edinburgh

Chick J R 1975 Occupational therapy for the disabled child. British Journal of Occupational Therapy 38(Feb):25

Dubowitz V 1978 Muscular dystrophy. Journal of the Chartered Society of Physiotherapy

Field A 1970 The challenge of spina bifida. Heinemann, London

Finnie N R 1974 Handling the young cerebral palsied child at home. Heinemann Medical Books, London

Fox M 1977 Psychological problems of physically handicapped children. British Journal of Hospital Medicine 17(May):479–490

Gardner-Medwin D 1974 Children with neuromuscular disease. Muscular Dystrophy Group of Great Britain, London

Holt K S 1965 Assessment of cerebral palsy. Lloyd Luke (Medical Books), London

Illingworth R S 1975 The development of young children: Normal and abnormal. Churchill Livingstone, Edinburgh

Lorber J 1970 Your child with spina bifida. Association for Spina Bifida and Hydrocephalus, London

Muscular dystrophy handbook. Muscular Dystrophy Group of Great Britain, London

Nettles O R 1972 Growing up with spina bifida. Scottish Association for Spina Bifida, Edinburgh

Nettles O R 1972 The spina bifida baby. Scottish Association for Spina Bifida, Edinburgh

Nettles O R 1972 Equipment and aids to mobility. Scottish Association for Spina Bifida, Edinburgh

Nichols P J R 1976 Muscular dystrophy. British Journal of Occupational Therapy 39(June):149

Oswin M 1976 Behaviour problems amongst children with cerebral palsy. Wright & Sons, Bristol

Routledge L 1978 Only child's play. Heinemann Medical, London

Sheridan M 1975 The developmental progress of infants and young children. HMSO, London

Woods G E 1975 The handicapped child. Blackwell, Oxford.

Useful addresses

The Muscular Dystrophy Group of Great Britain, Nattrass House, 35 Macaulay Road, Clapham, London SW4 0QP

The Association for Spina Bifida and Hydrocephalus, Tavistock House North, Tavistock Square, London WC1H 9HJ

The Disabled Living Foundation, 346 Kensington High Street, London W14 8NS

The Spastic Society, 12 Park Crescent London W1N 4EQ

24

Parkinsonism

Parkinsonism is a chronic, progressive neuro-muscular disease caused by degenerative changes in the basal ganglia which are concerned with the control of muscle tone. It is common in the middle-aged and elderly, frequently manifesting itself between the age of 55 and 60 years.

Pathology and clinical features

Although first described by Dr James Parkinson in 1817 in *An Essay on the Shaking Palsy*, the pathology of the condition is still not clearly understood. However, recent research has shown it to be associated with a disturbance of the chemical transmittors and accompanying cell degeneration within the basal ganglia. This disturbance, which upsets the balance between the cholinergic and dopaminergic transmission systems, results in a variety of symptoms amongst which tremor, rigidity and reduced, poor movement patterns are the most dominant. Of these three symptoms one may predominate, although all three are usually present. The condition is often slow and insidious in its onset so that the sufferer finds it difficult to say when his symptoms first appeared. Although not fatal in itself, death usually occurs from intercurrent infection.

Tremor. This usually begins in the upper limbs. It commonly affects the forearm and elbow muscles, and the characteristic 'pill-rolling' tremor between the thumb and fingers may also be present. Initially, the tremor may only appear periodically. Later it can affect the lower limb, trunk, face, lip, tongue and neck muscles. The tremor occurs at rest and disappears during voluntary movement and sleep, and may therefore not affect activity. The tremor may be unilateral or bilateral.

Rigidity. A uniform and increased muscle tone within the limbs causes generalised rigidity in all muscle groups of the affected areas. The neck, trunk and forearm muscles are commonly affected early on, and such rigidity leads to a characteristic posture in which, particularly during walking, the neck is held flexed, the spine is rigid and the arm swing is lost. If the facial muscles are affected the patient has a mask-like, fixed expression which responds slowly, for example when smiling or eating. The person's writing may be small and tremulous.

The rigidity may be accompanied by the 'cogwheel' phenomenon, i.e. a series of jerky 'giving' movements if the limb is stretched passively, or be of the 'lead-pipe' type in which there is slow, smooth, resisted movement during passive stretching. Rigidity is increased by concentration and anxiety.

Hypokinesia. Slowness and poverty of movement resulting from muscle weakness and fatigue are perhaps the most disabling features of the condition. The patient's general activity level is reduced and he becomes slow in his actions and has difficulty in maintaining his independence, for although activity may begin adequately, movement becomes poor and ineffectual as he progresses. For this reason, every activity becomes laboured and mobility is affected. The patient may have difficulty, for example, in rising from a chair, bed or bath, and he tends to fall easily. He develops an accelerated gait (festination), and walks with short, shuffling steps. He may have difficulty in initiating activity and, indeed, there is frequently a delay between the stimulus and response. When walking, he may be slow in stopping the motion, in turning to the right or left, passing through doors or sitting down on a chair.

Because of the slowness and weakness of movement the actions of cutting and chewing food are also affected, and the patient may lose weight while still ambulant because he cannot take in an adequate diet. This weight, however, may be regained as he becomes less active or is confined to a wheelchair. The patient often dribbles from the mouth. His voice becomes weak, loses tone and may be reduced to a whisper. His speech may become incomprehensible. This poverty of movement, combined with rigidity, can lead to incoordination.

Mentally, there appear to be no major changes although mental processes slow down and many patients become depressed.

Causes

Idiopathic Parkinsonism (paralysis agitans), which is of unknown origin, is the commonest type in the United Kingdom. There appears to be some familial trend and the condition is usually progressive over a period of years. More men than women are affected. Tremor is often the first sign. Drug-induced Parkinsonism may occur in those taking large doses of phenothiazine drugs such as chlorpromazine and trifluoperazine. Anticholinergic drugs such as benzhexol, orphenadrine and procyclidine are often administered routinely along with these drugs in order to reduce the Parkinsonian symptoms. Parkinsonism as a sequel of encephalitis is now becoming rarer, as few cases of encephalitis lethargica have been reported since the 1917–27 epidemic. Rigidity is the main feature of this type of Parkinsonism and there are frequently accompanying behavioural and mental disorders. Other causes of Parkinsonism are cerebral tumours affecting the basal ganglia, toxic effects of carbon monoxide, copper and other poisons and severe head injuries or continuous cerebral contusion as seen in boxers (the 'punch drunk' syndrome).

Treatment

Parkinsonism can be treated by drug therapy and rehabilitation.

Drug therapy. Because of the imbalance of the dopaminergic and cholinergic transmission systems, L-Dopa can be prescribed to replace the deficient dopamine. Similarly, anticholinergic drugs such as benzhexol, orphenadrine and procyclidine can be given in order to inhibit the cholinergic agent. In this way an attempt is made to redress the balance of these two systems and thus reduce symptoms. For some patients the administration of drugs has brought dramatic relief from the disabling symptoms of Parkinsonism, although the therapist should be aware that not all patients respond so favourably. Because L-Dopa has a short active life it is often given in conjunction with a decarboxylase inhibitor, e.g. carbidopa, in order to prolong its action.

Rehabilitation. Occupational therapy, physiotherapy and speech therapy are given in order to increase and maintain the patient's highest level of functional ability.

THE ROLE OF THE OCCUPATIONAL THERAPIST

The progressive nature of Parkinsonism will mean that the occupational therapist is likely to maintain contact with the patient and his family over a period of many months or years. Obviously, it is impractical and unnecessary for the patient to receive continuous treatment throughout his illness, and often, following an initial period of assessment and treatment, the patient will receive short periods of intensive therapy at regular intervals in order to increase and/or maintain his functional ability. Such help can be given either at home or in the hospital on an in- or out-patient basis.

The therapist should be aware that the condition will produce a wide variation in the degree of disability. Some patients may only have minor symptoms and may never become severely affected, whereas others with severe disability may need full nursing care. Obviously, the treatment required will vary and the therapist must maintain a realistic outlook as to the progression of the condition when organising her treatment programme. Some cases of Parkinsonism (for example those attributed to arteriosclerosis) will gain little benefit from rehabilitation, although help and advice for relatives should still be offered. By contrast, some patients with idiopathic Parkinsonism will respond extremely well to treatment with drugs such as L-Dopa.

The therapist may be asked to participate in the assessment of the patient's level of function before and after treatment with anti-Parkinsonism drugs or, less commonly, stereotactic surgery.

The aims of occupational therapy are:

1. to maintain the patient at his maximum functional level in all activities of daily living

2. to increase and maintain the patient's level of mobility and coordination

3. to aid the patient's confidence and morale, and give support and advice to both him and his family

4. to assist with social and/or work activities and improve communication

5. to assist in the assessment of drug/operative treatment.

Independence in activities of daily living

Owing to the patient's rigidity, poverty of movement and tremor, activities of daily living become tiring and difficult to complete. Because of his slowness and fatigue both the patient and his relatives frequently find that by giving assistance with personal activities frustration and disruption of family routine appear to be minimised. Thus, it becomes easier for a relative to dress, wash and feed the patient, than to let him struggle slowly to complete these activities independently. In this situation, the occupational therapist must discuss with the patient and his family the advantages of gaining a balance between dependence and independence in personal activities. Complete dependence on others for these activities will reduce the patient's self-respect and limit his mobility through inactivity. On the other hand, a fruitless struggle will leave him exhausted and unable to participate in social or recreational interests. The therapist, patient and his family must organise their routine to encourage a degree of independence, yet still conserve energy, especially where relatives feel it is their duty to help the disabled person and when both parties find comfort in such assistance.

Dressing. This should be done in a warm, light room so that the slow patient is as comfortable as possible. He should sit on a firm seat with both feet on the floor and his back supported. Because of his slowness the patient will need plenty of time to complete his dressing, but he should not be allowed to continue to the point of exhaustion. Clothing should be easy to handle. Lightweight, warm and stretchy fabrics are advisable. Where possible wool, cotton or cotton-polyester mixtures should be used, for they have all these properties, yet can be smart, comfortable and easily laundered. Styles with wide openings and a minimum of front or side fastenings should be recommended. Fastenings need to be easy to use, well positioned and easily seen. As few garments as necessary for warmth and comfort will reduce dressing and undressing time. Aids such as elastic laces and shoe horns, and combined garments like bra-petticoats or slipper-socks can also reduce effort.

Eating. Slowness in eating and difficulty with chewing and dribbling may lead to a reduced food intake. A high-protein; high-calorie diet of easily managed food can be recommended. The patient should eat little and often, taking one course of his main meal at midday and the second course in the evening, where practical, or tackling a small portion of the meal at each sitting. If the patient is a slow eater the food can be kept warm in insulated plates and mugs, or a portion of the meal can be kept in the oven or over a saucepan while a first small amount is being eaten. Padded and/or light-weight cutlery, plate guards and stablising mats may be necessary. In order to avoid stress or embarrassment caused by slowness, it may be advisable for the patient to begin his meals slightly ahead of the rest of the family so that he does not feel he is holding everybody up by being the last to finish. If tremor is a particular problem it is often advisable that mugs be only half filled; weighted bracelets may help, provided they are not too heavy. Mugs and cups that can be easily held in both hands, such as Peto mugs, are especially helpful.

Correct positioning is particularly important during eating. It may be useful to reduce the distance between the hands and mouth, for example by raising the table or plate, or by positioning the patient so that his elbows can be used as a pivot in order to assist hand movements (Fig. 24.1).

Home safety and management. If patients are inclined to fall, either due to fatigue and failure of righting mechanisms or because of their small, shuffling steps, home safety is especially important. Floor coverings should be as even as possible, and non-slip polishes can be used. Grab rails can be fitted where patients are particularly at risk, for instance on the wall next to an internal step, by the bath or near the toilet.

If the patient himself usually performs the main household chores a planned, but flexible routine will help to conserve energy. Once he can no longer continue as home maker, the services of a home help, Meals on Wheels and other community agencies may be required. Heavy tasks, such as laundry and shopping, should be kept to a minimum. If practical, a weekly or monthly shopping expedition can replace more frequent trips to the shops. When household items are being replaced, non-iron and drip-dry fabrics should be considered as these reduce the ironing load. Fabric softener can obviate, or at least minimise, ironing, especially of woollen and some nylon garments. Sheets, towels and pillowcases, if folded carefully when taken off the line or out of the drier, may not need ironing.

Carrying aids, such as a light box or net bag clipped to the walking frame, and a trolley or an apron with large pockets all reduce the danger of tripping. For those who may be left alone an alarm system or telephone can be installed.

Bathing. Particular attention should be paid to safety in the bathroom. If an able relative or friend cannot supervise the patient in the bath, a bed bath, strip wash or help from the district nurse should be considered. Where lack of mobility is a problem, bath aids or a shower can be useful; a commode/shower chair which can be wheeled into the shower or over the W/C may be appropriate.

Beds. Turning over in bed can present a prob-

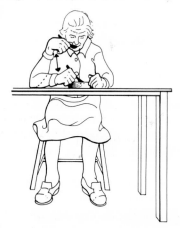

Fig. 24.1 Good positioning to allow control of the upper limbs (Note: one elbow is used as a pivot)

lem for some patients, and practice on the hard surface of the gym or department floor can be followed by supervised attempts on a mattress later on. If the mattress is very soft, boards placed between it and the bed frame will provide a firmer surface. A grab rail by the bed can help, and a point of focus at each side of the bed, for example a luminous alarm clock, a night light or a light left on in the hallway, can help the patient to fix his gaze and therefore steady his head when turning.

Mobility. Once the patient has deteriorated to a point where he can no longer be independently mobile at home, support and help for the family in the form of a hoist, wheelchair, ripple bed or similar aid should be considered. A reclining wheelchair may be necessary if balance is very poor, and some patients may need the additional support of restraining straps. Should the management of a severely disabled person be too great a strain on family resources, some kind of long-term care must be discussed.

Mobility and coordination

Rigidity and weakness gradually affect the mobility of patients with Parkinsonism. Poor movement and increasing fatigue often result in the fading out of an activity shortly after it has begun. For example, a patient asked to tap with hands or feet will initiate the action, but movement will deteriorate and disappear after a few attempts.

The therapist must aim to help with balance, transfers and gait. Delay in initiating movement should also be treated. Liaison between the physiotherapist and occupational therapist is vital as both must be aware of the methods used and results obtained by the other.

Gait. Steps are small and shuffling because the patient finds it difficult to lift his feet off the floor. Treatment should therefore aim to improve size and rhythm of the walking pattern. Large, rhythmical bilateral non-resisted movements have been found to improve gait. Activities such as work on the bicycle fretsaw, sitting treadling at the potters' wheel and walking practice using foot outlines (Fig. 24.2) or lines marked on the floor at paced intervals (Fig. 24.3) are all suitable. Activities which encourage walking should be included in the programme, as they will give the patient the

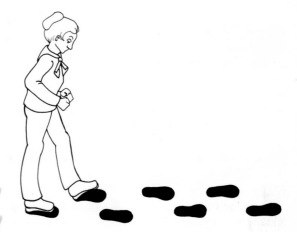

Fig. 24.2 Encouraging a good gait by using foot markers or outlines

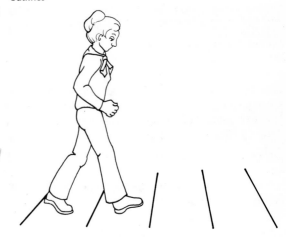

Fig. 24.3 Walking over spaced lines to increase the length of the step

opportunity to practise his walking under supervision.

Balance. Activities which encourage good posture and make gradually increasing demands can be used to improve balance. Work at a balance table, either standing with the hips supported or seated with the back supported, can be used initially. Mirrors may help the patient to correct his sagging posture. Later, activities which encourage side flexion and rotation, such as printing or collating work, can be introduced. The patient should also be taught and encouraged to bend and stoop, where this is feasible and activities such as gardening and skittles may be considered. Occasionally wedged shoes or weighted clothing have been tried to help overcome balance problems, but these have not always been successful. Raised chairs or beds and inclined seats reduce the risk of over-balancing when rising.

Initiating movement. Several methods have to be tried to help the patient who has difficulty with initiating movement. When rising from sitting or walking from standing still, a rocking motion, which can initially be started by the therapist, but later by the patient himself, may help him to gain enough impetus. Such action can be accompanied by a verbal stimulus, such as 'One, two, three, go!' To take a step backwards before attempting to walk forward may also help. Auditory and visual stimuli have proved useful in helping the patient to initiate an activity. For example, one patient found that if he became 'stuck' when walking, he could start moving again by dropping a screwed-up piece of paper in front of his feet. This gave him something to step over, and he was able to continue on his way.

Similarly auditory and visual stimuli can help patients to continue an activity. Paper 'stepping stones' on the floor, or a trolley or wheeled walking aid pushed in front of him may help the patient. Verbal stimuli in the form of counting, marching and music, or rhythmic encouragement such as 'Step and step and ...' appear to help some patients by transmitting the control of the action from a subcortical to a cortical level. The visual stimulus received when climbing up stairs often makes this activity easier than walking on level ground.

Transfers. Surfaces should be stable, firm and of optimum height for the patient. Rocking may help to initiate the impetus required for standing up, and a grab rail may assist with balance. Again, verbal stimulation can be tried. It may be helpful to raise the back legs of a chair slightly. A firm wedged cushion or a rocking motion may also help the patient to rise from sitting. If the patient tends to lean backwards a grab rail placed in front of him or a steady arm or hand to pull up on may offer considerable help, as this encourages the head to come forward over the feet and thus assists a forward and upward motion. It should be emphasised, however, that the patient must not pull up on an unstable object such as a walking aid or trolley. For those with great difficulty in transferring a Renray turntable may be the answer.

Coordination. Coordination can be hampered by rigidity and poverty of movement, especially in the upper limbs. Treatment to improve coordination should include large bilateral and rhythmic activities with little resistance. As coordination improves, the time spent on each activity can be increased and the size of movement decreased. A patient may begin by sanding a large surface (such as a transfer board) and progress to smaller items such as a stool frame. Similarly, he may commence pottery with actions requiring large movement, such as wedging clay, and progress to rolling and modelling coil pots. If artistically inclined, he may try large painting, or painting to music and later potato printing or spokeshave work.

Regular practice of writing and writing patterns can improve upper limb coordination while at the same time assisting communication.

Support for the patient and his family

As the therapist is likely to stay in touch with the patient and his family over a considerable period of time, it is important that a good relationship is established by giving sound and appropriate help and advice. The therapist should reassure the family that, even when their relative is not receiving active treatment, they can feel free to contact her should any problem arise. She should help the patient and his family to be realistic in their expectations, neither too optimistic so that the patient becomes exhausted and frustrated by attempting to ignore his condition, nor too pessimistic so that he becomes dependent, immobile and cannot plan for the future. If the patient and his family can discuss his condition realistically with the therapist, it will be easier to arrange a flexible programme of treatment. In this way problems can be anticipated; advice, e.g. to slow down activity or to lessen responsibility, can be given at the appropriate time, and major aids such as a hoist or wheelchair may be accepted rationally rather than being seen as a failure. Where possible, the patient should be encouraged to undertake household duties which he will be able to continue even as his condition deteriorates. Chores such as washing up, preparing vegetables, and dusting can be useful in helping the patient to maintain a useful role in the family.

If the patient's highest level of social and physical function is maintained and his home made safe and easy to live in, he will be able to retain his confidence for as long as possible. Community help, holiday relief and similar schemes to support the patient and his family will ease the strain of coping with a disabled member. The family should not expect the patient to perform activities beyond his capability, but emphasise those he can do.

Social activities, work and communication

As speech and mobility deteriorate, the patient may become isolated and depressed. During treatment sessions, the therapist should slowly introduce the patient to working in small groups, both to avoid isolation and to assist communication. A high proportion of patients with Parkinsonism are depressed, and this must be explained to relatives and remembered by the therapist, as it will greatly affect her approach to the patient. When dealing with a depressed patient, the therapist must make treatment sessions positive and purposeful so that the relevance of activities is easily seen by the patient. Activities should be familiar and interesting, and a wide variety of stimuli in the form of colour, sound and touch should be included. The therapist should work within the concentration span of the patient.

Lack of communication can frustrate both the patient and his relatives and, therefore, activities which specifically encourage this skill should be included in the treatment. It is important to explain to relatives that frequently an apparent lack of response may stem from a combination of slow thought processes, depression and weak facial movement. The patient should be given ample time to reply to direct questions, and allowances should be made for his slowness during conversation. Some patients with very slow and weak speech benefit from the use of a word chart, as the impatience of relatives will only further inhibit his responses. Activities to encourage speech control may be used, and positive efforts to increase the volume of speech, to swallow saliva, to breathe deeply and to break up sentences or even words into short sections should be encouraged. Singing, board games, quizzes, discussion groups and work with others will also encourage speech.

The patient may be very upset by his loss of writing ability (Figs. 24.4 and 24.5). Formal exercises may prove rather inhibiting, and the use of a blackboard or large poster-sized sheets of paper may reduce his self-consciousness and fears of failure. Later, rhythmical writing patterns using widely spaced lines can be introduced to encourage a more legible script. Progression to writing letters and words should follow (Figs. 24.6 & 7). All attempts should be kept as a record and also as positive reinforcement for the patient. Writing aids such as padded pens, writing boards and paper stabilisers may be supplied, and some patients may find that a felt tip pen is easier to handle than a fountain or ball-point pen.

Where possible, social contact should be maintained through hobbies, pastimes, visits and outings. Attendance at a day centre, lunch club or day hospital may be acceptable, and the therapist should ensure that help with transport, e.g. mobility allowance or orange parking disc, is also given if the patient is eligible. In some areas, Parkinson's Clubs have been established.

If the patient is of working age, part-time work or less responsibility at work may be considered. It is unwise for the patient to persist with work to the point where he becomes exhausted and possibly unsafe. Weakness, dribbling at the mouth, tremor and speech problems may cause embarrassment in the company of colleagues or when using the telephone. Retraining is unlikely if the patient cannot continue his former job, and lighter work with the same employer, work in an advisory capacity or an early retirement may be indicated. Sheltered employment could also be considered.

Assessment of drug treatment

If an assessment of the effect of drug treatment is required the occupational therapist may be asked to contribute by assessing the degree of functional improvement. It is usual for the doctor to assess the physical manifestations of the condition, such as tremor, rigidity and dribbling.

In arranging such an assessment, the therapist must remember that any activities used must be easily repeatable. She must, for instance, use the same equipment, in the same place, preferably at the same time of day; where possible assessment

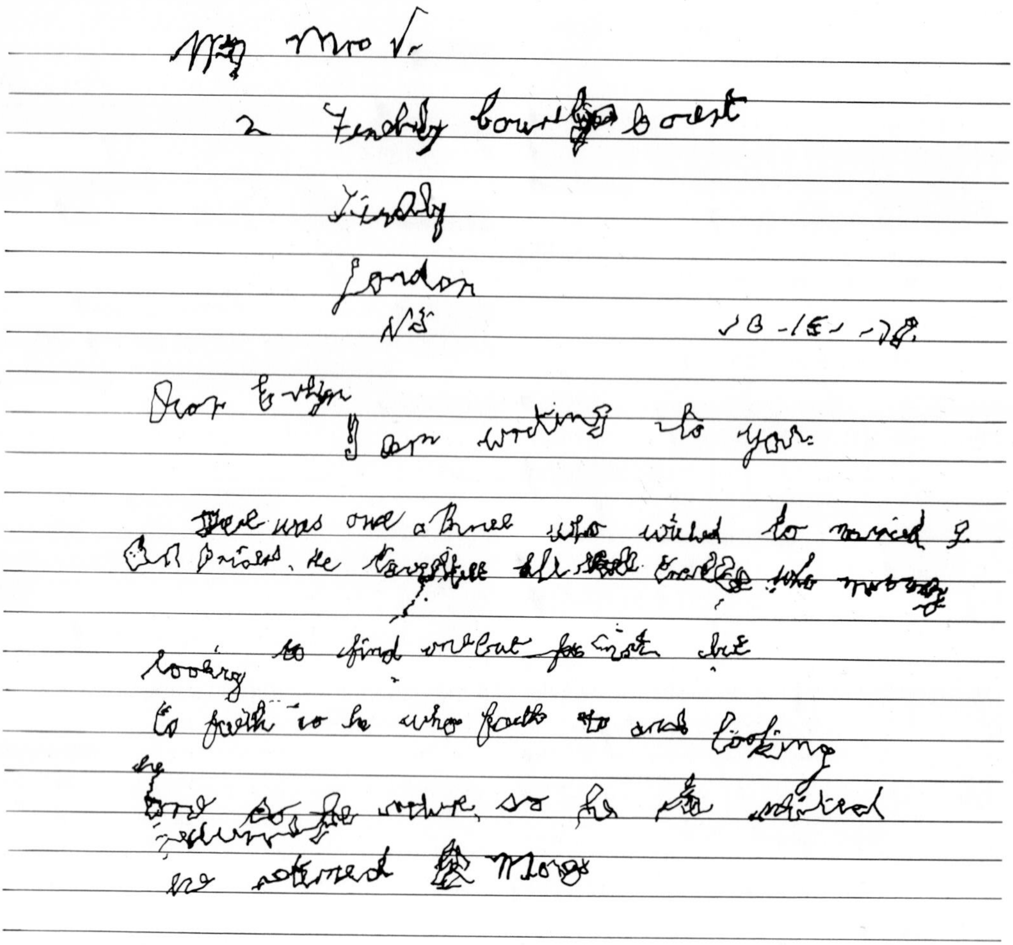

Fig. 24.4 Letter written by a patient, aged 63

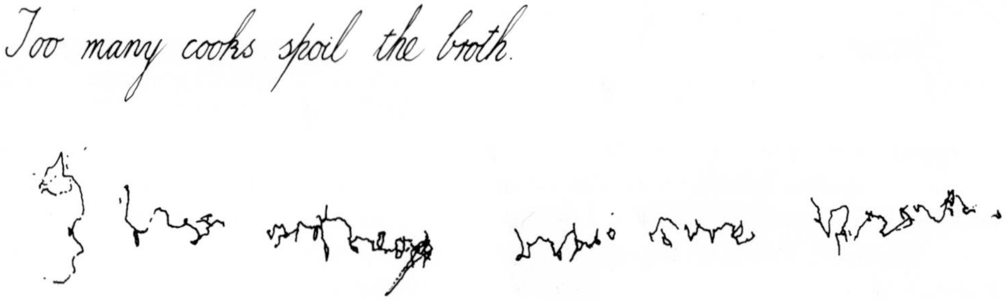

Too many cooks spoil the broth.

Fig. 24.5 Attempt to copy writing

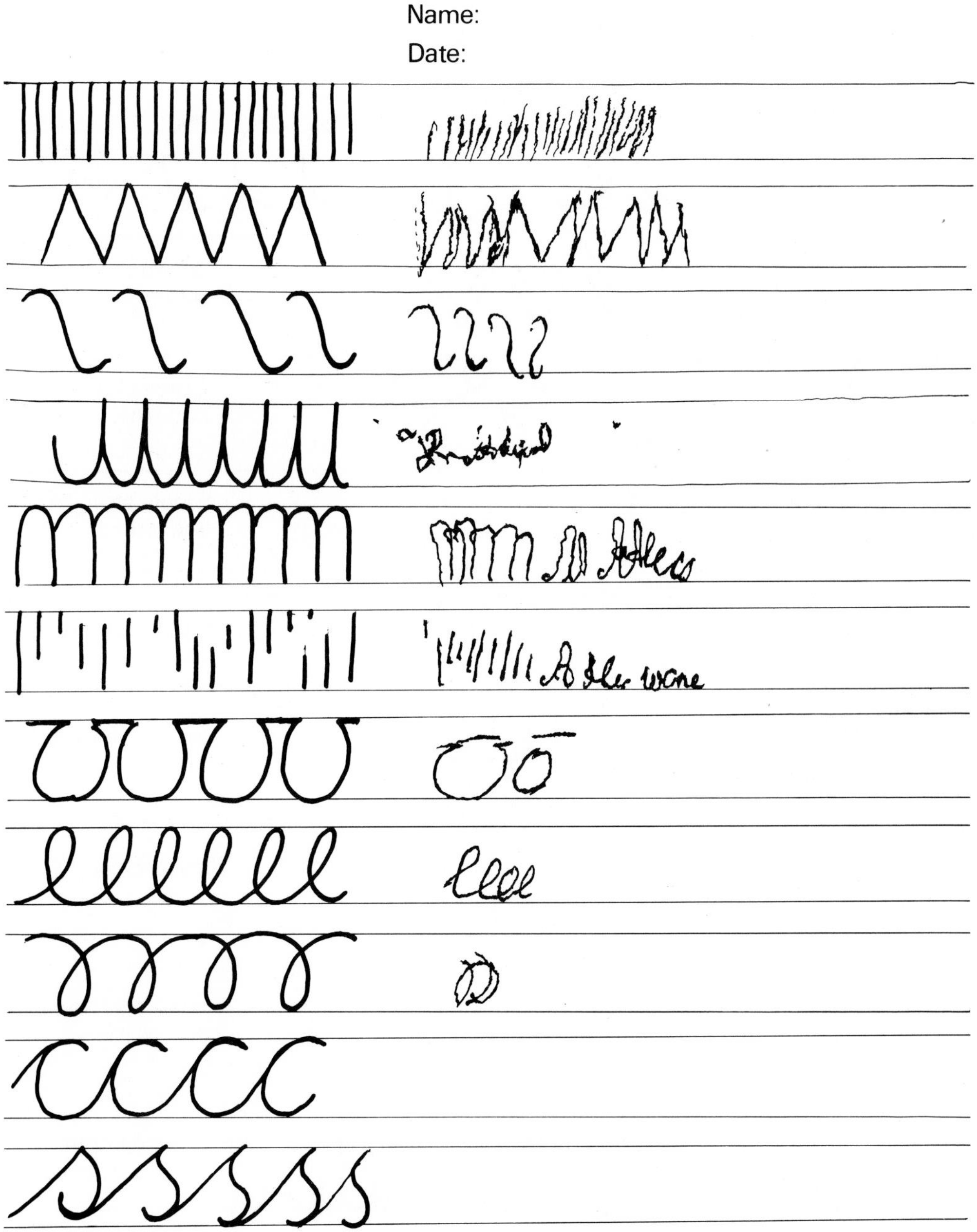

Name:

Date:

Fig. 24.6 Rhythmical writing patterns

should be carried out by the same person each time. In this way the patient's peformance can be exactly compared to his previous attempt. Precision is of great importance, especially when activities are performed against time or with a set number of moves or pieces of equipment, for if they are recorded wrongly or inaccurately results become meaningless. The assessment activities should always take place in the same order, and clear instructions should be given each time.

The following activities may be used for a functional assessment:

Upper limb function. Easily repeatable activities which involve as many of the movements and

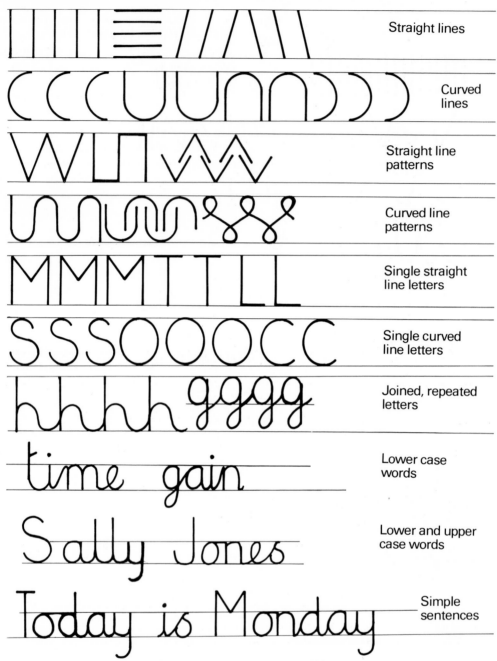

	Straight lines
	Curved lines
	Straight line patterns
	Curved line patterns
	Single straight line letters
	Single curved line letters
	Joined, repeated letters
	Lower case words
	Lower and upper case words
	Simple sentences

Fig. 24.7 Writing patterns progressing to letters and words

functions of the upper limb as possible can be used. Tasks such as threading a set number of beads onto a wire, posting bricks into a box, placing discs over a tall pole or pouring liquid from cup to cup are suitable, for each activity can be performed against time and recorded accordingly.

Coordination levels and the rate of 'falling off' of activity should also be assessed. Activities include hand clapping (number of successful actions recorded), writing the alphabet in a continuous stream, maze following or other similar tests (Fig. 24.8). The right and left arm should be assessed separately, where appropriate.

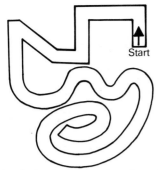

The patient is asked to draw a line along the path of the maze

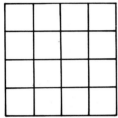

The patient is asked to mark each square with a dot

Fig. 24.8 A maze and dot test to assess coordination

Mobility. A set mobility course can be arranged so that the therapist can record the time taken by the patient to complete it, or the distance travelled if completion is impossible. Activities can include rising from a chair, manoeuvring around objects placed on the floor, climbing up and down steps, stepping over low objects, walking between straight lines and sitting down in a chair. These actions can be easily repeated as required, and the therapist can note any particular problems encountered.

Daily functional activities. Such an assessment is difficult to repeat with accuracy. For example, with dressing activities the therapist must ensure that the same clothes are worn each time. This may be possible if the patient is asked to wear the same coat, cardigan or shoes for each session so that the time taken to take them off or put them on can be directly compared. Alternatively, a garment such as a jacket or jumper may be kept in the department for use during such a test. Other functions which could be assessed include cutting food (bread or lumps of cheese), peeling vegetables (two or more carrots) or climbing into the bath and sitting down.

The therapist must ensure that a standard recording system is used, so that subjective variations in grading are eliminated. For example, activities which cannot be timed or actions which cannot be counted can be recorded on a three-point scale:
1. completed activity without difficulties
2. completed activity but with difficulties
3. failed to complete activity.

In this way the tester's observation is objectively recorded and she does not have to rely on a subjective 'Fair', 'Good' or 'Difficult' opinion. The therapist must ensure that accurate records are kept to show the difference in response when a variety of drugs are used. In each case, results achieved before the drugs are taken, once an optimum level has been reached and also at follow-up should be recorded.

The occupational therapist has much to offer the patient with Parkinsonism, and with continuous assessment, encouragement, and realistic treatment, she can help to make his life more comfortable and purposeful.

REFERENCES AND FURTHER READING

Macdonald E M 1971 Occupational therapy in rehabilitation, 4th edn. Balliere, Tindall & Cassell, London, ch 9
Marks J 1974 The treatment of Parkinsonism with L-Dopa. Lancaster Medical and Technical Publishing
Messiha F S, Kenny A D 1976 Parkinson's Disease. Plenum Press, New York

25

Peripheral nerve lesions

When peripheral nerves are injured, both motor and sensory functions are affected. There is always deformity and sensation loss, and assessment and treatment need to be based on detailed anatomical knowledge.

Causes

1. Direct trauma. This is a cut or injury directly to the nerve and its sheath. It is most common at the wrist with a cut to the ulnar and median nerves.

2. Stretching. The nerve is stretched in a dislocation or other injury where the limb is pulled. The nerve separates, but the sheath may remain intact. This injury occurs most commonly around the shoulder with damage to the brachial plexus.

3. Pressure. When heavy pressure is applied to the nerve, transmission may be affected temporarily. This is most common at the shoulder, e.g. in 'crutch' palsy when the patient leans on his crutches, and in 'Saturday night' palsy when the patient has slept with his arm over the back of a chair.

There are different degrees of nerve damage. In *axonotmesis* the nerve separates, but the sheath remains intact. The prognosis is good. In *neurotmesis* both the nerve and the sheath are severed. The prognosis is poor. In *neuropraxia* the damage is due to pressure, causing only a transient block in transmission.

Repair

Except in neuropraxia, the nerve distal to the injury dies and is removed by scavenger cells in the blood. Degeneration also occurs above the injury back to the last node of Ranvier. If the sheath is separated this is repaired surgically. The nerve may have retracted and suture must then be preceded by exploratory surgery. Primary suture is done immediately after injury whenever possible, e.g. when there is no open wound or when the wound is sterile. Secondary suture may be done after the wound has healed when there is less danger of secondary infection.

Recovery

Full functional recovery depends on the type of injury, the level of injury and on rehabilitation.

Neuropraxia has the best and shortest recovery rate. Neurotmesis takes the longest time and has the worst prognosis. Lesions at the elbow will take longer to recover than lesions at the wrist because of the distance between the injury and the end organ. After trauma to the elbow, therefore, there is a longer time to keep the limb in good condition while awaiting regeneration of the nerve and reinnervation of its motor and sensory areas. This period of time lessens the chances of full recovery.

If rehabilitation starts on the day of injury there is more chance of full recovery. If rehabilitation involves the whole limb with emphasis on the affected joints, recovery is better. Sensory stimulation from the beginning greatly enhances the chances of full sensory and motor return. If the patient fully cooperates in his own rehabilitation recovery is faster and more complete.

To assess the degree of recovery tap along the course of the nerve moving from the distal to the proximal end, until the patient reports a tingling sensation (Tinel's sign). Tingling is at its greatest at the level of the growth cone. The area of sensory loss will gradually diminish. Regular testing and plotting of this area indicates the speed of recovery. Check muscle reinnervation. Individual muscles progress from total paralysis, to a flicker of movement and then to full range of movement and to full strength. An electromyelogram will indicate which muscles are innervated.

Rate of regrowth

The nerve regrows at approximately one millimetre a day. A severed nerve and sheath may regrow splendidly, but to an inappropriate end organ. If a sensory nerve regrows to the wrong sensory nerve ending the patient has to be re-educated in its new function. If a sensory nerve regrows to a motor end organ it dies back and restarts. On average, an injury to the shoulder takes two to three years to recover fully; an injury to the elbow six months to one year; an injury to the wrist takes three to six months and leg injuries usually take longer. In the hip or pelvis recovery will usually take three to four years and in the knee one to two years.

OCCUPATIONAL THERAPY

The therapist must obtain a clear picture of the person and his injury before starting treatment. Treatment tends to be highly specific as well as general and functional, and may last many months. The better the relationship between patient and therapist the more successful the treatment.

Assessment

The area of sensory loss needs to be tested first. The skin is touched with cotton wool and gentle pin pricks, and the patient is asked to close his eyes and indicate when he can feel the touch. The areas of sensory loss are then mapped and dated (Fig. 25.1).

The active and passive range of movement needs to be assessed for the whole limb. Full passive range needs to be maintained in the absence of muscle power. Active range needs accurate recording to indicate recovery. This is tested on the recommended five-point scale as described in Chapter 2. It is important that each patient is always measured by the same member of the team.

Precautions

Where sensation is lost, the skin may be in poor condition, easily injured and will recover slowly. The patient may not realise he has injured himself. He will smell his flesh burning before he realises the cause of the smell. Smoking and cooking are the most hazardous activities. Both patient and

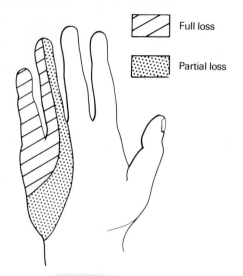

Full loss

Partial loss

Fig. 25.1 A diagrammatic record of an area of sensory loss

therapist must be constantly aware of the desensitised area, and the patient must be taught to check it twice daily.

Non- or partially-innervated muscles are weak. Like weak elastic, they must not be overstretched, nor should they be fully contracted. Thus, if the triceps is weak the elbow should not be fully flexed or extended against resistance until the muscle has reached grade four.

Aims of treatment

Once the assessment has been completed and the precautions explained, the treatment can be planned. The patient should be seen daily for as long as necessary. Patients who are cooperative and understanding can be asked to attend only two or three times a week in the knowledge that home activities will back up the treatment. Weekly attendance is necessary for all patients to check for damage and to record progress.

Sensory retraining

Early sensory stimulation reduces the possibility of ignoral and facilitates motor recovery. It is used most commonly in lesions to the brachial plexus and to the median and ulnar nerves. Any activity that involves touching and handling can be used. Making bread, stool seating, collating, pottery, gardening, typing, composing print and wood-

work all stimulate the hands. The vibration from sawing, hammering and sanding, and work at the bicycle fretsaw and lathe are good for desensitised skin. Remedial games with handles of different shape, size and texture can be used for more specific stimulation. Objects of different size, shape and texture can be felt (with the eyes closed) for identification. Initially, the articles should be easy to recognise, e.g. milk bottles, a pair of scissors and a hair brush. Later, the patient can be asked to discriminate between a piece of writing paper and a post card, a paper clip and a safety pin, a two-pence and a five-pence piece.

Whole-limb movement

Especially in the early stages, it is vital to maintain as full a range of movement and as much strength as possible in the whole limb. If the injured area is surrounded by a strong limb with good circulation it stands a better chance of regaining function. Activities should be bilateral and wide to give cross stimulation and therefore more facilitation to the injured area; they should offer maximal resistance. Support should be given if there is pain or danger of dislocation, for example by the OB help arm. Activities for the legs can be foot games, work on the bicycle fretsaw, rug loom using foot pedals, lathe or treadle fretsaw and activities involving standing and walking, such as skittles, archery and gardening. For the arms remedial games, weaving, stool-seating using soft cord or nytrim, printing, sanding and polishing table tops, cross-cut sawing and handling large off-cuts can be used. These last two provide good general movements for both lower and upper limbs.

The prevention of deformity

Splints are usually necessary to prevent deformity and encourage function. The splint is fitted individually and worn from the time of injury until recovery begins. As soon as the paralysed muscles have some innervation the splint is taken off for increasing lengths of time to allow active unassisted movements. The process of gradually withdrawing the splint should be closely monitored by the therapist and its importance explained to the patient. A splint discarded too early will encourage the deformity it was meant to prevent. If discarded too late the splint will have discouraged returning strength by doing the work for the weak muscles.

Strength and function

Rebuilding strength is achieved by any activity that gives the greatest resistance compatible with the patient's strength. This needs to be finely adjusted to all stages of recovery. The weight that was lifted yesterday should not be today's poundage. In the final stages, static muscle work can be used: lathe work for the hands and the standing leg, sawing for the gripping hand, writing for the wrist and composing for the hand holding the stick. Rebuilding function needs to be relevant to each person; it includes increasing manipulation and dexterity. Activities can be graded gradually from large draughts to composing print, from cross-cut sawing to marquetry. The patient's discharge may be delayed by his inability to perform a particular action, and details of jobs and hobbies should therefore be discussed earlier in the treatment. For instance, a railway labourer needed full finger extension to put his hand between two blocks so close together that only an extended hand would fit in. Because he had forgotten this one vital movement, the therapist worked for grip and strength, and an extra fortnight was needed to return full extension to those fingers.

Finally, as the recovery rate of nerve lesions is slow, activities and exercises at home should be encouraged to follow up the treatment. These should be worked out jointly by the occupational therapist and the physiotherapist so that reinforcement can be given and duplication avoided.

Brachial plexus lesions

The patient will at worst present with a totally flail limb and a poor prognosis. After a shoulder injury it is difficult to tell whether the plexus has been badly bruised or the nerves actually severed. If severed, the nerves have a long way to regrow, and after two years recovery may only just be beginning. In nerve-root lesion no recovery can be expected. Splintage is used in the form of a sling to prevent dislocation at the shoulder (Fig. 25.2).

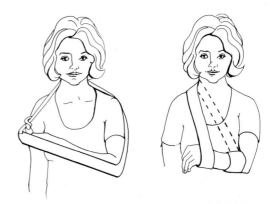

Fig. 25.2 Slings used to prevent dislocation or subluxation of the shoulder joint

This is removed for treatment and replaced by the OB help arm or similar aid. Later, a combination of radial, median and ulnar splints may be used. Sensory stimulation needs to be continuous or the whole arm will be forgotten. Whole-arm bilateral movements with maximal resistance are needed, with as much variety as possible to maintain interest and function throughout the treatment period. Collating, weaving, cooking, industrial assembly, macramé, cane work, stool seating, collage, cane seating, drawing, sanding and polishing may be used. Large draughts, chess or other games on a large board are also suitable. The patient should be encouraged to get a job during this long period. The therapist may have to undertake a work assessment as resettlement is usually necessary. Home activities are encouraged within the patient's capabilities. One patient completely redecorated his home as a complementary activity to the specific occupational therapy. It is important that the patient does not suffer boredom and the resultant loss of morale. If the limb is still flail after two years, amputation may be suggested. In the arm this is usually at mid-shaft of the humerus with arthrodesis of the shoulder in slight flexion and slight abduction. After six weeks of immobilisation, scapular and trunk movements are encouraged. The prosthesis will be powered by the opposite shoulder muscles and the occupational therapist will be involved in prosthetic training. Should recovery occur, specific retraining of movement and muscle strength is needed. Returning muscle power and sensation must be carefully monitored by one member of the treatment team and needs to be relayed to the others. Recovery will take between six months and two years. The length of time is a challenge to the therapist's relationship with the patient and to her ability to maintain his interest and morale.

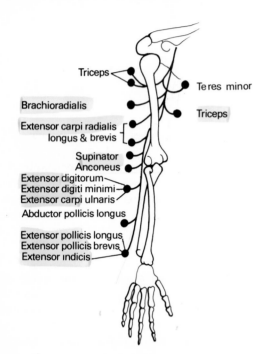

Fig. 25.3 Muscles supplied by the radial nerve

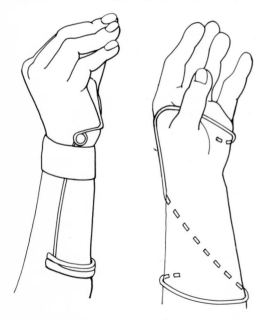

Fig. 25.4 Wrist extension splint

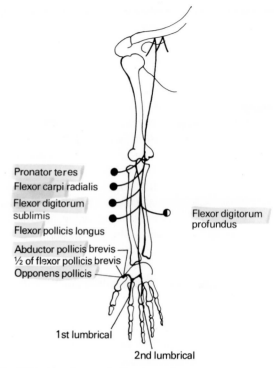

Fig. 25.5 Muscles supplied by the median nerve

Radial nerve lesions

These occur most commonly where the nerve runs in the radial groove of the humerus. The muscles involved are shown in Fig. 25.3. The patient presents with weak elbow extension and no supination or extension of wrist, thumb or fingers. There is a small area of sensory loss over the dorsum of the thumb web. If there is much deformity a splint should be fitted to hold the wrist in extension while allowing flexion (Fig. 25.4). This prevents the contraction of the flexors and the overstretching of the paralysed extensors. Outriders to the fingers are usually unnecessary as the fingers will extend on wrist flexion. This method of obtaining finger extension is a so called 'trick movement' and should be taught; as soon as power returns to the extensors it should be specifically discouraged. Whole-arm movements are used in the early stages. Once recovery occurs, specific activities are used to encourage supination, and wrist and finger extension. As there is a common extensor origin, recovery of these movements should occur simultaneously. Coil pottery, pastry making, work using large scissors (e.g. collage work and dressmaking), bagatelle, karam, large draughts and solitaire, and a wide shuttle for weaving and macramé can be used. The rubber-band game involves hooking the fingers under bands and placing them over nails in patterns. These are all gentle activities and can be followed by more resisted actions as strength returns and the extensors can no longer be overstretched by strong flexion. Later activities include stool seating with a wide shuttle and a large FEPS wheel attached to weaving or printing. Velcro on draughts also necessitates resisted extension. The FEPS roller can be used to strengthen the wrist extensors. As dexterity returns, cat's cradles or Indian string games can also be used. Home activities to be encouraged include window cleaning, polishing, playing cards, pastry or bread making, wall papering and painting ceilings.

Median nerve lesions

This injury usually occurs at the wrist and the patient presents with a 'monkey' hand. The thumb is flat and adducted, and there is wasting of the thenar eminence. The first two digits tend to hyperextend at the metacarpophalangeal joint due to weakness of the lumbricals. The muscles affected are shown in Figure 25.5. Areas of sensory loss are shown in Figure 25.6. This loss is most disabling and combined with the weak pincer grip renders the hand both clumsy and lacking in function. If a splint is needed it should hold the thumb in opposition and abduction while allowing free movement (Fig. 25.7). Sensory stimulation should take place daily. Should the area of sensation supplied by the radial nerve extend to the edge or over the palmar surface of the thenar eminence, this can also be used. Activities should be for the whole arm in the early stages. As recovery occurs others should be added to encourage tripod grip and coordination, e.g. weaving and stool seating, pastry and bread making, glove puppets, weeding, greenhouse gardening, polishing, macramé, cane work and cane seating, collating and assembling case notes. For finer coordination use composing and clay modelling. Static work such as sawing, writing and gripping activities can be used in the final stages. Home

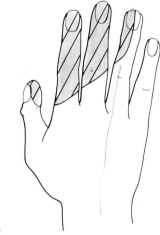

Dorsum

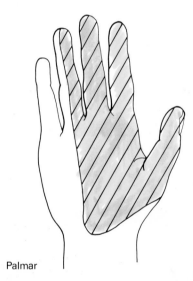

Palmar

Fig. 25.6 Sensory loss following a median nerve lesion

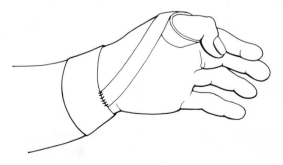

Fig. 25.7 Thumb opponens splint

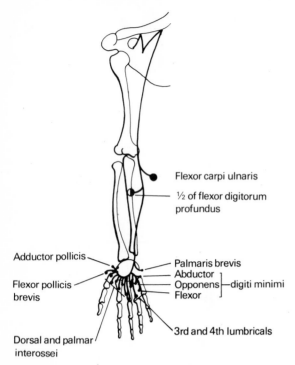

Flexor carpi ulnaris

½ of flexor digitorum profundus

Adductor pollicis

Flexor pollicis brevis

Dorsal and palmar interossei

Palmaris brevis
Abductor
Opponens ⎤—digiti minimi
Flexor ⎦

3rd and 4th lumbricals

Fig. 25.8 Muscles supplied by the ulnar nerve

activities include sewing, dressmaking, gardening and model making.

Ulnar nerve lesions

These occur most commonly at the wrist; the muscles involved are shown in Figure 25.8 and the areas of sensory loss in Figure 25.9. The patient presents with a 'claw' hand. The medial side is flat, there is wasting of the hypothenar eminence, and the third and fourth fingers hyperextend at the metacarpophalangeal joint due to the imbalance caused by the weak third and fourth lumbricals. Paralysis of all interossei and the thumb's adductor results in weakness of the whole hand. The grip is present, but weak. Almost all the fine movements of the hand are weak or absent. The splint shown in Figure 25.10 will correct hyperextension at the metacarpophalangeal joints and restore the arch of the hand while allowing free movement. Sensory retraining is necessary, as the area of sensory loss is at risk when rubbing over rough surfaces or resting on a hot plate. Activities should be for the whole arm in the early stages and as recovery occurs should encourage opposition of the thumb

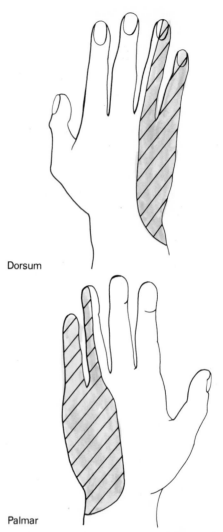

Dorsum

Palmar

Fig. 25.9 Sensory loss following an ulnar nerve lesion

to the third and fourth fingers, metacarpophalangeal flexion and coordination. These movements can be encouraged by games such as draughts using the thumb and little finger, by sharpening plane blades or using a scraper, with a FEPS wheel attached to printing or weaving, or the dried peas game (Fig. 25.11) in a race with another patient, by papier maché work and by pulling up (rather than down) on a printing adaptation, e.g. a cotton reel attached to the press handle and running through a pulley immediately below it. Macramé, making nail pictures (holding the hammer in the injured hand or the string between thumb and little finger), pastry and bread making, pottery and wood carving are all suitable. The static grip can

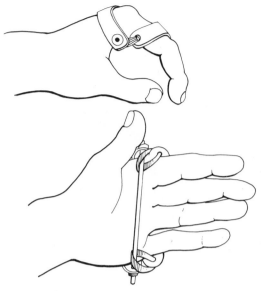

Fig. 25.10 Ulnar nerve lesion splint to encourage metacarpophalangeal flexion

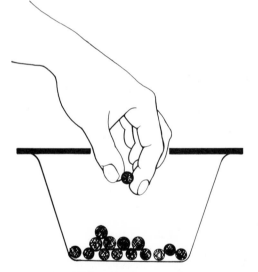

Fig. 25.11 The 'dried peas' game encourages metacarpophalangeal flexion

be used later, for instance on the lathe or when cross-cut sawing or hedge-cutting. Home activities include general housework and cooking, gardening, playing a musical instrument, or any crafts activity in which the person is already interested.

Lateral popliteal lesions

This nerve is usually injured where it winds round the head of the fibula. The muscles affected are

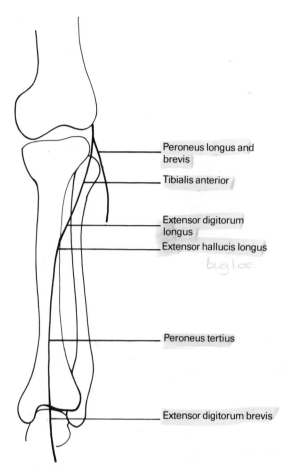

Peroneus longus and brevis

Tibialis anterior

Extensor digitorum longus

Extensor hallucis longus

big toe

Peroneus tertius

Extensor digitorum brevis

Fig. 25.12 Muscles supplied by the lateral popliteal (common peroneal) nerve

shown in Figure 25.12 and the area of sensory loss in Figure 25.13. The patient presents with a dropped foot with lack of eversion and may walk with a high-stepping or 'steppage' gait, lifting his dragging toe to clear the ground. A temporary foot-raise should be fitted (Fig. 25.14). If no recovery occurs this may have to be worn permanently. The sensory loss should be considered in precautionary measures and foot care. The feet should be washed daily and carefully dried, and clean socks should be worn each day. Skin should be checked for rubbing or bruising and the cause removed before further damage occurs. No retraining should be necessary. Activities should be for the whole leg in the early stages. Once recovery occurs activities are also needed for active dorsiflexion and eversion. There are not many such activities and great reliance is placed on the

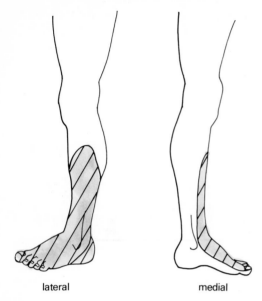

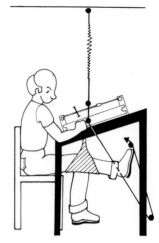

Fig. 25.15 Weaving adapted to encourage dorsiflexion

Fig. 25.13 Sensory loss following a lesion to the lateral popliteal nerve

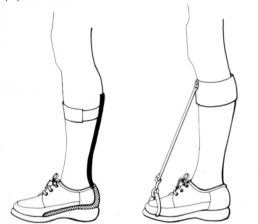

Fig. 25.14 Temporary foot-raises

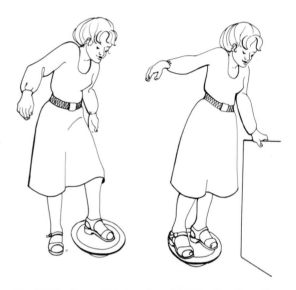

Fig. 25.16 The wobble board used to strengthen the ankles

passive movements given in whole-leg activities. However, active movements must not be neglected, or the dorsiflexors and evertors will not regain their full strength. Activities encouraging active dorsiflexion are the PIED switch (see Ch. 9) and foot draughts (played with the foot hooking a draught to move it). The Camden treadle fretsaw gives a little active movement, as do the weaving adaptation shown in Fig. 25.15, walking round tyres and the ankle rotator. Squatting, for instance with archery and gardening, should also be encouraged. Activities for eversion include the wob-

ble board (Fig. 25.16), walking over rough ground as when digging, the ankle rotator and various games made specially for this movement. These include an in/evertor table marble game, described in Occupational Therapy Journal, September 1978, and a footmaze which resembles the wobble board, but is played sitting; all movements of the ankle are needed to control the maze and guide the ball. The passive range can be extended by blocking the foot plates of the treadles with wedges. Home activities include all walking and running games. General mobility can be encouraged by good walking patterns, cycling and swimming. The patient should be taught to keep the sole of the foot flat on the ground and not let it fall into inversion. Specific eversion and dorsiflexion exercises should be taught by one member of the treatment team.

Other peripheral nerves can be damaged, but the lesions described above are certainly the most common. The circumflex nerve may be injured in the shoulder giving rise to deltoid palsy. Specific abduction then needs retraining. If the femoral nerve is damaged the whole leg needs to be retrained, especially the quadriceps muscle group. However, the principles described above apply to all peripheral nerve injuries and treatment can be adapted accordingly to the site of the lesion.

The middle stage of each treatment period is the most exciting, demanding the most specific work the occupational therapist is ever asked to do. Because of this it is also the most challenging and the most rewarding.

REFERENCES AND FURTHER READING

Medical Reasearch Council 1943 Aids to investigation of peripheral nerve injuries. HMSO, London
Shopland A et al 1979 Refer to occupational therapy. Churchill Livingstone, Edinburgh
Wynn-Parry C B 1973 Rehabilitation of the hand, 3rd edn. Butterworths, London

26
Rheumatoid arthritis

Rheumatoid arthritis is a chronic or subacute process of inflammation of unknown origin, usually affecting the joints in a symmetrical fashion and causing swelling, pain and deformity. The small joints are often affected first (i.e. the wrist, fingers and feet), but not to the exclusion of larger joints. Other tissues and organs of the body may be involved as a result of inflammation of blood vessels, the presence of rheumatoid nodules or as a result of pressure on nerves.

Rheumatoid arthritis occurs world-wide. It can start at any age, but onset is most commonly between the age of 35 and 55. Women are affected more often than men; the incidence is approximately 6 per cent of the female and 2.5 per cent of the male population.

Causes. These are still unknown. However, theories have included (a) infection and (b) abnormalities in the immunological system. At the present time it is though that some agent, possibly a virus, precipitates a chain of intense immunological activity. Eventually this leads to destruction of cartilage and bone. The reason why this should occur in some people and not others is unknown. Several factors may precipitate the onset of the disease, but cannot be regarded as causative (e.g. emotional or physical stress). The condition tends to run in families, but no hereditary factor has yet been found.

Course. The disease is widely varying in its severity and many patients probably never need medical care. In the more common forms it runs a course of exacerbations and remissions, eventually leading to some degree of deformity.

It may, however, follow a milder course, sometimes episodic, with relatively little functional impairment. In some cases it pursues a malignant course with gross disability resulting in 12 to 18 months. It may be surprising to discover that about 25 to 50 per cent of patients seen in hospital are left with only a relatively mild loss of function.

Pathology. The synovial lining becomes oedematous (influx of fluid) and the lining cells multiply rapidly; later many new blood vessels form in the synovial membrane. This is followed by an infiltration of chronic inflammatory cells (plasma cells and lymphocytes). The synovial membrane, usually a thin diaphanous layer, becomes a thickened vascular and cellular tissue. There is usually an associated increased secretion of synovial fluid resulting in an effusion into the joint. The fluid is viscous and has the features of inflammation with many thousands of white blood cells and a high protein content. It may contain the rheumatoid factor.

It is thought that enzymes are released which are capable of eroding cartilage and bone. The bones in proximity to the joint become osteoporotic and there is muscle wasting. Eventually secondary degenerative changes may occur and varying degrees of fibrous ankylosis. — movements restricted by fibrous bands/ malformation or actual union of bone.

Symptoms and signs

The disease can be mono- or polyarticular. The patient complains of feeling unwell with general malaise; he is often anaemic. Early morning stiffness and pain are common features especially after a period of immobility. Any or all of the peripheral joints may be involved in a symmetrical fashion.

There is swelling of the joints due to synovial thickening and effusion, limited range of movement and joint instability. Later, various deformities of the joints develop.

Cervical spine. Involvement of the cervical spine may lead to dizziness, and to paraesthesia (pins and needles) in the hands which causes loss of function if untreated. Subluxation in the upper cervical spine results in compression of the cord, and tetraplegia or sudden death can occasionally occur.

Shoulders. In the upper limb there may be restriction of movement at the shoulder, flexion deformity at the elbow and inability to rotate the forearm. The carpal tunnel syndrome is an early sign of the involvement of the wrist. Later, the lower end of the ulna may become prominent and tender; the extensor tendon may rupture. There is ulnar drift and palmar subluxation; fusion may occur.

Hands. The hands are frequently involved. Early signs are swelling of the proximal interphalangeal and metacarpophalangeal joints. Later, ulnar drift as a result of metacarpophalangeal subluxation becomes apparent. Palmar subluxation, swan-neck deformities and Boutonniere deformities are other characteristic signs. Tendons, especially of the extensors, may rupture and tendon sheath involvement will cause thickening in the flexor tendon sheaths and consequent poor grip. Nodules may form in the flexor tendons, causing trigger finger.

Dorsal and lumbar spine. Rheumatoid arthritis is unlikely to produce clinical manifestations in the dorsal and lumbar spine. Problems may arise with osteoporosis. This is more likely if the patient is on long-term steroid therapy. Osteoporosis causes pain and it may lead to the collapse of vertebrae.

Hips. Involvement of the hip may lead to flexion deformity and limitation of range of movement in untreated patients. Effusion into the knee with synovial hyperplasia is an early sign of involvement. Later, flexion deformity (weak quadriceps muscles), popliteal cysts, lateral instability and rotation deformity (usually external) may develop.

Ankles and feet. The ankles and feet are usually involved at an early stage. First signs are pain and swelling. Later signs include subluxed metatarsal heads (patients feel they are walking on pebbles) and valgus deformity of the feet if the subtalar joints are involved.

Other features sometimes associated with rheumatoid arthritis are:

1. Subcutaneous nodules, particularly just below the elbow and along the tendons of the fingers and toes.

2. Sjögrens syndrome. The patient complains of dry eyes and a dry mouth. This is caused by failure of secretion of the lacrimal and salivary glands.

3. Felty's syndrome. This is characterised by an enlarged spleen and a low white cell count. It is often associated with leg ulcers.

4. vascular lesions. These may be seen as nail-fold lesions. They can affect any system in the body, but are most common in the peripheral nerves (peripheral neuropathy).

Other forms of connective tissue disease

Psoriatic arthritis. This usually affect the sacro-iliac joints and the terminal interphalangeal joints of the hands. The rheumatoid factor is absent, as are subcutaneous nodules. About eight per cent of the population with psoriasis also develop arthritis. There is no female predominance.

Reiter's disease. This almost always affect men. The main features are urethritis, conjunctivitis, lesions of the skin and nails (keratoderma blennor-rhagica) and inflammatory arthritis affecting the weight-bearing joints, particularly the knees and the sacro-iliac joint. There may be oral and genital ulceration. The disease is usually sexually trans-mitted, but may follow epidemic dysentry.

Ankylosing spondylitis. This is much more com-mon in young men than women. The onset is usually in the late teens or early twenties. The main changes are seen in the spine and the sacroiliac joints. About one fourth of patients develop iritis.

Occasionally arthritis is associated with in-flammatory bowel disease, i.e. ulcerative colitis and Crohn's disease.

Systemic sclerosis (formerly known as scleroder-ma). This is characterised by a thickening of the skin. It is commonly seen in the hands. Raynaud's phenomenon is seen early in the disease; later the skin becomes tight, thick and shiny. The hands are very painful and stiff and eventually necrosis of the distal phalanges may occur. The mouth may be-come tight and puckered, making it difficult to open it fully. Telangiectasia (small red lines) are seen on the nose and cheeks. Dysphagia is also common. If there is widespread systemic involve-ment the long-term prognosis is poor.

Systemic lupus erythematosus. The disease is mainly seen in women, starting in the child-bearing years. Many organs of the body may be involved. It is characterised by the butterfly rash seen on the cheeks and over the bridge of the nose. There is no set pattern of the disease and it may be difficult to diagnose.

TREATMENT

The general aims of treatment are relief of pain and stiffness, maintainance of function, prevention and correction of deformities, modification of the dis-ease process and management of extra-articular features and complications of therapy. Educational and psychological support may also be needed.

As the cause of the disease is unknown, treat-ment must be to relieve symptoms and maintain or restore function. This can be achieved by bed rest, resting individual joints, drug therapy and occupa-tional and physiotherapy. Continual reappraisal and assessment is important. Surgery may be necessary.

Note: As the disease presents a constantly changing picture in each patient, modifications in management are required throughout the course of treatment. The severity of the disease and the extent of joint damage will determine future man-agement. The psychological state of the patient must be borne in mind. Sinking into a state of dependency takes a long time and it is unreason-able to expect a sudden return to normal. The patient's own ambition should equal that of the team treating him.

Drugs

These play an important part in the treatment of the patient with rheumatoid arthritis. By giving the right drug at the right time relief can often be obtained from pain and stiffness, and the progress of the disease can be affected.

The most commonly used drugs are discussed below in the order in which they are usually prescribed.

1. *Analgesics.* Paracetamol is the most com-monly used simple pain reliever. It may be given in combination with dextropropoxyphene (Dis-talgesic).

2. *Analgesic anti-inflammatory drugs.* These are pain-relieving drugs with an anti-inflammatory action. Aspirin is the most commonly used drug in this group, but it can have side effects, such as gastrointestinal bleeding, if taken in large doses over a long time. Indomethacin (Indocid) can be taken by mouth or as a suppository. Other non-steroid anti-inflammatory drugs which are widely

used are ibuprufen (Brufen) and ketoprofen (Orudis).

3. *Corticosteroids.* These have a powerful action and must always be prescribed with care because of the numerous and serious side effects which can occur. They play a large part in the treatment of progressive arthritis. Prednisolone (prednisone) is one of the most commonly used in this group. The side effects of steroids taken in large doses over a long time include osteoporosis, fluid retention, Cushing syndrome (giving rise to a moon face appearance), peptic ulcer, excess facial hair, thin atrophic skin, delayed healing, cataracts, redistribution of body fat, increased susceptibility to infection, hypertension and psychosis.

An exacerbation of severe rheumatoid arthritis may be treated with adrenocorticotrophic hormone (ACTH), injected in a reducing course. This stimulates the patient's adrenal glands to overproduce the natural hormones. Although ACTH has the potential to produce the same long-term side effects as prednisolone, these are not seen as frequently.

If arthritis is limited to only one or two joints, local intra-articular injections, often of hydrocortisone, may be given to relieve symptoms. Prolonged use can cause osteoporosis.

4. *Immunosuppressive drugs.* Penicillamine is given in small doses initially. If the drug is well tolerated this is very gradually increased to a maintainance dose. Side effects are indigestion, loss of taste, skin rashes and albuminuria. The white cell and platelet count can fall, and regular fortnightly blood test are therefore necessary. The urine is tested for albumin daily for three weeks, and thereafter weekly.

5. *Gold.* A course of intramuscular gold injections may be given at weekly intervals in increasing doses. Benefits will not be felt until halfway through the course. Side effects such as albuminuria and skin rashes may occur, in which case the injections are stopped immediately. Blood and urine analysis is carried out regularly. White cell and platelet counts can fall and bone marrow activity suppressed. More than one course can be given, but subsequent treatments are usually less beneficial.

6. *Antimalarial drugs.* Chloroquine is given orally and the indications for its use are the same as for gold, namely progressive disease. Retinal damage may occur as the result of long-term treatment.

7. *Chemical synovectomy.* This is sometimes considered if conventional treatment is unsuccessful. Radioactive yttrium is injected into the knees or shoulders. Complete bed rest is necessary for 72 hours after the injection, and resting plaster back shells are provided. The patient is usually allowed home after five days.

Cytotoxic drugs such as cyclophosphamide may also be given. The white cell and platelet count must be checked.

Surgery

This plays an increasingly important role in the treatment of patients with rheumatoid arthritis and is sometimes undertaken as a prophylactic measure. It is fortunate that surgery is now being used in the earlier rather than later stages of the disease, as the benefits will be only slight if the patient is already crippled or deformed. Factors to be taken into consideration when contemplating surgery are pain, loss of movement, deformity, progressive disease, home circumstances, personality and motivation.

The most common procedures are fusion of the cervical spine and of the wrist; synovectomy of the shoulder, elbow and metacarpophalangeal joints of the hand, and of the knee and ankle; excision of the humeral or radial head and of the lower end of the ulna; arthrodesis of the shoulder, thumb, knee or ankle; forefoot arthroplasty and amputation of the toes. Total joint replacement can be performed at the shoulder, hip, knee and ankle, and partial replacement at the shoulder (humeral head), elbow (hinge replacement) and at the hand (sylastic replacements). Excision arthroplasty may be performed at the hip (Girdlestone) and a tibial osteotomy at the knee.

Routine laboratory tests

All patients with rheumatoid arthritis require certain investigations and tests.

Blood tests.

(a) Haemoglobin (HB). The normal HB is about 14 grams per 100 millilitres. Many patients with arthritis are anaemic. This is related to the disease activity and may be aggravated by the side effects of some drugs.

(b). White blood count (WBC). A normal WBC is 5000–10 000 per mm^3. The action of some drugs may alter the number of white cells. In Felty's syndrome and in systemic lupus erythematosus there is a fall in the WBC, whereas infective arthritis may be associated with an increase in white cells.

(c). Erythrocyte sedimentation rate (ESR). The normal value is about 10mm per hour in men and about 14mm per hour in women. It reflects the activity of the inflammatory process.

(d). Platelets. The normal count is 200 000–400 000 per mm^3. It may be much higher in patients with active rheumatoid arthritis. Gold or penicillamine treatment can suppress platelet formation and this may lead to purpura and bleeding. Immediate action must be taken as this can be fatal.

(e). Rheumatoid factor. Patients with rheumatoid arthritis have certain proteins in their serum which are not usually detected in other patients. These proteins belong to the IgM class of immunoglobulins and are often referred to as rheumatoid factor.

(i) Sheep cell agglutination test (SCAT). When red sheep cells coated with rabbit anti-sheep cell globulin are allowed to react with patient serum containing rheumatoid factor agglutination occurs.

(ii) Rheumaton slide test. This is used as a screening test to decide whether a more elaborate SCAT should be carried out. One drop of the patient's serum is mixed with rheumaton reagent and is observed for agglutination after two minutes. If the rheumatoid factor is absent from the serum of rheumatoid patients, the prognosis is better. Higher concentrations usually indicate a less favourable prognosis.

Urine tests. Albuminuria can be caused by certain drugs, e.g. gold and penicillamine, and if this happens the drug must be discontinued, as permanent kidney damage may result. Other tests can be carried out to differentiate the diagnosis from other diseases such as gout.

Nursing procedures

Ideally, patients with rheumatoid arthritis should be cared for in special units where treatment is geared toward their needs.

Caring for these patients requires empathy and understanding, and the nursing staff on a rheumatology unit should give as much support as possible. The nurse is often the first person a patient sees after admission, and the first impression made on the often apprehensive patient is important. The ward should be equipped to encourage self help with Hi-Lo beds, firm mattresses, light but warm bedclothes, bed cages and named wardrobes and lockers.

All the patient's own drugs should be handed in and charted, and the kardex filled in. A brief assessment of his ability to carry out basic activities of daily living should be made at this stage. The position of the patient's bed is important, not only for psychological reasons, but also to ensure that patients on diuretics are close to the toilet. Showers or bath aids can relieve the nurse of having to lift patients, but where this is not realistic hoists should be provided.

It is important that all nursing staff are aware of the roles of the other paramedical services and of the aims of treatment for each patient. Nursing staff see far more of the patient than anyone else, and any spare time should be spent talking to the patient and observing him. It is of no benefit to the patient if, in order to save time, a nurse assists him with activities which he is well able to do himself. Walking aids and other personal aids issued to the patient should be used by him. If he has difficulty in handling them the therapist should be informed.

Nursing in the acute phase

Attention to the skin and a daily blanket bath are important. If the patient is obese special care must be taken that the skin folds are dry to prevent sores. Frequent repositioning or turning is necessary to prevent bed sores. If a patient is treated with steroids the skin is especially vulnerable, and care must be taken that it is in no way bumped or bruised. If there is oedema in the ankle or leg the foot of the bed should be raised and bed cradles provided.

The temperature, pulse, respiration and blood pressure must be carefully checked, especially after surgery.

Physiotherapy

The aims of treatment are to improve joint range and muscle power by physical means and thereby allow greater independence:

Heat. Damp heat appears to be most effective for patients with rheumatoid arthritis.

1. Hydropacks. These help to relieve stiff, painful joints. They are heated in water, wrapped in cloths and applied to one or several joints as required. In order to preserve the heat the packs and towels are wrapped in a waterproof covering. They are left in position for 20 to 30 minutes. Frail patients may find these packs too heavy. If there is known loss of sensation the area must be tested first to avoid burning.

2. Hydrotherapy. Ideally, the pool should be 98°F. The warmth and buoyancy of the water help the muscles to relax and make exercises easier to perform. Very disabled patients can be lowered into the water on hoists and more mobile patients can perform exercises whilst sitting on stools. Re-education of walking will often be started in the pool. Patients will be asked to perform a series of general exercises and others related to specific areas of disability.

The chlorine in the water may cause a rash. Hydrotherapy is also contraindicated in patients with ulcers and sores.

3. Wax baths. The hands, elbows and feet are frequently treated in wax baths. The paraffin wax is heated to blood temperature and five layers are applied to the joint and this is left for 10 minutes. The wax is then peeled off and the patient asked to work through a series of exercises. Alternatively, shallow trays of liquid wax can be used. The patient puts his hands in the wax and then continues with the exercises which add resistance as the wax hardens:

(a). Place hands into the liquid wax with fingers fully extended

(b). Flex and extend fingers at metacarpophalangeal joints while the wax is still soft

(c). Form the wax into one large ball or two smaller ones and compress; watch grip

(d). Make two balls and pinch off small pieces, opposing thumb to index and middle fingers

(e). Make two balls, pinch off small pieces between thumb and each finger in turn

(f). Make small pyramids by pinching up from a flat piece

(g). Make two coils; using fingers like scissors cut off pieces between index and middle finger, middle and ring finger and so on

(h). Make two coils large enough to be gripped by both hands, roll alongside each other and pull apart, or pull apart with pinch-type grip from either end.

(i) Make small rolls, four for each hand, and pull between thumb and first metacarpophalangeal joint and between proximal phalangeal joints of both hands.

Alternate exercises between both hands. They may take anything from two to twenty minutes. The sequence may have to be altered to suit individual patients, e.g. exercise (g) may have to be performed before exercise (d) in the early stages of treatment.

4. *Infra-red lamps.* Heat in this form can be applied to the neck, shoulders and back for twenty minutes; it is then followed by massage.

Shortwave diathermy is rarely used for patients with rheumatoid arthritis as little benefit is derived.

Serial splints. These are used to treat flexion contractures of the knee. After exercising in the pool, a plaster of Paris cylinder is applied to the leg from groin to ankle. This is done by two therapists. The plaster is left in position for 48 hours and the exercise then repeated until maximum extension is obtained. The back shells can be used for walking and are bandaged on at night so that the correction gained is not lost.

Re-education in walking. If the patient has not walked for some time, this may start in the pool. A high gutter frame with wheels is often used in the beginning to give the patient confidence, but this is usually impracticable for home use because of its width. Other walking aids in common use are the Zimmer frame, Delta walking aid, gutter crutches and sticks. Axilla and elbow crutches are not encouraged as the weight is thrown onto the elbows, wrists and hands.

Exercises. Ideally, these should follow heat treatment. Patients should put their joints through a full range of movement every day. Class work should be done whenever possible, as this is less demanding on the physiotherapist's time and is enjoyed by the patients. Assisted exercises should be done three times a day and quadriceps exercises as regularly as possible. Patients should be encouraged to lie in a prone position as this will help to prevent hip and knee flexion deformities.

Splints. These are worn to prevent deformity, immobilise painful joints and to assist movement by putting the joint in a good position.

1. Collars. These must fit well and care should be taken that they do not rub. Different types of collars are available; the Ll. Williams and Dolls collars for cervical collapse; the Zimmer and Camp collars if a hard collar is needed, and inflatable and Sorbo-rubber collars for night-time use.

2. Back supports. Plaster of Paris slab with tubigrip, followed by a made-to-measure light-weight Aertex support with Velcro fastenings may be provided.

3. Futura wrist supports or leatherette made to measure (Taylor's of Walsall) with Velcro fastenings are very satisfactory, as they give the wrist support when working and are not unattractive to look at. Polythene supports can be worn if it is likely that the hands will get wet, but they are rigid and can be difficult to put on independently.

4. Elastic knee supports are easy to put on, but for more support a cinch splint may be necessary. Elastic supports and Hartshill heel cups can be used for the ankle.

5. Shoes. Plastazote boots are easy to make and can be made with holes to accommodate pressure lesions. They are not very robust and therefore not suitable for outside wear, and tend to be hot. Drushoes are more attractive. If a 'D'-ring is attached to the fastening the shoes can be taken off and put on independently with a dressing stick. Metatarsal buttons and plastazote insoles can be put into shoes for support and metsox also give support.

6. Resting splints are made from plaster of Paris which is economical to use. When making these for the hand, the wrist should be in slight extension with the fingers slightly flexed at the metacarpophalangeal joints. These splints should be worn alternately during rest periods and at night to prevent further deformity. Knee cylinders can be worn at night to prevent and correct flexion deformity.

Ozone. An ion ozone machine which vapou-rises distilled water using ultraviolet light is flashed across the vapour and then applied at a nine-inch distance for 10 minutes. Arachis oil is often rubbed into the surrounding tissue to keep the skin in good condition.

Psoriasis is treated with cold tar baths during which the affected areas are scrubbed. This is followed by general ultraviolet light, and dithranol is rubbed carefully into the affected area. The course lasts one month with daily treatments.

Oedematous hands, wrists, feet and ankles can be treated with Flotron boots. The limb must be elevated and the boots can be left on for any length of time. The alternate pressure and relaxation increases blood flow and helps to disperse waste materials. Vasculitis is treated in a tunnel bath by radiant heat, which improves the circulation. It is followed by Berger's exercises.

OCCUPATIONAL THERAPY

The aims of the occupational therapist should be directed to helping the patient to reattain the level of function necessary to cope adequately within his environment. It should be remembered that rheumatoid arthritis is a progressive condition and that, therefore, constant reassessment and reappraisal is necessary.

The importance of establishing a good rapport early on cannot be emphasised too much, as much of the success of treatment depends on the relationship between patient and therapist. Many patients have deep-seated anxieties and problems which will only be brought to light if the therapist takes the time to listen and to show genuine concern for the patient and his problems.

If time permits, a pre-admission visit to the patient's home can often be of great value. By seeing the patient in his own home, a true assessment of his limitations can be made. Not all patients will require this service, but by reading through a case sheet, the following points should be noted as a guide for those who do: widespread deformities and limitation of movement, isolation of home in relation to the rest of the community, living alone, of advanced age. Obvious depression and deterioration may also be an indication for a home visit. A short letter should be sent to the

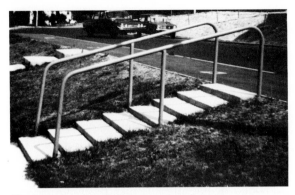

Fig. 26.1 Firm handrails by a set of outdoor steps

patient notifying him of the reason for the visit, and of the date and approximate time that the visit is to be made.

The following features should be noted during this or any later home visit:

Situation of the house in relation to the rest of the community (town centre or outskirts, estate, small town, village or on its own)

Terrain (flat or hilly)

Position (e.g. on main or side road, in the middle of an estate or on a track)

Access (path and its state of repair, garden gate, number and depth of steps, handrail — Fig. 26.1)

Type of house (detached, semi-detached, terraced, bungalow, cottage, maisonette, high-rise building or tenement, level of flat)

Size and state of garden.

Inside the house, the position of toilet and bath should be checked (e.g. upstairs, downstairs or outside), the type of toilet (flush type or Elsan) and whether aids and adaptations have already been provided. Some patients may not have a bath. If there is a coal fire enquire who is responsible for carrying the coal, laying the fire and tending to it. What is the main form of heating (electric or gas fires, central heating), is there an immersion heater? Other points to remember are inside steps, number of rooms in use and floor coverings (e.g. fitted carpets, mats, linoleum or quarry tiles).

Check who is at home with the patient and whether he or she is working. If this is so, ask if they are home for lunch and what hours they work, whether from 9 to 5 or on a shift system. If the patient himself works, a detailed job analysis is needed.

After getting these details from the patient a picture should start to emerge of his lifestyle, and it is now necessary to complete a full assessment covering all areas which might pose problems. Even though a patient may appear fairly mobile it is still necessary to go through this check-list as some patients will make light of their problems and try to gloss over them.

Daily living

To avoid repetition later in the chapter, solutions to problems which may present will be noted after each activity. Some of these may not be dealt with until the patient is admitted to hospital.

Feeding. Difficulties in using cutlery and holding a cup may be caused by poor grip, limitation of pronation/supination and by restriction of shoulder or elbow movement. Often, the weight of the cup causes a problem. Large-grip and extended cutlery may be considered either of the Red Cross (now being deleted) or the Sunflower range and also Manoy cutlery, plates and mugs, or rubbazote handles. Handles can also be made from clear perspex rod and covered with pimple rubber for easier holding. The Skyline cheese and tomato knives have sharp cutting edges and are often forgotten as useful aids. An Insulex mug or cup is suitable for some patients, as it is lightweight, insulated and has a large handle. Alternatively, Polytemp mugs and Pyrex Drink-up mugs can be used or, if grip is very poor, a feeding strap.

Dressing. All items of clothing can present difficulties, depending on limitation of movement. It should be established which areas of dressing cause problems to the patient.

With shoulder and elbow involvement it may be difficult to put clothes over the head and around the shoulders, and to fasten top buttons, back zips, braces and bras. If hips and knees are involved putting on pants and trousers, tights, stockings, socks and shoes, and skirts and waist petticoats may cause problems. If the hands are involved it may be difficult or impossible to fasten buttons and belts, to handle clothes generally and to pull them up because of the weakened grip.

Ask the patient how long it usually takes him to get dressed, whether he needs help and whether he already has any dressing aids.

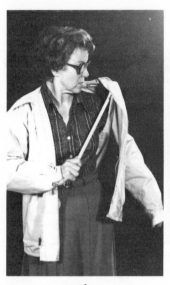
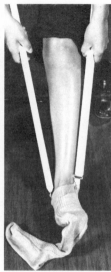

A   B

Fig. 26.2   Dressing aids of particular value to the patient with rheumatoid arthritis. (A) Dressing stick (B) Sock sticks

The dressing stick made out of half-inch dowelling (or a coat-hanger) is one of the best and most versatile aids for patients with rheumatoid arthritis (Fig. 26.2A). Other aids in common use are long-handled shoe horns, stocking gutter or sock sticks, or the Downes stocking aid (Fig. 26.2B): zip-pulls or rings on zippers, a Helping Hand, Cee-Vee Reacher or Lazy Tongs and buttons hooks. The therapist may also give advice on suitable clothing and alterations.

Hair care and hygiene. Limitation of shoulder and elbow movement and rotation will cause problems in reaching round the back of the neck and head. Some severely disabled patients have difficulty in washing their hands and cleaning their teeth not only because of joint limitation, but also because of poor hand function. Check who cuts and washes the patient's hair.

Useful aids are spontex mops, available from hardware shops, as they have thickened handles and can be bent in hot water, For washing between the toes a Twixtik can be used. Other popular aids are toothbrush extensions or straps in the Sunflower range, towelling mitts, long-handled brushes and combs, and flannels, towelling or loofahs on loops.

Hand activities. Poor hand and upper limb function, and restriction of pronation/supination can obviously limit a wide variety of activities.

These include the ability to write, to pick up small objects and to switch on lights. When opening doors both lever and ball handle types may be difficult, as may taps, cooker controls, plugs and keys. Unlocking doors, especially with a Yale-type key, can present problems because of the inside knob. Not all of the activities will be relevant to each patient, and it is therefore important that the therapist establishes which of these tasks the patient will need to master and whether he can perform them independently or not.

Padded or felt-tip pens may be useful for patients with writing difficulties. A reconditioned electric typewriter is often invaluable. Other useful aids include a Helping Hand, Cee-Vee Reacher or Lazy Tongs to pick up objects, and a dressing stick with a cup hook on one end for switching on lights. A Jubilee clip with lever extension is useful for Yale keys and a metal or wood extension for other keys. Two keys can be riveted together for better leverage. Lever adaptations for cooker controls are available, and the Gas Board will assist with this as well as with problems with gas fires. Plugs can be pulled out with an extractor plug handle and adapted three-pin plugs are available.

Transfer and mobility

Chairs. Most modern chairs are too soft and too low for many patients who often try to overcome this problem by piling extra cushions onto the seat. This, however, will only tend to squash and thus minimise any assistance to rising given by chair arms. Further joint damage can occur when a patient rocks backwards and forwards several times in an attempt to rise. It is important that the patient is made aware of the correct sitting position and that alterations to the height of the chair (hips and knees at 90 degrees, if possible, with feet flat on the floor) are being made for his own well-being.

In the majority of cases advice will need to be given on raising a chair. Correct measurement should be taken with the patient sitting so that the seat of his chair is depressed when measuring the height from the floor (Fig. 26.3A).

1. Raising blocks. Unless a one-inch or two-inch raise is needed, blocks are not a very safe way of permanently raising a chair. They are, however,

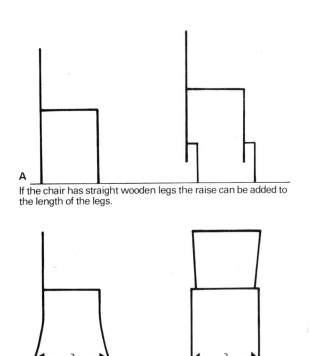

If the chair has straight wooden legs the raise can be added to the length of the legs.

Distance between front & back legs   Width between legs

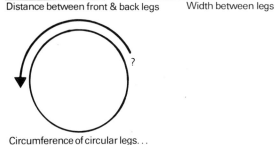

Circumference of circular legs...

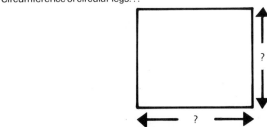

or length & depth of rectangular legs

Chair leg   Chair leg

Height of raise required

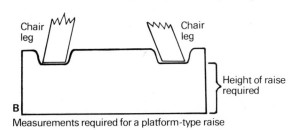

Measurements required for a platform-type raise

Fig. 26.3 Methods of raising a chair to the appropriate height for the patient

useful to assess the correct height. The blocks can either be made in the occupational therapy department or obtained commercially (e.g. the Homecraft Ladywell Sleeves).

2. Permanent raises. These should be measured, made and fitted by an occupational therapy technician or a professional joiner. If a chair has wooden legs the raise can be bolted on. If the patient has an armchair, a box-like construction will have to be made with the raise varnished, stained, or covered in a matching material (Fig. 26.3B).

If the services of a technician or joiner are not available it is possible to raise the chair by using raising blocks with a safety bar between the legs (from front to back) to prevent slipping.

3. Ejector Cushions. These must have a firm base and should not be used by very old or confused patients or where there is a danger that the patient could inadvertently lean forward and fall off. Some ejector cushions only operate with a lever, but this requires good hand function and good balance.

4. Ejector Chairs. These have the advantage that they look like an ordinary high-seat chair and the user himself decides whether to use the ejector action (Powell, Shackleton). (Fig. 26.4A).

5. Electric Chairs. Where all else fails this type of chair may have to be considered. At present not many types are available and some are more suitable for certain types of disability than others.

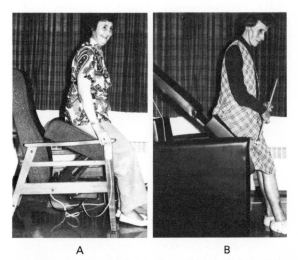

A   B

Fig. 26.4 Two types of electric chairs which assist the patient during transfer

Careful tuition is necessary, particularly for the patient with stiff knees where a skid-proof surface is essential. The Power Rise, Orthokinetic, Some-is essential. The Power Rise, Orthokinetic. The Somerford Chair are some examples (Fig. 26.4B).

6. Plywood bases. If several cushions are used to raise a chair and this appears satisfactory, a plywood base with a hole in the middle and placed between the cushions will often prevent them from being compressed too much.

Beds. Many modern beds, such as divans are too low and soft for the patient with rheumatoid arthritis and cause obvious problems in getting on and off. Some patients have morning stiffness and may find the weight of the bedclothes too heavy. They may also be unable to sit up in bed because of pain, stiffness and generalised weakness.

If the bed is too high and has wooden legs these can be cut off to the appropriate height. If a bed is too low and has wooden legs then a raise can be bolted on as in a chair or bed blocks can be made (Fig. 26.5). For those divan beds with screw-in legs divan bed raises provide up to a 4" raise. A permanent wooden made-to-measure raise can be made by the occupational therapy technician once the correct height has been ascertained (Fig. 26.6). In some cases a standard hospital bed with or without a monkey pole or an adjustable Kings Fund bed will have to be provided.

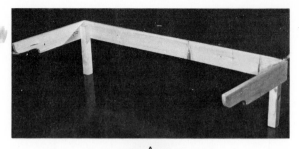

A

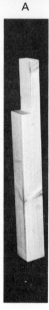

B

Fig. 26.6 A permanent bed raise. (A) One end of a platform bed raise (B) A separate raise may be used for each leg

If a mattress is too soft a piece of chip-board can be provided. A door can also be used. Some patients will require advice on the purchase of a new mattress and should be told that they may not always need to go to the expense of buying an orthopaedic mattress.

Other ideas or aids which could be helpful are continental quilts, electric over blanket, bed cradle, cellular blankets, rope ladder and bed aid.

Toilet. Most modern toilets are 15 to 16 inches high and this is often at least four inches too low for the rheumatoid patient with hip and knee involvement. Some patients will want to have something to hold on to, be it the wash-basin or a grab rail. Other problems which may occur are an inability to clean themselves because of restricted wrist supination, and insufficient pressure or reach to flush the toilet.

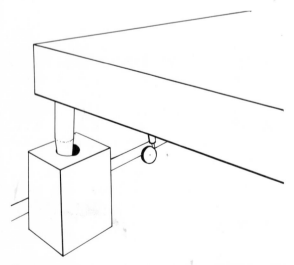

Fig. 26.5 Bed blocks to raise the bed to the appropriate height for the patient

A four-inch toilet raise will often solve many problems, and this must fit tightly so as to prevent any risk of slipping off. For those who are taller, or who have very stiff knees, a six-inch raise or the Carter's adjustable seat may be needed.

If the wash-basin is firmly fixed or if the bath is near these will often be suitable as support for a patient. Some patients hold on to the back of the door for support but this is not satisfactory. If a grab rail is contemplated this must obviously be atttached to an outside wall if internal walls are not brick built, and individual positioning is necessary, usually in a horizontal position. Renray have a large range of different types of rails and many firms make portable rails which do not need fixing. For those who cannot manage with ordinary toilet raises or rails there are ejector and power-assisted toilet raises.

Hygiene is often a very embarrassing topic for a patient, so the subject may have to be introduced tactfully. A toilet-paper holder can be easily made with coat hanger wire or old knitting needles at the desired length and angle. The Clos-o-mat toilet has a douching and drying action. Chemical toilets are sometimes provided through social services. They are usually of a fixed height. Commodes can be used where toilet access is impossible, but they are frequently too low. If a female rheumatoid patient has very limited abduction of the hips a urinal with a good-sized handle will be necessary. These are also often used during the night by patients who cannot get out of bed fast enough because of stiffness.

Baths. Do make sure that the patient has a bath before getting overenthusiastic about providing seats and rails. Remember also, that if a patient has leg ulcers or if he sleeps downstairs and the bath is upstairs an assessment will not be needed. Some patients will not have attempted a bath for years because of infirmity or disability, and in many cases it is wiser to leave things as they are.

Getting in and out of the bath is often the first area in which the patient loses independence. Enquire if the patient has a shower attachment over the bath or a separate shower.

Over-bath boards and half seats will help many patients (The measurements are shown in Figure 26.7). Often, it is advisable to encourage the patient to fill the bath higher and to stay on the half

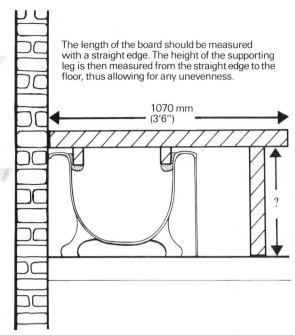

The length of the board should be measured with a straight edge. The height of the supporting leg is then measured from the straight edge to the floor, thus allowing for any unevenness.

1070 mm
(3'6")

?

Fig. 26.7 Measurements to be taken for an over-bath board

seat. It is easy enough to get down but not as easy to get up, since the leverage is wrong and the patient's arms may be weak. Rails over the taps will often not help these patients, as they often cannot pull. Grab rails on the wall and vertical poles can be used, as can non-slip mats, strips or flowers. A shower-ring and blow-up cushions also can be used.

Showers. It is not always necessary to go to the expense of a proper plumbed-in shower. The position of the tanks will have a bearing on water pressure and this must be checked. A simple shower attachment for the taps and a curtain and perhaps a bath board or a cheaper solution. If proper shower controls are to be fitted, these should be thermostatically controlled with lever controls. The shower base should not have too high a ledge, and a grab rail and/or a folding seat may be needed.

Some patients will never be independent in using the bath, however many aids are provided and it may be more practical to enlist the help of a bath attendant or district nurse.

General mobility

Try to assess the level of mobility, the distance

managed and the type of walking aid used. Patients will have different needs; pottering around the house might be sufficient for an elderly widow, but not for a young mother with a growing family or for the wage earner. If the patient is bed-bound, try to assess the real motivation to walk. If there is an adoring family to dance attendance the aims of treatment will need to be modified.

Stairs. If a patient sleeps downstairs and is going to continue doing so, there is no need to measure the depth of tread, position of bannister and number of stairs. To the patient with rheumatoid disease the inability to climb stairs can cause great misery. Many will have to be levered or lifted up by relatives. Many will find their own ways, such as descending backwards or sliding down on their bottoms. Check on the mode of ascent and descent and the time taken. A turn at the top of the stairs where there is no bannister can often cause problems. If there is a bannister, make sure the patient can grip it properly. Many council houses have bannisters with closed-in sides which are difficult to grip. If the patient has a stair lift, make sure that this is suitable for his needs.

Steps. The maximum and minimum depth of these should be noted, whether inside or outside the house, and the presence or otherwise of a hand-rail.

Wheelchair. Many rheumatoid patients benefit from having a chair for outside use, as frequently they will be unable to walk far and may become even more isolated by not going out. Note, however, that no matter how great the disability, some patients will not accept a chair because of pride and self-consciousness. When ordering the chair, always order a three-inch cushion with it for comfort. In some cases an electric wheelchair will be needed.

Car. Check if the patient drives or if he is a passenger and if there are problems in getting in and out and using the controls. Check whether he is already in receipt of a car parking disc, Invacar, private car allowance or war-disabled person's car.

Kitchen activities. Enquire how much meal preparation the patient needs or wants to do, and look at the kitchen, noting continuous working surfaces, cupboard heights and type of cooker. The usual problems encountered are difficulty in peeling and straining vegetables, making pastry and cakes, standing and bending down to the oven and low cupboards. Reaching up to cupboards and shelves, carrying pans and plates, and lifting and pouring kettle and teapot can cause problems, as can opening windows, opening tins, bottles, jars and taps. Many very disabled patients will do little or no cooking and may only need to make themselves a drink. Check who cooks for them and what the usual arrangements are throughout the day. Exhaustion after very little effort is common.

If a patient appears to live on sandwiches or snacks his diet may need to be checked once he is admitted to hospital.

Valuable kitchen aids are vegetable peelers, chip baskets for straining vegetables, wall or electric can openers and bottle and jar openers. Trolleys (Fig. 26.8A) help with general mobility as well as with carrying. Food mixers, pastry blenders, alterations to cooker knobs, kitchen stools (Fig. 26.8B), non-slip mats and convenience foods are other possible solutions to problems in the kitchen.

Housework. Remember that everyone has varying standards and that although a house may look as if it needs a good clean, this does not necessarily indicate that there is no one to do it.

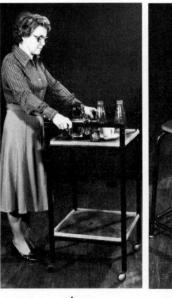
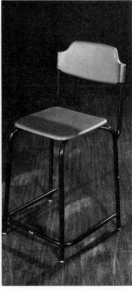

A   B

Fig. 26.8 Kitchen aids of particular use to the patient with rheumatoid arthritis (A) Trolley (B) Stool

Arthritis may prevent a patient from doing housework as he may be unable to stand for long, and tire after little effort. The patient's mental state may be a contributory factor.

Check what help is given by family or friends and whether the patient is receiving the services of a home help or has a private cleaner. Common difficulties are dusting and polishing (because of the pressure required), cleaning brasses, hoovering, washing floors and windows and moving furniture.

Long-handled dustpan and brush, a Minit Mop and spray polish are valuable household aids. The services of the home help service may be required.

Shopping. Ask who usually does this. In some areas there is a delivery service or a mobile van. Frequently a friend or relative will do the weekly shopping in a supermarket, leaving the patient to deal only with small day-to-day requirements. Obviously a deep freeze is a great advantage.

The usual problems are the inability to carry shopping or handle money, difficulty in walking and/or standing and loading purchases into the car. There may also be transport difficulties, e.g. problems with getting on a bus.

Shopping trolleys or a Zimmer bag on pulpit walking aid are obviously very useful and a deep freeze will reduce the need for daily shopping.

Laundry. Although some patients now have fully automatic washing machines, there may still be problems in loading and unloading the machine and in operating the controls. Some patients do their personal washing, but send the sheets and towels to the laundry. There is often a problem in wringing clothes and in hanging them out. Standing to iron is particularly tiring and some patients adapt to sitting down. Many patients reduce their ironing load by extensive use of synthetic fabrics.

Lightweight irons, stools to sit on while ironing, dolly pegs and spin dryers may be the answer to some of these problems.

Benefits.

These might already have been discussed in the course of conversation, but surprisingly many patients have no idea of their entitlements. At present age limits some of the benefits so be certain of the patient's age beforehand. At present the following benefits are available: attendance allowance, mobility allowance, sickness and invalidity benefit and non-contributory invalidity pension for married women. Also check if the patient has or needs contact with the social services departments, a health visitor, district nurse, Meals on Wheels, a home help, assistance from the Disabled Resettlement Officer (DRO). He may profit from attendance at a day centre, a wheelchair, the help of the community physiotherapist or a sitter service.

Hobbies and Interests

Many patients find that they cannot continue lifelong hobbies such as sewing and knitting, but have found nothing to put in their place apart from reading and watching television. Some patients will be so exhausted by the end of the day that they will have no energy to do anything else.

There will often be an underlying depression, and when you ask 'Do you have days when things get you down?', be prepared for a sudden onset of tears which often follows the frustration of not being able to manage and inability to come to terms with the disease.

Throughout the visit it is important to try to assess motivation. It is of little value to help the patient to attain a high level of function whilst in hospital, only to realise that once discharged he will not be allowed to maintain this level. Some patients will be apprehensive about coming into hospital, and this is a good opportunity to explain about the ward, its staffing and the type of treatment they are likely to have. If immediate action needs to be taken, such as the provision of aids, referral to the appropriate social services department can be made, particularly if the patient is not to be admitted fairly soon. All the information taken should be clearly set out in the notes, ideally on a separate occupational therapy form, so that all members of the treatment team can see what the problems are and what they should be aiming for (Fig. 26.9).

If a patient has not been seen prior to admission, he should be assessed on admittance. If transfers seem to be a problem the home heights can be sent for; if a patient needs rehousing this can be initiated whilst he is still in hospital with a suitable letter of support from the consultant in charge.

Name .... Reg. No. ....Date of Admission ....

Housing

Social

Worst joints
Recommendations to solve any problems

Signed ....
Occupational Therapist

O.T. – Aids given in hospital

Aids requested through Social Services

Adaptations requested

Physio – Splints given in Hospital

Splints ordered via Derwen/Taylors or others (please specify)

	Date	
Home help		
Meals of wheels		
Rehousing		
Wheelchair		
Attendance allowance		
Mobility allowance		
Non-contributory allowance for married women		
British Rheumatism and Arthritis Association (if Shrewsbury area patient)		

D.R.O.

Community nursing requests

Fig. 26.9 Preadmission report form as used at the Robert Jones and Agnes Hunt Orthopaedic Hospital, Oswestry

Specific remedial treatment

Although, perhaps, re-education in activities of daily living is the area in which the occupational therapist really comes into her own, there is a definite place for remedial treatment when time allows. This should aim at building up muscle strength and range of movement, so leading to greater independence.

Frequent rest periods and correct seating and posture must be observed and the treatment time should be graded. Activities should not be static or too hard. Canework, ceramics and remedial games can be used and some of these can be continued as a home interest. New methods of gardening can be taught with advice on tools and other equipment. Where there is a heavy workshop, group projects can be initiated, and this will also help with socialisation. If the patient is likely to have to change his job the Disablement Resettlement Officer should be informed early, and a job simulation or assessment may need to be carried out by the occupational therapist. Early contact should be made with the patient's employer.

Provision of aids. These should be issued with care. It is to be hoped that after physiotherapy and/or surgery many functional problems will have been resolved, and reassessment can be done at a later date. Some aids will have to be made if not commercially available.

Joint preservation. This is beginning to play an increasingly large part in some units, and advice is given on easier ways of performing day-to-day tasks. The patient should be instructed to avoid activities which push the hands into ulnar deviation. Alternative methods of lifting can be shown and good posture should be encouraged (see also Ch. 3).

Sexual Counselling.

Rheumatoid arthritis will obviously lead to restrictions in sexual activities because of stiffness, joint deformity and pain. There will often be reluctance to talk freely about this and maybe lack of understanding and tolerance by the partner. Hip replacements requested by younger women who have had difficulty in hip abduction have been performed with good results. Counselling of both partners by the occupational therapist, social worker and/or doctor can be of value.

Hand Assessments

These may be requested for several reasons:
1. As part of a routine assessment
2. To assess whether deterioration is taking place
3. As a base line for treatment
4. To assess whether splintage is necessary
5. Preoperative assessment
6. Post-operative assessment
7. To assess whether surgery is indicated
8. To assess patients ability to cope with their employment
9. Prior to advice on joint preservation

Method. Check on hand dominance. Observe how the patient uses his hands in everyday situations and when pursuing hobbies. If a patient is working a job breakdown should be done. Ascertain how long the hand has been involved as distinct from the onset of the disease, and the order of progression and involvement of different joints.

Look for obvious deformities, such as swanneck, boutonniere, ulnar or radial deviation, ruptured extensor tendons in the fifth finger or nodules. Check the colour and texture of the skin, its condition (hot, cold, clammy) and note any sutures or swelling.

Many patients will be self-conscious and ashamed of the appearance of their hands and may request surgery for cosmetic reasons, whereas there are those who do not mind how their hands look, as long as they can use them.

Activities to assess

1. Dressing. Fasten/unfasten buttons, tie laces, fasten hooks/press studs, fasten suspenders, buckles, belts

2. Eating. Cutting food, lifting cup or glass, buttering bread

3. General activities. Writing, turning key in lock, turning knobs, squeezing toothpaste, winding watch, dialling telephone numbers, turning pages of book/paper, cutting and filing nails, striking match and operating lighter, cleaning spectacles, picking up and handling money, fastening and unfastening safety pins

4. Kitchen activities. Turn on/off taps, wash

dishes, dry dishes, clean saucepan, lift pan/teapot, open/close screw top jar, open a tin, crack an egg, beat egg/cake, cut bread, make and roll pastry, peel fruit/vegetables, turn on gas/electricity, wring clothes, polish/dust

5. Hobbies. Embroidery, sewing, knitting, photography, driving a car.

These activities must be related to the patient's needs, and careful recording should be made noting speed, compensation and trick movements, pain, normal pattern of use, inability to perform a task and general dexterity.

Tracings can be made using odstock wires so that grip and individual movements of the fingers can be recorded, i.e. pinch and power grip, lateral pinch. Ask the patient to try to flex his fingers (a) to the base of the metacarpophalangeal joints (b) to the wrist crease. A comparison must be made with the other hand, ideally by the same therapist doing the assessment at the same time of the day. In order that an accurate record can be made, sufficient time must be allowed.

Guidelines for the occupational therapist

All treatment must be purposeful, and close liaison is necessary between the occupational therapist and physiotherapist so that the patient's day is well balanced. After the initial assessments, a patient may need a period of concentrated physiotherapy to improve joint range of movement and stiffness.

Dressing and feeding practice can be done on the ward. Nursing staff should be made aware of what aids the patient is using and how much help he needs.

Some rheumatology units are specially equipped to encourage self care and have Kings Fund beds, high chairs, toilet and bath aids and laundry facilities. The occupational therapist may need to advise on this or to suggest ward planning and furnishing.

Ideally, ward meetings should be held regularly to discuss specific problems and treatment in general. Other relevant personnel, such as the social worker and the Disablement Resettlement Officer, should be invited to attend if necessary.

Reassessment of problem areas noted in the preadmission visit or initial assessment should be carried out, incorporating any specific treatment.

The patient should observe frequent rest periods, as mobility might have been very limited before admittance.

Occupational therapy plays an increasingly large part in the later stages of the patient's treatment, when longer sessions will be needed for meal preparation, simulation of home duties and other activities.

If there is doubt as to whether a patient can manage at home, he should be taken home for part of the day to see if he can cope. This could be an ideal time to see relatives. Often an overprotective role is adopted by families, and by inviting them to attend a treatment session instruction and counselling can be given.

Some occupational therapy departments have a self-contained flat where a patient in the final stages of treatment can live. If he normally receives Meals on Wheels he can now get his meals from the hospital kitchen, so that the home circumstances are simulated as far as possible.

When the patient is to be discharged, a discharge report should be written noting the areas of improvement and the aids of adaptations which have been issued or requested through the social services department. The patient and his relatives should be encouraged to telephone or write for help if needed in the future. They can also be put in touch with the Arthritis and Rheumatism Council and local day centres.

Follow-up Visits. Selected patients should be visited at home, usually before the first outpatient appointment. This can be done with any member of the relevant community services who should be encouraged to liaise with the hospital occupational therapist if any specific rheumatological problems arise.

It has been found very beneficial to take student nurses from the ward on visits with the therapist, as they gain a far greater insight into the patient, the problems he has to face and his home circumstances. As well as checking the patient's general mobility and progress since discharge, the use of splints and reaction to drugs should be noted. A report can then be put in the case notes.

It is essential that treatment is documented, since a patient's condition will fluctuate over the years, and the success of all treatment is often reflected in the patient's continued ability to be independent. If a patient is readmitted a reassessment should be made to compare function.

Acknowledgements

Dr D. J. Ward, M.B. Ch.B. F.R.C.P.; Mrs Jean Archer, Senior Physiotherapist, Rheumatology Unit; Miss Marian Wisdom, Senior Occupational Therapist, Rheumatology Unit, Sister D. Hughes, Rheumatology Unit S.O.H.; Mr David Jones, Senior Medical Photographer — all from Robert Jones & Agnes Hunt Orthopaedic Hospital, Oswestry, Shropshire.

REFERENCES AND FURTHER READING

Boyle A C 1974 A colour atlas of rheumatology. Wolfe Medical, London
Brattstrom M 1977 Principles of joint protection in chronic rheumatoid disease. Wolfe Medical, London
Dixon A 1965 Progress in clinical rheumatology J & A Churchill, London
Jayson M I V, Dixon A 1974 Rheumatism and arthritis. Pan, London
Macfarlane H 1970 Arthritis help in your own hands. Thorsons, London
Office of health economics 1973 Rheumatism and arthritis in Britain. Office of Health Economics, London
Wright V, Haslock I 1977 Rheumatism for nurses and remedial therapists. Heinemann, London

27
Spinal cord injuries

Serious road traffic accidents are on the increase, but with improved rescue techniques many accident victims now survive. Some of these will have sustained damage to their spinal cords. This is a serious injury and requires specialist treatment to complete successful rehabilitation and resettlement.

At present, there are some 12 Spinal Injuries Units in England, Scotland and Wales, varying in size from 20 to 200 beds. Each unit covers a certain catchment area which has a common boundary with its neighbour. Each unit has a highly specialised team of doctors, nurses, physiotherapists, occupational therapists and social workers, and they may also call upon the services of other specialists in the local community. There is close liaison between the various units at each level of staff.

It is essential that a patient with a spinal cord injury be transferred as soon as possible following injury to one of these units so that he may benefit from the specialist knowledge and facilities available. Important complications may thus be avoided, and a comprehensive rehabilitation and resettlement programme can be offered.

Unless one has actually experienced a spinal cord injury with the resulting paralysis and loss of sensation, it is impossible to fully understand the true extent and implication of such a condition. Sensations have been described in many vivid ways. One patient likened it to the feeling of sitting on a rubber sack filled with ice-cold water, over which he had no control; another described the amazement he felt on suddenly realising, after some time, that the body and legs the nurses were busy washing and moving about the bed were in fact his own, and of feeling completely detached from them. Some patients say that there was no one moment when they realised the full implication and seriousness of their injury, but more 'a gradual acceptance of the obvious'. For others there may be the moment of harsh reality when the future has to be faced.

Functional anatomy

The spinal column consists of seven cervical, twelve thoracic, five lumbar and five sacral vertebrae, and the coccyx. Each vertebra articulates with its neighbours and is separated from them by intervertebral discs. The vertebrae are held together by strong ligaments running posteriorly and anteriorly and are further supported by the powerful back muscles. The spinal cord is situated within the protective bony structure of the spinal canal formed by the vertebrae. The cord at the top of the neck is about the size of a man's little finger, decreasing in diameter until, at the level of L1–L2, it forms the cauda equina (horse's tail). It consists of thousands of separate nerve fibres enclosed in specially adapted tissue, protected in the spinal canal by the colourless cerebrospinal fluid (CSF).

In cross-section the cord shows a central grey butterfly-shaped area and outer white matter. The nerve fibres are divided within the cord into groups of fibres called tracts. These tracts usually run vertically up and down the cord, except where they cross over to supply the opposite side of the body. The ascending tracts lying posteriorly carry sensory nerve fibres and the descending tracts lying anteriorly motor nerve fibres. The spinal cord gives off nerve roots on either side corresponding to each vertebra. These are called spinal nerves and supply both motor and sensory function to particular muscle groups and skin areas (dermatomes). The cord has its own blood supply. Branches of the vertebral arteries run into the main posterior and anterior spinal arteries.

There are 30 segments in the spinal cord — 8 cervical, 12 thoracic, 5 lumbar and 5 sacral segments. Roots C1 to C7 leave the spinal cord above the appropriate vertebral body, but from

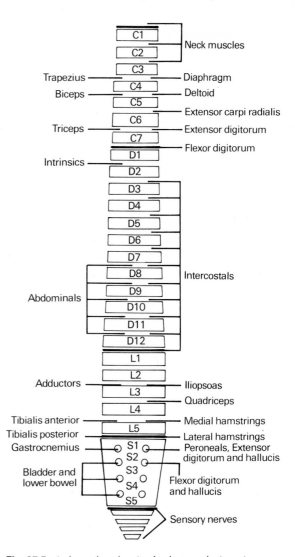

Fig. 27.5 Independent dressing for the paraplegic patient

root C8 downwards they leave below the appropriate vertebral body (Fig. 27.1).

Terminology. The spinal cord is part of the central nervous system. Damage to it above the level of L1 produces the symptoms of an upper motor neurone lesion with no regeneration of the cord. Below L1 (cauda equina), damage or injury may produce symptoms characteristic of a lower motor neurone lesion.

Tetraplegia or quadriplegia refers to any lesion of the spinal cord in the region of the cervical vertebrae (a neck injury).

Paraplegia refers to any lesion of the spinal cord

within the region of the thoracic (dorsal), lumbar or sacral vertebrae (a back injury).

A complete lesion is one in which there is no muscle function or body sensation below the level of lesion. In an incomplete lesion some fibres of the spinal cord remain intact and functioning so that there may be muscle power or sensation below the level of the lesion.

Level of the lesion. For example, C6 tetraplegia, may appear as the official diagnosis. This means that C6 spinal nerve is the last functioning nerve above the lesion.

Causes There are two main causes of damage to the spinal cord — traumatic and non-traumatic.

Traumatic causes involve a direct force or impact on the spinal column which causes disruption of the vertebral bodies, tearing of the ligaments and damage to the spinal cord. Common causes are: road traffic accidents (including car, motorbike and push-bike drivers/passengers and pedestrians), accidents at work, for example falling from heights, being crushed by falling weights or mining injuries; sporting accidents, for example mountaineering falls, diving and pot-holing injuries, trampoline accidents, horse-riding falls and rugby injuries; falls, particularly of the elderly with spondylitic changes of the spine. Because of the sudden hyperextension of the cervical spine the cord is 'pinched' in the narrowed spinal canal. Suicide attempts such as jumping from a height; complications after spinal surgery, for example laminectomy, and penetrating injuries such as those resulting from stab or gunshot wounds are other causes of trauma.

Non-traumatic causes of spinal cord damage are: infection, for example an abscess, poliomyelitis, polyneuritis, tuberculosis of the spine or transverse myelitis and benign or malignant tumours. If malignant the tumour is usually a secondary from a primary focus somewhere else in the body. Thrombosis (commonly of a spinal artery) or haemorrhage, spondylosis of the spine or intervertebral disc lesions and multiple sclerosis may also cause spinal cord damage. It may be of psychological origin, as in hysterical paralysis, and can be accidental, i.e. due to radiation myelopathy or surgical injection. Spinal cord damage may also be congenital as in spina bifida, scoliosis, lordosis or kyphosis.

Signs and symptoms

The most common clinical features are loss of voluntary muscle power and sensation to all modalities below the level of the lesion and loss of sphincter control of the bladder and bowels. There is also loss of vasomotor and temperature control and disruption of sexual function.

Spinal shock. This condition is temporary, starting immediately after transection of the spinal cord. It can best be described as isolation of the spinal cord with total disruption of transmission between the brain and the cord. The duration of spinal shock varies. Some reflex activity may appear in three to four days, but may take as long as eight weeks. As reflex activity returns, spasticity and muscle tone appear. The full extent of the lesion cannot be assessed until spinal shock has subsided and bruising abated. It is usual for signs of recovery, if there are to be any, to appear fairly early, but there may be a delay of several weeks. Apparent late recovery may be due to damaged nerve roots recovering.

Care of the acute spinal-injured patient

Treatment techniques vary between Units but the principles of early nursing care are similar.

Day 1. Admission. Supervision from stretcher to electric Stoke Egerton Turning Bed or other prepared bed with necessary pillows and sand bags.

Medical examination: family history, full history of accident, full physical examination including motor and sensory loss, and other injuries. Radiological examination includes anterior, posterior, lateral, oblique and 'swimmer's' views.

Shave head if cervical injury.

Cervical traction (Crutchfield calipers or Gardner Wells tongs) with approximately six to ten pounds weight if fracture reduced. Unreduced fractures are reduced under X-ray supervision.

Intravenous fluids if there is shock or paralytic ileus. Ryles tube may be required for paralytic ileus (temporary loss of peristalsis leading to abdominal distension and vomiting).

No solid food or liquid, moisten lips only and take care of oral hygiene.

Bladder management. Continuous catheter

drainage or eight-hourly intermittent catheter regime.

Observations. Blood pressure, temperature, pulse, respiration, girth measurements.

Full blood count, urea and electrolytes, blood gases if necessary, ward urine test.

Physiotherapy. Attention to chest and passive movements.

Trained-staff turns two-hourly day and night. Care and observation of pressure areas (heels, malleoli, knees, trochanters, buttocks, natal cleft, sacrum, spine, scapulae, shoulders, head).

Controlled analgesics for relief of pain, for example diazepam (Valium).

Confirm that next of kin have been informed. Check possessions.

Day 2. Anticoagulant therapy to counteract the risk of deep vein thrombosis (DVT), subject to other injuries, for example head injury, limb and rib fractures.

If fluids allowed (paralytic ileus subsiding) amount will be gradually increased from sips to 60 mls hourly, or 1500 mls over 24 hours.

Daily blanket baths.

Four-hourly observations continued.

Day 3. Bowel management is commenced, alternate days with suppositories and manual evacuation.

Light diet introduced, e.g. soup, ice cream.

Three-hourly turns by trained staff.

The patient's condition should continue to improve and by day 7 full diet can be introduced, three-hourly turns continue, skin, bladder and bowel care are all continued. Complications during early days are deep vein thrombosis, paralytic ileus, rise in level of lesion and pulmonary embolus.

Week 6–8. Skull traction removed if clinical examination and X-ray are satisfactory (position of spine maintained with evidence of 'bony bridging'). Collar fitted. The patient is transferred to an ordinary hospital bed with manual turns. Hair wash and bath.

Week 9–12. Sitting up in bed, first against a wedge at 45° then into chair. Hypotension with lightheadedness and nausea may become evident as the body learns to adjust to lack of vasomotor control. Fresh air, deep breathing and reassurance may suffice; if symptoms persist, ergotamine tar-

trate (Ephedrine) may be prescribed half to one hour before getting up.

Continuing nursing care through rehabilitation programme

Care of the skin. When the patient is in bed the nursing staff continue to turn him every three hours. When up in a wheelchair he is taught to relieve pressure by lifting up 15 seconds every 15 minutes, to check his own skin with a mirror on returning to bed for signs of redness or skin abrasion and to inspect underwear and bed sheets for signs of bleeding or discharging areas.

Rehabilitating paraplegics and tetraplegics are transferred to a Hi-Lo bed with lifting pole and chain with handle or sling. The nursing staff teach the paraplegic to turn himself in bed and to reposition pillows correctly, while the tetraplegic patient can learn to assist with turning by using the lifting pole. Many patients, both paraplegics and tetraplegics, try prone-lying in bed, and if satisfactory may sleep all night in this position, thus removing the need for turning. For many tetraplegics who require turning by relatives every night, the supply of a continually moving electric turning bed or other special mattress gives both the patient and family a good night's sleep. Many social services departments will provide a similar bed or mattress for use at home by the patient.

Care of the bladder and bowel.

The care of bladder and bowel is of paramount importance in the rehabilitation programme, and a satisfactory outcome is often the key to a long and active life. With the onset of spinal paralysis, a patient loses awareness of bladder or bowel fullness and does not have the ability to voluntarily empty them in a normal way. Urine and faeces are both waste products of the body and as such should be removed as quickly and efficiently as possible to prevent any subsequent ill-effects such as infections or constipation.

Bladder. After a spinal cord injury, the effect on the bladder depends on the level of the injury, the amount of cord damage and the length of time since injury. During the period of spinal shock the bladder is affected by flaccid paralysis, resulting in acute retention of urine. A catheter is passed and the urine drains into a collecting bag or bottle at the bedside. This is called continuous catheterisation.

In a lesion above L1 reflex activity returns as spinal shock subsides. In a lesion above the conus (T11–L1) the spinal micturitional reflex is intact, and an automatic bladder can be developed with training, the bladder emptying spontaneously as it fills with urine. In lesions below L1, where paralysis is flaccid, the spinal micturitional reflex is disrupted and bladder function is obtained by increasing internal pressure due to filling of the bladder, which stimulates the stretch reflexes in the detrusor muscles of the bladder and allows urine to flow past the sphincter by overflow incontinence.

Following continuous catheterisation, the catheter is removed and the patient's fluid intake is restricted. Every eight hours a catheter is passed into the bladder and urine is drained off. This is intermittent catheterisation. The bladder eventually learns to respond to the filling and manual emptying by spontaneously voiding when the bladder is full of urine (return of the spinal micturitional reflex). As this involuntary voiding becomes more efficient, the catheterisations are reduced and stopped.

Residual urine (the amount of urine remaining in the bladder after voiding) is measured and considered in relation to the amount voided in order to estimate the efficiency of the 'automatic bladder'.

The flaccid bladder is trained in a similar fashion, but voiding is assisted by manual pressure, tapping or expressing of the lower part of the abdomen. This is a 'straining bladder'.

Men who become bladder trained achieve further independence by wearing a urinary appliance. This consists of a leg bag with emptying tap or spigot which fastens around the calf, under the trousers, with a connecting pipe attached to the penis by means of a condom or sheath. The urine collects in the leg bag which, when full, can be emptied via the tap by the patient or helper.

A woman is unable to wear such an appliance. Women are bladder-trained using the principles mentioned earlier, but the bladder is 'emptied' every two or three hours on a toilet or commode, by abdominal pressure or tapping to stimulate voiding. Initially, the nurses will do this, but the patient is taught to express her own bladder, to learn its frequency and relate this to her own personal requirements during the day and night.

Toileting facilities need to be accessible for female patients, although many carry a bedpan for emergencies and wear protective clothing in case of 'accidents'.

Routine urine tests. A sample of urine is sent regularly for laboratory analysis. Any organisms present are identified and drug sensitivity or resistance determined and appropriate therapy prescribed. Blood urea tests are carried out to check efficient renal functioning. Urine acidity is checked. Infections are less likely to develop in an acid urine and salts less likely to deposit forming calculi (bladder stones). Intravenous pyelogram (IVP) is a routine X-ray technique for identifying abnormalities or deficiencies in the genito-urinary tract. An opaque fluid (contrast medium) is injected into a vein in the arm; it circulates in the bloodstream and is excreted by the kidneys through the ureters, bladder and urethra. As this occurs it is monitored on an X-ray screen with the contrast outlining the various structures. Other bladder function tests which identify deficiencies or particular difficulties are cystograms and ice-water Desa tests.

Antibiotics may be prescribed to combat urinary infection and examine hippurate (Hiprex) or G500 to maintain urine acidity. Commonly, drugs are needed to improve reflex contractions of the bladder in voiding by assisting detrusor muscle function. Propantheline (Pro-Banthine) and other antispasmodics may be used to lessen excessive spasticity of the detrusor muscle.

Several difficulties may arise:

1. High residual urine with repeated bouts of infection. If there is no response to bladder expression or drug therapy, bladder-neck or sphincter surgery may be required (transurethral resection — TUR).

2. Continuous catheter drainage may need to be retained, but leads to complications such as blocking, bleeding and eventual by-passing.

Tetraplegic women who become bladder-trained require assistance throughout the day and night, never becoming independent.

When management is difficult, or there are problems with the urinary system and the possibility of kidney damage, a urinary diversion may be used, that is the ureter or bladder opening out directly onto the abdominal wall (uterostomy/ ileostomy) with the urine collected in a special bag with an emptying tap.

Hyperreflexia accompanied by pounding headache, sweating, hypertension and bradycardia is usually associated with bladder function difficulties in the tetraplegic patient. A patient presenting any of these symptoms should be immediately checked for voiding difficulties, for example a twisted tube or condom, or for a blocked catheter.

Bowel care. Routine in time-keeping and method forms the basis of the training programme for bowel function so that this becomes effective, efficient and reliable.

During early care the bowels are managed by the nursing staff, usually by manual evacuation. A suppository is passed into the rectum, lubricating the faeces which can then easily be removed. The bowel gradually learns to respond to this stimulus. When the patient starts to get up and begins to learn transfers, bowel evacuation occurs while sitting on the toilet, which is a more natural position and procedure. The nursing staff initially assist the patient, but eventually he learns to do this himself either by a straining action or by continued use of suppositories.

For others, such as tetraplegic patients, the method chosen for bowel care depends on the situation at home. If independent toilet transfer is not possible a 'Sanichair' or hoist may be used, or the easier bed evacuation method continued, particularly if the district nurse is to assist.

A certain routine is important. Evacuation should occur at the same time (morning, or evening if out at work all day) every other day to ensure that constipation does not develop. The patient must take care with his diet and include bran and other roughage if difficulties are experienced. Changes in diet or routine, for example on holiday, may lead to embarrassing faecal incontinence.

Sexual function

There is disruption of normal sexual function, often associated with worry and anxiety. It is important that all staff, medical or paramedical, are aware of this. They should be able to discuss this problem with the patient and his family and to offer practical advice if requested. Some people still find it embarrassing, and even impossible, to talk about their difficulties, while others will discuss them openly and frankly. Women eventually menstruate normally. Internal or external protection can be used and extra care should be taken with hygiene at this time. They can conceive, but without abdominal and pelvic floor muscles there is a danger of miscarriage. If a baby is carried to full term, birth may be normal or by Caesarian section if felt more suitable or safer. Subject to normal considerations and care, spinal cord-damaged patients can use standard methods of contraception. Many male patients continue to achieve erections, but in many the sperm count is low and fatherhood may often be impossible.

There is much assistance and support to be gained from the many books available on sex and sex aids, as well as from the organisation 'Sexual Problems of the Disabled' (SPOD). Experimenting is of great importance for couples where one partner is disabled. An important fact to remember is that no form of sexual practice, if acceptable to both partners and capable of providing pleasure and satisfaction, should be considered abnormal. Considerable research is being carried out in the field of artificial insemination techniques for disabled couples, and with the introduction of 'test-tube' babies the scope is ever widening.

Training of relatives

The nursing staff should undertake the tuition of relatives in all aspects of patient care. Much care and understanding is required in teaching and encouraging safe handling of a person unable to feel or move independently, and many relatives, understandably, are frightened of this.

In our unit, the relatives of all tetraplegic and some paraplegic patients spend one or two nights in a side room on the ward with the patient. They are shown how to handle the patient, how to turn, dress and bath him, how to transfer him and how to manage bladder and bowels. Once shown, they are encouraged to actually perform the procedures for themselves under staff supervision.

This nursing practice is also useful to assess the relative's attitudes and understanding of all that the disability entails. While most relatives gain in confidence and ability through this tuition, for some the prospect of all that is entailed, and the commitment required, is too great. It is better to find out that a family cannot cope during the early days, rather than after house alterations have been completed and much unnecessary expense and stress caused.

After this nursing practice and an initial home visit the patient may commence weekends at home if a bed can be moved downstairs and a commode supplied. This is an invaluable settling-in period when the patient, family and neighbours can become accustomed to the necessary change in routine and care. If a weekend at home is not possible because of hospital treatments or home architecture, a week-end in the A.D.L. Unit flat may be suggested for the patient and his relatives.

Review. Following discharge, a patient will continue to attend the unit on an out-patient or limited in-patient basis for a regular check or review of all aspects of his care.

An IVP is carried out together with routine urine and blood investigations. A physical examination will be completed and a check on how the patient is settling at home. If there are difficulties with regard to house alterations, transport, work, calipers or independence, appropriate action can be taken or advice given.

Muscle Charting. The doctor will keep a regular record of muscle function and sensory level from the day of admission in order to assess improvement or deterioration. This will provide an overall record of muscles functioning and reflect on balance, which can be related to treatment aims and expectations. Muscle function can be graded according to the Oxford scale:

0 No power.
1 Slight flicker.
2 Movement present, but with gravity eliminated.
3 Movement present against gravity.
4 Movement present against gravity and resistance.
5 Normal power.

Some doctors use plus or minus signs to indicate some degrees of function.

PHYSIOTHERAPY

Physiotherapy commences with a patient's admission to the unit. After the initial medical examination and necessary nursing care, the physiotherapist will check the patient's respiratory function and condition of limbs and joints.

Chest care. A patient's vital capacity (VC) is measured regularly with a spirometer and recorded in the case notes so that any deterioration or improvement may be noted immediately. The vital capacity is related to the patient's physical and mental condition, his cooperation, and his body size and occupation. For example, a sedentary worker will have a lower VC than a labourer or sportsman. Tetraplegic patients and some higher level lesion paraplegics without use of the intercostal and upper abdominal muscles will be unable to cough. If secretions are excessive, as with heavy smokers, assisted coughing will be required to remove these and so reduce the likelihood of chest infections and respiratory distress. Assisted coughing may be necessary throughout the whole of the day and night and is most effective if carried out before and after the turning of the patient. If the vital capacity falls below an acceptable level, or diaphragm function diminishes, tracheostomy or respirator assistance may be necessary with its associated nursing and physiotherapy care.

Passive movements. Each joint and group of muscles is put through a full range of passive movements at least twice a day. This prevents contractures by preserving muscle length and tone, and assists in the return of blood from the lower limbs where flow is sluggish and susceptible to deep vein thrombosis (DVT). Particular attention is paid to the range of movement and mobility at the shoulders, elbows, wrists and fingers, as these may develop stiffness, pain and oedema and prohibit independent wheelchair propulsion, transfers and personal independence in later rehabilitation. Existing muscle function can be improved by active assisted and resisted movements.

Sitting balance. When the patient is first transferred to a wheelchair he may need several days to become accustomed to the upright position. Paralysis of the trunk muscles affects balance, and patients often find this disturbing. When sitting up, many patients experience the effects of hypotension, that is, light-headedness and nausea. A patient usually adapts to this vasomotor instability, but if he has continued difficulty, the tilt table may be used to gradually acclimatise the patient to the upright position.

Swimming. Exercise in the swimming pool is useful and enjoyable. The water supports a patient's limbs and allows active muscles to function more easily. Air rings and jackets may be used for safety and to increase the patient's confidence. If a patient is nervous and apprehensive the therapist should take care to place the reassuring hand support where there is sensation. From an early therapeutic means of exercise swimming may develop into an enjoyable pastime.

Gym work. Active rehabilitation in the gym and its associated strenuous exercises are included to develop and fully use innervated muscles. Resisted exercises, springs and weights, press-ups and rope climbing are some of the exercises used. Mat work, with the patient lying on the floor, strengthens trunk muscles and increases tone in the paravertebral muscles which lead to an improved sitting balance and posture. It also assists with the control of excess spasticity in these muscles which subsequently contributes to improved functioning of the bladder and bowels. All patients practise rolling exercises and are taught, where possible, to sit up unassisted. Further balance may be developed by sitting on the side of the bed or plinth and maintaining body position, using a mirror to check it. Learning to catch a ball also improves his ability.

Wheelchair management. Practice is given in manoeuvring the wheelchair with confidence; this includes passing through doorways and negotiating rough ground, slopes and kerbs. Back-wheel balancing can be taught to assist with this mobility.

Standing. It is important that tetraplegic and paraplegic patients should be 'stood up' regularly. This is not ony excellent for morale and confidence, but relieves pressure on the sacrum and buttocks, assists with moderating muscle tone in the trunk and lower limbs, helps to combat any tendency to flexion deformity at the hips, knees and ankles, encourages efficient kidney drainage and bladder and bowel function, and plays its part

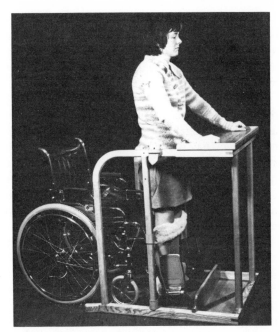

Fig. 27.2 Oswestry standing frame

in the prevention of osteoporosis and pathological fractures. The Oswestry standing frame (Fig. 27.2) provides an easy method of achieving this supported standing position. The sheepskin lined straps act as braces and the table permits activity during standing. The higher-lesion tetraplegic patient may need an under-arm chest strap and the central strut may have to be increased in length to accommodate this. These frames can be supplied for home use. The frame is normally used for patients with lesions above T12, as many patients with lower lesions are likely to achieve more benefit from walking exercises with leg calipers.

Walking exercises. Some patients who are trained to use calipers in hospital will find space limiting and caliper fitting tedious once they are at home. For others it is a worthwhile and rewarding activity which greatly increases independent access and function, and increases self-confidence. The will to succeed is important for success, which also depends on age, body weight and existing muscle function. Swing-to and swing-through gaits, using elbow crutches, are the most successful techniques.

Transfers. The muscles of the arm, shoulder and trunk must be developed as fully as possible to facilitate transfers, which must be achieved without dragging the buttocks. A standing transfer is an easy and efficient method of transferring a paraplegic or tetraplegic patient not otherwise capable of transfer. Relatives should be shown how to manage this transfer confidently (see Ch. 4).

Choice of wheelchair. A wheelchair suitable for the requirements of each patient must be selected and ordered. Ideally, a patient should be assessed for a wheelchair when starting to sit up in the early stages of rehabilitation. There is, however, many months' delay in the supply of chairs, so in most cases a wheelchair needs to be ordered soon after admission, anticipating the individual's eventual requirements.

A knowledge of models and accessories available through the Department of Health and Social Security (DHSS) and other suppliers is essential. The patient's age, body size, height and weight, the probable prognosis and its implications, and the expected future use of the chair determine the choice of wheelchair. Detachable, swinging footrests and adjustable-height or desk-type detachable arms are standard requirements. Drop-back back extension, wheelchair table and extended brake levers are also commonly needed. The most suitable cushion is a four-inch one with a fleecy, sheepskin cover, with or without a wooden board at the base. Electric chairs and a separate chair for employment purposes can be ordered later.

Different staff may be responsible for ordering the wheelchair in each hospital, but, if possible, this decision should be made by the treatment team after discussion.

SOCIAL WORK

The social worker is an important member of the treatment team and her job covers many different and varied aspects. When the patient is first admitted to hospital, contact is made with both the patient and his relatives. Assistance is often required with travelling expenses and with dealing with the many DHSS forms regarding sickness or industrial benefits, social security and war or disability pensions. The tetraplegic patient, who is unable to sign relevant documents and to deal with financial matters, will be helped by the social worker.

Contact with the patient's local social services department should be made as soon as possible and a good working relationship established. There is close liaison with social workers from the admitting hospital (if appropriate) and from the patient's home area, and contact is made with the patient's own general practitioner. This full cooperation allows home resettlement to be smoother. Where a return home is not possible, the social worker, on receiving the referral from the doctor in charge, will make the necessary applications for a bed in long-term care, in a Cheshire Home, or to a local geriatrician.

Many patients from abroad pass through a spinal unit's rehabilitation programme, and there has to be close liaison with the relevant embassy for language assistance, newspapers, travel arrangements (often using the services of the British Red Cross Society), and obtaining approval for the purchase of a wheelchair, calipers and any other equipment or aids. The social worker may also need to deal with the appropriate authority and relevant legislation for children who are in care or for patients on probation.

The social worker may be asked to give advice or assistance on a wide variety of topics, including methods of applying for Constant Attendance Allowance (CAA), Mobility Allowance and the Orange Badge for cars; supplying addresses of firms of solicitors from which the patient can select one regarding any legal claim; giving advice, if desired, to relatives and patients on sexual matters and dealing with any marital difficulties; applying for a reconditioned, electric typewriter for a patient if recommended by the occupational therapist.

The social worker is often asked about problems which trouble a patient or relative, and she will liaise closely with all other departments and treatment team members, particularly the occupational therapist with her extensive source of reference and practical, commonsense approach. It is important that the therapist in turn is aware of the exact role of the social worker.

OCCUPATIONAL THERAPY

The occupational therapist is an essential member

of the treatment team in the successful rehabilitation and resettlement of the patient with a spinal cord injury. Together with the physiotherapist she strengthens and uses innervated muscles, encourages her patients to positive thinking and stresses their capabilities above all else.

The tetraplegic patient has more difficulties to overcome than the paraplegic, who normally has full use of his upperlimbs. Treatment tends to be individual, but group activities are important in encouraging social interaction and allowing the personality to adjust to the sympathy proffered by able-bodied people.

Usually, the patient must lie flat and immobile for about 8 to 12 weeks. The occupational therapist begins her work as soon as the patient emerges from the initial intensive nursing care. She can do much to alleviate and prevent many of the problems which may arise as a direct result of the enforced, prolonged inactivity associated with bed rest.

A good relationship must be established with the patient, relatives and friends. This forms the foundation on which a successful and enjoyable rehabilitation programme is based. The therapist can do much to reassure her patients by helping them to understand some of the anxieties which arise and often appear threatening at this time. The recognition of depression, boredom, aggression and fear, and their causes, are of paramount importance. Reassurance must also include the relatives, many of whom will have had frank and distressing discussions with medical staff regarding the implications and prognosis, and may have to shield the patient from this knowledge.

The provision of aids at an early stage will increase a patient's awareness and interest in his immediate surroundings. A bed mirror allows a patient to view the ward, to maintain contact with his neighbours during the continual turning process, and to identify previously heard but unseen noises in the ward. Before providing a mirror, the therapist should make sure that the patient will be able to accept the often dramatic sight of a shaven head and skull traction *in situ*.

A reading aid, whether made in the department or electrical, gives the patient the opportunity to spend many pleasurable, informative hours reading books or newspapers. A perspex sheet sup-

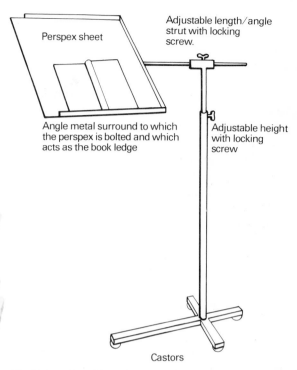

Fig. 27.3 Adjustable reading frame made in the occupational therapy department

ported on a movable stand will accommodate any size of book or paper, the pages of a letter, or a hand of playing cards. This aid adjusts to fit over any size of bed and can be used in any position (Fig. 27.3). The most popular electrical aid is a cassette, or 'talking book', which allows the patient to listen in comfort to a favourite novel without having to wear uncomfortable spectacles. Prismatic glasses allow the recumbent patient to observe activity in the ward, to look out through a nearby window, to watch television and to read with the book in a more comfortable position.

Useful remaining muscle function should be used constructively and strengthened through an activity suitable not only for the existing power, but also for the necessary horizontal position in bed. Relatives should take part in the choice of activity and should be encouraged to assist with the provision of materials and in the various processes involved. This not only helps the therapist, but encourages a feeling of inclusion and purpose, which is much appreciated by many relatives.

Once the patient becomes mobile in a wheelchair, a more active rehabilitation programme may commence. The actual 'sitting' in a wheelchair, whilst being an exciting and long-awaited event, often brings with it the realisation of the extent and meaning of the disability. To sit in a wheelchair and yet not feel it, or the body, to be unable to balance and to feel dependent can be both difficult and demoralising. Purposeful activity, a positive realistic approach to problems, and encouragement and support are invaluable in overcoming these problems. To ensure a good sitting and working position in the chair the footrests may require adjusting, heel- or toe-retainer straps may need to be fitted and brake-handle extensions added to ensure independent operation.

Once the patient has progressed from care in bed to his wheelchair, the occupational therapist will follow the broad outline of aims listed below:
● to further consolidate and establish rapport with the patient and relatives
● to assist the patient to achieve maximum independence in the activities of daily living
● to provide any necessary aids, adaptations or splints needed for independence
● to strengthen innervated muscles and encourage the development of 'trick' movements to compensate for absent function
● to teach awareness of the problems associated with loss of sensation in all body areas
● to increase strength of trunk muscles and improve balance and general posture in wheelchair
● to increase manoeuvrability and functioning in a wheelchair

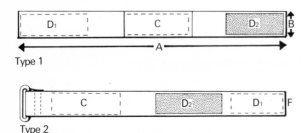

Type 1

Type 2

Fig. 27.4 Two types of hand straps. A. Standard total length 30.5 cm (width around palm + 7.5 cm) B. Width of strap 2.5 cm C. Pocket stitched on three sides, width 7.5 cm D. Velcro 7.5 cm overlap E. 'D'-ring. The benefit of type 2 is that one end (F) can be left threaded, enabling the tetraplegic patient to fasten and release the velcro by using his teeth, thus removing or applying the strap independently

● to encourage social contacts and increase self-confidence.
● to assist with resettlement at home and provide information and advice to relatives and others
● to assist with resettlement at work
● to encourage independence with transport
● to ensure patients and relatives have information on the various allowances
● to encourage hobbies and interests which can be continued after discharge
● to encourage a positive, realistic attitude to changed circumstances.

Activities of daily living

After extended bed rest and dependence upon nursing staff for all care, the achievement of independence in self-care activities is of prime importance. Initially, considerable adaptations may be necessary to achieve independence, but these should be re-assessed frequently as to their continued usefulness. As patients strive for independence they become stronger and more competent and need fewer gadgets.

Feeding. Cutlery handles may be adapted, increased in size, or lengthened to enable the patient to feed independently. The simplest, yet most effective, adaptable and inconspicuous aid, is a narrow leather strap (Fig. 27.4) which fits around the hand and fastens with velcro. An ordinary spoon or fork slots into the palm or pocket of the strap. A plate surround and non-slip mat may also assist independent feeding.

Drinking. Lack of sensation and muscle function in the hands and body makes it impossible to use an ordinary cup with safety. A lightweight, insulated mug with a wide handle through which a thumb or fingers may be slotted, provides a safe alternative.

Hair. A brush with a handle is always easier and more successful to use than a comb.

Hair washing. Hair washing must always be carried out under supervision, particularly if the front wash method is used. The paralysed patient, leaning forward into the basin to rinse his hair, can slip face down into the water and be unable to lift himself out again. The use of a spray or the back-wash technique is advisable.

Teeth. A toothbrush will slot easily into the

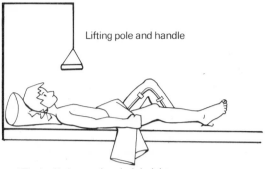

a) The bed is lowered to chair height

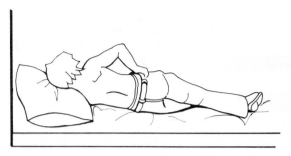

d) Rolling from side to side to pull lower garments over the hips

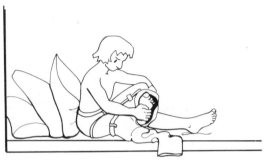

b) The heaviest or most difficult leg is dressed first

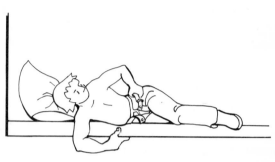

e) Holding under the bed side to assist rolling

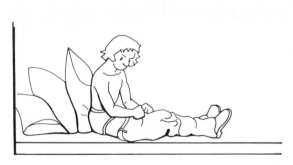

c) Garments are pulled up as high as possible above the knees

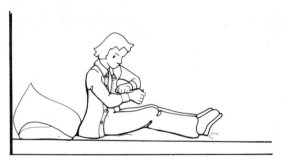

f) Top garments may be put on whilst sitting on the bed or in the wheelchair

Fig. 27.5   Independent dressing for the paraplegic patient

palmar pocket of a hand strap. Electric or battery operated toothbrushes have proved to be useful for many patients. The toothpaste tube can be held between both palms and the top removed with the teeth; paste is then squeezed onto the brush using palmar pressure.

Shaving. Electric or battery-operated razors are easier and safer to use than other types. If there is a likelihood of the razor slipping from between the hands, a leather razor pouch with hand-retaining strap can easily be made. A mirror should always be used and the patient taught to move the face across the razor, as well as the more traditional 'razor across the face' technique. For a wet shave a safety razor must be used; this can easily slip into the pocket of a hand strap.

Make-up. Lipstick and eye make-up containers can be adapted for use with a hand strap for female patients.

Washing. The tetraplegic patient will manage to

wash his hands, face and body front independently, using a flannel mitt either with a soap pocket or in conjunction with 'soap-on-a-rope' around the tap. A loofah or towel with tapes enables him to reach the back of his body.

Dressing

Paraplegic patients should learn to become independent in dressing if shown one of the basic methods and given daily practice and encouragement. They will invariably discover their own methods and techniques later. Age, body weight and size, pain or excessive spasticity in the legs, or a lack of perseverance may be limiting factors in achieving this independence.

Method A (Fig. 27.5). The urinary appliance is connected, checked and attached to the inside leg with Velcro tapes. Modesty towel or sheet should always be in position. The patient then sits up in bed, initially supported by pillows. He lifts one leg at a time, using his hands, and crosses it over the other, leaving the heel clear of the mattress for easy dressing. Underpants and trousers/skirt are put on and pulled up to thigh level. Socks/tights and shoes are put on. The patient then lies flat and rolls from side to side to pull garments up. Trousers are fastened, the leg bag connecting pipe is checked for position (that it has not become trapped) and transfer made into the wheelchair.

Upper limb garments may be put on while in bed or after transfer into the wheelchair. Shirts and jumpers are more easily managed over the head rather than in the more conventional way.

Method B. As above, but the legs remain extended and the feet are reached by increased forward trunk flexion.

Method C. The patient remains lying in the bed, or slightly propped up with pillows. Each leg is lifted in turn up and across the body to bring feet within reach and put on clothes. With this method there is no pain as a result of trunk flexion or difficulty with balance.

If a urinary appliance is worn the patient must be shown how to fix this himself and how to check it periodically throughout the day.

For many paraplegics it is an advantage to eventually learn to dress from a wheelchair. This method does not only provide more body support,

but also fits more easily into a bath and toilet routine.

Tetraplegic patients with lesions at the level of C6 and below can be taught to dress independently, but this is an exhausting process and must be seen in relation to the rest of their day's proposed activity. It is of little value if a patient manages to dress independently, but takes hours to complete the process and is then too exhausted to carry out a day's work. It may, however, be purposeful to show and explain the principles of self dressing to some patients so that they can manage in an emergency. Upper-half garments are most easily managed over the hed, and if small shirt or blouse buttons are replaced with velcro, or a button hook is used, and if a loop is attached to the zip-pull, independence can be achieved.

Clothing. Advice may be given on suitable material and styles. If excessive perspiration is a problem synthetic fibres, although easily washable, are to be avoided and cotton fabrics should be selected. Rough seams and tight-fitting styles, although fashionable, are not to be recommended. Shoes should be a size larger than previously worn to accommodate possible oedema.

Transfers

Wheelchair transfers to bed, toilet, bath, car and armchair are taught. Paraplegics learn to become independent in these transfers, while tetraplegics can be shown how to manage with minimum assistance. Relatives can be instructed in these techniques. Care must be taken that the patient with insensitive skin is not dragged during a transfer, or lifted by his trouser tops.

Bed transfers. The bed should be the same height from the floor as the wheelchair with cushion.

1. The chair is positioned alongside the bed with brakes applied and the nearest armrest removed. The wheel is covered with a sheet, pillow or towel to provide a protective and useful 'bridge'. The seated patient lifts himself across the mattress and into the chair, then lifts his legs carefully down on to the footplates and replaces the armrest.

2. If long sitting is too difficult or painful a similar transfer may be used, but the legs are

swung over the bedside and onto the footrests before the patient sits up. Once he has lifted himself into the chair and repositioned his legs, the armrest is replaced.

3. The chair, with footplates swung back against the wheels, is placed at right angles to the bed. The patient transfers backwards from the mattress into the chair, eases the chair away from bed to reposition footplates and lifts the legs carefully onto them.

Toilet transfers. A standard household toilet is usually lower than a wheelchair, and this makes transferring onto it easy, but returning to the chair difficult. The toilet should be raised to wheelchair height with a raised toilet seat, or by permanent raising from floor level. The seat should be protected with a fitted, inflatable rubber ring to guard against abrasion. If the patient has difficulty with self cleaning, a section of the side covering of some raised toilet seats can be removed. A fixed wall rail or overhead chain may prove useful.

1. A sideways transfer is the easiest method where space and bathroom design permit the chair to reverse in. The wheel can be padded with a towel, brakes should be securely engaged. A fixed wall rail provides stability and security.

2. There are two ways of making a forward transfer (a) the wheelchair is positioned close to the toilet and, if possible, at a slight angle. Footrests may need to be removed. A fixed rail on the wall towards which transfer is to be made is useful. The transfer involves a lifting, swinging, rotating action, (b) the patient remains seated facing the wall and transfers directly onto the toilet.

3. A backward transfer through a specially adapted chair back with zip fastening or straps and buckles is another possibility. Transfer by this method is easy, for the paralysed legs follow the body. On the return transfer, however, the legs require lifting forward.

A Sanichair or hoist used with a toilet sling may be recommended for use by tetraplegic patients, in conjunction with district nurse requirements. Bidets or Clos-o-mat toilets may be useful in the management of many spinal-injuries patients. A low-positioned wall mounted cistern is most suitable, as it can be an aid to balance.

Most paraplegic patients are trained to manage their own bowel routine. Tetraplegic patients need to rely upon the services of the district nurse or relatives for this very personal task. If a tetraplegic patient has sufficient finger function he can be trained to insert the suppository himself, using a specially adapted inserter and a mirror. A great deal of research is being done in this area of self help, including tampon inserters for tetraplegic women. Independence in these personal activities is very desirable.

Bath transfers. Bath transfers may be achieved independently by a paraplegic, and with assistance or mechanical device by a tetraplegic.

1. Sideways into the bath. The chair is positioned alongside the bath, brakes applied and nearest armrest removed. The legs are lifted over the bath side and the bottom transferred onto the bath back or side. The patient then lowers himself carefully into the bath.

2. The approach is made from the end of the bath. The footrests are swung out of the way, the legs lifted onto the end of the bath and the chair manoeuvred against the bath edge. The patient then eases forward, transfers to the back of the bath and down into it as above.

Difficulties may arise due to inability, or lack of muscle strength, to make the transfer back out of the bath and into the chair without marking the skin or slipping. Possible solutions are the provision of bath aids such as a well-covered bath board and/or a bath seat, the provision of a shower attachment to be used from bath taps and in conjunction with a bath seat or the replacement of the bath with a shower unit. (See also Ch. 4)

Shower transfers. Many showers with rimmed troughs or bases make access for a wheelchair user difficult and often necessitate transfer to a suitable shower chair left permanently inside the base. This must be well padded for protection, waterproof, rust-free and provide support. Shower controls must be accessible, easily used and thermostatically controlled. A shower in which the cold-water flow is affected when water is used elsewhere in the building, is dangerous. Shower units designed for the disabled are available, although expensive. Bathroom and toilet floors should be carpeted or have a non-slip surface.

Car transfers. The use of a transfer board or padded wheel facilitates this transfer, although many paraplegics require no aids at all.

Before rehabilitation is complete, a transfer board allows a patient to transfer safely and confidently on his own. When used by relatives with a tetraplegic patient it provides a more comfortable, easy sliding transfer, than the difficult lifting method. The basic technique described below is followed with or without the use of the board.

Approach the car seat as closely and as far forward as possible without damaging the car paintwork (a piece of carpet over the sill prevents this); brakes are applied and the armrest removed. The board is slipped under the patient's bottom and rests on the seat. The legs are placed into the front of the car and the body eases onto the board. The hand positions are altered, the head bends down into the car and the body slides along the board and onto the seat. The sitting position can be adjusted and legs positioned comfortably. Lastly, the seat belt is fastened.

For the return transfer, the process is reversed with the legs remaining in the car until last.

Aids to transferring into a car include mobile hoists, revolving passenger seats and roof-top hoist for the car. A standing transfer may also be used.

Armchair transfers. Many patients appreciate the change of position and comfort provided by a favourite armchair. Transfer to the chair is achieved by a forward angled transfer, with or without the use of a board. Most armchairs are low and comfortable with deep soft cushioning, which makes the return transfer difficult. Suggestions to overcome this include raising the chair to wheelchair height by blocks attached to the legs, adding a second cushion to provide the extra height required, placing a wooden board under the cushion to provide a firm base and advising the patient on other suitable high chairs available.

Transfer aids

1. Sliding or transfer board (Fig. 27.6).

(a). Standard transfer board. Dimensions 76.5 cm × 20 cm × 2.2 cm (30 in × 8 in × ⅞ in). When made of hardwood the edges are rounded and all surfaces well sanded and finished in beeswax. The finish is maintained with furniture polish. When made of plywood, 12 cm (½ in) board is used. The edges and surfaces are sanded and completely covered with self-adhesive vinyl (Fig. 27.6A).

(b). A smaller board can be made (61 cm × 20

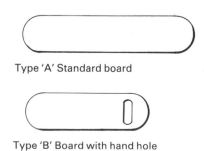

Type 'A' Standard board

Type 'B' Board with hand hole

Fig. 27.6 Sliding/transfer boards

cm — 24 in × 8 in) from 12 mm plywood with a hole cut out, thus enabling the patient to lift the board after transfer (Fig. 27.6B).

2. Hoists. A suitable hoist should be capable of being manoeuvred and operated by one person with easily understood instructions. The rear castors should have a braking device and be low enough to pass under a chair, bath or other furniture. A hoist which dismantles and stows into a car boot is useful for holidays and weekends (see also Ch. 4).

Communication

It is important that a disabled person is given the opportunity to express his thoughts on paper as well as verbally. Even a patient disinterested in typing should be encouraged to try writing his name, essential for signing documents. For cheques a signature must be 'written' and accepted by the bank if it has changed greatly. This signature can be simply an attempt or mark by the disabled person, or an authorised signature of another person on his behalf.

Writing is difficult to perfect and requires interest, practice, patience and perseverance by both the patient and therapist. Gripping and controlling a pen is difficult without finger flexion. The pen has to be moved across the paper with movement from the shoulder, elbow and wrist instead of the fingers.

The pen can be held in the usual position between the fingers with an adapted holder, or with an aid which fits into a hand strap (Fig. 27.7). It can also be held between both palms or intertwined between the fingers, which requires no aids. A fine felt-tip pen should be used, as this requires little pressure and can be used in any position. The paper should be held firmly on a clipboard, and shapes and capital letters should be

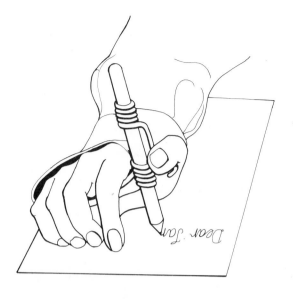

be used with a subsequent increase in speed. Simple, non-electric machines are useful for paraplegics learning to type and an advantage when considering future resettlement and employment.

Other means of communication to be considered and practised include the telephone (dialling, managing the receiver, coin box operation, and information on aids available), money (practice in handling coins, purses, pockets and coin organisers) and environmental control through the provision of Possum equipment for the severely handicapped person at home. This is available on recommendation and approval by the assessor through the DHSS. An alarm-bell system, front-door intercom and door-lock release, telephone adaptations, television control and channel change, and control over other electrical appliances provide a much wider field of independence within the home.

Homecraft

Kitchenwork, laundry, ironing and cleaning as well as repositioning of furniture cupboards and shelves, and removal of loose mats must all be considered, and practice, encouragement and advice given throughout treatment.

Kitchenwork. Men and women should all be encouraged to spend and enjoy some time in the kitchen, learning how to manage hot dishes and liquids safely and gaining in confidence and strength (Fig. 27.8).

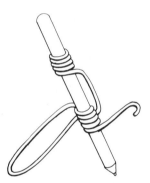

Fig. 27.7 Simple pen holder for a tetraplegic patient made of copper wire. It slots into the pocket of the hand strap

practised before script. Plenty of encouragement should be given, as the childlike efforts initially produced can be very demoralising. Many tetraplegic patients eventually confirm that their writing can be improved, due no doubt to the extra care taken in forming letters.

An electric typewriter provides an easily manageable means of communication. If the patient cannot use any of his fingers on the keys, a short stick inserted into a hand strap provides an accurate and simple method of striking letters. Balance, neck position, and muscle power and control must be considered when positioning the typewriter. With increased knowledge of the keyboard and improved balance, two hands may

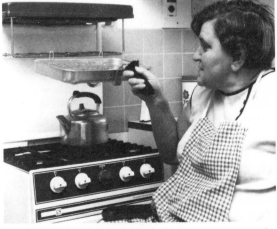

Fig. 27.8 A paraplegic housewife practises using a gas cooker by preparing a meal in the department

Preparation of food should include beverages, snacks, baking, vegetable preparation, meals and oven use. Activities should relate to the family requirements at home. The patient should be instructed in the use of aids and standard kitchen equipment such as a spike board or an electric mixer with all its accessories.

Adaptation of existing equipment may be necessary for safe management, e.g. extended stove control knobs for controls situated at rear of hob. The doors of the cupboard under the sink may be opened to allow footplate entry during a forward approach. It is important to make the best possible use of accessible storage areas for regularly-used ingredients and equipment. A 'Helping Hand' is useful for reaching higher shelves.

Menu planning and advanced meal preparation should be incorporated, and if this is too exhausting or time-consuming instant, frozen and pre-packaged foods may be considered.

Laundry. Washing machines remove much of the arduous task of laundering. The most suitable type is a top-loading fully-automatic machine. Controls may need the addition of a non-slip surface to facilitate turning. Washing smaller articles of clothing by hand should be practised. Hanging out clothes is simplest on a rotary line and 'Dolly' pegs can be used even with a weakened grip, as they have no springs. The ironing board should permit footrest access, otherwise an ordinary table can be used.

Cleaning and tidying. Practice should be given in day-to-day dusting, carpet sweeping or use of a vacuum-cleaner, even though heavier cleaning and polishing may be done by relatives or the home help service. Feather dusters and cylinder-type cleaners are useful. An easy solution to the difficulties of access during bedmaking is the use of continental quilts on beds. These only require a daily shake and replacement.

Departmental activity

Attendance at the occupational therapy department is an integral part of the treatment programme. It does not only provide a welcome break from the ward, but also entails working to a timetable and encourages social interaction with other patients, staff and visitors.

Activities are selected to strengthen and use innervated muscles to maximum benefit and to encourage further independence. Occupational therapy, whilst being specific and planned, should also be enjoyable. A relaxed patient participates with more enthusiasm and effort in all rehabilitation activities.

Specific activities including pottery, resisted sanding, puff football, activities involving the use of FEPS, and other general dexterity exercises are used for strengthening specific muscles or encouraging a particular movement, for example wrist extension. Pottery is a useful activity as clay can be made as pliable and easy to mould as required. Resisted sanding with a bilateral grip on the block is a good progressive activity for all levels of disability. Tetraplegics, using soft leather hemi-gloves to obtain a 'grip', strengthen all muscles of the arm, shoulder and neck, and appreciate the weight-grading progression. It can also be used to improve trunk stability and general balance.

General activity includes various crafts which are purposeful, remedial and absorbing, produce a pleasing result and give the patient a sense of achievement and pride in his work. Tetraplegic patients learn to use remaining muscle function to adapt to the movements and processes involved in a particular craft, for example canework, which is usually used to encourage finger movements by weaving the cane in and out of the stakes. The tetraplegic patient can adapt to an absence of finger power by hooking the cane over the hand and 'lifting it' around the upright stakes. A cane guillotine made in the department enables them to cut their own stakes, and the use of a table vice to hold the base enables the stakes to be threaded through the holes. Ceramics, leather thonging, printing, wood-block art and painting are examples of other suitable crafts. The hand strap with its pocket is once again a useful aid in many craft activities, for example for holding a brush for paint or glue.

Table height and a good working position are important for ease of performance, balance and general comfort. Adjustable or desk wheelchair arms are an advantage, as they will fit under most tables. Some tables may need to be placed on blocks to ensure free passage for the knees.

Remedial games provide a competitive range of

activities, social contact with an opponent and enjoyment, and can require a wide range of movements, strength, dexterity and coordination. Draughts, dominoes, chess, solitaire and cards are the most popular. These may be played with a normal board and pieces, using a different technique for moving them across the board (for example sliding instead of lifting) or with an adapted board and/or pieces, for example cotton reels replacing flat draughts, clothes pegs on a raised board for solitaire or an upturned brush forming a makeshift card holder.

Sport begins within the hospital environment as a means of increasing muscle strength and coordination, the determination to better a personal performance or to beat an opponent, and for the pleasure and enjoyment they provide. A plan for sport is normally arranged jointly between the rehabilitation staff.

Swimming, archery and table tennis are often the first sports included. The bow or table tennis bat is bandaged to the tetraplegic's hand, and in archery the bow string is pulled back and released

by means of a special hook attached to the hand. Bowls (carpet bowls for tetraplegics), basketball, field events, snooker (Fig. 27.9), weightlifting, fencing, and wheelchair slalom and races can all be included.

Many patients find sport so enjoyable that they wish to continue with it after discharge. This they may do through their own unit's sports club, through a local disabled sports group or preferably alongside able-bodied sportsmen. Suitable sports in this latter group include in particular archery, table tennis and snooker.

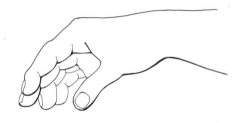

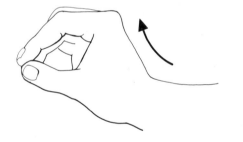

Fig. 27.10 Tenosesis action at the wrist enables the hand to perform a weak pincer grip

Tenodesis or automatic grip. This is one of the 'trick' movements which can be taught to a tetraplegic and which can greatly increase independence. When the wrist is extended the fingers curl towards the palm (Fig. 27.10) and come into contact with the upward travelling thumb either at the finger tips, or with the side of the index finger. While wrist extension is maintained, so too is this contact, and this can be used as a gripping agent. Practice in picking up objects of varying shapes, weights and textures should be given and the patient made fully aware of the real significance of this 'grip'. This movement is possible for a tetraplegic patient with a C6 lesion.

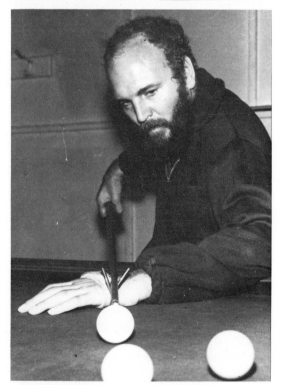

Fig. 27.9 A tetraplegic patient controls a snooker cue with a simple aid made in the department

Loss of sensation

It is essential to make the patient aware of the dangers arising from loss of body sensation. Many of these precautions are common sense.

Cigarettes, if allowed, should only be smoked using a holder. Hot pipes, kitchen stoves, fires and car heaters must all be approached and used with care. Hot water bottles should not be used.

Sitting areas should be carefully inspected for stray articles before use; buttons on trouser back pockets should be removed; rough seams and tight clothing should be avoided and fabric choice carefully considered. On a cold day, warm clothing should be worn. A cold, able-bodied person 'shivers' to become warm, and peripheral vessels constrict to retain body heat. If muscle function is absent with an associated loss of vasomotor control, as for instance in tetraplegic patients, these reactions do not occur. Body temperature drops and hypothermia occurs. There may be reverse difficulties associated with extreme heat and sunlight.

The body position in the wheelchair should be altered at regular intervals. The patient should be taught to 'lift up' in the chair for 15 seconds every 15 minutes, regardless of any activity in progress.

Work surfaces and tool care should be observed.

Splinting

The amount of splinting practised varies considerably and depends upon the therapist's skills, time available, and the consultant's opinions of splinting values. Early splinting can be used alongside physiotherapy's passive movements to maintain a functional position of wrist, fingers and elbows. Night splinting is particularly useful for the active patient as daytime splints limit chair propulsion and general activity. During sleep, spasticity eases and deformity is more easily corrected. The two splints commonly used in the above way, depending on physical requirements, are a soft leather boxing-glove type and the paddle splint.

For daytime use, and as an aid to independence the following splints are useful:

1. Wrist extensor splint for support where these muscles are non-functioning or weak

2. Chair-pushing mitts to protect the hands and provide a friction surface for chair propulsion

3. Ball-bearing arm supports, available through the DHSS.

Some departments may also be responsible for the manufacture and application of neck collars and trunk supports.

The material used must provide the required support, but be capable of a smooth finish to prevent body abrasion. The splints must be carefully fitted, pressure points should be checked and all splint areas and straps well-lined. The simpler the design of a splint, the more effective it usually is, and easy application is appreciated by nursing staff.

Social contacts

The development of self-confidence and social contacts begins from the date of admission. Relationships are formed between patients, staff and

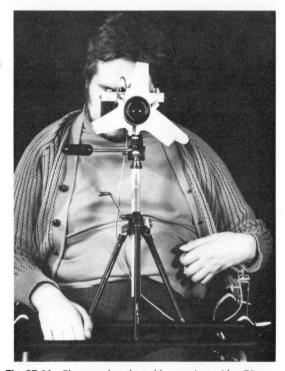

Fig. 27.11 Photography adapted for a patient with a C5 lesion. A special frame has been made to hold the camera and tripod. Extended lens aperture and focusing controls have been made out of Darvic. The extra-long shutter release cable is operated from the arm rest with pressure from the hand. This patient also operates a cine camera and his own darkroom

visitors within the ward and then widened to include others attending a department for treatment. Shopping trips, parties and other outings into the nearby community provide a first contact with the outside world, and weekends spent at home provide a link with old and new acquaintances.

A disabled person must learn to become independent and achieve, wherever possible, a satisfying quality of life in his new-found circumstances. It is important that he is taught and encouraged to develop a considerate and thoughtful personality. While expecting a certain amount of consideration from others, he must also learn to accept people's often misplaced sympathy, embarrassment and excessive assistance graciously and to refuse help if not required, but in such a manner that it will not offend or prevent that person from offering assistance to any other disabled person.

Comments are often passed on the happy, cheerful atmosphere which is so often evident on a spinal injuries unit. As therapists, we must continue to encourage the development of positive and realistic, forward-thinking personalities with a real enjoyment of life.

Hobbies and interests

Hobbies or interests which can be continued after discharge home should be encouraged and developed. While in hospital, a patient's day is planned for him with constant company around. At home, there are many empty hours without company. Access around the house may be difficult, thereby making outings tiresome and frustrating. Craftwork, typing, gardening, television and radio, reading, study of stocks and shares, painting, photography (Fig. 27.11), dressmaking, wine-making, card and table games, watching football matches and participating in sport are some of the many varied interests followed by patients at home.

Resettlement at home

A patient's relatives are usually made aware of the probable prognosis and its implications by the doctor during the first few weeks of treatment. This

enables some early investigation to be made into the home environment to which the patient is to return. Once the patient is using a wheelchair and progressing realistically with rehabilitation, a date should be chosen for a day-visit home. The patient's general practitioner and representatives from the local social services department (including the domiciliary occupational therapist), community nursing service and, if appropriate, housing department should be notified of the intended visit and invited to attend in order to meet the patient, relatives, hospital occupational therapist and aftercare nursing officer and discuss and assess what nursing help, alterations and aids will be required. It is very important to carry out this visit with the patient and his family present. It is not only their house and premises under discussion, but family feelings and cooperation must be considered and obtained. It is also only by actually trying a wheelchair through doorways, for example, that many difficulties become obvious. A list of common problems and possible solutions is given below:

1. An upstairs flat or very small, totally unsuitable downstairs facilities: Rehousing, taking into consideration family feelings, friends and possible support from neighbours
2. Steps at access: (A) alternative entrance such as rear door or French window (b) ramping if approach area permits suitable gradient (concrete is preferable to wood; a safety rim or sloping sides should be provided)
3. Door step or 'sill' into the house: A bevelled piece of wood fixed to the floor to accommodate step height
4. Doors too narrow (average wheelchair width 28 in): (A) widen door to at least 30 in (b) remove wheel-pushing rims and decrease chair width by three inches
5. Door opening difficult or space-reducing: Replace with sliding door
6. Limited turning area between rooms necessitating removal of footplates: Widen doors or replace with sliding doors; reposition or reangle door frame, remove wall angle
7. Bedroom, bathroom and toilet upstairs or inaccessible: (A) if upstairs and suitable, access may be provided by a direct inter-floor lift or a platform stair lift (b) a purpose-built extension

8. Toilet access limited and transfer difficult: If bathroom adjoining, it may be incorporated into one larger room

9. Bathroom fittings difficult to reach: Toilet pedestal may be reangled, wash-basin made into accessible vanity unit or the bath replaced with a shower

10. Access to garden, road and car-transferring area difficult: (A) widen concrete pathways or areas (b) car port

11. Kitchen access and management difficult: Adjust working height and reposition cupboards; provide knee access under kitchen sink and lever taps; split-level cooker

12. Dependence on relatives: Provide necessary aids and equipment. (a) Daily or twice-daily district nurse for bowel and bladder care, bathing and dressing (b) home help service (c) adjustable hospital bed with a lifting pole; ripple mattress; water mattress; a turning bed (e.g. Steeper Co-Ro bed) or a Mecalift hoist

13. Need for environmental control and independence: Possum equipment, telephone, reading aids, electric wheelchair

14. Need for further or continued treatment and outside social contact: Outpatient treatment at a local hospital, attendance at a day hospital or craft centre; contact with local disabled groups, for example Disabled Drivers' Association, Physically Handicapped and Able Bodied (PHAB) groups.

Consideration should also be given to the ability to manage plugs, light switches, taps, and gas or electric appliances.

Resettlement at work

A disabled person should, wherever possible, return to some form of employment. Age, physical capabilities, mental attitude, interests, possibilities in the home area and pending compensation claims may all influence this resettlement. There should always be close liaison with the Disablement Resettlement Officer (DRO). The therapist is able to assess fully a patient's aptitudes, capabilities and attitudes with regard to the working situation. By referring a patient to the DRO, she can ensure a smooth return to employment. The patient's job with his previous employer must be considered and its physical and mental demands related to his present condition, working position, overall ability and safety. If it is not possible for him to return to his previous job alternative work with the same employer should be considered. Failing this, similar work with another employer should be investigated. Re-training, further education or assessment may be necessary. Correspondence courses and home study can be arranged.

Factors such as access to and within the premises, including toilets; facilities at work, including work processes, work load and rate; the employer's and patient's interest, and the distance of work from home and method of transport must all be considered.

Through the DRO the Manpower Services Commission (MSC) can currently:

● pay for all aids required, and up to 50 per cent of alterations to premises to a maximum of £5000
● pay a patient's wages during a training period, with the employer contributing as this progresses
● give assistance with fares if a patient cannot use public transport or drive a car
● offer retraining facilities with an employer or Employment Rehabilitation Centre (ERC — assessment only), at a Skills Centre or Residential Training College (RTC) or at a normal college of further education for vocational courses
● arrange a job introduction scheme with an employer uncertain of a patient's ability by offering the firm £30 a week for a six-week trial period
● apply for assistance from the Motability scheme

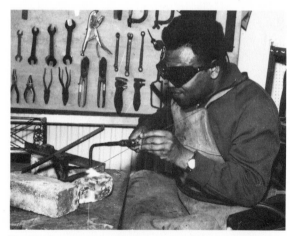

Fig. 27.12 Pre-work training and assessment. A paraplegic patient practises welding and brazing in the heavy workshop as a preliminary to a period of retraining with his former employer in bench work

for a patient who has not officially received an application form, but requires a car for attending work or training.

The employer should be kept informed of the patient's progress during hospitalisation so that he is already knowledgeable and interested when work resettlement is considered and an early visit to the works can be arranged.

The therapist and DRO liaise closely regarding assessment results, adaptation to tools, machinery and premises, work safety and general work potential (Fig. 27.12). A patient's daily attendance in the department and adherence to a timetable, his ability to follow written and/or verbal instructions and pride taken in his work are all important considerations.

Transport

Most paraplegic, and many tetraplegic patients with lesions of C5/6 and below, should consider becoming independent in driving and should be given information and advice on suitable cars, hand controls, details of cost, licence and insurance requirements, and organisations for the disabled driver. Muscle strength, balance, available finance and general interest shown by the patient must be noted before realistic discussion can take place, and the doctor will often indicate his opinion as to a candidate's suitability.

An automatic car with a single-hand control lever (Fig. 27.13) connected to accelerator and brake is the easiest car to drive, but a manual

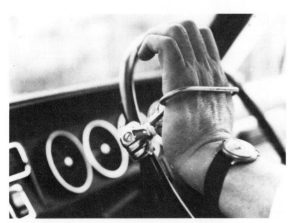

Fig. 27.13 A tetraplegic patient with a C6 lesion uses existing wrist extension to slip his hand into the driving aid shown

gear-change car may also be adapted. A converted car still retains the foot pedals and may be driven by an able-bodied person. The make and type of car to be recommended depends not only on cost, but also on the patient's preference in terms of comfort, ease of transfer and steering control. He may select a two- or four-door saloon or estate model with adequate boot storage area. Self-loading of his wheelchair, other drivers and other uses of the car such as business requirements or pets must be taken into account, as must local suppliers and servicing facilities. Visits from outpatients who drive and are willing to offer advice to others are invaluable.

A driver holding a full licence, need not retake the driving test, but it is always advisable to become accustomed to using hand controls with another driver in the car. The vehicle licensing authority at Swansea must under law be informed of a disability and will send an appropriate medical form to be completed before reissuing the licence. Insurance companies must also be notified.

A Mobility Allowance should be applied for, subject to age restrictions, by both disabled drivers and passengers. Following recent legislation the road fund licence is now free to disabled drivers who are in receipt of a Mobility Allowance.

Treatment for patients with incomplete lesions

If there is any remaining muscle function in the lower limbs the occupational therapist, in conjunction with the physiotherapist, should consider this aspect in her treatment plan. The general prognosis will provide guidelines as to the usefulness of this function, and treatment should be formulated accordingly. It should increase muscle strength and standing tolerance and reinforce a correct walking pattern through practice with the aids provided. The function should obviously relate to independence and home and work resettlement.

All the above activities can be completed from a standing position, or by using bench slings or the standing frame for support.

The electric cycle may be used specifically and the therapist should remember to:

a. pad the seat well as protection for any loss of sensation in the legs and buttocks

b. check the position of the leg drainage bag and its connecting tube, which may become trapped between the saddle and leg

c. take care with the raising and lowering technique

d. take care if there is increased spasticity in the lower limbs.

The cycle is useful for breaking down some patterns of spasticity but may be contraindicated if it induces greater spasticity and clonus. This activity strengthens muscles, reinforces a walking pattern and can be visibly graded. Treadle lathes and fretsaws can also be included in the treatment programme.

Any patient walking safely with aids in physiotherapy should be encouraged to abandon his wheelchair (and sit on ordinary suitable chairs), walk around the department and eventually to and from the ward.

Information

The occupational therapist has access to a great deal of information and literature. For this reason, she continues in the role of an 'information officer' long after her patients have been discharged. Information about holidays, including suitable addresses for wheelchair users, is a common query, and apart from providing available information, the therapist may be able to provide direct contact with another patient who has recently returned from a similar holiday.

Complications

Pressure sores. These may be a direct result of spending too much time lying or sitting in one position. This leads to disruption of blood flow and subsequent death of tissues. The sores may be skin abrasions caused by transferring awkwardly, or through contact with rough or sharp surfaces. They may be due to sweating with skin maceration, for example in the natal cleft, or may be directly linked to abscesses, septic spots or urinary infections.

The only effective treatment is to keep the body weight off the area with bed rest and good nursing care. An infected sore can infect underlying bone. Any sore should be seen and attended to. Excision of tissue may be necessary to produce a fresh bleeding and healing area; antibiotics may be prescribed, with plenty of protein in the diet, and the blood haemoglobin level should be checked. Skin grafting may be necessary in severe cases. It is important to identify the cause of the sore so that, wherever possible, the cause can be removed or a method altered to avoid recurrence. Extremes of temperature may also cause skin lesions, for example burns and frostbite.

A certain degree of spasticity is beneficial in maintaining muscle tone and bulk, and some spasms may indeed be useful. For example, extension spasm in the lower limbs may assist with standing. Increased spasticity, however, may cause problems such as severe pain, an inability to retain a satisfactory sitting position in a wheelchair, which is often associated with sacral 'skin off' area, and difficulty with transfers or self-help, as strong extensor spasm of the lower limb can prohibit independent dressing. Incomplete lesions may be associated with more severe spasms than complete lesions, and this can mask useful voluntary power.

Drugs such as diazepam (Valium) or dantrolene sodium (Dantrium) may be prescribed to inhibit spasticity, but further investigation of other possible causes should always be made. Contributory factors are chest or urinary infection, pressure sore or skin abrasion, constipation, insufficient physiotherapy, (weight-bearing and exercise often inhibit spasticity), anxiety and increased tension. These should be resolved and a further assessment of the spasticity made before prescribing further drugs.

Infections. Chest and urinary tract infection, including catheter blockage are common complications. All unit staff learn to recognise symptoms associated with urinary infection. The patient complains of sweating, often with a pounding headache, and a feeling of nausea sometimes associated with rigor and pyrexia. Urine may be clouded and 'bitty' and may smell offensive. If a specimen has not recently been sent for analysis, this must be done immediately. The patient should be treated with antibiotics. A catheter is usually inserted into the bladder and a high fluid intake encouraged. The patient is nursed in bed, with cooling fans if necessary. An infection should be treated immediately to prevent spread to the ureters and kidneys. Patients sent home with a catheter *in situ* (and their families) should be advised what to do in case of a blockage. It may also be necessary for them to have a sterilised catheter and changing pack in the house so that the attending nurse or doctor is well-equipped and able to deal with the situation.

Chest infections and colds must also be treated promptly, particularly if already-restricted breathing and coughing becomes difficult. Analysis of sputum samples will indicate appropriate antibiotic treatment and chest physiotherapy may be prescribed together with the use of a humidifier to ease breathing.

Ascending myelopathy. Most spinal cord injuries are stable, once satisfactory rehabilitation has been completed. In some cases where the cause is doubtful, or where circulatory or progressive neurological disease has been diagnosed, there may be a gradual rise in the level of the lesion with associated muscular and sensory losses. In some patients, often several years after injury, there is a progressive loss of higher spinal cord function with associated 'one-sided' symptoms. There is numbness or 'pins and needles' and loss of function. This is diagnosed as post-traumatic syringomyelia, which is thought to be caused by a type of cavity or cyst in the central grey matter of the cord.

Chronic pain. Some patients complain of constant 'stabbing or burning' pain in their lower limbs, around the level of the lesion, and to a lesser extent in the arms and hands. There are usually no obvious causes for this pain, although in some cases the site of pain originates from the actual lesion, or associated trapped nerve roots. For some patients reassurance by medical staff, and assistance in dealing with any major worries, has a pain-reducing effect. Others respond to increased physiotherapy and exercise, while for some the only answer may be a nerve block with phenol or alcohol injections, or in more drastic cases, surgery.

Contractures. Prevention of contractures is important not only early in treatment, but throughout the whole of a paralysed person's life. The limbs should be moved passively through a full range of movement once a day, either by the patient himself or by a relative. This can be carried out most conveniently before getting out of bed in the morning, or on getting into bed at night. Particular attention should be paid to fingers, wrists, elbows and shoulders, hips, knees, ankles and toes. The position of joints at night in bed is also important. Care should be taken with the position of the feet on the footrests, as 'foot drop' with increased dorsiflexion can become a problem. Contractures may respond to increased movement, to serial splinting or antispasmodic drugs. In very severe cases, surgery may need to be considered.

Osteoporosis. In the paralysed extremities there is often marked osteoporosis of the bones with loss of calcium and protein. Osteoporosis is more marked in the flaccid lesion, as when spasticity is present the involuntary movement maintains more of the bone substance. Secondary to this osteoporosis pathological fractures may occur. Fractures of the lower limb, in particular the femur, are most common, often following sudden movement or a fall from the chair. With the absence of pain, diagnosis is usually made from the history, swelling at site of the injury, increased spasticity and finally by X-ray examination.

Para-articular heterotopic ossification (PAO). In this condition bone is laid down around a joint, beginning between the muscle layers. Diagnosis is by radiological examination together with the observed limitation of range of movement at the affected joint. Treatment is usually conservative, although if function is grossly affected, surgery may be necessary. Treatment with adrenocorticotrophic hormone (ACTH) is sometimes effective.

Oedema. There is often oedema of the feet and legs when a patient sits in a wheelchair, and this is particularly evident at the end of the day. This gravitational oedema responds best to elevation of the affected limb and to the wearing of supportive stockings. To a much lesser extent, oedema may affect the hands and fingers of tetraplegic patients, particularly those used to hard physical work. Exercise and elevation relieve this considerably, and care must be taken to prevent or counteract deformity.

Circulatory disturbance. This occurs chiefly in the lower limbs below the knee. Circulation is sluggish with blood tending to 'pool' in the feet and lower leg. The leg appears purple and blue with the skin becoming shiny and thin. In extreme cases, there may be gangrene of the toes and foot. Prevention may be aided by elevation of the limbs, warm loose clothing and shoes, and in some cases prescribed circulatory drugs. Cold rooms and cold weather may produce hypothermia with associated lethargy, inactivity and, in extreme cases, paranoid symptoms.

Psychological problems. A certain amount of depression and anxiety is to be expected with any disability as severe as spinal cord injury. Reassurance from staff and family, and a positive approach to the patient and his capabilities, do much to alleviate symptoms. It is important to spend time usefully and purposefully, allowing little time for contemplation and morbid thought.

A fear of the future and the implications of the disability, an unrealistic attitude towards the disability and proffered help, an aggressive manner, or constant complaining of secondary symptoms and ailments may all be signs of emotional upset. Time, understanding and encouragement to overcome problems are of paramount importance.

Prognosis

The time at which to discuss the future prognosis of a disability and its implications varies. Some patients ask penetrating questions from the early days and require more direct answers than may be given to others at this time. Generally, some indication is given formally when the patient is more mobile. He can do more to counteract this news when he is mobile, than when lying flat and immobile in bed. Hope should never be completely extinguished, for while there is some hope, a person will strive to gain maximum ability and achievement. Unrealistic hope, however, must be discouraged as this only delays progress with rehabilitation and inhibits satisfactory resettlement at home. Once the prognosis has been discussed with a patient by the doctor, the rest of the team members can reinforce the positive achievements and attainments possible. Prognosis is usually discussed with relatives long before the patient is involved, but this discussion often passes unheeded in the stress of the early days and may need to be reinforced at a later date.

Life expectancy

Where adequate care is available and circumstances permit satisfactory functioning and supervision, the life expectancy of patients with paraplegia and tetraplegia is no different from that of anyone else.

It is well known that people cared for at home generally survive longer than patients living in hospital. This is not mainly related to nursing care received, but to the love and companionship which exist in the home.

Causes of death may be chest infections (pneumonia, inhalation of vomit) and renal failure (hydronephrosis, renal calculi, anylordosis, pyelonephritis). Sepsis from multiple or deep pressure sores involving bone and tissues can also lead to death, and cardiac arrest may occur due to the general stress and strain of spinal injury.

Patients with spinal cord injuries often ask about their life expectancy, and this question is also of great importance in legal claims for compensation. To put a figure in terms of the number of years a person is expected to survive, is difficult and can be distressing to the person concerned. The best tonic for a patient is to have the opportunity to converse with another similarly disabled person who has spent a considerable time in a wheelchair, has looked after himself well and leads a full and interesting life. This may strengthen his determination to strive and enjoy each year of his life.

Compensation claims

Claims for compensation often follow a spinal cord injury. A patient with a case pending should be encouraged to contact a solicitor early in his treatment programme so that as little time as possible is wasted in this lengthy and often protracted procedure. The police may be involved when statements have to be obtained.

Unfortunately, many solicitors advise patients not to consider return to work and to limit their range of activities and independence in order to enhance their case and increase the amount of compensation payment. These cases often take many years to reach a settlement by which time the inclination to work has often disappeared. For many patients this is a frustrating time.

Understandably, they feel entitled to financial compensation for the accident and its effect upon their lives. Financial hardship is usually greatest in the first year after the accident, when housing may be impossible, local authorities unhelpful, or a new car required, and not in three to five years' time, when the claim may be settled. Once the reason for a case has been established and liability admitted, it is often possible for an advance payment to be arranged.

Accurate medical information should be written clearly at the time of admission and thereafter throughout rehabilitation, so that medical reports are available when necessary.

Acknowledgements Dr Francis Jones and all nursing and paramedical staff of the Midland Spinal Injuries Unit, Oswestry. In particular: Sister P. Jones, Senior Unit Sister; Sister P. Griffiths, Unit Sister (now School of Nursing) Oswestry; Miss A. Evans, Senior Physiotherapist, Spinal Injuries Unit; Mrs B. Spicer, Social Worker, Spinal Injuries Unit; Mr D. Jones, Senior Medical Photographer; Mr S. Clarke, Disablement Resettlement Officer; Miss L. Barrington, occupational therapy student, for some illustrations; Mrs B. K. Stewart, secretarial staff, occupational therapy department; School of Nursing staff.

Useful Organisations/Publications

Spinal Injuries Association, 5, Crowndale Road, London NW1 1TU. Annual subscription, regular newsletter and information sheet. Research into particular aspects of care. Advice on any topic etc.

Disabled Drivers Association (D.D.A.): local groups throughout the country. Main office: Ashwellthorpe Hall, Norwich, Norfolk NR16 1EX. Annual subscription. Publication *The Magic Carpet* on all aspects of disability.

Disabled Drivers Motor Club (D.D.M.C.), 9 Park Parade, London W3 9BD. Annual subscription. Publication *The Flying Mat.*

The Cord. International Journal for Paraplegics. Annual subscription. Available from Stoke Mandeville Sports Stadium, Harvey Road, Aylesbury, Buckinghamshire.

British Paraplegic Sports Association. Stoke Mandeville Sports Stadium, Harvey Road, Aylesbury, Buckinghamshire. Information on all sport for the disabled and local clubs.

Royal Association for Disability and Rehabilitation (R.A.D.A.R.) Annual subscription. Regular publication *The Bulletin*: up to date information/legislation for all disabilities.

Disabled Living Foundation Information Service, 346 Kensington High Street, London W14.

Holidays for the Physically Handicapped Published by R.A.D.A.R. Available at W. H. Smith.

REFERENCES AND FURTHER READING

Bromley I 1976 Tetraplegia and paraplegia. A guide for physiotherapists. Churchill Livingstone, Edinburgh
Burke, D, Duncan Murray D 1975 Handbook of spinal cord medicine. Macmillan, London
Fallon B 1975 So you're paralysed. Spinal Injuries Association, London
Fallon B 1979 Able to work. Spinal Injuries Association, London
Ford J, Duckworth B 1974 Physical management for the quadriplegic patient. Davies, Philadelphia
Guttman L 1973 Spinal cord injuries, 8th edn. Blackwell, Oxford
Hardy A, Rossier 1975 Spinal cord injuries. Littleton, U.S.A.
Hardy A, Elson R 1976 Practical management of spinal injuries, 2nd edn. Churchill Livingstone, Edinburgh
Malick M, Meyer C 1978 Manual on management of the quadriplegic upper extremity. Harmarville Rehabilitation Centre, U.S.A.
Powell, M 1976 Orthopaedic nursing 7th edn. Churchill Livingstone, Edinburgh, ch 16
Walsh J J 1964 Understanding paraplegia. Dolphin Book Co, Oxford

28

Upper limb injuries

Although not the world's fastest, strongest or most agile inhabitant, man can surely lay claim to having developed a greater combination of dexterity, coordination and sensation in his upper limbs than any other creature. With this combination he is able to work by grasping, pushing, pulling and lifting; to play by throwing, catching, fingering and creating; to explore his environment by reaching, touching, handling and feeling and to express himself through writing, gesticulating, miming and drawing.

When the upper limb is injured or loses function in any way, a wide range of activities is curtailed because of the inability to use the upper limb and hand as a purposeful unit. Clearly, it is difficult to separate the functional use of the upper limb from that of the hand, as the two must work together in order to perform efficiently. The hand has already been discussed in detail in Chapter 17. This chapter therefore aims to consider the functions and treatment of the other components of the upper limb, these being the shoulder and shoulder girdle, the elbow, forearm and wrist.

Whatever the joint or condition being treated in the upper limb, there are several general rules which the therapist must remember when planning her treatment programme.

1. The purpose of the shoulder girdle and upper limb is to place the hand in a correct and stable position for the activity it is going to perform. If, therefore, there is loss of movement or normal structure in the upper limb, hand function will be severely affected, no matter how mobile and strong the hand itself may be. However, compen-

satory movements may be possible. For example, where pronation of the forearm is limited (as in cross-union between the radius and ulna), shoulder abduction can be substituted with reasonable success; similarly, where shoulder joint movement is lost (for instance following arthrodesis or in severe cases of rheumatoid arthritis), trunk, scapular and shoulder girdle movements can be encouraged.

2. Because the arm and hand normally function as a unit, it is important for the therapist to treat the whole of the upper limb, rather than just the joint directly affected.

3. Oedema must be reduced as soon as possible (by elevated and 'pumping' activities for example), as its presence can cause pressure on nerves and vessels, as well as restricting the range of movement.

4. During the period of immobilisatiion following injury or surgery, it is important to encourage active movement in all parts of the limb which are not immobilised in order to prevent disuse atrophy and joint stiffness.

5. For any given condition there are often several different treatment regimes, and the therapist should ensure that she always treats her patient according to the preference of the doctor in charge of each patient.

6. Accurate measurement and records are vital during treatment; they should be kept regularly and written up clearly.

7. When treating a limb following injury or disease, some degree of pain can be expected as more movement is attempted. However, the therapist can help to reduce this pain by using rhythmical and bilateral activities in a warm and relaxed atmosphere. It is important, should any signs of infection or excessive pain occur, that these be reported immediately.

8. If it has been necessary to immobilise the limb, the joints above and below the site of damage are included wherever possible and both, therefore, will be affected by stiffness and weakness after healing. It is likely, however, that the joint distal to the damage will be more severely affected because of the presence of oedema and the possibility of damage to muscles and other soft tissues supplying the joint as they cross the site of injury.

9. Because of the function of the upper limb, mobility is perhaps the prime consideration during treatment.

10. When strength is being increased activities offering maximum resistance in the mid-range of movement should be used.

THE SHOULDER JOINT AND SHOULDER GIRDLE

As mentioned earlier, the function of the shoulder joint and shoulder girdle is to help in positioning and stabilising the hand. Because of its wide range of movement the shoulder can help to place the hand in a large area above, below, to the front of and behind the trunk. For extremely fine work, such as threading a needle, the normal muscular action of stabilising the shoulder, limb and hand may be complemented by taking a deep breath in to fix the chest wall and ensure complete stillness of the shoulder.

Problems occur if shoulder movement is weak or the shoulder joint stiff or fixed. If the shoulder is weak the hand cannot be stabilised and therefore coordination and smoothness of movement are affected. Similarly, the weak shoulder cannot place the hand within the normal range and hand activity is therefore affected. Finally, a weak shoulder is more at risk from dislocation or subluxation, as slack muscles, tendons and capsule may not be able to hold the head of the humerus in the glenoid cavity against resistance. By contrast, the stiff joint, unless surgically arthrodesed, is often painful and the patient will therefore move it only reluctantly. Again, movement may be slow and limited, and activities of daily living present an especial problem. Although these may be overcome adequately if the elbow, wrist and hand are mobile, it often happens that these joints are also affected, for example in rheumatoid arthritis or stiffness following a bony or soft tissue injury such as a burn.

Conditions treated

Many conditions may present to the occupational therapist for treatment:

1. *The results of trauma,* such as fractures

around the shoulder, shoulder girdle and in the upper arm; dislocations and subluxations, and spinal and peripheral nerve injuries (e.g. of the nerve supplying the deltoid muscle).

2. *Other conditions*

(a). The arthropathies. For those with rheumatoid arthritis, ankylosing spondylitis and other related conditions gentle activities designed to increase and maintain the range of movement can be used.

(b). Progressive and other muscular weakness. For adults with motor neurone disease, syringomyelia, muscular dystrophy or other progressive conditions, activities designed to maintain the range of movement can be used. Children with progressive conditions should be treated according to the principles described in Chapter 23.

(c). Non-traumatic conditions. These include specific soft-tissue damage such as tendonitis and bursitis, and those covered under the general term of frozen shoulder.

Complications following injury to the shoulder may arise if a fracture fails to unite, or if union is delayed, if the radial nerve is damaged in a fracture to the upper shaft of the humerus, if the brachial artery is damaged leading to Volkmann's ischaemia or if there is recurrent dislocation. 'Frozen shoulder' may itself be considered a complication arising after injury to another part of the upper limb, and the long head of biceps may rupture following a fracture of the humerus.

Treatment principles

Initially the therapist must assess the patient's shoulder, both physically and functionally. Any problems associated with the activities of daily living must be investigated and the shoulder then treated by specific activities. In the early stages of treatment, gentle activities to increase general movement should be used, with abduction and flexion being especially emphasised. To assist these activities the shoulder can be aided by supporting the limb in a sprung or counterbalanced sling system, such as an OB help arm, in order to relieve the muscles from the effort of both supporting and moving the limb (Fig. 28.1A). Similarly, the patient can be treated whilst lying prone on a plinth or bed so that the shoulder

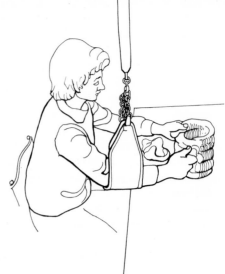

A Upper limb supported in a sprung sling

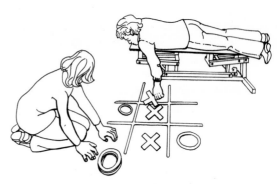

B Shoulder movement assisted by gravity

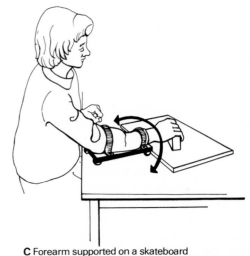

C Forearm supported on a skateboard

Fig. 28.1 Treating the shoulder in the early stages

automatically falls into flexion, assisted by gravity (Fig. 28.1B), or seated at a table with the forearm supported on a 'skateboard' (Fig. 28.1C). From any of these positions a selection of lightweight, rhythmical activities working in mid-range can be used, such as solitaire, draughts, pottery, artwork, sanding, correlating, origami or weaving. Bilateral activities will help avoid compensatory trunk movement.

As movement increases, the range of activities can be widened and support to the shoulder decreased. Thus, where a counterbalance system is used the number of weights should be reduced, and in a sprung sling system a spring with lower poundage should be used. Activities previously worked at waist height can be raised to chest, then shoulder level to encourage abduction and flexion, and those requiring extension and rotation, such as use of the long handle on the wire twister, planing or circular sanding, can be gently encouraged. The range of movement and resistance offered by activities can be increased and, therefore, printing, stool seating, elevated and large remedial games, basketry, macramé, bread making and weaving can be used. Where possible, bilateral activities should be given to avoid compensatory movements.

Finally, activities offering both a wide range of movement and resistance (necessary for strengthening muscles and therefore stabilising the shoulder) can be introduced. Such activities can include printing adapted with an overhead bar, work on the upright rug loom, coathanger making on an elevated jig, wire twisting with the long handle and wall-mounted stool seating or remedial games. As all these activities are tiring they should be attempted for short periods only when first introduced and may be alternated with the familiar and less demanding activities previously used. At this stage, a static sling apparatus can be used to encourage rotation where this is particularly desirable. The apparatus may be set up in conjunction with weaving, painting, sanding, adapted games or any similar lightweight activity (Fig. 28.2). Where appropriate, the patient should be encouraged to participate in leisure activities which will assist his shoulder function, such as swimming, archery, table tennis and billiards. Home decorating and window cleaning, although

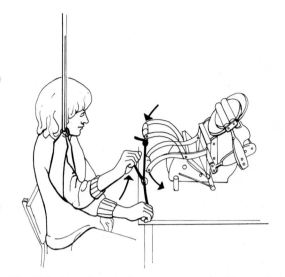

Fig. 28.2 Use of a static sling to encourage shoulder rotation

hardly leisure activities, will also maintain and increase shoulder function.

THE ELBOW AND FOREARM JOINTS

The elbow and forearm find their main task in helping to place the hand. Good function is especially important for activities of daily living, for without a mobile elbow it is impossible to bring the hand to the mouth — a fairly vital action for survival. Similarly, if supination is limited the patient will be greatly hindered by being unable to present his hand palm uppermost, as this is essential when holding a large, flat object, such as a tray or pile of ironing, making a bed or receiving change! It is important to remember that, because of the proximity of the head of the radius to the elbow joint, pronation and supination are often affected when elbow function is disturbed and that flexion and extension of the elbow can be affected following forearm injury. It is essential, therefore, that elbow and forearm movements are assessed and treated simultaneously.

As the elbow and forearm themselves are relatively stable joints, weakness usually occurs when either the muscles or the nerves supplying the movement to the joints are affected, as may happen following a nerve lesion or in muscular degeneration. This weakness affects hand function, especially where a degree of force is required, as the elbow cannot be stabilised except when lock-ed into full extension. This may, however, not be practical or possible. Similarly, a weak elbow and forearm will inhibit coordination in the upper limbs. If the joints are stiff or fixed the previously mentioned problems of getting the hand to the face or presenting it palm upwards will appear. Follow-ing injury a patient will often present with stiff and weak joints. As the elbow joint must never be forced into passive extension because of the risk of myositis ossificans, the therapist should treat these joints gently, especially in the beginning, and remember that results may be slow.

Conditions treated

The following conditions are most frequently tre-ated by the occupational therapist:

1. *The results of trauma*, such as fractures of the lower end of the humerus, those affecting the elbow joint, and fractures of the proximal and mid-shaft of the forearm; fracture dislocations; peripheral and spinal nerve injuries and burns.

2. *Other conditions*

(a). Arthropathies. Gentle rhythmical activities can be used to help maintain as full a range of movement as possible.

(b). Progressive and other muscular weakness. Lightweight activities to help maintain a full range of movement can be used.

(c). Non-traumatic conditions. These include 'tennis elbow' (inflammation of the common ex-tensor origin) and 'golfer's elbow' (inflammation of the common flexor origin). Treatment of the elbow joint is particularly important for patients with below-elbow amputations.

Complications following injury around the elbow and forearm can arise if there is delayed or non-union of a fracture, if there is cross-union between the radius and ulna, or if there is ulnar nerve involvement (leading to the characteristic 'claw hand'). Median nerve damage may occur, especially following a supracondylar fracture (common in children), resulting in a 'monkey hand', and damage to the brachial artery can lead to Volkmann's ischaemia. If the patient does not move the non-immobilised joints of the limb while the damaged joints are in plaster, or fails to respond to treatment afterwards, a frozen shoulder

or disuse atrophy can occur. If the elbow is forced into extension myositis ossificans (post-traumatic ossification) can also result. Some permanent loss of function is not uncommon.

Treatment principles

Following a physical and functional assessment of the upper limb, the therapist should aim to solve any problems in the activities of daily living which have been caused by the disturbance of elbow and forearm function.

Specific treatment should initially include gentle activities to encourage flexion and extension as well as pronation, supination and grip, which may also have been affected. Increase in the range of movement should be the prime objective of treat-ment, along with the reduction of any oedema. Strength and coordination can then be increased once the limb is more mobile. Of the movements affected, the therapist should particularly encour-age extension at the elbow using activities which require a light 'pushing' action (such as rolling clay and pastry or light elevated sanding) in order to increase the strength in the extensors. In the forearm, the treatment of supination may take priority over the return of pronation, as not only is its loss more inhibiting and difficult to compensate for, it is also often slower to return. Where practi-cal, activities should be planned in order to alter-nate those encouraging elbow and forearm move-ment.

Early treatment, therefore, may include activi-ties such as painting, pastry making, sanding, weaving, pottery (especially making coil pots), use of FEPS or large remedial games, as these can encourage all required movements. If the limb is especially weak or swollen, it may be treated in a sprung sling. It is especially important at this stage to emphasise that the patient should not force the elbow joint into extension either consciously by trying to push or pull it straight, or unconsciously by carrying heavy loads. The reason for this should be explained.

As the joints improve, activities should be altered to offer more resistance, and a full range of movement may now be encouraged. For alternate flexion and extension the following activities may be used: the upright rug loom, stool seating, printing (initially unadapted and later using the overhead bar), work with the stand drill, cord knotting and the long handle attached to the wire twister. For encouraging pronation and supination adapted disc-shaped remedial games (see Ch. 10), FEPS using the disc handle (see Ch. 9), the wire twister (using the spade or disc handle), table football, jacks (also known as 'Five stones' or 'Dibs'), table tennis and work with a screwdriver can be incorporated into treatment. Should the therapist find that the patient is compensating with excessive use of shoulder movement during these activities, forearm movement can be isolated by placing a piece of card between the patient's arm and chest wall so that he must hold the shoulder adducted in order to prevent the card slipping out (Fig. 28.3).

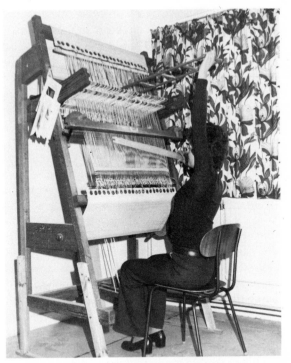

Fig. 28.4 The upright rug loom set to encourage elbow extension

The therapist should also encourage the patient to participate in activities in his own time, which will maintain and increase his elbow and forearm function. Swimming, badminton, gardening, carpentry, cookery, skittles, window cleaning and home decorating can all be attempted and are especially important in view of the length of time which may be involved before optimum function is reached.

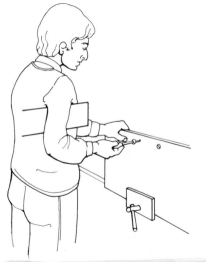

Fig. 28.3 A card placed between the arm and chest prevents shoulder movement when treating the forearm

Finally, where a full range of movement and resistance are required, activities such as sawing, planing, archery and wrought iron work can be introduced. Previous activities can be continued and upgraded. For example, stool seating can now be done using a pattern and cord offering more resistance, and a longer shuttle can be used to increase extension; the upright rug loom can be set to encourage full elbow extension when reaching for the shed bar, and a long shuttle and wide warp will also encourage full movement (Fig. 28.4). Resistance on both printing and the wire twister can be increased.

THE WRIST JOINT

As with the shoulder, elbow and forearm joints, the wrist joint is vital in helping to place the hand ready for action. However, rather than simply placing it in the correct location the wrist is concerned with the finer positioning and angling of the hand by a combination of flexion, extension, radial and ulnar deviation. As with the elbow, it is impossible to separate the function of the wrist from that of the forearm with which it articulates at its distal end and thus, when either the wrist or forearm are damaged, the function of the other joint is invariably affected.

Moreover, the wrist itself plays an active part in hand function, for not only do many of the structures supplying the hand pass over the wrist, it also is impossible for the hand to grip strongly if the wrist is not stable and extended. For this reason, it is essential that basic hand functions (that is grip, coordination and movement) are treated when the wrist is damaged.

Conditions treated

Conditions of the wrist most commonly requiring treatment by the occupational therapist:

1. *The results of trauma,* such as fractures to the mid- and distal shafts of the radius and ulna and of the carpus and metacarpals; tendon or nerve lesions (especially of the radial nerve); crush injuries, burns or any open wound resulting in soft tissue damage around the wrist.

2. *Other conditions*

(a). The arthropathies, for which lightweight, rhythmical activities can be given to help maintain as full a range of movement as possible.

(b). Progressive and other muscular weaknesses. These can be treated as the arthropathies.

(c). Non-traumatic conditions affecting the wrist include ganglions and disruption of normal tendon function such as tenosynovitis. Carpal tunnel syndrome may also occur.

Complications following injury to the wrist joint include delayed or malunion of the fracture; cross-union between the radius and ulna or failure of the fracture to unite. The fingers as well as the wrist and forearm often suffer some degree of stiffness and weakness, and if the shoulder has not been moved a 'frozen shoulder' can result. Where the wrist and hand have been damaged and the shoulder has subsequently stiffened the term 'shoulder-hand syndrome' may be applied. If swelling is severe around the carpal tunnel, the median nerve may be compressed, or the nerve may have been severed by a deep wound at the wrist. Sudek's atrophy and rupture of the extensor pollicis longus tendon may also occur, as could prolonged or permanent stiffness, even following rehabilitation.

Treatment principles

Damage around the wrist invariably causes oede-

ma in the hand and fingers, and as fractures in this area occur frequently in elderly people who slip and fall onto their hand, it is particularly important that the need for maintaining mobility in the hand, shoulder and, if not also immobilised, the elbow is emphasised. As some elderly people may be reluctant to move the damaged limb, or discover their independence is curtailed, it is not uncommon to find that they are referred for treatment while the wrist is still immobilised.

Where this occurs, assistance with the activities of daily living is important, and equipment to stabilise items or cutlery with enlarged handles can often help. Advice on dressing and washing may be necessary and aids to help with cutting food while one hand is temporarily out of action can be supplied. The patient will probably have been shown exercises at the outpatient clinic or in the physiotherapy department, which he should perform at least once an hour in order to ensure that his limb remains mobile, and the therapist should satisfy herself that the patient has remembered these and understands their importance. Where necessary she may additionally encourage the patient to squeeze a soft woollen or rubber ball, roll of foam or lump of Plasticine in order to help maintain hand mobility and reduce oedema in the hand. Should further supervised treatment be necessary, gentle shoulder and elbow activities may be given.

Once the wrist is free to move, activities should be given which encourage flexion and extension of the wrist, pronation and supination of the forearm, and grip with wide range of movement in the hand. Radial and ulnar deviation at the wrist are rarely treated specificially.

To ensure mobility in the other joints of the upper limb specific activities for the wrist can be given once an assessment has been made. Should any joints other than the wrist be affected they must be treated simultaneously.

Again, mobility is of prime importance and gentle general activities should be given initially. Those which encourage flexion and extension include the use of FEPS or the wire twister with the roller handle, sanding or spoke-shave work on a curved surface, printing unadapted for wrist extension, kneading dough or rolling pastry for wrist extension and remedial games played on a high shelf or over long poles for wrist flexion (see Ch. 10 — Remedial Games). To encourage pronation and supination, activities such as the use of FEPS or the wire twister using the spade or disc handle, jacks, pottery and playing cards can be used. Grip will also be encouraged during most of these activities. It may be advisable at this stage to encourage the patient to use activities in warm water at home, and he may find that squeezing or kneading Plasticine in a sink of water or 'wringing' a facecloth or sponge while in the bath may serve as a useful 'warming-up' exercise.

As wrist and hand function improve, activities should encourage a larger range of movement and greater resistance. At this stage, therefore, activities such as printing, wire twisting and the use of FEPS can be upgraded, and the programme can be extended to include carpentry (hammering, sawing, fretsaw work, sanding and work with a screwdriver), cookery (beating, pastry and bread making can be used both during treatment sessions and at home), artwork (collage to encourage the use of scissors, potato printing, screen printing and origami for example), remedial games such as table and puff football, and stool seating using cotton cord or nytrim.

Finally, activities offering greater resistance to increase stability and strength can be introduced. Printing using a bell-rope adaptation or wrist-extension board, (Fig. 28.5), carpentry and remedial games can be continued and upgraded, and clay wedging, heavy sawing, stool seating with nylon cord or seagrass and wrought iron work may be included where it is felt appropriate. In many cases treatment may not continue into this final stage as many patients find that, once movement and strength have begun to return to the wrist, normal occupational or household duties will finally strengthen and mobilise the joint. However, for those with especially heavy or demanding jobs this final period of strengthening may be essential. I remember, for example, treating an

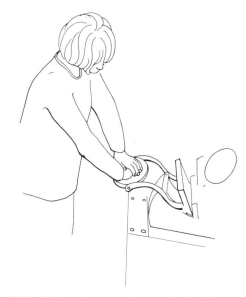

Fig. 28.5 Printing using the wrist-extension board

upholsterer and self-employed plasterer with wrist injuries, both of whom were anxious to return to work. However, within a week of being discharged with reasonable movement and strength, both had returned to the department for further treatment as their wrists could not withstand the rigours of piecework or plastering ceilings.

REFERENCES AND FURTHER READING

Adams J C 1978 Outline of fractures, 7th edn. Churchill Livingstone, Edinburgh
Adams J C 1981 Outline of orthopaedics, 9th edn. Churchill Livingstone, Edinburgh
Jones M, Jay P, 1977 An approach to occupational therapy, 3rd edn. Butterworths, London
MacDonald E M 1976 Occupational therapy in rehabilitation, 4th edn. Balliere Tindall, London
Shopland A 1980 Refer to occupational therapy, 2nd edn. Churchill Livingstone, Edinburgh
Trombly C A, Scott A D 1977 Occupational therapy for physical dysfunction. Williams & Wilkins, Baltimore

Appendices

Appendices

Appendix 1

ASSOCIATIONS GIVING GENERAL HELP AND INFORMATION

Age Concern, Bernard Sunley House, 60 Pitcarn Road, Mitcham, Surrey CR4 3LL

Association for Disabled Professionals, The Stables, 73 Pound Road, Banstead, Surrey SM7 2HU

British Council for the Rehabilitation of the Disabled (REHAB), Tavistock House (South), Tavistock Square, London WC1H 9LB

British Red Cross Society, 9 Grosvenor Crescent, London SW1X 7EJ

Central Council for the Disabled, 34 Eccleston Square, London SW1

Centre on Environment for the Handicapped, 126 Albert Street, Camden, London NW1 7NF

Community Health Councils — for help in local cases. For address see local telephone directory.

Disabled Living Foundation, 346 Kensington High Street, London W14 8NS

Disablement Income Group(DIG), Attlee House, Toynbee Hall, 28, Commercial Street, London E1 6LR

Disability Alliance, 1 Cambridge Terrace, London NW1 4JL

Distressed Gentlefolks Aid Association, Vicarage Gate House, Vicarage Gate, London W8 4AQ

The Family Fund, Joseph Rowntree Memorial, PO Box 50, York, YO1 1UY

Help the Aged, 32 Dover Street, London W1A 2AP

King Edward's Hospital Fund for London, Kings Fund Centre, 126 Albert Street, London NW1 7NF

Leonard Cheshire Foundation, 7 Market Mews, London W1Y 8HP

Medic-Alert Foundation, 9 Hanover Street, London W1R 9HE

Naidex (National Aids for the Disabled Exhibitions) Conventions Ltd, Temple House, 36 High Street, Sevenoaks, Kent, TN13 1JG

National Association of Leagues of Hospital Friends, 565 Fulham Road, London SW6 1ES

National Bureau for Handicapped Students, 40 Brunswick Square, London WC1N 1AZ

National Association of Citizens Advice Bureau, 110 Drury Lane, London WC2B 5SW

National Fund for Reasearch into Crippling Diseases, Vincent House, 1 Springfield Road, Horsham, West Sussex, RH12 2PN

Open University, Richard Tomlinson, Adviser for Disabled Students, Open University Walton Hall, Milton Keynes MK7 6AA

Possum Users Association, 14, Greenvale Drive, Timsbury, Bath BA3 1HP

Rehabilitation Engineering Movement Advisory Panels (REMAP), Thames House North, Millbank, London SW1P 4QG

The Royal Association for Disability and Rehabilitation (RADAR), 25 Mortimer Street, London W1N 8AB

Sexual and Personal Relationships of the Disabled (SPOD), % RADAR, 25 Mortimer Street, London W1N 8AB

The Shaftesbury Society, 112 Regency Street, Westminster, London SW1P 4AX

Sue Ryder Foundation, Sue Ruder Home Cavendish, Suffolk CO10 8AY

National Federation of Women's Institutes, 39 Eccleston Street, London SW1W 9NT

Women's Royal Voluntary Service, 17 Old Park Lane, London W1

ASSOCIATIONS RELATED TO SPECIFIC CONDITIONS

Arthritis and Rheumatism Council for Research, 8/10 Charing Cross Road, London WC2H 0HN

Association for Spina Bifida and Hydrocephalis (ASBAH), Tavistock House North, Tavistock Square, London WC1H 9HJ

Association to Combat Huntington's Chorea, Lyndhurst, Lower Hampton Road, Sudbury-on-Thames, Middlesex, TW16 5PR

British Arthritis and Rheumatism Association, 1 Devonshire Place, London W1N 2BD

British Association for the Hard of Hearing, 16 Park Street, Windsor, Berkshire SL4 1LU

British Association for Rheumatology and Rehabilitation, Royal College of Physicians, 11 St Andrews Place, Regents Park, London NW1 4LE

Brittle Bone Society, 63 Byron Crescent, Dundee DD3 6SS

British Deaf Association, 38 Victoria Place, Carlisle, CA1 1HU

British Diabetic Association, 10, Queen Anne Street, London W1M 0BD

British Dyslexia Association, 4, Hobart Place, London SW1W 0HU

British Epilepsy Association, Crowthorne House, New Wokingham Road, Wokingham, Berkshire

British Heart Foundation, 57 Gloucester Place, London W1H 4HP

British Polio Fellowship, Bell Close, West End Road, Ruislip, Middlesex, HA4 6LP

Chest, Heart and Stroke Association, Tavistock House (North), Tavistock Square, London WC1H 9JE

Cystic Fibrosis Research Trust, 5 Blyth Road, Bromley, Kent, BR1 3RS

Friedreich's Ataxia Group, Bolsover House, 5-6 Clipatone Street, London W1

Jewish Blind Society, 1 Craven Hill, London W2 3EW

Multiple Sclerosis Action Group, 71 Grays Inn Road, London WC1X 8TR

Multiple Sclerosis Society of Great Britain and Northern Ireland, 286 Munster Road, London SW6 6AP

Muscular Dystrophy Group of Great Britain, Nattrass House, 35 Macaulay Road, Clapham, London SW4 0QP

National Ankylosing Spondylitis Society, (NASS) 12 Holly Mount, Hampstead, London NW3

National Society for Epilepsy, Chalfont Centre for Epilepsy, Chalfont St Peter, Gerrards Cross, Bucks SL9 ORJ

Parkinson's Disease Society, 81 Queens Road, Wimbledon London SW19 8NR

Perthes Disease Group, 61 Wickfield Road, Hackenthorp, Sheffield

Royal National Institute for the Blind, 224-6-8 Great Portland Street, London W1N 6AA

Royal National Institute for the Deaf, 105 Gower Street, London WC1E 6AH

Society for the Aid of Thalidomide Children, 28 Four Acres Walk, Hemel Hempstead, Hertfordshire

Society for Skin Camouflage, Wester Pitmenzier, Auchtermuchty, Fife, Scotland

Spastics Society, 12 Park Crescent, London W1N 4EQ

Spinal Injuries Association, 5 Crowndale Road, London NW1 1TU

ASSOCIATIONS OFFERING HELP FOR DISABLED CHILDREN

Child Poverty Action Group, 1 Macklin Street, London WC2

The Girl Guides Association, 17-19 Buckingham Palace Road, London SW1W 0PT

Handicapped Adventure Playground Association, Fulham Palace, Bishops Avenue, London SW6 6EA

Invalid Children's Aid Association, 126 Buckingham Palace Road, London SW1W 9SB

Lady Hoare Trust for Physically Disabled Children, 7 North Street, Midhurst, West Sussex, GU29 9DJ

National Association for the Welfare of Children in Hospital, Exton House, 7 Exton Street, London SE1 8VE

National Deaf Children's Society, 45 Hereford Road, London W2 5AH

National Society for Brain Damaged Children, 35 Larchmere Drive, Birmingham, B28 8JB

Physically Handicapped and Able Bodied Association (PHAB), 42 Devonshire Street, London W1N 1LN

The Scout Association, Baden Powell House, Queens Gate, London SW7 5JS

Toy Libraries Association, Seabrook House Wyllyotts Manor, Darkes Lane Potters Bar EN6 2HL

SPORTS AND LEISURE ASSOCIATIONS FOR THE DISABLED

Association of Swimming Therapy, 10 West Way, Wheelock, Cheshire CW11 9LQ

British Library of Tape Recordings for Hospital Patients, 12 Lant Street, London SE1 1QR

Disability Training Centre, The British School of Motoring Ltd, 102 Sydney Street, Chelsea, London SW3 6NJ

British Sports Association for the Disabled, Hayward House, Sir Ludwig Guttman Sports Centre for the Disabled, Stoke Mandeville, Harvey Road, Aylesbury, Buckinghamshire HP21 8PP

Committee for the Promotion of Angling for the Disabled, 18-19 Claremont Crescent, Edinburgh EH7 4QD

Disabled Campers Club, 28 Coote Road, Bexley Heath, Kent, DA7 4PR

Disabled Drivers Association, Ashwellthorpe Hall, Ashwellthorpe, Norwich NR15 1HP

Disabled Drivers Insurance Bureau, 292 Hale Lane, Edgware, Middlesex HA8 8NP

Disabled Drivers Motor Club Ltd, 9 Park Parade, Gunnersbury Avenue, Acton, London W3 9BD

Homebound Craftsmen Trust, 29 Holland Street, London W8 4NA

Jigsaw Puzzle Loan Club, 16 Bucks Avenue, Watford Heath, Hertfordshire

Motability, Boundary House, 91–93 Charterhouse Street, London ECIM 6BT

National Association of Swimming Clubs for the Handicapped, 93 The Downs, Harlow, Essex

National Association of Visually Handicapped Bowlers, 28 Brook Street, Barry, South Glamorgan

National Library for the Blind, 35 Great Smith Street, Westminster, London SW1

National Listening (Library Talking Books for the Handicapped) 49 Great Cumberland Place, London W1H 4LH

Riding for the Disabled Association, Avenue R, National Agricultural Centre, Kenilworth, Warwickshire, CV8 2LY

Photography for the Disabled, 190 Secrett House, Ham Close, Ham, Richmond, Surrey

Society of One Armed Golfers, 48 Fairby Road, Lee Green, London SE12 8JR

Wheelchair Dance Association, 8 Starvecrow Close, Shipbourne Road, Tonbridge, Kent

Wireless for the Bedridden, 81b Corbets Tey Road, Upminster, Essex RH14 2AJ

Appendix 2

Common Medical Abbreviations

If you wish to test your knowledge of the following abbreviations, cover the right-hand column with a blank sheet of paper on which you can write your answers.

1. Related to people and departments

ALAC	Artificial Limb and Appliance Centre
CSSD	Central Sterile Supply Department
OAP	Old Age Pensioner
RG	Remedial Gymnast
Pt	Patient
DRO	Disablement Resettlement Officer
FRCS	Fellow of the Royal College of Surgeons
OT	Occupational Therapist
OPD	Out Patients' Department
FRCP	Fellow of the Royal College of Physicians
GP	General Practitioner
PNO	Principal Nursing Officer
A and E	Accident and Emergency
MCSP	Member of the Chartered Society of Physiotherapists
MSW	Medical Social Worker
SEN	State Enrolled Nurse
PT	Physiotherapist
RMN	Registered Mental Nurse
SCM	State Certified Midwife
ST	Speech Therapist

2. Related to facts recorded during the examination of a patient

CNS	Central Nervous System
C/O	Complained of
DA	Doctors appointment
DOA	Date of admission
DOB	Date of birth
DNA	Did not attend
FH	Family history
NAD	Nothing abnormal discovered
OE	On examination
NFA	No further appointment
PH	Past history
ROM	Range of movement
TCI	To come in
△	Diagnosis

3. Related to specific diagnoses

CP	Cerebral Palsy
CVA	Cerebral Vascular Accident
OA	Osteoarthrosis
PUO	Pyrexia of Unknown Origin
PID	Prolapsed Intervertebral Disc
RA	Rheumatoid Arthritis
CCF	Congestive Cardiac Failure

4. Related to limbs

AK	Above knee
BK	Below knee
FWB	Full weight bearing
SLR	Straight leg raising
NWB	Non-weight bearing
PWB	Partial weight bearing
MCP	Metacarpal phalangeal joint
DIP	Distal interphalangeal joint
PIP	Proximal interphalangeal joint
CMC	Carpo metacarpal joint

5. Related to drug therapy

AC	Before meals (ante cibos)
BD	Twice a day (bis in die)
MAOI	Mono amine oxidase inhibitors
Nocte	At night
PC	After meals (post cibos)
OD	Once a day (omni die)
PRN	As required (pro re nata)
QDS	Four times a day (quater in die sumendum)
TID	Three times a day (ter in die sumendum)

6. Related to tests performed to aid diagnosis

A & P	Anterior and Posterior (X-ray view)
CSF	Cerebro Spinal Fluid
ECG	Electro cardiogram
ESR	Erythrocyte sedimentation rate
FBC	Full blood count
Hb	Haemoglobin count
LP	Lumbar puncture
EEG	Electroencephalograph

7. Related to treatment

GA	General anaesthetic
POP	Plaster of Paris
TLC	Tender loving care
DXR	Deep X-ray
MUA	Manipulation under anaesthetic

8. Related to bladder and bowel

BO	Bowels open
PU	Passed urine
PR	Per rectum

Index

Index